Order your own copy of

Drug Identification Bible

This page can be removed without damaging the book.

D1478660

Ordered by:

Name (Please print or type)

Title

Phone Number (include area code)

Purchase Order Number

Ship to:

Name (Agency/Department)

Attention

Street Address (Orders are shipped UPS)

City State Zip Code

Quantity Ordered	Description	Price Each	Total
	Drug Identification Bible - Second Edition	$29.95*	
		Shipping $4.50 per order	$4.50
		Total Amount	

Payment Method:

❑ Check Enclosed

❑ VISA

❑ MasterCard

❑ Bill Governmental Agency

Note: Billings issued only to governmental agencies

*Quantity discounts available - please call for quotes.

Card Number

Name of card holder (please print)

Expiration Date (Mo./Yr.)

Mail, Phone or Fax To:

Drug Identification Bible
Box 480244
Denver, CO 80248

Phone 1-800-772-2539
Fax 1-800-852-7870

Order your own copy of

Drug Identification Bible

This page can be removed without damaging the book.

Ordered by:

Name (Please print or type)

Title

Phone Number (include area code) | Purchase Order Number

Ship to:

Name (Agency/Department)

Attention

Street Address (Orders are shipped UPS)

City | State | Zip Code

Quantity Ordered	Description	Price Each	Total
	Drug Identification Bible - Second Edition	$29.95*	
		Shipping $4.50 per order	$4.50
		Total Amount	

Payment Method: ❑ Check Enclosed

❑ VISA ❑ MasterCard

❑ Bill Governmental Agency

Note: Billings issued only to governmental agencies

*Quantity discounts available - please call for quotes.

Card Number

Name of card holder (please print) | Expiration Date (Mo./Yr.)

Mail, Phone or Fax To:

Drug Identification Bible
Box 480244
Denver, CO 80248

Phone 1-800-772-2539
Fax 1-800-852-7870

Order your own copy of

Drug Identification Bible

This page can be removed without damaging the book.

Ordered by: ______________________________

Name (Please print or type)

____

Title

______________________________ ______________________________

Phone Number (include area code) Purchase Order Number

Ship to: ______________________________

Name (Agency/Department)

____

Attention

____

Street Address (Orders are shipped UPS)

____

____

City State Zip Code

Quantity Ordered	Description	Price Each	Total
	Drug Identification Bible - Second Edition	$29.95*	
		Shipping $4.50 per order	$4.50
		Total Amount	

Payment Method: ❑ Check Enclosed

❑ VISA ❑ MasterCard

❑ Bill Governmental Agency

Note: Billings issued only to governmental agencies

*Quantity discounts available - please call for quotes.

Card Number

______________________________ ______________________________

Name of card holder (please print) Expiration Date (Mo./Yr.)

Mail, Phone or Fax To:

Drug Identification Bible
Box 480244
Denver, CO 80248

Phone 1-800-772-2539
Fax 1-800-852-7870

DRUG IDENTIFICATION BIBLE®

Second Edition

Tim Marnell, Editor

Published by:

Drug Identification Bible®
Box 480244
Denver, Colorado 80248
TEL 1-800-772-2539
FAX 1-800-852-7870

Drug Identification Bible®
Second Edition

Published and distributed by:
Drug Identification Bible®
Box 480244
Denver, Colorado 80248
TEL 1-800-772-2539
FAX 1-800-852-7870

ISBN 0-9635626-0-6

Library of Congress Catalog Card No. 94-093967

The purpose of this publication is to serve as a quick field identification aid. While every effort has been made to reproduce the drugs pictured throughout this book in an accurate manner, variations in size and color may exist because of the photographic reproduction or printing processes. There is always the possibility of transposition and/or typographic error. Information provided is advisory only and not intended to replace clinical opinion. There is no substitute for an accurate chemical analysis of an unknown drug by an authorized laboratory. The editors do not assume any responsibility for any use the reader makes of the information provided herein. Any application of this publication is at the readers risk.

ACKNOWLEDGMENTS

Appreciation is extended to the following individuals, without whom this project could not have been completed:

Dwight and Ruth Kinnett

Casey Clark R.Ph.

Mel Galbraith R. Ph.

Duke Fleetfoot

Sandy Marnell

Harry Toto

And especially to my wife, Kathy, for her loving patience and tireless work

TABLE OF CONTENTS

INTRODUCTION

Controlled drugs appear in hundreds of different forms. Nowhere could we find a complete publication which attempted to fully document the current drug scene with the use of color photos, combined with information on street prices, purities, packaging, methods of use, slang, and other factual information.

This void lead to the production of this book. Where were parents, educators, law enforcement personnel, and individuals with a personal interest in drugs to locate answers to the questions "What is it", "What does it look like", and "What does it do"? Hopefully the reader will find the Drug Identification Bible to be of help in answering those questions.

Two sections of the Drug Identification Bible are devoted to the identification of tablets and capsules. The section on Controlled Prescription Drugs shows full color/ actual size photos of 654 prescription tablets and capsules which are controlled by the DEA. The section on non-controlled and over-the-counter drugs lists marking and logo information on approximatley 9,000 items.

All major illicit drugs are included in the photo and text sections. Where possible, the pictorial path is shown for each drug: how it is grown, produced, distributed, packaged for sale on the street, paraphernalia associated with its use, methods of ingestion, etc. Each of the illicit drugs are discussed in detail in the text section.

The last section, slang, deals with communication with and between drug users.

The word "drug" often evokes an emotional response from different sectors. In this book, every effort has been made to present factual information to the reader in an unbiased and truthful manner.

The editors will strive to make future editions of the Drug Identification Bible the most complete and up-to-date text available.

▮

THE CONTROLLED SUBSTANCES ACT (CSA)

The CSA is the federal law which places all controlled substances into one of five categories, or schedules, according to the drugs potential for abuse, physical and psychological dependence liability, and current accepted medical use. Schedule I, the most strictly controlled category, includes heroin, LSD, marijuana, and other drugs considered to have a high abuse potential and no recognized medical use in the United States. Schedule II drugs, which include morphine, methadone, and amphetamines, are primarily different from Schedule I drugs in that they have some currently accepted medical uses. The manufacture and distribution of these drugs are controlled by production quotas, security regulations, import and export controls, and nonrefillable prescription requirements. Schedule III, IV, and V drugs are considered in descending order to have less abuse potential and dependence liability.

The CSA provides a mechanism for substances to be controlled, or added to a schedule; decontrolled, or removed from control; and rescheduled or transferred from one schedule to another.

Proceedings to add, delete, or change the schedule of a drug or other substance may be initiated by the Department of Health and Human Services (HHS), by the DEA, or by petition from any interested person: the manufacturer of a drug, a medical society or association, a pharmacy association, a public interest group, a state or local government agency, or an individual citizen. When a petition is received by the DEA, the agency begins its own investigation of the drug.

The DEA may also begin an investigation of a drug at any time based upon information received from law enforcement laboratories, state and local law enforcement and regulatory agencies, or other sources of information.

Once DEA has collected the necessary data, the Administrator of DEA requests from HHS a scientific and medical evaluation and recommendation as to whether the drug or substance should be controlled or removed from control. HHS solicits information from the Food and Drug Administration, evaluations and recommendations from the National Institute on Drug Abuse, and on occasion from the scientific and medical community at large. HHS compiles the information and transmits back to DEA a medical and scientific evaluation regarding the drug or other substance, a recommendation as to whether the drug should be controlled, and in what schedule it should be placed.

The medical and scientific evaluations are binding on DEA with respect to scientific and medical matters. The recommendation on scheduling is binding only to the extent that if HHS recommends that the substance not be controlled, DEA may not control the substance.

Once DEA has received the scientific and medical evaluation from HHS, DEA will evaluate all available data and make a final decision whether to propose that a drug or other substance should be controlled and into what schedule it should be placed.

The threshold issue is whether the drug or other substance has abuse potential. If a drug does not have a potential for abuse, it cannot be controlled. Although the term potential for abuse is not defined in the CSA, there is much discussion of the term in the legislative history of the CSA. The following items are indicators that a drug or other substance has a potential for abuse:

THE CONTROLLED SUBSTANCES ACT (CSA)

(1) There is evidence that individuals are taking the drug or drugs containing such a substance in amounts sufficient to create a hazard to their health or to the safety of other individuals or of the community; or

(2) There is significant diversion of the drug or drugs containing such a substance from legitimate drug channels; or

(3) Individuals are taking the drug or drugs containing such a substance on their own initiative rather than on the basis of medical advice from a practitioner licensed by law to administer such drugs in the course of his professional practice; or

(4) The drug or drugs containing such a substance are new drugs so related in their action to a drug or drugs already listed as having a potential for abuse to make it likely that the drug will have the same potentiality for abuse as such drugs, thus making it reasonable to assume that there may be significant use contrary to or without medical advice, or that it has a substantial capability of creating hazards to the health of the user or to the safety of the community. Of course, evidence of actual abuse of a substance is indicative that a drug has a potential for abuse.

In determining into which schedule a drug or other substance should be placed, or whether a substance should be decontrolled or rescheduled, certain factors are required to be considered:

(1) The drug's actual or relative potential for abuse.
(2) Scientific evidence of the drug's pharmacological effects.
(3) The state of current scientific knowledge regarding the substance.
(4) Its history and current patterns of abuse.
(5) The scope, duration, and significance of abuse.
(6) What, if any, risk there is to the public health.
(7) The drug's psychic or physiological dependence liability.
(8) Whether the substance is an immediate precursor of a substance already controlled.

After considering the above listed factors, the DEA Administrator must make specific findings concerning the drug or other substance. This will determine into which schedule the drug or other substance will be placed. These schedules are established by the CSA. They are as follows:

Schedule I
- The drug or other substance has a high potential for abuse.
- The drug or other substance has no currently accepted medical use in treatment in the United States.
- There is a lack of accepted safety for use of the drug or other substance under medical supervision.

THE CONTROLLED SUBSTANCES ACT (CSA)

Schedule II

- The drug or other substance has a high potential for abuse.
- The drug or other substance has a currently accepted medical use in treatment in the United States or a currently accepted medical use with severe restrictions.
- Abuse of the drug or other substance may lead to severe psychological or physical dependence.

Schedule III

- The drug or other substance has a potential for abuse less than the drugs or other substances in Schedules I and II.
- The drug or other substance has a currently accepted medical use in treatment in the United States.
- Abuse of the drug or other substance may lead to moderate or low physical dependence or high psychological dependence.

Schedule IV

- The drug or other substance has a low potential for abuse relative to the drugs or substances in Schedule III.
- The drug or substance has a currently accepted medical use in treatment in the United States.
- Abuse of the drug or other substance may lead to limited physical dependence and psychological dependence relative to the drugs or other substances in Schedule III.

Schedule V

- The drug or other substance has a low potential for abuse relative to the drugs or other substances in Schedule IV.
- The drug or other substance has a currently accepted medical use in treatment in the United States.
- Abuse of the drug or other substances may lead to limited physical dependence or psychological dependence relative to the drugs or other substances in Schedule IV.

When the Administrator of DEA has determined that a drug or other substance should be controlled, decontrolled, or rescheduled, a proposal will be published in the Federal Register setting forth the schedule for which control is proposed, or that a substance should be decontrolled, and inviting all interested persons to file comments with DEA. Affected parties may also request a hearing with DEA. If no hearing is requested, DEA will evaluate all comments received and publish a final order in the Federal Register, controlling the drug as proposed or with modifications based upon the written comments filed. This order will set the effective dates for imposing the various requirements imposed under the CSA.

If a hearing is requested, DEA will enter into discussions with the party or parties requesting a hearing in an attempt to narrow the issue for litigation. If necessary, a hearing will then be held before an Administrative Law Judge. The Judge will take evidence on factual issues and hear arguments on legal questions regarding the control of the drug. Depending on the scope and complexity of the issues, the hearing may be brief or quite extensive. The Administrative Law Judge, at the close of the hearing, prepares findings of facts and conclusions of law and a recommended decision which is submitted to the DEA. The DEA will review these documents, as well as the underlying material, and prepare his own findings of fact and conclusions of law (which may or may not be the same as those drafted by the Administrative Law Judge). The Administrator then publishes a final order in the Federal Register either scheduling the drug or other substance or declining to do so.

THE CONTROLLED SUBSTANCES ACT (CSA)

Once the final order is published in the Federal Register, interested parties have 30 days to appeal to a U.S. Court of Appeals to challenge the order. Findings of fact by the DEA Administrator are deemed conclusive if supported by "substantial evidence". The order imposing controls is not stayed during the appeal, however, unless so ordered by the Court.

EMERGENCY OR TEMPORARY SCHEDULING

In 1984, the CSA was amended by the Comprehensive Crime Control Act of 1984. This Act included a provision which allows the Administrator of DEA to place a substance, on a temporary basis, into Schedule I when necessary to avoid an imminent hazard to the public safety.

This emergency scheduling authority permits the scheduling of a substance which is not currently controlled, is being abused, and is a risk to the public health while the formal rule making procedures described in the CSA are being conducted. This emergency scheduling applies only to substances with no accepted medical use. A temporary scheduling order may be issued for one year with a possible extension of up to six months if formal scheduling procedures have been initiated. The proposal and order are published in the Federal Register as are the proposals and orders for formal scheduling.

CONTROLLED SUBSTANCES ANALOGS

A new class of substances was created by the Anti-Drug Abuse Act of 1986. Controlled substance analogs are substances which are not controlled substances, but may be found in the illicit traffic. They are structurally or pharmacologically similar to Schedule I or II controlled substances. A controlled substance analog has no legitimate medical use. A substance which meets the definition of a controlled substance analog that is intended for human consumption is treated under the CSA as if it were a controlled substance in Schedule I.

∎

HOW TO USE THE IMPRINT SECTION

The drug imprint list is a preliminary identification aid for tablets and capsules with unique imprints. Unless indicated by the word "CONTROLLED", these items are not controlled by the DEA and are not included in the color photograph section. Those that are controlled have either a corresponding page number which shows an actual size/full color photograph of the drug, or lists the drugs pertinent information, such as ingredients, Schedule classification, etc.

This section is divided into two groups: (1) tablets and capsules with an imprint that starts with a number; and (2) tablets and capsules with an imprint that starts with a letter. The drugs are sorted in alphabetical and numerical order.

For tablets which have an imprint on both sides, each side is separated by a slash (/). For instance, if a tablet has "071" on one side and "300" on the other side, the imprint would be represented as "071/300", or "300/071". The brand name or generic name, and the strength are listed next to the imprint, along with the manufacturer or marketer. The imprints in this section do not include score marks or slashes.

Keep in mind that although this is a very extensive list, not every drug manufactured is included in this section, and several manufacturers may have the same markings for different drugs.

Imprint	Ingredient/Brand Name	Manufacturer
001	Acetaminophen 500 mg	West-ward Inc.
009 [logo]	Chlor-Trimeton 12 mg	Schering Corp
0021-V	Acetaminophen 80 mg	Vintage
0031 [logo]	Nystatin	Savage Labs
0032-1204	Vitamins	Reid-Rowell
0057	Docusate Sodium 100 mg, Casanthranol 30 mg	Granutec
0063 1390	Reserpine, Hydralazine, Hydrochlorothiazide	Reid-Rowell
0063 1393	Reserpine, Hydralazine, Hydrochlorothiazide	Reid-Rowell
0063 3006	Erythromycin 250 mg	Reid-Rowell
0063 4001	Medroxyprogesterone 10 mg	Reid-Rowell
0063 4410 25/25	Hydralazine 25 mg, Hydrochlorothiazide 25mg	Reid-Provident
0063 4420 50/50	Hydralazine 50 mg, Hydrochlorothiazide 50mg	Reid-Provident
0085-V	Chlorpheniramine Maleate 4 mg	Vintage
0093 HY-PAM 25mg	Hy-Pam 25	Lemmon Pharm
0093 HY-PAM 50mg	Hy-Pam 50	Lemmon Pharm
010	Allopurinol 100 mg	West-ward Inc.
013	Allopurinol 300 mg	West-ward Inc.
016/R	CONTROLLED - SEE PAGE 192	
018/R	CONTROLLED - SEE PAGE 197	
020	Aminophylline 100 mg	West-ward Inc.
023/R	CONTROLLED - SEE PAGE 196	
025	Aminophylline 200 mg	West-ward Inc.
026/R	CONTROLLED - SEE PAGE 186	
027/R	CONTROLLED - SEE PAGE 225	
028/R	CONTROLLED - SEE PAGE 186	
029/R	CONTROLLED - SEE PAGE 225	
031/R	CONTROLLED - No Photo - Alprazolam 1 mg - Blue, round tablet - DEA Schedule IV	Purepac Pharm
045	Amitriptyline 10 mg	West-ward Inc.
046	Amitriptyline 25 mg	West-ward Inc.
047	Vitamins/Minerals	West-ward Inc.
048	Vitamins /Minerals	West-ward Inc.
049	Amitriptyline 100 mg	West-ward Inc.
050	Amitriptyline 50 mg	West-ward Inc.
051/R	CONTROLLED - SEE PAGE 191	
052/R	CONTROLLED - SEE PAGE 206	
053/R	CONTROLLED - SEE PAGE 210	
062	Aspirin 325 mg	West-ward Inc.
063	Aspirin 650 mg	West-ward Inc.
063/R	CONTROLLED - SEE PAGE 191	
064	Aspirin 500 mg	West-ward Inc.
070	Vitamins	West-ward Inc.
073	Bisacodyl 5 mg	West-ward Inc.
076	Vitamins	Amide Pharm
077	Vitaplex Plus	Amide Pharm
078/R	CONTROLLED - SEE PAGE 210	
080	Ascorbic Acid 100 mg	West-ward Inc.
083/R	CONTROLLED - SEE PAGE 207	
085	Ascorbic Acid 250 mg	West-ward Inc.
085/R	CONTROLLED - SEE PAGE 208	
087	Vitamins	West-ward Inc.
087	Chlorpromazine 100 mg	West-ward Inc.
090	Ascorbic Acid 500 mg	West-ward Inc.
090	Chlorpromazine 200 mg	West-ward Inc.
092	Caffeine, Ephedrine, Phenylpropanolamine	Unknown
095	Aspirin 325 mg	West-ward Inc.

Imprint	Ingredient/Brand Name	Manufacturer
0114 1405	Tetracycline 250 mg	Richlyn Labs
0115 1110	Diphenhydramine 25 mg	Richlyn Labs
0115 1111	Diphenhydramine 50 mg	Richlyn Labs
0115 1142	Ephedrine Sulfate 3/4 gr	Richlyn Labs
0115 1374	Quinine Sulfate 325 mg	Richlyn Labs
0115 1398	Tetracycline 100 mg	Richlyn Labs
0115 1400	Tetracycline 250 mg	Richlyn Labs
0115 1402	Tetracycline 500 mg	Richlyn Labs
0115 1405	Tetracycline 250 mg	Richlyn Labs
0115 2150	Aminophylline 100 mg	Richlyn Labs
0115 2158	Aminophylline 200 mg	Richlyn Labs
0115 2390	Sulfisoxazole, Phenylazodiaminopyridine	RichlynLabs
0115 2758	CONTROLLED - SEE PAGE 221	
0115 2760	CONTROLLED - SEE PAGE 223	
0115 2762	CONTROLLED - SEE PAGE 220	
0115 2790	Chloroquine Phosphate 20 mg	Richlyn Labs
0115 2810	Chlorpheniramine Maleate 4 mg	Richlyn Labs
0115 2920	Cortisone Acetate 25 mg	Richlyn Labs
0115 3030	Dehydrocholic Acid 250 mg	Richlyn Labs
0115 3100	Dexamethasone 0.75 mg	Richlyn Labs
0115 3250	Pepsin 250 mg, Pancreatin 300 mg, Bile Salts 150 mg	Richlyn Labs
0115 3585	Folic Acid 1 mg	Richlyn Labs
0115 3660	Hydralazine 25 mg	Richlyn Labs
0115 3662	Hydralazine 50 mg	Richlyn Labs
0115 3670	Hydrochlorothiazide 25 mg	Richlyn Labs
0115 3675	Hydrochlorothiazide 50 mg	Richlyn Labs
0115 3677	Hydrochlorothiazide 100 mg	Richlyn Labs
0115 3685	Hydrocortisone 20 mg	Richlyn Labs
0115 3706	Isoniazid 100 mg	Richlyn Labs
0115 3875	Meclizine 25 mg	Richlyn Labs
0115 3888	CONTROLLED - SEE PAGE 194	
0115 3890	CONTROLLED - SEE PAGE 197	
0115 3900	Methocarbamol 500 mg	Richlyn Labs
0115 3902	Methocarbamol 750 mg	Richlyn Labs
0115 3976	Methenamine Mandelate 500 mg	Richlyn Labs
0115 3977	Methenamine Mandelate 1000 mg	Richlyn Labs
0115 3982	CONTROLLED - SEE PAGE 206	
0115 3984	CONTROLLED - SEE PAGE 194	
0115 3986	CONTROLLED - SEE PAGE 206	
0115 4214	CONTROLLED - SEE PAGE 185	
0115 4233	CONTROLLED - SEE PAGE 186	
0115 4252	Piperazine Citrate 250 mg	Richlyn Labs
0115 4280	Prednisolone 5 mg	Richlyn Labs
0115 4294	Prednisone 5 mg	Richlyn Labs
0115 4302	Probenecid 500 mg, Colchicine 0.5 mg	Richlyn Labs
0115 4306	Promethazine 25 mg	Richlyn Labs
0115 4308	Propantheline Br 15 mg	Richlyn Labs
0115 4322	Propylthiouracil 50 mg	Richlyn Labs
0115 4331	Pseudoephedrine 60 mg, Triprolidine 2.5 mg	Richlyn Labs
0115 4332	Pseudoephedrine 60 mg	Richlyn Labs
0115 4334	Phenazopyridine 100 mg	Richlyn Labs
0115 4336	Phenazopyridine 200 mg	Richlyn Labs
0115 4380	Quinidine Sulfate 200 mg	Richlyn Labs
0115 4400	Rauwolfia Serpentina 50 mg	Richlyn Labs
0115 4404	Rauwolfia Serpentina 100 mg	Richlyn Labs
0115 4428	Reserpine 0.25 mg	Richlyn Labs

Imprint	Ingredient/Brand Name	Manufacturer
0115 4631	Sodium Flouride 2.21 mg	Richlyn Labs
0115 4711	Sulfadiazine 2.5 mg, Sulfamerazine 2.5 mg, Sulfamethazine 2.5 mg	Rich
0115 4714	Sulfadiazine 500 mg	Richlyn Labs
0115 4747	Sulfisoxazole 500 mg	Richlyn Labs
0115 4824	Thyroid 1 grain	Richlyn Labs
0115 4825	Thyroid 1 grain	Richlyn Labs
0115 4826	Thyroid 2 grains	Richlyn Labs
0115 4827	Thyroid 2 grains	Richlyn Labs
0115 4829	Thyroid 3 grains	Richlyn Labs
0115 4840	Triamcinolone 4 mg	Richlyn Labs
0115 4860	Trichlormethiazide 4 mg	Richlyn Labs
0115 4871	Tripelennamine 50 mg	Richlyn Labs
0115 6537	Diethylcarbamazine Citrate 200 mg	Richlyn Labs
0115 6540	Diethylcarbamazine Citrate 400 mg	Richlyn Labs
0118	Folic Acid, Iron	Copley Pharm
0124	Docusate Sodium 100 mg	R.P. Scherer
0129	Docusate Sodium 250 mg	R.P. Scherer
0131 20/08	Chlorpheniramine 2 mg, Pseudoephedrine 30 mg, Acetaminophen 325 mg	Central Pharm
0140	Vitamin D 50,000 units	Richlyn Labs
0149 0008	Macrodantin 50 mg	Norwich Eaton
0149 0009	Macrodantin 100 mg	Norwich Eaton
0149 0412	Entex 5 mg/45 mg/200 mg	Norwich Eaton
0149 0436	Entex LA 75 mg/400 mg	Norwich Eaton
0149 0444	Comhist 2 mg/25 mg/10 mg	Norwich Eaton
0149 0446	Comhist LA 4 mg/50 mg/20 mg	Norwich Eaton
0157	Prenatal 1 mg/60 mg	Copley Pharm
0158	Vitamins, Fluoride 0.5 mg	Copley Pharm
0159	Vitamins, Fluoride	Copley Pharm
0230	Doxycycline 100 mg	Rugby
0250	Erythromycin 250 mg	Rugby
0265	Erythromycin 500 mg	Rugby
0280	Doxycycline 50 mg	Rugby
0310 [logo logo]	Magnesium Salicylate 600 mg	Ascher & Co
0340	Doxycycline 100 mg	Rugby
0345 1032	CONTROLLED - No Photo - Propoxyphene HCl 65 mg, Aspirin 389 mg, Caffeine 32.4 mg - DEA Schedule IV	Lemmon
0390	Doxcycline 50 mg	Rugby
0524/0405	Allopurinol 100 mg	UDL Labs
0524/0410	Allopurinol 300 mg	UDL Labs
0527 1179	CONTROLLED - SEE PAGE 209	
0527/1552	CONTROLLED - No Photo - Butalbital 50 mg, Aspirin 325 mg, Caffeine 40 mg - Green capsule - DEA Schedule III	Lannett
0628	Ferrous Fumarate 150 mg, Docusate Sodium 100 mg	R.P. Scherer
0665	Lithium Carbonate 300 mg	Reid-Rowell
0665-1393	Reserpine 0.1 mg, Hydralazine 25 mg, Hydrochlorothiazide 15 mg	Reid
0665-4001	Medroxyprogesterone Acetate 10 mg	Reid-Rowell
0665-4120	Valproic Acid 250 mg	Scherer
0665 4160	Lithium Carbonate 300 mg	Reid-Rowell
0665-4410 25/25	Hydralazine 25 mg, Hydrochlorothiazide 25 mg	Reid-Rowell
0665-4420 50/50	Hydralazine 50 mg, Hydrochlorothiazide 50 mg	Reid-Rowell
0822	Sodium Fluoride 2.2 mg	Pharmafair
0822 0405	Allopurinol 100 mg	Boots Labs
0822 0410	Allopurinol 300 mg	Boots Labs
0822 0430	CONTROLLED - SEE PAGE 198	
0822 0545	Hydrochlorothiazide 25 mg	Boots Labs

Imprint	Ingredient/Brand Name	Manufacturer
0822 0550	hydrochlorothiazide 50 mg	Boots Labs
0866	Docusate Calcium 240 mg	R.P. Scherer
0878	Docusate Potassium 100 mg	R.P. Scherer
0882 0576	Meclizine 25 mg	Boots Labs
0882 0841	Sodium Fluoride 2.2 mg	Boots Labs
0882 1259	l-Thyroxine 0.1 mg	Boots Labs
0882 1530	l-Thyroxine 0.2 mg	Boots Labs
0882 1531	l-Thyroxine 0.3 mg	Boots Labs
0891	Docusate Potassium 100 mg, Casanthranol 30 mg	R.P. Scherer
0895	Docusate Calcium 60 mg, Yellow Phenolphthalein 65 mg	R.P. Scherer
0897	Docusate Sodium 100 mg	R.P. Scherer
0898	Docusate 10 mg	Scherer
0920 [logo]	Dilatrate-SR 40 mg	Vitarine Pharm
01001	Pancreatin 425 mg	Viobin
1	Choloxin 1 mg	Flint
1	Nitrogard 1 mg	Parke-Davis
1/841	Haloperidol 1 mg	Searle Pharm
1 APAP	Acetaminophen 500 mg	Magno-Humphries
1 APAP 500	Acetaminophen 500 mg	Magno Humphries
1 D 50	Diphenhydramine 50 mg	Magno-Humphries
1P 211	Pseudoephedrine 60 mg, Chlorpheniramine Maleate 4 mg, Acetaminophen 650 mg	Econolab
1/WYETH	CONTROLLED - SEE PAGE 196	
2	Nitrogard 2 mg	Parke-Davis
2	Choloxin 2 mg	Flint
2	Panwarfin 2 mg	Abbott
2 1/2 [logo]	Zaroxolyn 2.5 mg	Pennwalt Corp
2/851	Haloperidol 2 mg	Searle Pharm
2 LL L12	Levothyroxine Sodium 0.2 mg	Lederle Labs
2 VALIUM/ROCHE	CONTROLLED - SEE PAGE 193	
2/WYETH	CONTROLLED - SEE PAGE 195	
3	Nitrogard 3 mg	Parke-Davis
3/CIBA	CONTROLLED - SEE PAGE 209	
3M/107	Aluminum Hydroxide	3M
3M/221	Orphenadrine 100 mg	3M
3M/ALU-CAP	Aluminum Hydroxide	3M
3M/SR 200	Theophylline 200 mg	3M
3M/SR 250	Theophylline 250 mg	3M
3M/SR 300	Theophylline 300 mg	3M
3M/SR 500	Theophylline 500 mg	3M
3M/TR 150	Flecainide Acetate 150 mg	3M
4	Ibuprofen 400 mg	LuChem Pharm
4	Dextrothyroxine Sodium 4 mg	Boots Labs
4	Acetaminophen 325 mg	Bristol-Myers
4 [logo]	Choloxin 2 mg	Flint Labs
5	Panwarfin 5 mg	Abbott
5 C33	Leucovorin Calcium 5 mg	Lederla Labs
5 GGG	Acetaminophen 500 mg	Granutec
5 [logo]	Zaroxolyn 5 mg	Pennwalt Corp
5 VALIUM ROCHE	CONTROLLED - SEE PAGE 206	
6	Dextrothyroxine Sodium 6 mg	Boots Labs
6	Ibuprofen 600 mg	LuChem Pharm
6 6/LEMMON	CONTROLLED - SEE PAGE 211	
7/41 LuChem	Phenylpropanolamine 75 mg, Guaifenesin 400 mg	LuChem Pharm
8	Ibuprofen 800 mg	LuChem Pharm
8 [heart logo] [heart logo]	CONTROLLED - SEE PAGE 225	

Imprint	Ingredient/Brand Name	Manufacturer
10	Panwarfin 10 mg	Abbott
10	Pyrilamine	Unknown
10/78 2	Melleril 10 mg	Sandoz Pharm
10 78-212	Metaproterenol 10 mg	Sandoz Pharm
10 88/SOLVAY	CONTROLLED - SEE PAGE 204	
10/93 911	Isoxsuprine 10 mg	Lemmon Pharm
10-267 [logo]	Caffeine, Ephedrine,Phenylpropanolamine	Unknown
10/832	Chlorpromazine HCl 10 mg	Pharm Basics
10/871	Haloperidol 10 mg	Searle Pharm
10-1356 [logo]	Caffeine, Ephedrine,Phenylpropanolamine	Unknown
10 1362	Caffeine	Unknown
10 [logo]	Zaroxolyn 10 mg	Pennwalt Corp
10 LL C12	Leucovorin Calcium 10 mg	Lederle Labs
10 VALIUM/ROCHE	CONTROLLED - SEE PAGE 209	
11 11/GYNEX	CONTROLLED - SEE PAGE 199	
11/[triangle]	Akineton 2 mg	Knoll Pharm
12.7	Caffeine	Unknown
13/308	K-Lease 750 mg	Adria Labs
13 411	Magnesium Salicylate 650 mg	Adria Labs
13/503	Modane Soft 120 mg	Adria Labs
13 511	Docusate Sodium 100 mg	Adria Labs
13/807	Caffeine	Unknown
14 01/SEARLE	CONTROLLED - SEE PAGE 199	
14 [triangle logo]	Quadrinal 65 mg/24 mg/ 320 mg/24 mg	Knoll
16-665 [star]	Caffeine, Ephedrine, Phenylpropanolamine	Unknown
16 807	Caffeine, Ephedrine, Phenylpropanolamine	Unknown
16 856	Caffeine	Unknown
16 865	Caffeine	Unknown
16 870	Caffeine, Ephedrine, Phenylpropanolamine	Unknown
16 907	Caffeine, Ephedrine, Phenylpropanolamine	Unknown
17 865	Caffeine, Ephedrine, Phenylpropanolamine	Unknown
17 906	Caffeine, Ephedrine, Phenylpropanolamine	Unknown
18-0010 [logo]	K-Norm 750 mg	Pennwalt Corp
18 356	Adapin 10 mg	Pennwalt Corp
18 357	Adapin 25 mg	Pennwalt Corp
18 358	Adapin 50 mg	Pennwalt Corp
18 359	Adapin 100 mg	Pennwalt Corp
18 361	Adapin 75 mg	Pennwalt Corp
18-361 [logo]	Doxepin	Pennwalt Corp
18-370 [logo]	Adapin 150 mg	Pennwalt Corp
18 704	Caffeine, Ephedrine, Phenylpropanolamine	Unknown
18 789	Caffeine, Ephedrine, Phenylpropanolamine	Unknown
18 845 [logo]	Caffeine, Ephedrine, Phenylpropanolamine	Unknown
18 850	Caffeine, Ephedrine, Phenylpropanolamine	Unknown
18 858	Caffeine, Ephedrine, Phenylpropanolamine	Unknown
18 875	Caffeine, Ephedrine, Phenylpropanolamine	Unknown
18 876	Caffeine, Ephedrine, Phenylpropanolamine	Unknown
18-892 [logo]	Tussionex 10 mg/5 mg	Pennwalt Corp
18-894/ [logo]	CONTROLLED - SEE PAGE 195	
18 895	Caffeine, Ephedrine, Phenylpropanolamine	Unknown
18-904[logo]	CONTROLLED - SEE PAGE 215	
18 906	Caffeine, Ephedrine, Phenylpropanolamine	Unknown
18 907	Ephedrine	Unknown
18 985	Caffeine, Ephedrine	Unknown
18C658	Caffeine, Ephedrine, Phenylpropanolamine	Unknown
19 80	Caffeine, Ephedrine, Phenylpropanolamine	Unknown

Imprint	Ingredient/Brand Name	Manufacturer
19 731	Caffeine	Unknown
19 795	Caffeine, Ephedrine, Phenylpropanolamine	Unknown
20	Hygroton 50 mg	USV Labs
20 20	Caffeine, Ephedrine, Phenylpropanolamine	Unknown
20/832	Chlorpromazine 20 mg	Pharm Basics
21	Hygroton 100 mg	USV Labs
22	Hygroton 25 mg	USV Labs
25	Dicumarol 25 mg	Abbott Labs
25 50	Caffeine, Pseudoephedrine	Unknown
25/323	Hydrolxyzine 25 mg	Barr Labs
29 02/SYNTEX	CONTROLLED - SEE PAGE 189	
30	Dyphylline 200 mg	Lemmon Pharm
30 30	Caffeine	Unknown
31	Regroton 50 mg/0.25 mg	USV Labs
32	Demi-Redroton 25 mg/0.125 mg	USV Labs
32/OP	CONTROLLED - SEE PAGE 210	
33/OP	CONTROLLED - SEE PAGE 202	
34/CIBA	CONTROLLED - SEE PAGE 205	
37	Dyphylline 400 mg	Lemmon Pharm
37/37	Dyphylline 400 mg	Lemmon Pharm
37 112/BUTISOL SODIUM	CONTROLLED - SEE PAGE 209	
37 113/BUTISOL SODIUM	CONTROLLED - SEE PAGE 212	
37 114/BUTISOL SODIUM	CONTROLLED - SEE PAGE 203	
37 115/BUTISOL SODIUM	CONTROLLED - SEE PAGE 207	
37 4401	Depen 250 mg	Wallace Labs
37 WALLACE 1001	CONTROLLED - SEE PAGE 197	
37 WALLACE 3001	CONTROLLED - SEE PAGE 207	
39 14/RUGBY	CONTROLLED - SEE PAGE 226	
40 [logo]	Verapamil 40 mg	Knoll
40 40	Caffeine	Unknown
44	Vicks Formula 44 Cold & Cough	Procot & Gamble
44-107	Diphenhydramine HCl 25 mg	LNK International
44-111	Pseudoephedrine 30 mg	LNK
44-156	Acetaminophen 325 mg, Phenyltoloxamine Citrate 30 mg	LNK
44-160	Aspirin 325 mg, Aluminum Hydroxide 50 mg, Calcium Carbonate 50 mg, Magnesium Hydroxide 50 mg	LNK
44-163	Phenylephrine 5 mg, Chlorpheniramine 2 mg, Acetaminophen 325 mg	LNK
44-165	Aspirin 325 mg, Aluminum Hydroxide 75 mg, Calcium Carbonate 75 mg, Magnesium Hydroxide 75 mg	LNK
44-184	Acetaminophen 80 mg	LNK
44-188	Pseudoephedrine 30 mg, Chlorpheniramine 2 mg, Acetaminophen 500 mg	LNK
44-189	Diphenhydramine 25 mg	LNK
44-191	Diphenhydramine 25 mg	LNK
44-197	Phenylpropanolamine 75 mg, Brompheniramine 12 mg	LNK
44-198	Dimenhydramine 50 mg	LNK
44 218	Aspirin 81 mg	LNK International
44-194	Pseudoephedrine 60 mg, Chlorpheniramine Maleate 4 mg	H.L. Moore
44-201	Aluminum Hydroxide 200 mg, Magnesium Hydroxide 200 mg	H.L. Moore
44 249	Aspirin 325 mg	UDL Labs
44 250	Aspirin 325 mg	UDL Labs
45	Arlidin 6 mg	USV Labs
45/USV	Arlidin 6 mg	Rorer
46	Arlidin 12 mg	USV Labs
46/USV	Arlidin 12 mg	Rorer

Imprint	Ingredient/Brand Name	Manufacturer
50	Dicumarol 50 mg	Abbott Labs
50/832	Chlorpromazine 50 mg	Pharm Basics
51/RP	CONTROLLED - SEE PAGE 205	
52/RP	CONTROLLED - SEE PAGE 205	
54 009	Propranolol 20 mg	Philips Roxane
54 010	Diflunisal 250 mg	Philips Roxane
54 012	Amitriptyline 25 mg	Philips Roxane
54 013	Leucovorin Sodium 25 mg	Phillips Roxane
54 019	Chlorpheniramine 4 mg	Philips Roxane
54 039	Naproxen 500 mg	Phillips Roxane
54 049	Dexamethasone 8 mg	Philips Roxane
54 050	Haloperidol 1 mg	Philips Roxane
54 053/300	Quinidine Sulfate 300 mg	Phillips Roxane
54 062	Propranolol 60 mg	Philips Roxane
54 063	Acetaminophen 325 mg	Philips Roxane
54 080	Prednisone 25 mg	Philips Roxane
54 090	CONTROLLED - SEE PAGE 196	
54 090/30	CONTROLLED - SEE PAGE 196	
54 092	Prednisone 1 mg	Philips Roxane
54 093	Diflunisal 500 mg	Philips Roxane
54 099	Amitriptyline 50 mg	Philips Roxane
54 103	Bisacodyl 5 mg	Philips Roxane
54 133	Calcium Carbonate 1250 mg	Philips Roxane
54 142	CONTROLLED - SEE PAGE 193	
54 143	Amitriptyline 100 mg	Philips Roxane
54 169	Haloperidol 0.5 mg	Philips Roxane
54 172	Isoxsuprine 10 mg	Philips Roxane
54 179	CONTROLLED - SEE PAGE 216	
54 180	Naproxen Sodium 275 mg	Phillips Roxane
54 183	Prednisolone 5 mg	Philips Roxane
54 210	CONTROLLED - SEE PAGE 187	
54 212	Neomycin 500 mg	Philips Roxane
54 213	Lithium Carbonate 150 mg	Philips Roxane
54 219	Sodium Docusate 250 mg	Philips Roxane
54 223	Diphenhydramine 50 mg	Philips Roxane
54 249	Propranolol 80 mg	Philips Roxane
54 252	Acetaminophen 500 mg	Philips Roxane
54 253	Sulfamethoxazole 400 mg, Trimethoprim 80 mg	Philips Roxane
54 259	Ferrous Sulfate 300 mg	Philips Roxane
54 262	CONTROLLED - SEE PAGE 191	
54 263	CONTROLLED - SEE PAGE 191	
54 280	Dihydrotachysterol 0.125 mg	Philips Roxane
54 293	Leucovorin 5 mg	Phillips Roxane
54 299	Dexamethasone 0.5 mg	Philips Roxane
54 302	Calcium Carbonate 1250 mg	Philips Roxane
54 303	Propantheline Bromide 15 mg	Philips Roxane
54 329	Indomethacin 50 mg	Philips Roxane
54 333	Propranolol 40 mg	Philips Roxane
54 339	Prednisone 2.5 mg	Philips Roxane
54 343	Prednisone 50 mg	Philips Roxane
54 360	Amitriptyline 75 mg	Philips Roxane
54 369	Loperamide 2 mg	Philips Roxane
54 372	Calcium Gluconate 500 mg	Philips Roxane
54 379	Sodium Docusate 50 mg	Philips Roxane
54 382	Haloperidol 10 mg	Philips Roxane
54 383	Methyldopa 500 mg	Philips Roxane

Imprint	Ingredient/Brand Name	Manufacturer
54 409	CONTROLLED - No Photo - Morphine Sulfate 30 mg - DEA Schedule II	Phillips Roxane
54 410	CONTROLLED - SEE PAGE 188	
54 412	CONTROLLED - SEE PAGE 192	
54 413	Aluminum Hydroxide 500 mg	Philips Roxane
54 422	Indomethacin 25 mg	Philips Roxane
54 450	Dexamethasone 0.125 mg	Philips Roxane
54 452	Lithium Carbonate 300 mg	Philips Roxane
54 463	Lithium Carbonate 300 mg	Philips Roxane
54 472	Piroxicam 10 mg	Phillips Roxane
54 479	Piroxicam 20 mg	Phillips Roxane
54 489	Dexamethasone 1 mg	Philips Roxane
54 492	Amitriptyline 150 mg	Philips Roxane
54 499	Hydrochlorthiazide 50 mg	Philips Roxane
54 503	CONTROLLED - SEE PAGE 185	
54 512	CONTROLLED - No Photo - Alprazolam 0.25 mg - DEA Schedule IV	Phillips Roxane
54 529	Thiethylperazine Maleate 10 mg	Philips Roxane
54 532	Pseudoephedrine 60 mg	Philips Roxane
54 533	Furosemide 80 mg	Philips Roxane
54 539	Ascorbic Acid 250 mg	Philips Roxane
54 542	CONTROLLED - SEE PAGE 200	
54 543	CONTROLLED - SEE PAGE 197	
54 570	Haloperidol 2 mg	Philips Roxane
54 572	CONTROLLED - SEE PAGE 188	
54 579	Isoxsuprine 20 mg	Philips Roxane
54 582	CONTROLLED - SEE PAGE 188	
54 583	Furosemide 40 mg	Philips Roxane
54 599	Alprazolam 0.5 mg	Phillips Roxane
54 603	Naproxen Sodium 550 mg	Phillips Roxane
54 609	CONTROLLED - SEE PAGE 188	
54 612	Prednisone 5 mg	Philips Roxane
54 613	CONTROLLED - SEE PAGE 188	
54 622	Methyldopa 250 mg	Philips Roxane
54 623	CONTROLLED - No Photo - Codeine Phosphate 30 mg, Acetaminophen 300 mg - DEA Schedule III	Phillips Roxane
54 643	Naproxen Sodium 250 mg	Phillips Roxane
54 650	Leucovorin Sodium 15 mg	Phillips Roxane
54 659	Pseudoephedrine 60 mg, Triprolidine 2.5 mg	Philips Roxane
54 662	Dexamethasone 2 mg	Roxane
54 663	Sodium Docusate 100 mg	Philips Roxane
54 680	Ascorbic Acid 500 mg	Philips Roxane
54 690	Haloperidol 20 mg	Philips Roxane
54 699	Niacin 50 mg	Philips Roxane
54 702	Lithium Carbonate 600 mg	Philips Roxane
54 703	Imipramine 50 mg	Philips Roxane
54 720	Sodium Docusate 100 mg, Casanthranol 30 mg	Philips Roxane
54 730	CONTROLLED - SEE PAGE 201	
54 733	CONTROLLED - SEE PAGE 187	
54 743	CONTROLLED - SEE PAGE 187	
54 760	Prednisone 20 mg	Philips Roxane
54 769	Dexamethasone 6 mg	Philips Roxane
54 772	Dihydrotachysterol 0.4 mg	Philips Roxane
54 773	Haloperidol 5 mg	Philips Roxane
54 779	CONTROLLED - SEE PAGE 192	
54 783	CONTROLLED - SEE PAGE 188	

Imprint	Ingredient/Brand Name	Manufacturer
54 810	Propranolol 90 mg	Philips Roxane
54 812	Hydrochlorothiazide 25 mg	Philips Roxane
54 819	Acetaminiophen 650 mg	Philips Roxane
54 822	Sulfamethoxazole 800 mg, Trimethoprim 160 mg	Philips Roxane
54 823	Pseudoephedrine 30 mg	Philips Roxane
54 840	Furosemide 20 mg	Philips Roxane
54 853	Methyldopa 125 mg	Philips Roxane
54 859	Aminophylline 100 mg	Philips Roxane
54 860	CONTROLLED - No Photo - Alprazolam 1 mg - DEA Schedule IV	Phillips Roxane
54 862/100	CONTROLLED - SEE PAGE 194	
54 880	Imipramine 25 mg	Philips Roxane
54 892	Dexamethasone 4 mg	Philips Roxane
54 899	Prednisone 10 mg	Philips Roxane
54 902	CONTROLLED - SEE PAGE 197	
54 903	Dihydrotachysterol 0.2 mg	Philips Roxane
54 930	Aminophylline 200 mg	Philips Roxane
54 933/60	CONTROLLED - SEE PAGE 193	
54 939	Imipramine 10 mg	Philips Roxane
54 942	Leucovorin Calcium 10 mg	Phillips Roxane
54 943	Dexamethasone 1.5 mg	Philips Roxane
54 960	Dexamethasone 0.75 mg	Philips Roxane
54 969/2	CONTROLLED - SEE PAGE 202	
54 970	Propranolol 10 mg	Philips Roxane
54 973/5	CONTROLLED - SEE PAGE 202	
54 979/200	Quinidine Sulfate 300 mg	Phillips Roxane
54 982/10	CONTROLLED - SEE PAGE 203	
54 983	Amitriptyline 10 mg	Philips Roxane
54 992	Naproxen 375 mg	Phillips Roxane
56-105	Symmetrel 100 mg	DuPont Pharm
56 70/RUGBY	CONTROLLED - SEE PAGE 225	
57/R	CONTROLLED - SEE PAGE 184 or 188	
57 [logo]	Zorprin 800 mg	Boots Pharm
58 [logo]	Ru-Tuss 25 mg/50 mg/8 mg	Boots Pharm
59/R	CONTROLLED - SEE PAGE 184 or 186	
60	Azolid 100 mg	USV Labs
60/R	CONTROLLED - SEE PAGE 225	
61/SEARLE	CONTROLLED - SEE PAGE 185	
62 51/AHR	CONTROLLED - SEE PAGE 201	
63 50/UAD	CONTROLLED - SEE PAGE 226	
64	Herbal Diuretic Tablets	Major Pharm
64/U	Provera 2.5 mg	Upjohn Comp
64 WYETH/A	CONTROLLED - SEE PAGE 189	
65 WYETH/A 2	CONTROLLED - SEE PAGE 192	
68-7	Norpramin 10 mg	Merrell Dow
71 71/LEMMON	CONTROLLED - SEE PAGE 199	
71/WYETH	CONTROLLED - SEE PAGE 186	
78-2	Mellaril 10 mg	Sandoz Pharm
78-3	Mellaril 25 mg	Sandoz Pharm
78-4	Mellaril 50 mg	Sandoz Pharm
78-5	Mellaril 100 mg	Sandoz Pharm
78-6	Mellaril 150 mg	Sandoz Pharm
78-7	Mellaril 200 mg	Sandoz Pharm
78-8	Mellaril 15 mg	Sandoz Pharm
78 8/15mg	Melleril 15 mg	Sandoz Pharm
78-27	Belladenal-S	Sandoz Pharm

Imprint	Ingredient/Brand Name	Manufacturer
78-28	Belladenal	Sandoz Pharm
78-31	Bellergal-S	Sandoz Pharm
78 66/SANDOZ	CONTROLLED - SEE PAGE 193	
78-71/SANDOZ	CONTROLLED - SEE PAGE 199	
78-212/10	Metaprel 10 mg	Sandoz Pharm
78-213/20	Metaprel 20 mg	Sandoz Pharm
82	Lozol 2.5 mg	USV Labs
85-WMH	Dexbrompheniramine 6 mg, Pseudoephedrine 120 mg	Schering
86 48/C	CONTROLLED - SEE PAGE 212	
86 62	Skelaxin 400 mg	Carnrick Labs
86 74/C	CONTROLLED - SEE PAGE 191	
861/5	Haloperidol 5 mg	Searle Pharm
91/GG	CONTROLLED - SEE PAGE 186	
92/2	Warfarin 2 mg	Lemmon Pharm
93 064	Tetracycline 250 mg	Lemmon Pharm
93 088	Sulfamethoxazole 400 mg, Trimethoprim 80 mg	Lemmon Pharm
93 089	Sulfamethoxazole 800 mg, Trimethoprim 160 mg	Lemmon Pharm
93 090	Carbamazepine 200 mg	Lemmon Pharm
93/2 1/2	Warfarin 2.5 mg	Lemmon Pharm
93/5	Warfarin 5 mg	Lemmon Pharm
93 7	Chlorpropamide 250 mg	Lemmon Pharm
93 10	Chlorpropamide 100 mg	Lemmon Pharm
93 21	Diltiazem HCl 60 mg	Lemmon Pharm
93 22	Diltiazem HCl 90 mg	Lemmon Pharm
93 23	Diltiazem HCl 120 mg	Lemmon Pharm
93 41	Clomiphene Citrate 50 mg	Lemmon Pharm
93 50/2	CONTROLLED - SEE PAGE 195	
93 93/COTRIM	Sulfamethoxazole 400 mg, Trimethoprim 80 mg	Lemmon Pharm
93 93/EPITOL	Carbamazepine 200 mg	Lemmon Pharm
93/93 778	Carbamazepine 100 mg	Lemmon Pharm
93 138	Diphenhydramine 25 mg	Lemmon Pharm
93 139	Diphenhydramine 50 mg	Lemmon Pharm
93 143	Warfarin Sodium 2 mg	Lemmon Pharm
93 144	Warfarin Sodium 2.5 mg	Lemmon Pharm
93 145	Warfarin Sodium 5 mg	Lemmon Pharm
93 150/3	CONTROLLED - SEE PAGE 195	
93 188	Sulfamethoxazole 400 mg, Trimethoprim 80 mg	Lemmon Pharm
93 189	Sulfamethoxazole 800 mg, Trimethoprim 160 mg	Lemmon Pharm
93 213	Tolmetin Sodium 400 mg	Lemmon Pharm
93 292	Carbidopa 10 mg, Levodopa 100 mg	Lemmon Pharm
93 293	Carbidopa 25 mg, Levodopa 100 mg	Lemmon Pharm
93 294	Carbidopa 25 mg, Levodopa 250 mg	Lemmon Pharm
93 307	Clemastine Fumarate 1.34 mg	Lemmon Pharm
93 308	Clemastine Fumarate 2.68 mg	Lemmon Pharm
93 311	Loperamide 2 mg	Lemmon Pharm
93 325	Desipramine 25 mg	Lemmon Pharm
93 326	Desipramine 50 mg	Lemmon Pharm
93 327	Desipramine 75 mg	Lemmon Pharm
93 328	Desipramine 100 mg	Lemmon Pharm
93 350/4	CONTROLLED - SEE PAGE 196	
93 431	Chlorthalidone 50 mg	Lemmon Pharm
93 433	Chlorthalidone 100 mg	Lemmon Pharm
93 484	Doxycycline 100 mg	Lemmon Pharm
93 486	Ibuprofen 200 mg	Lemmon Pharm
93 490	CONTROLLED -No Photo - Propoxyphene Napsylate 100 mg, Acetaminophen 650 mg - DEA Schedule IV	Lemmon Pharm

Imprint	Ingredient/Brand Name	Manufacturer
93 491	Ibuprofen 400 mg	Lemmon Pharm
93 492	Ibuprofen 600 mg	Lemmon Pharm
93 498	Ibuprofen 800 mg	Lemmon Pharm
93 541	Cephalexin 250 mg	Lemmon Pharm
93 542	Chlorzoxazone 500 mg	Lemmon Pharm
93 543	Cephalexin 500 mg	Lemmon Pharm
93 545	Chlorzoxazone 250 mg, Acetaminophen 300 mg	Lemmon Pharm
93 548	Amantadine 100 mg	Lemmon Pharm
93 585	Indo-Lemmon Pharm 25 mg	Lemmon Pharm
93 587	Indo-Lemmon Pharm 50 mg	Lemmon Pharm
93 613	Amoxicillin 250 mg	Lemmon Pharm
93 615	Amoxicillin 500 mg	Lemmon Pharm
93 617	Chlordiazepoxide 5 mg, Clidinium 2.5 mg	Lemmon Pharm
93 620	Propranolol 20 mg	Lemmon Pharm
93 628	Indomethacin 75 mg	Lemmon Pharm
93 637	Trazodone 50 mg	Lemmon Pharm
93 638	Trazodone 100 mg	Lemmon Pharm
93 640	Propranolol 40 mg	Lemmon Pharm
93 653	Doxycycline Hyclate 100 mg	Lemmon Pharm
93 665	Albuterol Sulfate 2 mg	Lemmon Pharm
93 666	Albuterol Sulfate 4 mg	Lemmon Pharm
93 670	Gemfibrozil 600 mg	Lemmon Pharm
93 686	CONTROLLED - SEE PAGE 222	
93 691	Propranolol 60 mg	Lemmon Pharm
93 692	Propranolol 80 mg	Lemmon Pharm
93 693	Propranolol 120 mg	Lemmon Pharm
93 694	Propranolol 160 mg	Lemmon Pharm
93 727	Papaverine 150 mg	Lemmon Pharm
93 728	Sulindac 150 mg	Lemmon Pharm
93 729	Sulindac 200 mg	Lemmon Pharm
93 741	CONTROLLED - SEE PAGE 215	
93 742	Doxy-Lemmon Pharm 50 mg	Lemmon Pharm
93 743	Doxy-Lemmon Pharm 100 mg	Lemmon Pharm
93 756	Piroxicam 10 mg	Lemmon Pharm
93 757	Piroxicam 20 mg	Lemmon Pharm
93 758/EPITOL	Epitol 100 mg	Lemmon Pharm
93 777	Hydrochlorothiazide 25 mg	Lemmon Pharm
93 779	Hydrochlorothiazide 50 mg	Lemmon Pharm
93 789	Perphenazine 2 mg	Lemmon Pharm
93 790	Perphenazine 4 mg	Lemmon Pharm
93 791	Perphenazine 8 mg	Lemmon Pharm
93 792	Perphenazine 16 mg	Lemmon Pharm
93 798	Indomethacin 25 mg	Lemmon Pharm
93 799	Indomethacin 50 mg	Lemmon Pharm
93 821	Reserpine 0.1 mg	Lemmon Pharm
93 824	Pseudoephedrine 60 mg	Lemmon Pharm
93 827	Reserpine 0.1 mg	Lemmon Pharm
93 828	Uninary Antiseptic No.3	Lemmon Pharm
93 835	Urinary Antiseptic Veterinary	Lemmon Pharm
93 841	Dicyclomine 10 mg	Lemmon Pharm
93 845	Urinary Antiseptic No. 2	Lemmon Pharm
93 848	Triphed 60 mg/2.5 mg	Lemmon Pharm
93 851	Metronidazole 250 mg	Lemmon Pharm
93 852	Metronidazole 500 mg	Lemmon Pharm
93 860	CONTROLLED - No Photo - Phentermine HCl 30 mg - Yellow capsule - DEA Schedule IV	Lemmon Pharm

Imprint	Ingredient/Brand Name	Manufacturer
93 891	Dicyclomine 20 mg	Lemmon Pharm
93 911/10	Isoxsuprine 10 mg	Lemmon Pharm
93 913/20	Isoxsuprine 20 mg	Lemmon Pharm
93 943	Nystatin 100,000 units	Lemmon Pharm
93 983	Nystatin Oral 500,000 units	Lemmon Pharm
93 DOXY	Doxycycline Hyclate 100 mg	Lemmon Pharm
94-44	Isoclor 8 mg/120 mg	Fisons Corp
100	Dicumarol 100 mg	Abbott Labs
100	Doxycycline 50 mg	Mutual Pharm
100/93 10	Chlorpropamide 100 mg	Lemmon Pharm
100/3027	Allopurinol 100 mg	Rugby
101	Indomethacin 25 mg	Mutual Pharm
101	Caffeine	Unknown
102	Aluminum Hydroxide 200 mg, Magnesium Hydroxide 200 mg	Guardian
103	Diphenhydramine 25 mg	Mutual Pharm
105	Doxycycline 100 mg	Mutual Pharm
106	Indomethacin 50 mg	Mutual Pharm
107	Dipyridamole 25 mg	West-ward Inc.
107	Diphenhydramine 50 mg	Mutual Pharm
109	Dipyridamole 50 mg	West-ward Inc
109 [star logo]	Uro-Kp-Neutral	Star Pharm
109 [logo]	Clofazimine 100 mg	Geigy
111	Dipyridamole 75 mg	West-ward Inc.
111	Prenatal 1 mg/1 mg	Copley Pharm
111/UAD	CONTROLLED - SEE PAGE 204	
113	R-Tannate	Copley Pharm
113	Chlorpheniramine 8 mg	West-ward Inc.
114	Chlorpheniramine 12 mg	West-ward Inc.
114	Procainamide 750 mg	Copley Pharm
115	Ferrous Gluconate 325 mg	West-ward Inc.
115/USV	Cerespan 150 mg	Rorer
117	Vitamin B Complex, Vitamin C	Freshlabs
122	Bismuth Subsalicylate 262 mg	Guardian
122	Loperamide 2 mg	Granutec
124 [logo]	Hydrochlorothiazide 50 mg	Heather Drug
126	Ferrous Sulfate 325 mg	West-ward Inc.
126	Calcium Carbonate 500 mg	Granutec
130	Ferrous Sulfate 325 mg	West-ward Inc.
130	Sodium Docusate 100 mg	West-ward Inc.
130/MYLAN	CONTROLLED - SEE PAGE 204	
131 05	Vitamins	Central Pharm
131 07	Prednisone 5 mg	Central Pharm
133 [logo]	Demazin 4 mg/20 mg	Schering Corp
134	Sodium Docusate 100 mg, Casanthranol 30 mg	West-ward Inc.
136	Diphenhydramine 25 mg	West-ward Inc.
136	Aspirin 500 mg	Granutec
137	Aspirin 325 mg	Granutec
137	Diphenhydramine 50 mg	West-ward Inc.
138	Aspirin 325 mg	Granutec
139	Aspirin 325 mg	Granutec
140	Vitamins	Marlop
141	Doxycycline 50 mg	West-ward Inc.
141 [logo]	Trilafon 8 mg	Schering Corp
141/SP	CONTROLLED - SEE PAGE 185	
142	Acetaminophen 325 mg	Granutec
142	Doxycycline 100 mg	West-ward Inc.

Imprint	Ingredient/Brand Name	Manufacturer
143	Salsalate 500 mg	Copley Pharm
143	Geocillin 382 mg	Pfizer Labs
144	Salsalate 750 mg	Copley Pharm
145	Ephedrine Sulfate 25 mg	West-ward Inc.
146	Brompheniramine 4 mg	West-ward Inc.
147	Imipramine 25 mg	West-ward Inc.
150 [triangle logo]	Rythmol 150 mg	Knoll
150	Imipramine 50 mg	West-ward Inc.
150	Aspirin 325 mg	West-ward Inc.
150 WALLACE 37-4001	Methacycline HCl 150 mg	Wallace
152	Vitamins	Copley Pharm
154	Phenylpropanolamine 25 mg	H.L. Moore
155/MYLAN	CONTROLLED - SEE PAGE 208	
160	Triprolidine 2.5 mg, Pseudoephedrine 60 mg	OHM
161 RIKER	Disipal	3M
165	Caffeine	Unknown
165	Caffeine, Ephedrine, Phenylpropanolamine	Unknown
165	Calcium Gluconate 640 mg	West-ward Inc.
166	Vitamins, Fluoride	Copley Pharm
167	Carbinoxamine Maleate 8 mg, Pseudoephedrine 120 mg	Econolab
169	Prenatal Rx	Copley Pharm
170	Calcium Gluconate 1000 mg	West-ward Inc.
170	Prenatal FA	Copley Pharm
174 [logo]	levo-Thyroxine 0.1 mg	Heather Drug
175	Vitamins	West-ward
175	Calcium Lactate 325 mg	West-ward Inc.
175	Caffeine, Pseudoephedrine	Unknown
175 [diamond logo]	Caffeine	Unknown
175 [logo]	levo-Thyroxine 0.2 mg	Heather Drug
177	Bromatapp Extended 12/75 mg	Superpharm Corp
178	Caffeine, Pseudoephedrine	Unknown
180	Calcium Lactate 650 mg	West-ward Inc.
182	Caffeine, Ephedrine, Phenylpropanolamine	Unknown
183	Chloropropamide 100 mg	West-ward Inc.
185	Chlorpropamide 250 mg	West-ward Inc.
187 [logo]	Prednisolone 5 mg	Heather Drug
188	Procainamide 500 mg	Copley Pharm
188 [logo]	Papverine 150 mg	Heather Drug
189 [logo]	Prednisolone 5 mg	Heather Drug
192	Metoclopramide 10 mg	Beecham Labs
193 [logo]	Methocarbamol 500 mg	Heather Drug
195	Chloroquine 250 mg	West-ward Inc.
196 [logo]	Methenamine 500 mg	Heather Drug
199	Bormatapp 12 mg/15 mg/15 mg	Copley Pharm
200	Chlorpheniramine 4 mg	West-ward Inc.
200 ZPP	Phenylpropanolamine 75 mg, Caramiphen Edisylate 40 mg	Pioneer
201	Colchicine 0.6 mg	West-ward Inc.
201/U U	CONTROLLED - SEE PAGE 201	
202	Cortisone Acetate 25 mg	West-ward Inc.
202 [logo]	Sulfisoxazole 500 mg	Heather Drug
203	Phenazopyridine 100 mg	Copley Pharm
203 [logo]	Tetracycline 500 mg	Heather Drug
204	Phenazopyridine 200 mg	Copley Pharm
205	Diphenhydramine 25 mg	Granutec
205	Chlorpromazine 25 mg	West-ward Inc.
206	Amitriptyline 10 mg	Copley Pharm

Imprint	Ingredient/Brand Name	Manufacturer
207	Chlorpromazine 50 mg	West-ward Inc.
207	Amitriptyline 25 mg	Copley Pharm
208	Amitriptyline 50 mg	Copley Pharm
208	Nitroglycerin 2.5 mg	West-ward Inc.
209	Chlorothiazide 250 mg	West-ward Inc.
209	Nitroglycerin 6.5 mg	West-ward Inc.
209	Amitriptyline 75 mg	Copley Pharm
209	Amitriptyline 75 mg	Copley Pharm
209 [logo]	Thyroid 1 grain	Heather Drug
210	Chlorothiazide 500 mg	West-ward Inc.
210	Oxytetracycline 250 mg	West-ward Inc.
210	Amitriptyline 100 mg	Copley Pharm
210/40	Furosemide 40 mg	Martec
211	Amitriptyline 150 mg	Copley Pharm
211/MYLAN	CONTROLLED - SEE PAGE 212	
212	Potassium Chloride	Copley Pharm
212 [logo]	Thyroid 2 grains	Heather Drug
213	Acetaminophen 500 mg	Granutec
214	Haloperidol 2 mg	Mylan
214 [logo]	Tetracycline 250 mg	Heather Drug
217	Chlorothiazide 250 mg, Reserpine 0.125 mg	West-ward Inc.
218	Caffeine 200 mg	P.L. Developments
218	Chlorothiazide 500 mg, Reserpine 0.125 mg	West-ward Inc.
224/2.5	Minoxidil 2.5 mg	Royce
225	Potassium Chloride 8 mg	Copley Pharm
225 [triangle logo]	Rythmol 225 mg	Knoll
225/10	Minoxidil 10 mg	Royce
225/105	Tolfrinic 600 mg/100 mg/0.025 mcg	Ascher & Co
225-250 [logo]	Ethaquin 100 mg	Ascher & Co
225 295 [logo]	Anaspaz 0.125 mg	Ascher & Co
225-356 [logo]	Mobigesic 325 mg/30 mg	Ascher & Co
225-450 [logo-logo]	CONTROLLED - SEE PAGE 201	
225 470/Adipost	CONTROLLED - SEE PAGE 213	
225-480 [logo]	Brompheniramine Maleate 12 mg, Pseudoephedrine 120 mg	Ascher
225 490	Docusate Na 230 mg, Phenolphthalein 130 mg	B.F. Ascher
226	Aspirin 325 mg	Granutec
227	Aspirin 500 mg	Granutec
228	Aspirin 80 mg	Granutec
229/0.5	Haloperidol 0.5 mg	Royce
230	Bisacodyl 5 mg	OHM
230/1	Haloperidol 1 mg	Royce
231/2	Haloperidol 2 mg	Royce
231 [logo]	Dexbrompheniramine Maleate 6 mg, Pseudoephedrine 120 mg	Schering
232/5	Haloperidol 5 mg	Royce
232/10	Haloperidol 10 mg	Royce
234/20	Haloperidol 20 mg	Royce
239	Dimenhydrinate 50 mg	West-ward Inc.
239 500	Chloroxazone 500 mg	Royce
239 [logo]	Chlorzoxazone 500 mg	Royce
240/0.5	CONTROLLED - No Photo - Lorazepam 0.5 mg - White, round tablet - DEA Schedule IV	Royce
241/1	CONTROLLED - No Photo - Lorazepam 1 mg - White, round tablet - DEA Schedule IV	Royce
242/2	CONTROLLED - No Photo - Lorazepam 2 mg - White, round tablet - DEA Schedule IV	Royce
243/barr	CONTROLLED - SEE PAGE 192	

Imprint	Ingredient/Brand Name	Manufacturer
244	Phenylpropanolamine 50 mg	H.L. Moore
244/barr	CONTROLLED - SEE PAGE 202	
247 2-10	Perphenazine 2 mg, Amitriptyline 10 mg	Royce
248 2-25	Perphenazine 2 mg, Amitriptyline 25 mg	Royce
248	Folic Acid	West-ward Inc.
249 4-10	Perphenazine 4 mg, Amitriptyline 10 mg	Royce
249	Furosemide 20 mg	West-ward Inc.
250 4-25	Perphenazine 4 mg, Amitriptyline 25 mg	Royce
250	Niacine 250 mg	Upsher Smith
250	Quinine Sulfate 192 mg	West-ward Inc.
250	Furosemide 40 mg	West-ward Inc.
250 125	Augmentin 250 mg/125 mg	Beecham Labs
250 MYSOLINE	Mysoline 250 mg	Ayerst Labs
251	Pseudoephedrine 30 mg	Granutec
252 0220	Thyroid 129.6 mg	Bowman Pharm
252 0400	CONTROLLED - SEE PAGE 187	
252 0401	CONTROLLED - SEE PAGE 189	
252 0494	Thyroid 32.4 mg	Bowman Pharm
252 0495	Thyroid 64.8 mg	Bowman Pharm
252/37	Sodium Fluoride 2.2 mg	Jones
252 1571	CONTROLLED - SEE PAGE 191	
252 3089	CONTROLLED - SEE PAGE 196	
253	Cold Decongestant Tablets	Granutec
253	Furosemide 80 mg	West-ward Inc.
254	Hydrocortisone 20 mg	West-ward Inc.
255	Quinine Sulfate 325 mg	West-ward Inc.
255	Chlorpheniramine Maleate 4 mg	Granutec
255/10	Baclofen 10 mg	Royce
256	Hydrochlorothiazide 25 mg	West-ward Inc.
256/20	Baclofen 20 mg	Royce
257	Hydrochlorothiazide 50 mg	West-ward Inc.
257	Isoxsuprine 10 mg	West-ward Inc.
257	Pseudoephedrine 60 mg, Tripolidine 2.5 mg	Granutec
258	Diphenhydramine 25 mg	Granutec
258	Afrinol 120 mg	Schering Corp
259	Isoxsuprine 20 mg	West-ward Inc.
260	Isoniazid 100 mg	West-ward Inc.
260	Acetaminophen 500 mg	Granutec
261	Isoniazid 300 mg	West-ward Inc.
262	Diphenhydramine 50 mg	Granutec
265 RIKER	Rauwiloid	3M
263	Hydrochlorothiazide 25 mg, Reserpine	West-ward Inc.
265	Hydrochlorothiazide 50 mg, Reserpine	West-ward Inc.
267	Chlorthalidone 25 mg	Barr Labs
268	Chlorthalidone 50 mg	Barr Labs
269	Hydralazine 25 mg	West-ward Inc.
271	Hydralazine 50 mg	West-ward Inc.
275	Meclizine 12.5 mg	West-ward Inc.
276	Meclizine 25 mg	West-ward Inc.
277/MYLAN	CONTROLLED - SEE PAGE 193	
281	Acetaminophen 500 mg	Granutec
282	Azatadine Maleate 1 mg	Schering Corp.
282 [logo]	Azatadine Maleate 1 mg	Schering
285	Sulfinpyrazone 200 mg	West-ward Inc.
285	Diphenhydramine 25 mg	Granutec
286	Dipyridamole 75 mg	Barr Labs

Imprint	Ingredient/Brand Name	Manufacturer
287	Acetaminophen 325 mg, Pseudoephedrine 30 mg	Granutec
290	Methocarbamol 500 mg	West-ward Inc.
290	Vitamins	West-ward Inc.
291	Metronidazole 250 mg	Barr Labs
292	Methocarbamol 750 mg	West-ward Inc.
294	Pseudoephedrine 60 mg, Chlorpheniramine maleate 4 mg	Granutec
295	Tetracycline 250 mg	West-ward Inc.
295	Metronidazole 250 mg	West-ward Inc.
296	Thioridazine 10 mg	West-ward Inc.
297	Thioridazine 15 mg	West-ward Inc.
297	Metronidazole 500 mg	West-ward Inc.
298	Thioridazine 25 mg	West-ward Inc.
299	Thioridazine 50 mg	West-ward Inc.
299	Caffeine 100 mg	Granutec
299	Hydroxyzine 50 mg	Barr Labs
300	Cimetidine 300 mg	Smith Kline
300	Hydroxyzine 100 mg	Barr Labs
300	Furosemide 20 mg	Watson Labs
300 [triangle]	Propafenone 300 mg	Knoll
300/3028	Allopurinol 300 mg	Rugby Labs
300 WALLACE 37-4101	Methacycline HCl 300 mg	Wallace
301	Furosemide 40 mg	Watson Labs
302	Thioridazine 100 mg	West-ward Inc.
302	Furosemide 80 mg	Watson Labs
302/50	Hydroxyzine 50 mg	Barr Labs
303	Indomethacin 25 mg	Watson Labs
303	Thioridazine 150 mg	West-ward Inc.
303 [logo]/325	Quinine Sulfate 324 mg	Royce
304	Thioridazine 200 mg	West-ward Inc.
304	Indomethacin 50 mg	Watson Labs
305	Iron/Vitamin B	Whitby
305	Propranolol 10 mg	Watson Labs
306	Propranolol 20 mg	Watson Labs
307	Trifluoperazine 1 mg	West-ward Inc.
307	Propranolol 40 mg	Watson Labs
308	Propranolol 80 mg	Watson Labs
309	Trifluoperazine 2 mg	West-ward Inc.
309 [logo]/10	Doxepin 10 mg	Royce
310	Trihemic 600 mg	Marlop
310 [logo]/25	Doxepin 25 mg	Royce
311	Trifuoperazine 5 mg	West-ward Inc.
311	Acetaminophen 500 mg	OHM Laboratories
311	Furosemide 20 mg	Watson Labs
311/ICN	CONTROLLED - SEE PAGE 197	
311 [logo]/50	Doxepin 50 mg	Royce
312	Vitamins	Marlop
312	Metoclopramide 10 mg	Watson Labs
313	Vitamins	Marlop
313	Trifluoperazine 10 mg	West-ward Inc.
317/barr	CONTROLLED - SEE PAGE 200	
320	Yellow Phenolphthalein 90 mg	OHM Laboratories
320	Hydroxyzine 25 mg	West-ward Inc.
321/M	CONTROLLED - SEE PAGE 185	
325	Hydroxyzine 50 mg	West-ward Inc.
330	Hydroxyzine 100 mg	West-ward Inc.
332 0.5/WATSON	CONTROLLED - SEE PAGE 184	

Imprint	Ingredient/Brand Name	Manufacturer
333 1.0/WATSON	CONTROLLED - SEE PAGE 188	
334 2.0/WATSON	CONTROLLED - SEE PAGE 190	
335	Caffeine, Ephedrine, Phenylpropanolamine	Unknown
335 [logo]/10	Piroxicam 10 mg	Royce
336	Indomethacin 25 mg	Barr Labs
336	Acetaminophen 325 mg	West-ward Inc.
336 [logo]/20	Piroxicam 20 mg	Royce
337	Indomethacin 50 mg	Barr Labs
339	Acetaminophen 500 mg	West-ward Inc.
342 3M	Theolair 125 mg	3M
344	Verapamil 80 mg	Watson Labs
345	Verapamil 120 mg	Watson Labs
345	Niacin 50 mg	West-ward Inc.
345 10	Hydroxyzine 10 mg	Royce
346/25	Hydroxyzine 25 mg	Royce
346	Verapamil 120 mg	Watson Labs
347	Propranolol 80 mg, Hydrochlorothiazide 25 mg	Rugby Labs
347	Diphenhydramine 25 mg	Granutec
347 50	Hydroxyzine 50 mg	Royce
348	Acetaminophen 500 mg, Diphenhydramine 25 mg	Granutec
349	chlorpropamide 100 mg	Barr Labs
350	Chlorpropamide 250 mg	Barr Labs
350	Niacin 500 mg	West-ward Inc.
352	Niacin 500 mg	West-ward Inc.
353	Pseudoephedrine 30 mg	Granutec
353/USV	CONTROLLED - SEE PAGE 194	
354/USV	CONTROLLED - SEE PAGE 198	
355	Caffeine, Ephedrine, Phenylpropanolamine	Unknown
357 MAGNUM	Caffeine	Unknown
358 [logo]	Propranolol 40 mg, Hydrochlorothiazide 25 mg	Rondex Labs
358 5-50	Amiloride 5 mg, Hydrochlorothiazide 50 mg	Royce
360 [logo]	Propranolol 80 mg, Hydrochlorothiazide 25 mg	Rondex Labs
360	Pseudoephedrine 30 mg	Granutec
361 5.4	Yohimbine 5.4 mg	Royce
361	Pseudoephedrine 30 mg, Chlorpheniramine 2 mg	Granutec
363	Acetaminophen 80 mg	Granutec
365	Docusate Calcium 240 mg	West-ward Inc.
371/b	CONTROLLED - SEE PAGE 184	
372/barr	CONTROLLED - SEE PAGE 189	
373/barr	CONTROLLED - SEE PAGE 205	
374 [logo]	Chlor-Trimeton 8 mg	Schering Corp
376	Acetaminophen 250 mg, Aspirin 250 mg, Caffeine 65 mg	Granutec
377-0008	Aminophylline 100 mg	Vale
377-0106	Chlorpheniramine 1 mg, Pyrilamine 12.5 mg, Phenylephrine 5 mg	Vale
377-0125	Guaifenesin 100 mg	Vale
377-0167	Pyrilamine Maleate 25 mg	Vale
377-0214	Rauwolfia Serpentina 50 mg	Vale
377-0215	Rauwolfia Serpentina 100 mg	Vale
377-0216	Phenylephrine 5 mg, Chlorpheniramine 2 mg, Salicylamide 250 mg,Acetaminophen150 mg	Vale
377-0217	Phenylephrine 2 mg, Chlorpheniramine 1 mg, Salicylamide 90 mg,Acetaminophen 60 mg	Vale
377-0238	Sodium Salicylate 324 mg	Vale
377-0240	Sodium Salicylate 324 mg	Vale
377-0242	Sodium Salicylate 324 mg	Vale

Imprint	Ingredient/Brand Name	Manufacturer
377-0272	Thyroid 30 mg	Vale
377-0277	Sulfadiazine 167 mg, Sulfamerazine 167 mg, Sulfamethazine 167 mg	Vale
377-0290	Diphenhydramine 50 mg	Vale
377-0311	Phenylephrine 5 mg, Chlorpheniramine 2 mg, Salicylamide 250 mg, Acetaminophen 150 mg, Guaifenesin 100 mg	Vale
377-0332	Pepsin 259 mg, Pancreatin 32 mg, Diastase 2 mg	Vale
377-0349	Magnesium Trisilicate 500 mg	Vale
377-0358	Pseudoephedrine 60 mg	Vale
377-0359	Guaifenesin 100 mg, Pseudoephedrine 30 mg	Vale
377-0396	Thyroid 65 mg	Vale
377-4280	Prednisolone 5 mg	Vale
377-4294	Prednisone 5 mg	Vale
381/b	CONTROLLED - SEE PAGE 188	
382/barr	CONTROLLED - SEE PAGE 192	
384	Diphenhydramine 12.5 mg, Pseudoephedrine 30 mg, Acetaminophen 500 mg	Granutec
386	Phenylpropanolamine 25 mg, Brompheniramine Maleate 4 mg	Granutec
393	Diabinese 100 mg	Pfizer
394	Diabinese 250 mg	Pfizer
394 [logo]	Reserpine 0.1 mg, Trichlormethiazide 4 mg	Schering
399	Caffeine 200 mg	Granutec
400 [logo]	Phenylpropanolamine 75 mg, Guaifenesin 400 mg	Abana
403	Pseudoephedrine 30 mg	OHM
403 [logo]	Sulfamethoxazole 500 mg	Heather Drug
404	Acetaminophen 648 mg	J.B. Labs
408	Bisacodyl 5 mg	G & W Labs
415	Ergoloid Mesylates 1 mg	Ascher & Co.
415 [logo]	Niloric 1 mg	Ascher & Co
420	Ibuprofen 200 mg	OHM
421	Covangesic 12.5 mg/7.5 mg/2 mg/275 mg	Wallace Labs
424	Ibuprofen 200 mg	OHM Laboratories
425	Verapamil 80 mg	Barr Labs
429	Florinef Acetate 0.1 mg	Apothecon
431	Pronestyl 250 mg	Princeton Pharm
431/WC	CONTROLLED - SEE PAGE 184	
434	Pronestyl 375 mg	Princeton Pharm
437 PM	Acetaminophen 500 mg	Perrigo
438	Pronestyl 500 mg	Princeton Pharm
446	Tamoxifen 10 mg	Barr Labs
450/MD	CONTROLLED - SEE PAGE 200	
453	Caffeine, Pseudoephedrine	Unknown
455	Verapamil 120 mg	Barr Labs
473	Prednisone 10 mg	West-ward Inc.
475	Prednisone 5 mg	West-ward Inc.
477	Prednisone 20 mg	West-ward Inc.
480	Propylthiouracil 50 mg	West-ward Inc.
481	Prednisone 50 mg	West-ward Inc.
485	Pseudoephedrine 60 mg	West-ward Inc.
485	Leucovorin calcium 25 mg	Barr
490	Pyridoxine 25 mg	West-ward Inc.
495	Pyridoxine 50 mg	West-ward Inc.
496 [logo]	Griseofulvin 500 mg	Schering
497	Pyridoxine 100 mg	West-ward Inc.
499	Ibuprofen 800 mg	Barr Labs
500	Niacin 500 mg	Upsher

Imprint	Ingredient/Brand Name	Manufacturer
500	Acetaminophen 500 mg	Amide Pharm
500 125	Augmentin 500 mg/125 mg	Beecham Labs
500 500	Aspirin 500 mg, Caffeine 32 mg	Whitehall Robins
500/RUSS	CONTROLLED - SEE PAGE 208	
501 [logo]	Methocarbamol 750 mg	Heather Drug
502	Propranolol 10 mg	West-ward Inc.
503 [logo]	Methenamine 1000 mg	Heather Drug
503	Propranolol 20 mg	West-ward Inc.
504	Propranolol 40 mg	West-ward Inc.
505	Propranolol 60 mg	West-ward Inc.
505 [logo]	Prednisone 10 mg	Heather Drug
506	Prednisone	Unknown
506	Propranolol 80 mg	West-ward Inc.
506 [logo]	Prednisone 20 mg	Heather Drug
510	Quinidine Sulfate 200 mg	West-ward Inc.
510 [logo]	Methylprednisolone 4 mg	Heather Drug
513 [logo]	Cortisone 25 mg	Heather Drug
514	Cephalexin 250 mg	Barr Labs
515	Cephalexin 500 mg	Barr Labs
518	Caffeine, Ephedrine, Phenylpropanolamine	Unknown
521 [hexagon]	Lufyllin 400 mg	Mallinckrodt Inc.
521/MYLAN	CONTROLLED - SEE PAGE 201	
524 HD	Cyproheptadine 4 mg	Halsey Drug
525/93	Amitriptyline 10 mg	Lemmon Pharm
527/93	Amitriptyline 25 mg	Lemmon Pharm
527/1043	Lanorinal 50 mg, 40 mg, 200 mg, 130 mg	Lannett
527 [logo]	Prednisone 50 mg	Heather Drug
529/93	Amitriptyline 50 mg	Lemmon Pharm
530	Reserpine 0.1 mg	West-ward Inc.
530	Nifedipine 20 mg	Novapharm
530/MD	CONTROLLED - SEE PAGE 209	
531/93	Amitriptyline 75 mg	Lemmon Pharm
531 [logo]	Furosemide 40 mg	Heather Drug
531/MD	CONTROLLED - SEE PAGE 204	
532 [logo]	Furosemide 20 mg	Heather Drug
532/MD	CONTROLLED - SEE PAGE 202	
533/93	Amitriptyline 100 mg	Lemmon Pharm
534 [logo]	Sulfamethoxazole 400 mg, Trimethoprim 80 mg	Heather Drug
535	Reserpine 0.25 mg	West-ward Inc.
535/93	Amitriptyline 150 mg	Lemmon Pharm
535 [logo]	Sulfamethoxazole 800 mg, Trimethoprim 160 mg	Heather Drug
535/MD	CONTROLLED - SEE PAGE 187	
538 [logo]	Doxycycline 100 mg	Heather Drug
539 [logo]	Doxycycline 100 mg	Heather Drug
540 [logo]	Doxycycline 50 mg	Heather Drug
541	Lufyllin-GG 200 mg/200 mg	Mallinckrodt Inc.
542	Amitriptyline	Unknown
555 0010	Tetracycline 500 mg	Barr Labs
555 0011	Tetracycline 250 mg	Barr Labs
555 0013	Erythromycin Stearate 250 mg	Barr Labs
555 0019	Hydrochlorothiazide 25 mg	Barr Labs
555 0020	Hydrochlorothiazide 50 mg	Barr Labs
555 0024	Sulfisoxazole 500 mg	Barr Labs
555 0026	Prednisone 5 mg	Barr Labs
555 0030	Colchicine 0.65 mg	Barr Labs
555 0057	Dimenhydrinate 50 mg	Barr Labs

Imprint	Ingredient/Brand Name	Manufacturer
555 0058	Diphenhydramine 25 mg	Barr Labs
555 0059	Diphenhydramine 50 mg	Barr Labs
555 0064	Hydralazine 25 mg	Barr Labs
555 0065	Hydralazine 50 mg	Barr Labs
555 0066	Isoniazid 100 mg	Barr Labs
555 0071	Isoniazid 300 mg	Barr Labs
555 0089	Propylthiouracil 50 mg	Barr Labs
555 0099	Bisacodyl 5 mg	Barr Labs
555 013	Erythromycin Stearate 250 mg	Barr Labs
555 065	Hydralazine 50 mg	Barr Labs
555 0106	Methocarbamol 500 mg	Barr Labs
555 0107	Methocarbamol 750 mg	Barr Labs
555 0114	Reserpine 0.125 mg, Hydrochlorothiazide 25 mg	Barr Labs
555 0115	Reserpine 0.1 mg, Hydralazine 25 mg, Hydrochlorothiazide 15 mg	Barr Labs
555 0116	Reserpine 0.125 mg, Hydrochlorothiazide 50 mg	Barr Labs
555 0126	Dicyclomine 20 mg	Barr Labs
555 0128	Dicyclomine 10 mg	Barr Labs
555 0129	Dexamethasone 0.25 mg	Barr Labs
555 0130	Dexamethasone 0.050 mg	Barr Labs
555 0131	Dexamethasone 0.75 mg	Barr Labs
555 0132	Dexamethasone 1.50 mg	Barr Labs
555 0157	Prednisone 20 mg	Barr Labs
555 0170	Furosemide 20 mg	Barr Labs
555 0172	Isosorbide Dinitrate 2.5 mg	Barr Labs
555 0173	Isosorbide Dinitrate 5 mg	Barr Labs
555 0174	Isosorbide Dinitrate 5 mg	Barr Labs
555 0175	Isosorbide Dinitrate 10 mg	Barr Labs
555 0176	Acetaminophen 325 mg	Barr Labs
555 0186	Isosorbide Dinitrate 20 mg	Barr Labs
555 0188	Quinidine Sulfate 200 mg	Barr Labs
555 0192	Hydrochlorothiazide 100 mg	Barr Labs
555 0203	Amitriptyline 25 mg	Barr Labs
555 0209	Amitriptyline 10 mg	Barr Labs
555 0210	Amitriptyline 50 mg	Barr Labs
555 0211	Amitriptyline 75 mg	Barr Labs
555 0212	Amitriptyline 100 mg	Barr Labs
555 0218	Ergoloid Mesylates 0.5 mg	Barr Labs
555 0227	Ergoloid Mesylates 1 mg	Barr Labs
555 0230	Erythromycin Estolate 250 mg	Barr Labs
555 0233	Prednisone 10 mg	Barr Labs
555 0241	Allopurinol 100 mg	Barr Labs
555 0242	Allopurinol 300 mg	Barr Labs
555 0251	Tolbutamide 500 mg	Barr Labs
555 0252	Dipyridamole 25 mg	Barr Labs
555 0255	Chlorzoxazone 250 mg, Acetaminophen 300 mg	Barr Labs
555 0259	Erythromycin Ethylsuccinate 400 mg	Barr Labs
555 0260	Thioridazine 10 mg	Barr Labs
555 0261	Thioridazine 25 mg	Barr Labs
555 0262	Thioridazine 50 mg	Barr Labs
555 0263	Thioridazine 100 mg	Barr Labs
555 0265	Spironolactone 25 mg, Hydrochlorothiazide 25 mg	Barr Labs
555 0266	Spironolactone 25 mg	Barr Labs
555 0267	Chlorthalidone 25 mg	Barr Labs
555 0268	Chlorthalidone 50 mg	Barr Labs
555 0271	Sulfinpyrazone 100 mg	Barr Labs

Imprint	Ingredient/Brand Name	Manufacturer
555 0272	Sulfinpyrazone 200 mg	Barr Labs
555 0276	Chlorpropamide 250 mg	Barr Labs
555 0277	Isosorbide Dinitrate 10 mg	Barr Labs
555 0279	Isosorbide Dinitrate 30 mg	Barr Labs
555 0281	Aminophylline 200 mg	Barr Labs
555 0282	Aminophylline 100 mg	Barr Labs
555 0285	Dipyridamole 50 mg	Barr Labs
555 0286	Dipyridamole 75 mg	Barr Labs
555 0291	Metronidazole 250 mg	Barr Labs
555 0292	Metronidazole 500 mg	Barr Labs
555 0295	DOXY-TABS 100 mg	Barr Labs
555 0296	DOXY-CAPS 50 mg	Barr Labs
555 0297	DOXY-CAPS 100 mg	Barr Labs
555 0298	Hydroxyzine 25 mg	Barr Labs
555 0299	Hydroxyzine 50 mg	Barr Labs
555 0300	Hydroxyzine 100 mg	Barr Labs
555 0301	Hydroxyzine 10 mg	Barr Labs
555 0314	Sulfamethoxazole 500 mg	Barr Labs
555 0321	Sulfamethoxazole 400 mg, Trimethoprim 80 mg	Barr Labs
555 0322	Sulfamethoxazole 800 mg, Trimethoprim 160 mg	Barr Labs
555 0326	Acetaminophen 500 mg	Barr Labs
555 0327	Thioridazine 150 mg	Barr Labs
555 0328	Thioridazine 200 mg	Barr Labs
555 0329	Thioridazine 15 mg	Barr Labs
555 0331	Disopyramide 100 mg	Barr Labs
555 0332	Disopyramide 150 mg	Barr Labs
555 0347	Chlorpropamide 100 mg	Barr Labs
555 0365	Propranolol 10 mg	Barr Labs
555 0366	Propranolol 20 mg	Barr Labs
555 0367	Propranolol 40 mg	Barr Labs
555 0383	Ergoloid Mesylates 1 mg	Barr Labs
555 0388	Hydralazine 10 mg	Barr Labs
555 0389	Hydralazine 100 mg	Barr Labs
555 0395	Phenylbutazone 100 mg	Barr Labs
555 0396	Phenylbutazone 100 mg	Barr Labs
555 0415	Tolazamide 100 mg	Barr Labs
555 0416	Tolazamide 250 mg	Barr Labs
555 0417	Tolazamide 500 mg	Barr Labs
555 0419	Ibuprofen 400 mg	Barr Labs
555 0420	Ibuprofen 600 mg	Barr Labs
555 0429	Trimethoprim 100 mg	Barr Labs
555 0434	Folic Acid 1 mg	Barr Labs
555 19	Hydrochlorthiazide 25 mg	Barr Labs
555 20	Hydrochlorthiazide 50 mg	Barr Labs
555 26	Prednisone 25 mg	Barr Labs
555 163/barr	CONTROLLED - SEE PAGE 190	
555 164/barr	CONTROLLED - SEE PAGE 209	
555 169	Furosemide 40 mg	Barr Labs
555 201	Amitriptyline 50 mg	Barr Labs
555 271	Sulfinpyrazone 100 mg	Barr Labs
555 278	CONTROLLED - SEE PAGE 197	
555 288	Isosorbide Dinitrate 40 mg	Barr Labs
555 293/Barr	CONTROLLED - SEE PAGE 206	
555 363/barr	CONTROLLED - SEE PAGE 205	
555 368	Propranolol 60 mg	Barr Labs
555 369	Propranolol 80 mg	Barr Labs

Imprint	Ingredient/Brand Name	Manufacturer
555 424	Metoclopramide 10 mg	Barr Labs
555 427	Propranolol 40 mg, Hydrochlorothiazide 25 mg	Barr Labs
555 428	Propranolol 80 mg, Hydrochlorothiazide 25 mg	Barr Labs
555 430	Trimethoprim 200 mg	Barr Labs
555 444	Triamterene 75 mg, Hydrochlorothiazide 50 mg	Barr Labs
555 477	Haloperidol 0.5 mg	Barr Labs
555 478	Haloperidol 1 mg	Barr Labs
555 479	Haloperidol 2 mg	Barr Labs
555 480	Haloperidol 5 mg	Barr Labs
555 481	Haloperidol 10 mg	Barr Labs
555 482	Haloperidol 20 mg	Barr Labs
555 483	Amiloride 5 mg, Hydrochlorothiazide 50 mg	Barr Labs
555 489	Trazodone 50 mg	Barr Labs
555 490	Trazodone 100 mg	Barr Labs
555 585	Chlorzoxazone 500 mg	
591-A	CONTROLLED - SEE PAGE 195	
591-B	CONTROLLED - SEE PAGE 192	
606	Naturetin 5 mg	Princeton
610/HD	CONTROLLED - SEE PAGE 200	
617	Caffeine, Pseudoephedrine	Unknown
618	Naturetin 10 mg	Princeton
622 HD	Iboprofen 800 mg	Halsey
630/HD	CONTROLLED - SEE PAGE 208	
632 HD	Fenoprofen Calcium 200 mg	Halsey
633 HD	Fenoprofen Calcium 300 mg	Halsey
634 HD	Fenoprofen Calcium 600 mg	Halsey
675	Caffeine, Ephedrine, Phenylpropanolamine	Unknown
680	Sulfinpyrazone 100 mg	West-ward Inc.
683	Sulfisoxazole 500 mg	West-ward Inc.
689	Theophylline 200 mg	West-ward Inc.
690	Theophylline 300 mg	West-ward Inc.
697	Caffeine	Unknown
711	Pseudoephedrine 30 mg, Acetaminophen 500 mg Dextromethorphan Hydrobromide 15 mg	Hall Labs
713	Raudixin 50 mg	Princeton
715	Thiamine 50 mg	West-ward Inc.
720	Thiamine 100 mg	West-ward Inc.
721	Caffeine, Pseudoephedrine	Unknown
734 [D logo]	Gyne-Lotrimin 100 mg	Schering Corp
735 [logo]	Theophylline 250 mg	Schering Corp.
750	Niacin 750 mg	Upsher-Smith
751 [logo]	Demazin 4 mg/25 mg	Schering Corp
754 93	Diflunisal 750 mg	Lemmon Pharm
755 93	Diflunisal 500 mg	Lemmon Pharm
756	Pronestyl 375 mg	Princeton Pharm
757	Pronestyl 500 mg	Princeton Pharm
758	Pronestyl 250 mg	Princeton Pharm
765	Isosorbide Dinitrate 2.5 mg	West-ward Inc.
767	Isosorbide Dinitrate 5 mg	West-ward Inc.
769	Isosorbide Dinitrate 5 mg	West-ward Inc.
771	Isosorbide Dinitrate 10 mg	West-ward Inc.
772	Isosorbide 20 mg	West-ward Inc.
773	Hyoscyamine Sulfate 0.125 mg	Marlop
775	Pronestyl-SR 500 mg	Princeton Pharm
776	Raudixin 100 mg	Princeton
787	Butalbital 50 mg, Acetaminophen 325 mg, Caffeine 40 mg	West-ward Inc.

Imprint	Ingredient/Brand Name	Manufacturer
812	Butalbital 50 mg, Acetaminophen 325 mg, Caffeine 40 mg	Marlop
812	Caffeine, Ephedrine, Phenylpropanolamine	Unknown
813	Caffeine, Ehpedrine, Phenylpropanolamine	Unknown
813 [logo]	Caffeine, Ephedrine, Phenylpropanolamine	Unknown
814	Ibuprofen	Marlop
815	Caffeine, Ephedrine, Phenylpropanolamine	Unknown
815 [logo]	Caffeine, Ephedrine, Phenylpropanolamine	Unknown
817	Caffeine, Ephedrine, Phenylpropanolamine	Unknown
817 [logo]	Caffeine, Ephedrine, Phenylpropanolamine	Unknown
819	Caffeine, Ephedrine, Phenylpropanolamine	Unknown
819 [logo]	Caffeine, Ephedrine, Phenylpropanolamine	Unknown
832 5	CONTROLLED - SEE PAGE 221	
832 10	CONTROLLED - No Photo - Chlordiazepoxide 10 mg - Green/Yellow Capsule - DEA Schedule IV	Pharm Basics
832 25	CONTROLLED - No Photo - Chlordiazepoxide 25 mg - Green/White Capsule - DEA Schedule IV	Pharm Basics
832/10	Chlorpromazine 10 mg	Pharm Basics
832/25	Chlorpromazine 25 mg	Pharm Basics
832/50	Chlorpromazine 50 mg	Pharm Basics
832/100	Chlorpromazine 100 mg	Pharm Basics
832/200	Chlorpromazine 200 mg	Pharm Basics
832 G359	CONTROLLED - SEE PAGE 211	
832 G463	Medroxyprogesterone Acetate 10 mg	Pharm Basics
832 G528C	CONTROLLED - No Photo - Phendimetrazine Tartrate 35 mg - Yellow tablet - DEA Schedule III	Pharm Basics
832 G531C	CONTROLLED - SEE PAGE 187	
832 G532C	CONTROLLED - SEE PAGE 186	
832 G533C	CONTROLLED - SEE PAGE 190	
832 G536C	CONTROLLED - No Photo - Phentermine 30 mg - Blue/clear capsule - DEA Schedule IV	Pharm Basics
832 L01	Levothyroxine Sodium 0.1 mg	Pharm Basics
832 L02	Levothyroxine Sodium 0.2 mg	Pharm Basics
832 L03	Levothyroxine Sodium 0.3 mg	Pharm Basics
832 L15	L-Thyroxine Sodium 0.15 mg	Pharm Basics
832 P-5C	CONTROLLED - SEE PAGE 214	
832 P-10C	CONTROLLED - SEE PAGE 220	
832 PPPC	Phenylpropanolamine 40 mg, Phenyltoloxamine Citrate 15 mg, Phenylephrine 10 mg, Chlorpheniramine maleate 5 mg	Pharm Basics
832 S500	Salsalate 500 mg	Pharm Basics
832 S750	Salsalate 750 mg	Pharm Basics
866 [logo]	Disophrol 6 mg/120 mg	Schering Corp
875	Caffeine, Ephedrine, Phenylpropanolamine	Unknown
879	CONTROLLED - SEE PAGE 185	
879 027	CONTROLLED - SEE PAGE 214	
879 0130	Propylthiouracil 50 mg	Halsey Drug
879 0155	CONTROLLED - SEE PAGE 215	
879 0158	Tetracycline 250 mg	Halsey Drug
879 0364	CONTROLLED - SEE PAGE 221	
879 0365	CONTROLLED - SEE PAGE 223	
879 0366	CONTROLLED - SEE PAGE 219	
879 113	Isoniazid 100 mg	Halsey Drug
879 129	Prednisone 5 mg	Halsey Drug
879 159	Tetracycline 500 mg	Halsey Drug
879 341	Isoniazid 300 mg	Halsey Drug
879 358	Quinidine Sulfate 200 mg	Halsey Drug
879 360	Triprolidine 2.5 mg, Pseudoephedrine 60 mg	Halsey Drug

Imprint	Ingredient/Brand Name	Manufacturer
879 452	Acetaminophen 500 mg	Halsey Drug
879 453	Acetaminophen 500 mg	Halsey Drug
879/501	Chlordiazepoxide 5 mg, Clidinium Bromide 2.5 mg	Halsey Drug
879 525	Doxycycline 50 mg	Halsey Drug
879 526	Doxycycline 100 mg	Halsey Drug
879 G594C	CONTROLLED - SEE PAGE 215	
879 G638	Folic Acid 1 mg	Halsey Drug
884 Miles 30	Adolat 30 mg	Miles
885 Miles 60	Adolat 60 mg	Miles
886 Miles 90	Adolat 90 mg	Miles
890/93	CONTROLLED - SEE PAGE 208	
900	Triprolidine, Pseudoephedrine	West-ward Inc.
901/RUSS	CONTROLLED - SEE PAGE 200	
902/RUSS	CONTROLLED - SEE PAGE 200	
903/RUSS	CONTROLLED - SEE PAGE 200	
917	Moduretic 5mg, 50mg	Merck
945	Caffeine, Ephedrine, Phenylpropanolamine	Unknown
945 [logo]	Caffeine, Ephedrine, Phenylpropanolamine	Unknown
948 [logo]	Griseofulvin 250 mg	Schering
950	Caffeine, Ephedrine, Phenylpropanolamine	Unknown
950 [logo]	Caffeine, Ephedrine, Phenylpropanolamine	Unknown
966	Acetaminophen 500 mg, Chlorpheniramine Maleate 2 mg, Pseudoephedrine 30 mg	Hall Labs
968 [logo]	Tindal 20 mg	Schering Corp
975	Caffeine, Pseudoephedrine	Unknown
975	Caffeine	Unknown
980/WC	CONTROLLED - SEE PAGE 208	
997	Chlorpheniramine Maleate 4 mg	Hall Labs
1001	Aminophylline 100 mg	Vortech
1004	Pseudoephedrine 30 mg	Hall Labs
1005	Phenylpropanolamine 18.7 mg, Chlorpheniramine 2 mg	Hall Labs
1006	Dimenhydrinate 50 mg	Hall Labs
1007	Pseudoephedrine 60 mg, Triprolidine 2.5 mg	Hall Labs
1008	Diphenhydramine 25 mg	P.L. Developments
1009	Digitoxin 0.2 mg	Vortech
1010 1010	Caffeine, Ephedrine, Phenylpropanolamine	Unknown
1016	Pseudoephedrine 60 mg, Chlorpheniramine 4 mg	Hall Labs
1031	Carbatapentane 60 mg, Chlorpheniramine 5 mg, Ephedrine 10 mgPhenylephrine 10 mg	Econolabs
1032	Reserpine 0.25 mg	Vortech
1033	Rauwolfia Serpentina 100 mg	Vortech
1043	Thyroid 2 gr	Vortech
1044	Thyroid 1 gr	Vortech
1045	Thyroid 1 gr	Vortech
1077	Chlorpheniramine Maleate 8 mg	Vortech
1079	Digitoxin 0.1 mg	Vortech
1086	Acetaminophen 325 mg, Chlorpheniramine Maleate 2 mg Pseudoephedrine 30 mg	Hall Labs
1093	Thyroid 2 gr	Vortech
1094	Penicillin G 250,000 units	Vortech
1098	Prednisone 5 mg	Vortech
1113 [logo]	Dilor 100 mg	Savage Labs
1115 [logo]	Dilor 200 mg	Savage Labs
1116 [logo]	Dilor 400 mg	Savage Labs
1124 [logo]	Dilor-G 200 mg/200 mg	Savage Labs
1167	Ephedrine	Unknown

Imprint	Ingredient/Brand Name	Manufacturer
1168	Caffeine, Ephedrine, Phenylpropanolamine	Unknown
1237	Pentaerylthritol Tetranitrate 20 mg	Vortech
1242	Prednisolone 5 mg	Vortech
1253	Vitamins	H.L. Moore
1276	Thyroid 1/2 gr	Vortech
1332	Chlorpheniramine Maleate 4 mg	Vortech
1339	Phenylpropanolamine 40 mg, Phenylephrine 10 mg, Phentoloxamine 15 mg, Chlorpheniramine 5 mg	Vortech
1342	Penicillin G 400,000 units	Vortech
1390	Sodium Levothyroxine 0.2 mg	Vortech
1463	Conjugated Estrogens 0.625 mg	Vortech
1531	Sulfasoxazole 500 mg	Vortech
1533	Digoxin 0.25 mg	Vortech
1603	Diphenhydramine 25 mg	Hall Labs
1779	Colchicine 0.65 mg	Vortech
1796 180 mg	Diltiazem HCl 180 mg	Marion
1797 240 mg	Diltiazem 240 mg	Marion
1798 300 mg	Diltiazem 300 mg	Marion
1806 0.5 G	CONTROLLED - No Photo - Lorazepam 0.5 mg - White, round tablet - DEA Schedule IV	Goldline
1807 1 G	CONTROLLED - No Photo - Lorazepam 1 mg - White, round tablet - DEA Schedule IV	Goldline
1808 2 G	CONTROLLED - No Photo - Lorazepam 2 mg - White, round tablet - DEA Schedule IV	Goldline
1812	Benzthiazide 50 mg	Vortech
1820	Tetracycline 250 mg	Rugby Labs
1830	Tetracycline 250 mg	Rugby Labs
1840	Nitrofurantion 50 mg	Vortech
1870	Tetracycline 500 mg	Rugby Labs
1886	Propantheline Bromide 15 mg	Vortech
1908	Orphenadrine Citrate 100 mg	Vortech
1915	Hydrochlorothiazide 50 mg	Vortech
1922	Brompheniramine 12 mg, Phenylephrine 15 mg, Phenylpropanolamine 15 mg	Vortech
1934 [logo]	Brexin L 8 mg/120 mg	Savage Labs
1945	Trichlormethiazide 4 mg	Vortech
1945	Ferrous Sulfate 50 mg	Nutro Labs
1975	Triprolidine 2.5 mg, Pseudoephedrine 60 mg	Vortech
1975	Caffeine, Pseudoephedrine	Unknown
1998	Methocarbamol 750 mg	Vortech
2013	Chlorpheniramine Maleate 4 mg	Bolar
2020	Caffeine 175 mg	B & M Labs
2095	Dioctyl Sodium Sulfosuccinate 100 mg	Vortech
2105	Ferrous Sulfate 65 mg	Nutro Labs
2130	Tripelennamine	Unknown
2130 [logo]	Tripelennamine	Unknown
2205	Ferrous Sulfate 65 mg	Nutro Labs
2428	Diphenylhydantoin Sodium 100 mg	Vortech
2472	Diphenhydramine 25 mg	Vortech
2473	Diphenhydramine 50 mg	Vortech
2525	Butalbital 50 mg, Aspirin 200 mg, Phenacetin 130 mg Caffeine 40 mg	Vortech
2715	Nitroglycerine 6.5 mg	Vortech
2718	Nitroglycerine 2.5 mg	Vortech
2768	Tetracycline 250 mg	Vortech
2867	Tetracycline 500 mg	Vortech

Imprint	Ingredient/Brand Name	Manufacturer
2874	Dicyclomine 10 mg	Vortech
3000	Quinidine Gluconate 324 mg	Philips Roxane
3061	Cefaclor 250 mg	Eli Lilly
3062	Cefaclor 500 mg	Eli Lilly
3125	Vancomycin 125 mg	Eli Lilly
3126	Vancomycin 250 mg	Eli Lilly
3591/RUGBY	CONTROLLED - SEE PAGE 191	
3592/RUGBY	CONTROLLED - SEE PAGE 205	
3593/RUGBY	CONTROLLED - SEE PAGE 209	
3642	Papaverine 150 mg	Vortech
3681 [logo]	Satric 250 mg	Savage Labs
3688 [logo]	Satric 500 mg	Savage Labs
3900	Theophylline 150 mg, Guaifenesin 90 mg	Pharmacaps Inc.
3937/RUGBY	CONTROLLED - SEE PAGE 196	
3961/RUGBY	CONTROLLED - SEE PAGE 189	
4005/R	CONTROLLED - SEE PAGE 192	
4006/R	CONTROLLED - SEE PAGE 195	
4285 [logo]	Chromagen 200 mg/250 mg/0.010 mg	Savage Labs
4350	Isoniazid 300 mg	Vitarine Pharm
4354	Isoniazid 100 mg	Vitarine Pharm
4556	Phenylpropanolamine 50 mg, Pheniramine 25 mg, Pyrilamine 25 mg	Eon
4841	Neomycin Sulfate 500 mg	Eon
4940/RUGBY	CONTROLLED - SEE PAGE 210	
4941/RUGBY	CONTROLLED - SEE PAGE 202	
4942/RUGBY	CONTROLLED - SEE PAGE 207	
5595/RUGBY	CONTROLLED - SEE PAGE 225	
5678/DAN	CONTROLLED - SEE PAGE 194	
5679/DAN	CONTROLLED - SEE PAGE 212	
6460	Rauwolfia Serpentina 50 mg	Bowman Pharm
6462	Rauwolfia Serpentina 100 mg	Bowman Pharm
7449	Robaxin-750	A.H. Robins
8642 [crescent moon]	Phrenilin 15 mg/325 mg/40 mg	Carnrick Labs
8650 [moon logo]	Phrenlin 50 mg/325 mg	Carnrick Labs
8652	Nolahist 25 mg	Carnrick Labs
8658	Ephedrine, Caffeine	Unknown
8666 [dot logo]	Sinulin 650 mg/4 mg/25 mg	Carnrick Labs
8671	Salflex 500 mg	Carnrick Labs
8672	Salflex 750 mg	Carnrick Labs
8797 360	Triprolidine, Pseudoephedrine	Unknown
9531	Methenamine 300 mg, Sodium Biphosphate 500 mg	Poythress
9532	Mudrane-2 195 mg/130 mg	Poythress Labs
9533	Aminophylline 130 mg, Guaifenesin 100 mg	Poythress
9550	Potassium Iodide 195 mg, Aminophylline 130 mg, Phenobarbital 8 mg, Ephedrine 16 mg	Poythress
9551	Aminophylline 130 mg, Ephedrine 16 mg, Phenobarbital 8 mg, Guaifenesin 100 mg	Poythress
19795	Caffeine, Ephedrine, Phenylpropanolamine	Unknown
23601	Caffeine	Unknown
33605	Haloperidol 0.5 mg	Searle Pharm
33635	Warfarin 2 mg	Lemmon Pharm
33636	Sominex 2 25 mg	Beecham Labs
43797-007	Hyoscyamine Sulfate 0.125 mg	Hauck
97209 63	Caffeine	Unknown
97209 63	Caffeine, Ephedrine, Phenylpropanolamine	Unknown
2432926	Caffeine, Ephedrine, Phenylpropanolamine	Unknown

Imprint	Ingredient/Brand Name	Manufacturer
2432926 [logo]	Caffeine, Ephedrine, Phenylpropanolamine	Unknown
51479007	Chlorpheniramine 4 mg, Pseudoephedrine 60 mg	Dura
A 002	Vitamins	Amide Pharm
A 003	Phenazopyridine 100 mg	Amide Pharm
A 004	Phenazopyridine 200 mg	Amide Pharm
A05	Potassium Chloride 300 mg	Eli Lilly
A06	Potassium Iodide 300 mg	Eli Lilly
A-018	Chlordiazepoxide 5 mg, Clidinium Bromide 2.5 mg	Amide Pharm
A 019	Amigesic 500 mg	Amide Pharm
A 020	Amigesic 750 mg	Amide Pharm
A 027	Amilic Antacid	Amide Pharm
A 031	Vitamins	Amide Pharm
A 038	Vitamins	Amide Pharm
A 040	Dimenhydrinate 50 mg	Amide Pharm
A 056	Chlorpheniramine Maleate 4 mg	Amide Pharm
A 058	Ami-Tex LA 75 mg/400 mg	Amide Pharm
A-059	Ami-tex 45 mg/5 mg/200 mg	Amide Pharm
A 088	Docusate Sodium 100 mg	Amide Pharm
A 089	Docusate Sodium 250 mg	Amide Pharm
A/2	Panwarfin 2 mg	Abbott Labs
A2C	Lanoxicaps 0.05 mg	Burroughs Wellcome
A/2 1/2	Panwarfin 2.5 mg	Abbott Labs
A/5	Panwarfin 5 mg	Abbott Labs
A10	Nifedipine 10 mg	Miles
A/10	Panwarfin 10 mg	Abbott Labs
A 11S	Caffeine	Unknown
A14	Thyroid 30 mg	Eli Lilly
A15	Thyroid 60 mg	Eli Lilly
A 19	Diethylstilbestrol 0.1 mg	Eli Liily
A/25	Dicumarol 25 mg	Abbott Labs
A31	Potassium Chloride 1000 mg	Eli Lilly
A33	Diethylstilbestrol 5 mg	Eli Lilly
A 40	Dimenhydrinate 50 mg	Amide Pharm
A/50	Dicumarol 50 mg	Abbott Labs
A 51/LL	CONTROLLED - SEE PAGE 227	
A 52/LL	CONTROLLED - SEE PAGE 227	
A 53/LL	CONTROLLED - SEE PAGE 227	
A 77/W[in box]	Aralen 500 mg	Winthrop-Breon
A/100	Dicumarol 100 mg	Abbott Labs
A 102	Sodium Bicarbonate 5 gr	Amide Pharm
A 103	Sodium Bicarbonate 10 gr	Amide Pharm
A 106	Guaifenesin 600 mg	Amide Pharm
A 110	Vitamins	Amide Pharm
A 111	Methenamine Mandelate 0.5 gr	Amide Pharm
A 113	Chlorpheniramine Maleate 60 mg, Pseudoephedrine 4 mg	Amide Pharm
A 116	Meclizine HCl 12.5 mg	Amide Pharm
A 117	Meclizine HCl 25 mg	Amide Pharm
A 121	Phenylpropanolamine 25 mg	Amide Pharm
A 122	Phenylpropanolamine 50 mg	Amide Pharm
A 124	Sodium Fluoride 0.25 mg	Amide Pharm
A 127	Sodium Fluoride 0.5 mg	Amide Pharm
A 128	Sodium Fluoride 1 mg	Amide Pharm
A200	Ibuprofen 200 mg	Sterling
A 512	Phenolphthalein 60 mg	Adria
A 513	Phenolphthalein 130 mg	Adria
A 515	Phenolphthalein 65 mg, Docusate Sodium 100 mg	Adria

Imprint	Ingredient/Brand Name	Manufacturer
A 554	Carbamazepine 200 mg	Lemmon
A 585	Carbidopa 25 mg, Levodopa 100 mg	Lemmon Pharm
A 587	Carbidopa 25 mg, Levodopa 250 mg	Lemmon Pharm
A/A	Vanex Forte 50 mg/25 mg/10 mg/4 mg	Abana
AA	Aspirin 800 mg	Able Labs
AA Logo/0310	Mobidin 600 mg	Ascher & Co
AA/310	Mobidin 600 mg	Ascher & Co
a AA	Chlorthalidone 25 mg	Abbott Labs
A [logo]	Phenylpropanolamine 75 mg, Brompheniramine Maleate 12 mg	P & G
A[logo] AA	Aquasol 7.5 mg	Armour Pharm
A[logo] AB	Aquasol 15 mg	Armour Pharm
AA [logo]	Chlorthalidone 25 mg	Abbott Labs
a AB	Chlorthalidone 50 mg	Abbott Labs
a AD	Peganone 250 mg	Abbott Labs
a AE	Peganone 500 mg	Abbott Labs
AAE/SCHERING	Chlor-Trimeton 12 mg	Schering Corp
a AF	Colchicine 0.6 mg	Abbott Labs
a AH	Oreticyl 25	Abbott Labs
a AI	Oreticyl 50	Abbott Labs
a AJ	Fero-Folic 500	Abbott Labs
a AK	Iberet-Folic 500	Abbott Labs
a AL	Tral 50 mg	Abbott Labs
a AM	Tridione 300 mg	Abbott Labs
a AN	Dicumarol 25 mg	Abbott Labs
a AO	Dicumarol 50 mg	Abbott Labs
AARP 205	Acetaminophen 325 mg, Chlorpheniramine Maleate 2 mg	Invamed
AARP 217	Acetaminophen 325 mg, Chlorpheniramine maleate 2 mg, Phenylpropanolamine 12 mg	Invamed
AARP 243	Aspirin 500 mg, Calcium Carbonate 165 mg, Magnesium Carbonate 30 mg, Magnesium Oxide 100 mg	Invamed
AARP 247	Aluminum Hydroxide 80 mg, Magnesium Trisilicate 20 mg	Invamed
AARP 251	Calcium Carbonate 280 mg, Magnesium Hydroxide 128 mg, Simethicone 20 mg	Invamed
AARP 267	Senna Concentrate 187 mg	Generic Sal
AARP 381	Aspirin 325 mg, Aluminum Hydroxide 50, Magnesium Hydroxide 50 mg	Invamed
AARP 540	Acetaminophen 250 mg, Aspirin 250 mg, Caffeine 65 mg	Invamed
AARP 552	Yellow Phenolphthalein 90 mg	Invamed
AARP 566	Acetaminophen 500 mg	J.B. Labs
AARP 3731	Aspirin 325 mg, Aluminum Hydroxide 75 mg, Magnesium Hydroxide 75 mg	Invamed
a AT	Vercyte 25 mg	Abbott Labs
AB [logo]	Chlorthalidone 50 mg	Abbott Labs
Abana 217	CONTROLLED - SEE PAGE 220	
Abana 250	Pseudoephedrine 90 mg, Guaifenesin 250 mg	Abana
Abana 500	CONTROLLED - SEE PAGE 213	
ABB/SCHERING	Meticorten 5 mg	Schering Corp
AC 75	Choline Magnesium Trisalicylate 750 mg	Able Labs
ACCUTANE 10 ROCHE	Accutane 10 mg	Roche Labs
ACCUTANE 20 ROCHE	Accutane 20 mg	Roche Labs
ACCUTANE 40 ROCHE	Accutane 40 mg	Roche Labs
a CE	CONTROLLED - SEE PAGE 214	
a CF	CONTROLLED - SEE PAGE 221	
a CH	CONTROLLED - SEE PAGE 214	
A[logo] CP	CVP 100 mg	Armour Pharm
AC Pediacare	Pediacare Cold Allergy	McNeil

Imprint	Ingredient/Brand Name	Manufacturer
ACTIDIL L2A	Actidil 2.5 mg	Burroughs Wellcome
ACTIFED	Actifed 60 mg/2.5 mg	Burroughs Wellcome
ACTIFED 12-HOUR	Actifed 120 mg/5 mg	Burroughs Wellcome
ACTIFED DAY	Acetaminophen 325 mg, Pseudoephedrine 30 mg	Burroughs Wellcome
ACTIFED M2A	Actifed 2.5 mg/60 mg	Burroughs Wellcome
ACTIFED NIGHT	Actifed Sinus Nighttime	Burroughs Wellcome
ACTIFED PLUS	Actifed 500 mg/30 mg/1.25 mg	Burroughs Wellcome
AD [logo]	Peganone 250 mg	Abbott Labs
Adams 0012	Humibid LA 600 mg	Adams Labs
Adams 0014	Deconsal 60 mg/200 mg	Adams Labs
Adams 0016	Deconsal Sprinkle 10 mg/200 mg	Adams Labs
Adams 0017	Guaifenesin 600 mg, Pseudoephedrine 60 mg	Adams Labs
Adams 0018	Guaifenesin 300 mg	Adams Labs
Adams 0021	Atrohist LA 4 mg/50 mg/120 mg	Adams Labs
Adams 0022	Atrohist Sprinkle 2 mg/25 mg/10 mg	Adams Labs
Adams 0030	Guaifenesin 600 mg, Dextromethorphan Hydrobromide 30 mg	Adams
ADAPIN 10	Adapin 10 mg	Pennwalt Corp
ADAPIN 25	Adapin 25 mg	Pennwalt Corp
ADAPIN 50	Adapin 50 mg	Pennwalt Corp
ADAPIN 75	Adapin 75 mg	Pennwalt Corp
ADAPIN 100	Adapin 100 mg	Pennwalt Corp
ADD/SCHERING	Demazin 10 mg/2 mg	Schering Corp
ADEFLOR/0.5	Adeflor	Upjohn Comp
ADEFLOR/1.0	Adeflor	Upjohn Comp
ADIPEX-P	CONTROLLED - No Photo - Phentermine HCl 37.5 mg - White capsule - DEA Schedule IV	Lemmon Pharm
Adria/130	Axotal 650 mg/50 mg	Adria Labs
Adria/200	Ilozyme	Adria Labs
Adria 217	Phenolphthalein 130 mg	Adria Labs
Adria/230	Octamide 10 mg	Adria Labs
Adria/231	Ilopan-Choline 50 mg/25 mg	Adria Labs
Adria/304	Kaon CL-10 750 mg	Adria Labs
Adria/307	Kaon CL 500 mg	Adria Labs
Adria/312	Kaon 1170 mg	Adria Labs
Adria/412	Magan 545 mg	Adria Labs
Adria 420	Magnesium Lactate 7mEq	Adria Labs
Adria 648	Cyclothiazide 2 mg	Adria Labs
Advil	Advil 200 mg	Whitehall Labs
ADX/SCHERING	Trilafon 8 mg	Schering Corp
AE [logo]	Peganone 500 mg	Abbott Labs
a EA	Erythromycin 500 mg	Abbott Labs
a EB	Erythromycin 250 mg	Abbott Labs
a EC	Ery-Tab 250 mg	Abbott Labs
a ED	Ery-Tab 500 mg	Abbott Labs
a EE	EES 400	Abbott Labs
a EF	EES 200	Abbott Labs
a EH	Ery-Tab 333 mg	Abbott Labs
a ES	Erythromycin 250 mg	Abbott Labs
a ET	Erythromycin 500 mg	Abbott Labs
AF-1	Acetaminophen 325 mg, Phenylpropanolamine 5 mg, Chlorpheniramine maleate 2 mg	Perrigo Company
AF 2	Sodium Fluoride 2.2 mg	Able Labs
AF ANACIN	Acetaminophen 500 mg	Whitehall Robins
AF [logo]	Colchicine 0.6 mg	Abbott Labs
AF Excedrin	Aspirin free Excedrin	Bristol-Myers
AFPM	Acetaminophen 500 mg, Diphenhydramine 25 mg	Whitehall Robins

Imprint	Ingredient/Brand Name	Manufacturer
AFRINOL	Afrinol 120 mg	Schering Corp
AH[logo]	Oreticyl 25	Abbott Labs
a HH	Depakene 250 mg	Abbott Labs
AHR	Dextromethorphan Hydrobromide 5 mg	A.H. Robins
AHR 0674	Allbee with C 300 mg	A.H. Robins
AHR 0677	Allbee C-800	A.H. Robins
AHR 0678	Vitamins	A.H. Robins
AHR 0689	Z-BEC	A.H. Robins
AHR 1 Tenex	Tenex 1 mg	A.H. Robins
AHR 2	Robinul Forte 2 mg	A.H. Robins
AHR 2/7840	Robinul-Forte 2 mg	A.H. Robins
AHR 10/REGLAN	Reglan 10 mg	A.H. Robins
AHR/21 17	Dimetane 4 mg	A.H. Robins
AHR 1535	Mitrolan 500 mg	A.H. Robins
AHR 1650	Dimacol 100 mg/30 mg/15 mg	A.H. Robins
AHR 1843	Brompheniramine Maleate 12 mg	A.H. Robins
AHR 1857	Brompheniramine Maleate 4 mg	A.H. Robins
AHR 1868	Brompheniramine Maleate 8 mg	A.H. Robins
AHR 2117	Phenylephrine 10 mg, Brompheniramine Maleate 4 mg	A.H. Robins
AHR 2245	Pseudoephedrine 30 mg	A.H. Robins
AHR 2248	Brompheniramine Maleate 4 mg	A.H. Robins
AHR 2250	Brompheniramine Maleate 4 mg	A.H. Robins
AHR 2254	Brompheniramine Mal. 4 mg, Phenylpropanolamine 25 mg	A.H. Robins
AHR 2255	Dimetapp Cold & Allergy Capsule	A.H. Robins
AHR 2279	Dimetapp Cold & Cough	A.H. Robins
AHR 2280	Dimetapp Cold & Flu Caplet	A.H. Robins
AHR 2290	Brompheniramine 1 mg, Phenylpropanolamine 6.25 mg	A.H. Robins
AHR 4649	Donnazyme	A.H. Robins
AHR 5049	Entozyme	A.H. Robins
AHR 5449	Exna 50 mg	A.H. Robins
AHR 5720 Micro-K	Micro-K 600 mg	A.H. Robins
AHR 5730 Micro-K	Micro-K 750 mg	A.H. Robins
AHR 5816	Pabalate 300 mg/300 mg	A.H. Robins
AHR 5883	Pabalate-SF 300 mg/300 mg	A.H. Robins
AHR 6207	Phenaphen 325 mg	A.H. Robins
AHR 6242	CONTROLLED - SEE PAGE 223	
AHR 6257	CONTROLLED - SEE PAGE 223	
AHR 6274	CONTROLLED - SEE PAGE 220	
AHR 6447	CONTROLLED - SEE PAGE 203	
AHR 7429	Robaxin 500 mg	A.H. Robins
AHR/7449	Robaxin 750	A.H. Robins
AHR 7824	Robinul 1 mg	A.H. Robins
AHR 8217	Robicillin VK 250 mg	A.H. Robins
AHR 8227	Robicillin VK 500 mg	A.H. Robins
AHR 8317	Robimycin 250 mg	A.H. Robins
AHR 8417	Robitet 250 mg	A.H. Robins
AHR 8427	Robitet 500 mg	A.H. Robins
AHR 8600	Robitussin Cold & Cough Capsules	A.H. Robins
AHR 8601	Guaifenesin 200 mg, Pseudoephedrine 30 mg	A.H. Robins
AHR 8602	Robitussin Cold, Cough & Flu Caplets	A.H. Robins
AHR 8831	Silain 50 mg	A.H. Robins
AHR 8871	Silain-Gel 141 mg/141 mg/85 mg/25 mg	A.H. Robins
AHR/ALLBEE C	Vitamins	A.H. Robins
AHR FEAC	Ascorbic Acid 150 mg, Vitamins	A.H. Robins
AHR/ROBAXIN	Robaxin 750	A.H. Robins
AHR/ROBAXIN 750	Robaxin-750	A.H. Robins

Imprint	Ingredient/Brand Name	Manufacturer
AHR/ROBITAB 8217	Robicillin VK 250 mg	A.H. Robins
AHR/ROBITAB 8227	Robicillin VK 500 mg	A.H. Robins
AHR/ROBITAB 8317	Robimycin 250 mg	A.H. Robins
AHR/SCHERING	Rela 350 mg	Schering Corp
AHR/Z-BEC	Vitamins	A.H. Robins
AHS	Caffeine	Unknown
AHT/SCHERING	Naquival 4 mg/0.1 mg	Schering Corp
a II	Phenurone 500 mg	Abbott Labs
AI [logo]	Oreticyl 50	Abbott Labs
AJ	Fero-Folic-500	Abbott
AJ [logo]	Fero-Folic 500	Abbott Labs
AK	Iberet-Folic-500	Abbott
AKG	Caffeine, Ephedrine, Phenylpropanolamine	Unknown
AK [logo]	Iberet-Folic 500	Abbott Labs
a KN	CONTROLLED - SEE PAGE 218	
AKS	Ephedrine Sulfate	Unknown
AKS[in box]	Caffeine, Ephedrine, Phenylpropanolamine	Unknown
AKS 18-789	Caffeine, Ephedrine, Phenylpropanolamine	Unknown
AKS 20 20	Caffeine, Ephedrine, Phenylpropanolamine	Unknown
AKS 789	Caffeine, Ehpedrine, Phenylpropanolamine	Unknown
AKS 50845	Caffeine, Ephedrine, Phenylpropanolamine	Unknown
AL	CONTROLLED - SEE PAGE 210	
AL 0.25/G	CONTROLLED - SEE PAGE 227	
AL 0.5/G	CONTROLLED - SEE PAGE 227	
AL 1.0/G	CONTROLLED - SEE PAGE 227	
AL [logo]	Tral 50 mg	Abbott Labs
ALDACTAZIDE 25	Aldactazide 25 mg	Searle Pharm
ALDACTAZIDE 50	Aldactazide 50 mg	Searle Pharm
ALDACTAZIDE/SEARLE 1011	Aldactazide 25 mg	Searle Pharm
ALDACTONE 25	Aldactone 25 mg	Searle Pharm
ALDACTONE 50	Aldactone 50 mg	Searle Pharm
ALDACTONE 100	Aldactone 100 mg	Searle Pharm
ALDACTONE/SEARLE 1001	Aldactone 25 mg	Searle Pharm
a LE	Tridione Dulcet 150 mg	Abbott Labs
a LF	Panwarfin 10 mg	Abbott Labs
a LK	Harmonyl 0.25 mg	Abbott Labs
Alka-Mints	Calcium Carbonate 850 mg	Miles Pharm
ALKA SELTZER	Alka Seltzer 324 mg/200 mg/1050 mg/1900 mg	Miles Pharm
ALKA SELTZER ANTACID	Alka Seltzer 958 mg/832 mg/312 mg	Miles Pharm
ALKA SELTZER EX S	Alka Seltzer 500 mg/1985 mg/1000 mg	Miles Pharm
ALKA SELTZER PLUS	Alka Seltzer 325 mg/2 mg/24.08 mg	Miles Pharm
ALKERAN A2A	Alkeran 2 mg	Burroughs Wellcome
a LL	Oreticyl Forte 25/0.25 mg	Abbott Labs
Allbee C AHR	Vitamins	A.H. Robins
ALLEREST	Chlorpheniramine Maleate 2 mg, Pseudoephedrine 30 mg	CIBA
ALLEREST 12	Chlorpheniramine Maleate 12 mg, Phenylpropanolamine 75 mg	CIBA
a LM	Panwarfin 2 mg	Abbott Labs
a LN	Panwarfin 2.5 mg	Abbott Labs
a LO	Panwarfin 5 mg	Abbott Labs
a LR	Panwarfin 7.5 mg	Abbott Labs
ALRA 215	Ibuprofen 200 mg	Alra
ALRA GN	CONTROLLED - SEE PAGE 212	
ALRA GT	CONTROLLED - SEE PAGE 204	
ALRA GX	CONTROLLED - SEE PAGE 211	
ALRA IF 400	Ibuprofen 400 mg	Alra
ALRA IF 600	Ibuprofen 600 mg	Alra

Imprint	Ingredient/Brand Name	Manufacturer
a LS	Enduronyl 5 mg/0.25 mg	Abbott Labs
a LT	Enduronyl Forte 5 mg/0.5 mg	Abbott Labs
ALTO 401	Zinc Sulfate 220 mg	Alto Pharm
ALTO[in box] 425-4	EFED II 200 mg	Alto Pharm
ALTO[in box] 425-5	EFED II 25 mg	Alto Pharm
ALTO 455-4	Caffeine, Ephedrine, Phenylpropanolamine	Unknown
a LU	Ogen 0.75 mg	Abbott Labs
ALUDROX/WYETH	Aludrox 375 mg	Wyeth Labs
a LV	Ogen 1.5 mg	Abbott Labs
a LX	Ogen 3 mg	Abbott Labs
a LY	Ogen 6 mg	Abbott Labs
AM	CONTROLLED - SEE PAGE 202	
AM [logo]	Tridione 300 mg	Abbott Labs
AMB 5/5401	CONTROLLED - SEE PAGE 226	
AMB 10/5421	CONTROLLED - SEE PAGE 226	Amesec Glaxo
Amesec 130 mg/25 mg	Glaxo Inc	
AMIDE 001	Vitamins	Amide Pharm
AMIDE 002	Vitamins	Amide Pharm
AMIDE 003	Phenazopyridine 100 mg	Amide Pharm
AMIDE 004	Phenazopyridine 200 mg	Amide Pharm
AMIDE 005	Pseudoephedrine 60 mg	Amide Pharm
AMIDE 009/10	Isoxsuprine 10 mg	Amide Pharm
AMIDE 0046	Tri-Tannate 25 mg/8 mg/25 mg	Amide Pharm
AMIDE 010/20	Isoxsuprine 20 mg	Amide Pharm
AMIDE 013	Ephedrine 25 mg, Theophylline 130 mg, Hydroxyzine 10 mg	Amide
AMIDE 014	Dexchlorpheniramine 4 mg	Amide Pharm
AMIDE 015	Dexchlorpheniramine 6 mg	Amide Pharm
AMIDE 022	Prenatal Vitamin w/Beta-Carotene	Amide Pharm
AMIDE 024	Phenylephrine 20 mg, Guaifenesin 300 mg	Amide Pharm
AMIDE 026	Vitamins	Amide
AMIDE/031	Vitamins	Amide Pharm
AMIDE 032	Yohimbine HCl 5.4 mg	Amide Pharm
AMIDE 035	Theophylline 118 mg, Ephedrine 24 mg, Phenobarbital 8 mg	Amide
AMIDE 039	Isometheptene Mucate 65 mg, Dichloralphenazone 100 mg, Acetaminophen 325 mg	Amide Pharm
AMIDE 043	Vitamins	Amide Pharm
AMIDE 045	Vitamins	Amide Pharm
AMIDE 053	Chlorzoxazone 250 mg	Amide Pharm
AMIDE 076	Vitamins	Amide Pharm
AMIDE 077	Vitamins	Amide Pharm
AMIDE 078	Vitamins	Amide Pharm
AMIDE 082	Cyclendelate 200 mg	Amide Pharm
AMIDE 083	Cyclendelate 400 mg	Amide Pharm
Amitone	Calcium Carbonate 350 mg	Perrigo Company
AMN/SCHERING	Drixoral 6 mg/120 mg	Schering Corp
A MO	Toprol XL 50 mg	Astra
AMOXIL 125	Amoxil 125 mg	Beecham Labs
AMOXIL 250	Amoxil 250 mg	Beecham Labs
AMOXIL 500	Amoxil 500 mg	Beecham Labs
AMP 25	Caffeine, Ephedrine, Phenylpropanolamine	Unknown
AMS	Toprol XL 100 mg	Astra
A MY	Toprol XL 200 mg	Astra
AN	CONTROLLED - SEE PAGE 193	
AN [logo]	Dicumarol 25 mg	Abbott Labs
ANACIN	Anacin 400 mg/32 mg	Whitehall Labs
A[pestle] NC	Nicobid 125 mg	USV Labs

Imprint	Ingredient/Brand Name	Manufacturer
ANCOBON 250	Ancobon 250 mg	Roche Labs
ANCOBON 400	Ancobon 400 mg	Roche Labs
ANCOBON 500	Ancobon 500 mg	Roche Labs
A[pestle] ND	Nicobid 250 mg	USV Labs
a ND	Janimine 10 mg	Abbott Labs
a NE	Janimine 25 mg	Abbott Labs
A[pestle] NE	Nicolar 500 mg	USV Labs
a NF	Tral 25 mg	Abbott Labs
ANF/SCHERING	Coricidin D 2 mg/12.5 mg/325 mg	Schering Corp
A[pestle] NH	Nicobid 500 mg	USV Labs
a NJ	Cefol	Abbott Labs
a NK	Eutron 25 mg/5 mg	Abbott Labs
a NL	Janimine 50 mg	Abbott Labs
a NM	Ktab 750 mg	Abbott Labs
a NR	Depakote 250 mg	Abbott Labs
a NS	Depakote 500 mg	Abbott Labs
ANSPOR 250 SKF	Anspor 250 mg	Smith,Kline & French
ANSPOR 500 SKF	Anspor 500 mg	Smith,Kline & French
a NT	Depakote 125 mg	Abbott Labs
ANTABUSE 250	Antabuse 250 mg	Ayerst Labs
ANTABUSE 500	Antabuse 500 mg	Ayerst Labs
ANTIVERT/210	Antivert 12.5 mg	Pfizer Labs
ANTIVERT/211	Antivert 25 mg	Pfizer Labs
ANTIVERT/212	Antivert 25 mg	Pfizer Labs
ANTIVERT/214	Antivert 50 mg	Pfizer Labs
ANTURANE 200	Anturane 200 mg	Ciba Pharm
ANX	Anxanil 25 mg	Econo Med
AO [logo]	Dicumarol 50 mg	Abbott Labs
AP/0812	Doxycycline 100 mg	Halsey Drug
AP/0814	Doxycycline 100 mg	Halsey Drug
AP/0837	Doxycycline 50 mg	Halsey Drug
AP 1	Phenazopyradine 100 mg	Able Labs
AP 2	Phenazopyradine 200 mg	Able Labs
AP/2461	Nadolol 20 mg	Bristol-Myers
AP/2462	Nadolol 40 mg	Bristol-Myers
AP/2463	Nadolol 80 mg	Bristol-Myers
AP/2464	Nadolol 120 mg	Bristol-Myers
AP/2465	Nadolol 160 mg	Bristol-Myers
AP/2472	Nadolol 40 mg, Bendroflumethiazide 5 mg	Bristol-Myers
AP/2473	Nadolol 80 mg, Bendroflumethiazide 5 mg	Bristol-Myers
APAP 325 TTC	Acetaminophen 325 mg	Trinity
APAP 500 TTC	Acetaminophen 500 mg	Trinity
APHRODYNE	Aphrodyne 5.4 mg	Star Pharm
Appedrine Appedrine	Phenylpropanolamine 25 mg	Thompson Medical
APRESAZIDE 25-25	Apresazide 25 mg	Ciba Pharm
APRESAZIDE 50-50	Apresazide 50 mg	Ciba Pharm
APRESAZIDE 50-100	Apresazide 100 mg/50 mg	Ciba Pharm
APSE	Pseudoephedrine 120 mg, Guaifenesin 600 mg	Amide Pharm
A[logo] Rd	Dialume 500 mg	Armour Pharm
ARGESIC-38130	Argesic 600 mg/30 mg	Econo Med
ARM	Allergy Relief Medicine 4 mg/37.5 mg	Menley & James Labs
AS	Isoclor 4 mg/60 mg	Fisons Corp
A/S	Comtrex-A/S 500 mg/30 mg/2 mg	Bristol-Meyers
AS 94-44	Isoclor 8 mg/120 mg	Fisons Corp
AS 94 51	Isoclor 4 mg/60 mg	Arnar Stone Labs
ASB	Arthritis Strength Bufferin	Bristol-Myers

Imprint	Ingredient/Brand Name	Manufacturer
ASBRON-G 78-202	Asbron-G 150 mg/100 mg	Sandoz Pharm
AS + NT	Brompheniramine Maleate 2 mg, Phenylpropanolamine 20 mg, Dextromethorphan Hydrobromide 10 mg	Miles Pharm
Aspirin	Aspirin 325 mg	Zee Medical
Aspirin 1	Aspirin 5 gr	Magno-Humphries
Aspirin/44 249	Aspirin 325 mg	LNK International
Aspirin 500	Aspirin 500 mg	Perrigo Company
Aspirin L	Aspirin 325 mg	Perrigo Company
Aspirin VA 74	Aspirin 325 mg	Vitech Corp.
ASTRA 725	Bricanyl 2.5 mg	Astra Pharm
ASTRA 750	Bricanyl 5 mg	Astra Pharm
AT 054	CONTROLLED - SEE PAGE 216	
AT 076	Chlordiazepoxide 5 mg, Clidinium Bromide 2.5 mg	American Ther
AT 083	Danazol 200 mg	American Therapeutic
AT 092	Phenazopyridine 100 mg	American Therapeutic
AT 093	Phenazopyridine 200 mg	American Therapeutic
AT 094	Sulfisoxazole 500 mg, Phenylazodiaminopyridine 50 mg	American Therapeutic
AT 096	Chlorzoxazone 250 mg, Acetraminophen 300 mg	American Ther
AT 100	Vitamins, Minerals	American Therapeutic
AT 101	Meclofenamate 50 mg	American Therapeutic
AT 102	Meclofenamate 100 mg	American Therapeutic
AT 109	CONTROLLED - SEE PAGE 222	
AT 121	Trazodone 50 mg	American Therapeutic
AT 125	Trazodone 100 mg	American Therapeutic
AT 133	Vitamins	American Ther
AT 135	Methocarbamol 500 mg	American Therapeutic
AT 137	Methocarbamol 750 mg	American Therapeutic
AT 141	Prednisone 5 mg	American Therapeutic
AT 142	Prednisone 10 mg	American Therapeutic
AT 143	Prednisone 20 mg	American Therapeutic
AT 145	Quinine Sulfate 260 mg	American Therapeutic
AT 146	Quinine Sulfate 325 mg	American Ther
AT 147	Fenoprofen Calcium 600 mg	American Ther
AT 148	Clonidine 0.1 mg	American Therapeutic
AT 149	Clonidine 0.2 mg	American Therapeutic
AT 150	Clonidine 0.3 mg	American Therapeutic
AT 151	Thiothixene 1 mg	American Therapeutic
AT 152	Thiothixene 2 mg	American Ther
AT 153	Thiothixene 5 mg	American Therapeutic
AT 154	Thiothixene 10 mg	American Therapeutic
AT 155	Thiothixene 20 mg	American Therapeutic
AT 156	CONTROLLED - SEE PAGE 209	
AT 157	CONTROLLED - SEE PAGE 207	
AT 158	CONTROLLED - SEE PAGE 207	
AT 164	Triamterene 75 mg, Hydrochlorothiazide 50 mg	American Therapeutic
AT 165	Metaproterenol Sulfate 10 mg	American Therapeutic
AT 166	Metaproterenol Sulfate 20 mg	American Therapeutic
AT 167	Maprotiline 25 mg	American Therapeutic
AT 168	Maprotiline 50 mg	American Therapeutic
AT 169	Maprotiline 75 mg	American Therapeutic
AT 172	Albuterol Sulfate 2 mg	American Ther
AT 174	Chloroxazone 500 mg	American Ther
AT 177	Albuterol Sulfate 4 mg	American Ther
AT 178	Fenoprofen Calcium 200 mg	American Ther
AT 182	Prazosin 1 mg	American Ther
AT 184	Prazosin 2 mg	American Ther

Imprint	Ingredient/Brand Name	Manufacturer
AT 187	Prazosin 5 mg	American Ther
AT 190	Fenoprofen Calcium 300 mg	American Ther
AT 201/2	CONTROLLED - SEE PAGE 194	
AT 4307	Vitamins, Fluoride	American Therapeutic
AT 4312	Vitamins, Fluoride	American Therapeutic
AT [logo]	Pipobroman 25 mg	Abbott Labs
ATARAX 10/560	Atarax 10 mg	Pfizer Labs
ATARAX 25/561	Atarax 25 mg	Pfizer Labs
ATARAX 50/562	Atarax 50 mg	Pfizer Labs
ATARAX 100/563	Atarax 100 mg	Pfizer Labs
A[pestle] TC	Armour Thyroid 1/4 grain	Armour Pharm
A[pestle] TD	Armour Thyroid 1/2 grain	Armour Pharm
A[pestle] TE	Armour Thyroid 1 grain	USV Labs
A[pestle] TF	Armour Thyroid 2 grains	USV Labs
A[pestle] TG	Armour Thyroid 3 grains	USV Labs
A[pestle] TH	Armour Thyroid 4 grains	USV Labs
A[pestle] TI	Armour Thyroid 5 grains	USV Labs
A[pestle] TJ	Armour Thyroid 1 1/2 grains	USV Labs
a TL/T	CONTROLLED - SEE PAGE 210	
a TM/T	CONTROLLED - SEE PAGE 203	
a TN/T	CONTROLLED - SEE PAGE 207	
A[pestle] TO	Armour Thyroid 1/2 grain	USV Labs
ATROMID-S 500	Atromid-S 500 mg	Ayerst Labs
a TX	CONTROLLED - SEE PAGE 209	
a TY	CONTROLLED - SEE PAGE 213	
a UC	CONTROLLED - SEE PAGE 189	
a UD	CONTROLLED - SEE PAGE 213	
AUF/SCHERING	Fulvicin-U/F 250 mg	Schering Corp
AUG/SCHERING	Fulvicin-U/F 500 mg	Schering Corp
AUH/SCHERING	Fulvicin 125 mg	Schering Corp
A[pestle] YC	Thyrolar 1/4 grain	USV Labs
A[pestle] YD	Thyrolar 1/2 grain	USV Labs
A[pestle] YE	Thyrolar 1 grain	USV Labs
AYERST 102	Diucardin 500 mg	Ayerst Labs
AYERST 250	Amoxicillin 250 mg	Ayerst Labs
AYERST 252	Vitamins	Ayerst Labs
AYERST 430	Mysoline 250 mg	Ayerst Labs
AYERST 431	Mysoline 50 mg	Ayerst Labs
AYERST 442	Grisactin 125 mg	Ayerst Labs
AYERST 443	Grisactin 250 mg	Ayerst Labs
AYERST 444	Grisactin 500 mg	Ayerst Labs
AYERST 461	Inderal 10 mg	Ayerst Labs
AYERST 464	Inderal 40 mg	Ayerst Labs
AYERST 500	Amoxicillin 500 mg	Ayerst Labs
AYERST 702	Diucardin 50 mg	Ayerst Labs
AYERST 752	Vitamins	Ayerst Labs
AYERST 783	Thiosulfil-A Forte 500 mg/50 mg	Ayerst Labs
AYERST 784	Thiosulfil-A 250 mg/50 mg	Ayerst Labs
AYERST 785	Thiosulfil 250 mg	Ayerst Labs
AYERST 786	Thiosulfil Forte 500 mg	Ayerst Labs
AYERST 790	Riopan 400 mg	Ayerst Labs
AYERST 791	Riopan 400 mg	Ayerst Labs
AYERST 809	Antabuse 250 mg	Ayerst Labs
AYERST 810	Antabuse 500 mg	Ayerst Labs
AYERST 817	Beminal Forte	Ayerst Labs
AYERST 824	Beminal 500	Ayerst Labs

Imprint	Ingredient/Brand Name	Manufacturer
AYERST 865	Premarin 2.5 mg	Ayerst Labs
AYERST 866	Premarin 1.25 mg	Ayerst Labs
AYERST 867	Premarin 0.625 mg	Ayerst Labs
AYERST 868	Premarin 0.3 mg	Ayerst Labs
AYERST 878	Premarin with Methyltestosterone 0.625 mg, 5 mg	Wyeth Ayerst
AYERST 879	Premarin with methyltestosterone 1.25 mg, 10 mg	Wyeth Ayerst
A[pestle] YF	Thyrolar 2 grains	USV Labs
AYGESTIN 5	Aygestin 5 mg	Ayerst Labs
A[pestle] YH	Thyrolar 3 grains	USV Labs
A[pestle] YJ	Thyrolar 5 grains	Armour Pharm
B	Sodium Chloride 250 mg	Blairex Labs
B	Bufferin 325 mg	Bristol-Meyers
b 010	Tetracycline 500 mg	Barr Labs
b 011	Tetracycline 250 mg	Barr Labs
b 058	Diphenhydramine 25 mg	Barr Labs
b 059	Diphenhydramine 50 mg	Barr Labs
B 01	Bisacodyl 5 mg	Butler Pharm
B1	Bisacodyl 5 mg	Butler Pharm
B 2	Pseudoephedrine 60 mg, Triprolidine 2.5 mg	Butler Pharm
B 3	Ferrous Sulfate 5 gr	Butler Pharm
B 4	Pseudoephedrine 60 mg, Chlorpheniramine Maleate 4 mg	Butler Pharm
B 5	Pseudoephedrine 60 mg	Butler Pharm
B 6	Acetaminophen 325 mg, Pseudoephedrine 30 mg, Chlorpheniramine maleate 2 mg	Butler Pharm
B 7	Acetaminophen325 mg	Butler Pharm
B 8	Dimenhydrinate 50 mg	Butler Pharm
B2C	Lanoxicaps 0.1 mg	Burroughs Wellcome
B21	Levlen 0.03 mg, 0.15 mg	Berlex
B28	Levlen 0.03 mg, 0.15 mg	Berlex
B60	Ergocalcitrol 50,000 Units	Eli Lilly
B 57	Zorprin 800 mg	Boots Labs
B 58	Ru-Tuss 25 mg/50 mg/8 mg/0.04 mg/0.19 mg	Boots Labs
B95	Tri-Levlen	
B96	Levonorgestrel 0.075 mg, Ethinyl Estradiol 0.04 mg	Berlex
B97	Levonorgestrel 0.125 mg, Ethinyl Estradiol 0.03 mg	Berlex
b 115	Reserpine 0.1 mg, Hydralazine 25 mg, Hydrochlorothiazide 15 mg	Barr Labs
b 128	Dicyclomine 10 mg	Barr Labs
B 130	Hyoscymine 0.125 mg	Barr Labs
b 170	Furosemide 20 mg	Barr Labs
b 172	Isosorbide Dinitrate 5 mg	Barr Labs
b 173	Isosorbide Dinitrate 5 mg	Barr Labs
b 200	Ibuprofen 200 mg	Barr Labs
b 203	Amitriptyline 25 mg	Barr Labs
b 209	Amitriptyline 10 mg	Barr Labs
b 218	Ergoloid Mesylates 0.5 mg	Barr Labs
b 230	Erythromycin Estolate 250 mg	Barr Labs
b 237	Perphenazine 2 mg, Amitriptyline 25 mg	Barr Labs
b 238	Perphenazine 4 mg, Amitriptyline 25 mg	Barr Labs
b 245	Perphenazine 2 mg, Amitriptyline 10 mg	Barr Labs
b 246	Perphenazine 4 mg, Amitriptyline 10 mg	Barr Labs
B 248	Methyldopa 500 mg	Barr Labs
b 252	Dipyridamole 25 mg	Barr Labs
b 259	Erythromycin Ethylsuccinate 400 mg	Barr Labs
b 260	Thioridazine 10 mg	Barr Labs
b 261	Thioridazine 25 mg	Barr Labs

Imprint	Ingredient/Brand Name	Manufacturer
b 262	Thioridazine 50 mg	Barr Labs
b 263	Thioridazine 100 mg	Barr Labs
b 273	Sulfinpyrazone 200 mg	Barr Labs
b 276	Chlorpropamide 250 mg	Barr Labs
b 277	Isosorbide Dinitrate 10 mg	Barr Labs
b 281	Aminophylline 200 mg	Barr Labs
b 282	Aminophylline 100 mg	Barr Labs
b 283	Nalidixic Acid 1000 mg	Barr Labs
b 284	Nalidixic Acid 500 mg	Barr Labs
b/285	Dipyridamole 50 mg	Barr Labs
b/286	Dipyridamole 75 mg	Barr Labs
b 288	Isosorbide Dinitrate 40 mg	Barr Labs
b 295	Doxycycline 100 mg	Barr Labs
b 297	Doxycycline 100 mg	Barr Labs
b 298	Hydroxyzine 25 mg	Barr Labs
b 301	Hydroxyzine 10 mg	Barr Labs
b 321	Sulfamethoxazole 400 mg, Trimethoprim 80 mg	Barr Labs
b 322	Sulfamethoxazole 800 mg, Trimethoprim 160 mg	Barr Labs
b 326	Acetaminophen 500 mg	Barr Labs
b 327	Thioridazine 150 mg	Barr Labs
b 328	Thioridazine 200 mg	Barr Labs
b 329	Thioridazine 15 mg	Barr Labs
b 331	Disopyramide 100 mg	Barr Labs
b 332	Disopyramide 150 mg	Barr Labs
b 347	Chlorpropamide 100 mg	Barr Labs
B 357	Methyldopa 125 mg	Barr Labs
B 358	Methyldopa 250 mg	Barr Labs
b 361	Methyldopa 500 mg, Hydrochlorothiazide 30 mg	Barr Labs
b 362	Methyldopa 500 mg, Hydrochlorothiazide 50 mg	Barr Labs
b 365	Propranolol 10 mg	Barr Labs
b 383	Ergoloid Mesylates 1 mg	Barr Labs
b 388	Hydralazine 10 mg	Barr Labs
b 389	Hydralazine 100 mg	Barr Labs
b 395	Phenylbutazone 100 mg	Barr Labs
b 396	Phenylbutazone 100 mg	Barr Labs
b 397	Clonidine 0.1 mg	Barr Labs
b 398	Clonidine 0.2 mg	Barr Labs
b 399	Clonidine 0.3 mg	Barr Labs
b 415	Tolazamide 100 mg	Barr Labs
b 416	Tolazamide 250 mg	Barr Labs
b 417	Tolazamide 500 mg	Barr Labs
b 419	Ibuprofen 400 mg	Barr Labs
b 420	Ibuprofen 600 mg	Barr Labs
b 442	Acetohexamide 250 mg	Barr Labs
b 443	Acetohexamide 500 mg	Barr Labs
b 458	Amitriptyline 150 mg	Barr Labs
b 477	Haloperidol 0.5 mg	Barr Labs
b 478	Haloperidol 1 mg	Barr Labs
b 479	Haloperidol 2 mg	Barr Labs
b 480	Haloperidol 5 mg	Barr Labs
b/484	Leucovorin Calcium 5 mg	Barr Labs
b/485	Leucovorin Calcium 25 mg	Barr Labs
B 527	Doxycycline Hyclate 100 mg	Barr Labs
b 545	Cephalexin 250 mg	Barr Labs
b 546	Cephalexin 500 mg	Barr Labs
b 572	Methotrexate 2.5 mg	Barr Labs

Imprint	Ingredient/Brand Name	Manufacturer
B 1008	Allopurinol 100 mg	Boots Labs
B 1009	Allopurinol 300 mg	Boots Labs
BACTRIM-DS	Bactrim-DS 160 mg/400 mg	Roche Labs
BACTRIM/ROCHE	Bactrim 80 mg/400 mg	Roche Labs
Barr 0010	Tetracycline 500 mg	Barr Labs
Barr 0011	Tetracycline 250 mg	Barr Labs
Barr 0013	Erythromycin Stearate 250 mg	Barr Labs
Barr 0019	Hydrochlorothiazide 25 mg	Barr Labs
Barr 0020	Hydrochlorothiazide 50 mg	Barr Labs
Barr 0024	Sulfisoxazole 500 mg	Barr Labs
Barr 0026	Prednisone 5 mg	Barr Labs
Barr 0030	Colchicine 0.65 mg	Barr Labs
Barr 0057	Dimenhydrinate 50 mg	Barr Labs
Barr 0058	Diphenhydramine 25 mg	Barr Labs
Barr 0059	Diphenhydramine 50 mg	Barr Labs
Barr 0064	Hydralazine 25 mg	Barr Labs
Barr 0065	Hydralazine 50 mg	Barr Labs
Barr 0066	Isoniazid 100 mg	Barr Labs
Barr 0071	Isoniazid 300 mg	Barr Labs
Barr 0089	Propylthiouracil 50 mg	Barr Labs
Barr 0099	Bisacodyl 5 mg	Barr Labs
Barr 010	Tetracycline 500 mg	Barr Labs
barr 011	Tetracycline 250 mg	Barr Labs
barr 033	CONTROLLED - SEE PAGE 223	
barr 058	Diphenhydramine 25 mg	Barr Labs
barr/059	Diphenhydramine 50 mg	Barr Labs
Barr 066/100	Isoniazid 100 mg	Barr Labs
Barr 071/300	Isoniazid 300 mg	Barr Labs
Barr 0106	Methocarbamol 500 mg	Barr Labs
Barr 0107	Methocarbamol 750 mg	Barr Labs
Barr 0114	Reserpine 0.125 mg, Hydrochlorothiazide 25 mg	Barr Labs
Barr 0115	Reserpine 0.1 mg, Hydralazine 25 mg, Hydrochlorothiazide 15 mg	Barr Labs
Barr 0116	Reserpine 0.125 mg, Hydrochlorothiazide 50 mg	Barr Labs
Barr 0126	Dicyclomine 20 mg	Barr Labs
Barr 0128	Dicyclomine 10 mg	Barr Labs
Barr 0129	Dexamethasone 0.25 mg	Barr Labs
Barr 0130	Dexamethasone 0.50 mg	Barr Labs
Barr 0131	Dexamethasone 0.75 mg	Barr Labs
Barr 0132	Dexamethasone 1.5 0 mg	Barr Labs
Barr 0157	Prednisone 20 mg	Barr Labs
Barr 0169	Furosemide 40 mg	Barr Labs
Barr 0170	Furosemide 20 mg	Barr Labs
Barr 0172	Isosorbide Dinitrate 2.5 mg	Barr Labs
Barr 0173	Isosorbide Dinitrate 5 mg	Barr Labs
Barr 0174	Isosorbide Dinitrate 5 mg	Barr Labs
Barr 0175	Isosorbide Dinitrate 10 mg	Barr Labs
Barr 0176	Acetaminophen 325 mg	Barr Labs
Barr 0186	Isosorbide Dinitrate 20 mg	Barr Labs
Barr 0188	Quinidine Sulfate 200 mg	Barr Labs
Barr 0192	Hydrochlorothiazide 100 mg	Barr Labs
Barr 0203	Amitriptyline 25 mg	Barr Labs
Barr 0209	Amitriptyline 10 mg	Barr Labs
Barr 0210	Amitriptyline 50 mg	Barr Labs
Barr 0211	Amitriptyline 75 mg	Barr Labs
Barr 0212	Amitriptyline 100 mg	Barr Labs

Imprint	Ingredient/Brand Name	Manufacturer
Barr 0218	Ergoloid Mesylates 0.5 mg	Barr Labs
Barr 0227	Ergoloid Mesylates 1 mg	Barr Labs
Barr 0230	Erthromycin Estolate 250 mg	Barr Labs
Barr 0233	Prednisone 10 mg	Barr Labs
Barr 0241	Allopurinol 100 mg	Barr Labs
Barr 0242	Allopurinol 300 mg	Barr Labs
Barr 0251	Tolbutamide 500 mg	Barr Labs
Barr 0252	Dipyridamole 25 mg	Barr Labs
Barr 0255	Chlorzoxazone 250 mg, Acetaminophen 300 mg	Barr Labs
Barr 0259	Erythromycin Ethylsuccinate 400 mg	Barr Labs
Barr 0260	Thioridazine 10 mg	Barr Labs
Barr 0261	Thioridazine 25 mg	Barr Labs
Barr 0262	Thioridazine 50 mg	Barr Labs
Barr 0263	Thioridazine 100 mg	Barr Labs
Barr 0265	Spironolactone 25 mg, Hydrochlorothiazide 25 mg	Barr Labs
Barr 0266	Spironolactone 25 mg	Barr Labs
Barr 0267	Chlorthalidone 25 mg	Barr Labs
Barr 0268	Chlorthalidone 50 mg	Barr Labs
Barr 0271	Sulfinpyrazone 100 mg	Barr Labs
Barr 0272	Sulfinpyrazone 200 mg	Barr Labs
Barr 0276	Chlorpropamide 250 mg	Barr Labs
Barr 0277	Isosorbide Dinitrate 10 mg	Barr Labs
Barr 0279	Isosorbide Dinitrate 30 mg	Barr Labs
Barr 0281	Aminophylline 200 mg	Barr Labs
Barr 0282	Aminophylline 100 mg	Barr Labs
Barr 0285	Depyridamole 50 mg	Barr Labs
Barr 0286	Dipyridamole 75 mg	Barr Labs
Barr 0291	Metronidazole 250 mg	Barr Labs
Barr 0292	Metronidazole 500 mg	Barr Labs
Barr 0295	DOXY-TABS 100 mg	Barr Labs
Barr 0296	DOXY-CAPS 50 mg	Barr Labs
Barr 0297	DOXY-CAPS 100 mg	Barr Labs
Barr 0298	Hydroxyzine 25 mg	Barr Labs
Barr 0299	Hydroxyzine 50 mg	Barr Labs
Barr 0300	Hydroxyzine 100 mg	Barr Labs
Barr 0301	Hydroxyzine 10 mg	Barr Labs
Barr 0302	Hydroxyzine Pamoate 50 mg	Barr Labs
Barr 0314	Sulfamethoxazole 500 mg	Barr Labs
Barr 0321	Sulfamethoxazole 400 mg, Trimethoprim 80 mg	Barr Labs
Barr 0322	Sulfamethoxazole 800 mg, Trimethoprim 160 mg	Barr Labs
Barr 0323	Hydroxyzine Pamoate 25 mg	Barr Labs
Barr 0324	Hydroxyzine Pamoate 100 mg	Barr Labs
Barr 0326	Acetaminophen 500 mg	Barr Labs
Barr 0327	Thioridazine 150 mg	Barr Labs
Barr 0328	Thioridazine 200 mg	Barr Labs
Barr 0329	Thioridazine 15 mg	Barr Labs
Barr 0331	Disopyramide 100 mg	Barr Labs
Barr 0332	Disopyramide 150 mg	Barr Labs
Barr 0347	Chlorpropamide 100 mg	Barr Labs
Barr 0365	Propranolol 10 mg	Barr Labs
Barr 0366	Propranolol 20 mg	Barr Labs
Barr 0367	Propranolol 40 mg	Barr Labs
Barr 0383	Ergoloid Mesylates 1 mg	Barr Labs
Barr 0388	Hydralazine 10 mg	Barr Labs
Barr 0389	Hydralazine 100 mg	Barr Labs
Barr 0395	Phenylbutazone 100 mg	Barr Labs

Imprint	Ingredient/Brand Name	Manufacturer
Barr 0396	Phenylbutazone 100 mg	Barr Labs
Barr 0415	Tolazamide 100 mg	Barr Labs
Barr 0416	Tolazamide 250 mg	Barr Labs
Barr 0417	Tolazamide 500 mg	Barr Labs
Barr 0419	Ibuprofen 400 mg	Barr Labs
Barr 0420	Ibuprofen 600 mg	Barr Labs
Barr 0429	Trimethoprim 100 mg	Barr Labs
Barr 0434	Folic Acid 1 mg	Barr Labs
barr 115	Reserpine 0.1 mg, Hydralazine 25 mg, Hydrochlorothiazide 15 mg	Barr
barr 158	CONTROLLED - SEE PAGE 228	
barr 159	CONTROLLED - SEE PAGE 219	
Barr 198/3	CONTROLLED - SEE PAGE 195	
Barr 214	Chlordiazepoxide 5 mg, Clidinium Bromide 2.5 mg	Barr Labs
Barr 219	Erythromycin Stearate 500 mg	Barr Labs
Barr 229/4	CONTROLLED - SEE PAGE 197	
Barr 230	Erythromycin Estolate 250 mg	Barr Labs
barr 248	Methyldopa 500 mg	Barr Labs
barr/259	Erythromycin Ethylsuccinate 400 mg	Barr Labs
Barr 264/3	CONTROLLED - SEE PAGE 197	
barr 272	Sulfinpyrazone 200 mg	Barr Labs
Barr 280/4	CONTROLLED - SEE PAGE 199	
Barr/286	Dipyridamole 75 mg	Barr Labs
Barr 294/2	CONTROLLED - No photo - Codeine Phosphate 15 mg, Aspirin 325 mg - White, round tablet - DEA Schedule III	Barr Labs
barr 302 50	Hydroxyzine Pamoate 50 mg	Barr Labs
barr 323 25	Hydroxyzine Pamoate 25 mg	Barr Labs
barr 324 100	Hydroxyzine Pamoate 100 mg	Barr Labs
barr 325	CONTROLLED - SEE PAGE 201	
barr 331	Disopyramide Phosphate 100 mg	Barr Labs
Barr 336	Indomethacin 25 mg	Barr Labs
Barr 337	Indomethacin 50 mg	Barr Labs
barr 349	Chlorpropamide 100 mg	Barr Labs
barr 350	Chlorpropamide 250 mg	Barr Labs
barr 357	Methyldopa 125 mg	Barr Labs
barr 358	Methyldopa 250 mg	Barr Labs
barr 378	CONTROLLED - SEE PAGE 217	
barr 404	Doxepin 25 mg	Barr Labs
barr 405	Doxepin 50 mg	Barr Labs
barr 406	Doxepin 75 mg	Barr Labs
barr 407	Doxepin 100 mg	Barr Labs
barr/419	Ibuprofen 400 mg	Barr Labs
barr/420	Ibuprofen 600 mg	Barr Labs
barr 425	Verapamil 80 mg	Barr Labs
barr 442	Acetohexamide 250 mg	Barr Labs
barr 443	Acethexamide 500 mg	Barr Labs
barr 446	Tamoxifen Citrate 10 mg	Barr Labs
barr 455	Verapamil 120 mg	Barr Labs
barr 481	Haloperidol 10 mg	Barr Labs
barr 482	Haloperidol 20 mg	Barr Labs
barr 483	Amiloride 5 mg, Hydrochlorothiaxzide 50 mg	Barr Labs
Barr 486	Chlorthalidone 50 mg	Barr Labs
barr/499	Ibuprofen 800 mg	Barr Labs
Barr 514	Cephalexin 250 mg	Barr Labs
Barr 515	Cephalexin 500 mg	Barr Labs
Barr 545	Cephalexin 250 mg	Barr Labs
Barr 546	Cephalexin 500 mg	Barr Labs

Imprint	Ingredient/Brand Name	Manufacturer
barr 550	Cephradine 250 mg	Barr Labs
barr 551	Cephradine 500 mg	Barr Labs
barr 554	Meclofenamate Sodium 50 mg	Barr Labs
barr 555	Meclofenamate Sodium 100 mg	Barr Labs
barr 584	Erythromycin 250 mg	Barr Labs
Bayer Select	Ibuprofen 200 mg	Par Pharm
B B	Bufferin Caplet	Bristol-Myers
BBA/SCHERING	Tindal 20 mg	Schering Corp
BC BC	Aspirin 325 mg, Salicylamide 95 mg, Caffeine 16 mg	Block Drug Co.
BCP 7400	Tolmetin Sodium 400 mg	Baker
BD	Sennosides A & B 6 mg	Mikart
BDA [logo]	Betamethasone 0.6 mg	Schering
B-D B-D	D-Glucose 5 gm	Becton-Dickinson
BEACH 1111	K-PHOS Original	Beach Pharm
BEACH 1112	UROQID-Acid 350 mg/200 mg	Beach Pharm
BEACH/1114	UROQID-Acid No. 2 500 mg/500 mg	Beach Pharm
BEACH/1115	Thiacide 500 mg/250 mg	Beach Pharm
BEACH/1125	K-PHOS Neutral 852 mg/155 mg/130 mg	Beach Pharm
BEACH 1132	Beelith 660 mg	Beach Pharm
BEACH/1134	K-PHOS No. 2 305 mg/700 mg	Beach Pharm
BEACH 1135	K-PHOS M.F. 155 mg/350 mg	Beach Pharm
BEACH 1136	Citrolith 50 mg/950 mg	Beach Pharm
Beecham 185	Penicillin V Potassium 250 mg	Beecham
Beecham 186	Penicillin V Potassium 500 mg	Beecham
BEECHAM FASTIN	CONTROLLED - SEE PAGE 218	
BEMINAL 500	Beminal-500	Ayerst Labs
BENTYL 10	Bentyl 10 mg	Merrell Dow Pharm
Bentyl 20	Bentyl 20 mg	Merrell Dow Pharm
BERLEX 100	Elixophyllin SR 125 mg	Berlex Labs
BERLEX 123	Elixophyllin 200 mg	Berlex Labs
BERLEX 129	Elixophyllin 100 mg	Berlex Labs
BERLEX 181	Deconamine 8 mg/120 mg	Berlex Labs
BERLEX 184	Deconamine 4 mg/60 mg	Berlex Labs
BERLEX 200	Elixophyllin SR 250 mg	Berlex Labs
BEROCCA PLUS/ROCHE	Berocca Plus	Roche Labs
BEROCCA ROCHE	Berocca	Roche Labs
Betapace Tablets 80 mg	Betapace 80 mg	Berlex
Betapace Tablets 160 mg	Betapace 160 mg	Berlex
Betapace Tablets 240 mg	Betapace 240 mg	Berlex
BI 6	Catapres 0.1 mg	Boehringer Ingelheim
BI 7	Catapres 0.2 mg	Boehringer Ingelheim
BI 8	Combipres 0.1 mg/15 mg	Boehringer Ingelheim
BI 9	Combipres 0.2 mg/15 mg	Boehringer Ingelheim
BI 10	Combipres 0.3 mg/15 mg	Boehringer Ingelheim
BI 11	Catapres 0.3 mg	Boehringer Ingelheim
BI 12	Dulcolax 5 mg	Boehringer Ingelheim
BI 17	Persantine 25 mg	Boehringer Ingelheim
BI 18	Persantine 50 mg	Boehringer Ingelheim
BI 19	Persantine 75 mg	Boehringer Ingelheim
BI 20	Serentil 10 mg	Boehringer Ingelheim
BI 21	Serentil 25 mg	Boehringer Ingelheim
BI 22	Serentil 50 mg	Boehringer Ingelheim
BI 23	Serentil 100 mg	Boehringer Ingelheim
BI 25	Mesoridazine 25 mg	Boehringer
BI 28	Torecan 10 mg	Boehringer Ingelheim
BI 48	Respbid 250 mg	Boehringer Ingelheim

Imprint	Ingredient/Brand Name	Manufacturer
BI 49	Respbid 500 mg	Boehringer Ingelheim
BI 50	Mesoridazine 50 mg	Boehringer
BI 62	CONTROLLED - SEE PAGE 208	
BI 64	CONTROLLED - SEE PAGE 220	
BI 66 Mexitil 150mg	Mexitil 150 mg	Boehringer Ingelheim
BI 67 Mexitil 200mg	Mexitil 200 mg	Boehringer Ingelheim
BI 68 Mexitil 250mg	Mexitil 250 mg	Boehringer Ingelheim
BI 72	Alupent 20 mg	Boehringer Ingelheim
BI 74	Alupent 10 mg	Boehringer Ingelheim
BI 76	Thalitone 25 mg	Boehringer Ingelheim
BI 77	Chlorthalidone 15 mg	Boehringer
BI 100	Mesoridazine 100 mg	Boehringer
Big Red	Caffeine	Unknown
biocraft 01	Amoxicillin 250 mg	Biocraft Labs
biocraft/02	Dicloxacillin Sodium 250 mg	Biocraft Labs
biocraft/03	Amoxicillin 500 mg	Biocraft Labs
biocraft 04	Dicloxacillin Sodium 500 mg	Biocraft Labs
biocraft/05	Ampicillin 250 mg	Biocraft Labs
biocraft/06	Ampicillin 500 mg	Biocraft Labs
biocraft 12	Oxacillin 250 mg	Biocraft Labs
biocraft 14	Oxacillin 500 mg	Biocraft Labs
BIOCRAFT 16	Penicillin V Potassium250 mg	Biocraft Labs
Biocraft 20	Imipramine 25 mg	Biocraft Labs
Biocraft 21	Imipramine 50 mg	Biocraft Labs
Biocraft 22	Amitriptyline 10 mg	Biocraft Labs
Biocraft 23	Amitriptyline 25 mg	Biocraft Labs
Biocraft 24	Amitriptyline 50 mg	Biocraft Labs
Biocraft 25	Amitriptyline 75 mg	Biocraft Labs
Biocraft 26	Amitriptyline 100 mg	Biocraft Labs
biocraft 28	Cloxacillin Sodium 250 mg	Biocraft Labs
biocraft 30	Cloxacillin Sodium 500 mg	Biocraft Labs
Biocraft 32	Sulfamethoxazole 400 mg, Trimethoprim 80 mg	Biocraft Labs
biocraft 33	Sulfamethoxazole 800 mg, Trimethoprim 160 mg	Biocraft Labs
biocraft 34	Trimethoprim 100 mg	Biocraft Labs
Biocraft 38	Chloroquine 250 mg	Biocraft Labs
biocraft 40	Disopyramide Phosphate 100 mg	Biocraft Labs
biocraft 41	Disopyramide Phosphate 150 mg	Biocraft Labs
Biocraft 49	Penicillin V Potassium 500 mg	Biocraft Labs
Biocraft 71	Clonidine 0.1 mg	Biocraft Labs
Biocraft 72	Clonidine 0.2 mg	Biocraft Labs
Biocraft 73	Clonidine 0.3 mg	Biocraft Labs
Biocraft 93	Metoclopramide 10 mg	Biocraft Labs
BIOCRAFT 94	Cyclacillin 250 mg	Biocraft Labs
BIOCRAFT 95	Cyclacillin 500 mg	Biocraft Labs
biocraft 112	Cephradine 250 mg	Biocraft Labs
biocraft 113	Cephradine 500 mg	Biocraft Labs
Biocraft 114	Cefadroxil 500 mg	Biocraft Labs
biocraft 115	Cephalexin 250 mg	Biocraft Labs
biocraft 117	Cephalexin 500 mg	Biocraft Labs
Biocraft 134	Minocycline 50 mg	Biocraft Labs
Biocraft 135	Minocycline 100 mg	Biocraft Labs
biocraft 148	Clindamycin HCL 75 mg	Biocraft Labs
biocraft 149	Clindamycin HCL 150 mg	Biocraft Labs
biocraft 163	Cinoxacin 250 mg	Biocraft Labs
biocraft 164	Cinoxacin 500 mg	Biocraft Labs
Biocraft 185	Ketoprofen 25 mg	Biocraft Labs

Imprint	Ingredient/Brand Name	Manufacturer
Biocraft 187	Ketoprofen 50 mg	Biocraft Labs
Biocraft 192	Ketoprofen 75 mg	Biocraft Labs
BIPHET 12-1/2	CONTROLLED - SEE PAGE 224	
BIPHET 20	CONTROLLED - SEE PAGE 218	
BL 01	Amoxicillin	Biocraft Labs
BL 02	Dicloxacillin Sodium 250 mg	Biocraft Labs
BL 03	Amoxicillin 500 mg	Biocraft Labs
BL04	Dicloxacillin Sodium 500 mg	Biocraft Labs
BL 05	Ampicillin 250 mg	Biocraft Labs
BL 06	Ampicillin 500 mg	Biocraft Labs
BL/07	Penicillin G Potassium 200,000 units	Biocraft Labs
BL/09	Penicillin G Potassium 250,000 units	Biocraft Labs
BL/10	Penicillin G Potassium 400,000 units	Biocraft Labs
BL 12	Oxacillin 250 mg	Biocraft Labs
BL 14	Oxacillin 500 mg	Biocraft Labs
BL/15	Penicillin V Potassium 250 mg	Biocraft Labs
BL 16	Penicillin V 250 mg	Biocraft Labs
BL/17	Penicillin V Potassium 500 mg	Biocraft Labs
BL/18	Neomycin Sulfate 500 mg	Biocraft Labs
BL/19	Imipramine 10 mg	Biocraft Labs
BL 20	Pallace 20 mg	Bristol-Myers
BL/20	Imipramine 25 mg	Biocraft Labs
BL/21	Imipramine 50 mg	Biocraft Labs
BL/22	Amitriptyline 10 mg	Biocraft Labs
BL/23	Amitriptyline 25 mg	Biocraft Labs
BL/24	Amitriptyline 50 mg	Biocraft Labs
BL 25	Videx 25 mg	Bristol-Myers
BL/25	Amitriptyline 75 mg	Biocraft Labs
BL/26	Amitriptyline 100 mg	Biocraft Labs
BL 28	Cloxacillin 250 mg	Biocraft Labs
BL 30	Cloxacillin 500 mg	Biocraft Labs
BL/32	Sulfamethoxazole 400 mg, Trimethoprim 80 mg	Biocraft Labs
BL 33	Sulfamethoxazole 800 mg, Trimethoprim 160 mg	Biocraft Labs
BL 34	Trimethoprim 100 mg	Biocraft Labs
BL/35	Trimethoprim 200 mg	Biocraft Labs
BL 38	Chloroquine 250 mg	Biocraft Labs
BL 40	Pallace 40 mg	Bristol-Myers
BL 40	Disopyramide 100 mg	Biocraft Labs
BL 41	Disopyramide 150 mg	Biocraft Labs
BL/42	Thioridazine 10 mg	Biocraft Labs
BL/46	Thioridazine 100 mg	Biocraft Labs
BL 49	Penicillin V 500 mg	Biocraft Labs
BL 50	Videx 50 mg	Bristol-Myers
BL 52	Amiloride 5 mg, Hydrochlorothiazide 50 mg	Biocraft Labs
BL/53	Furosemide 12.5 mg	Biocraft Labs
BL/54	Furosemide 50 mg	Biocraft Labs
BL 71	Clonidine 0.1 mg	Biocraft Labs
BL 72	Clonidine 0.2 mg	Biocraft Labs
BL 73	Clonidine 0.3 mg	Biocraft Labs
BL 91	Salutensin 50 mg/0.125 mg	Bristol Labs
BL/92	Metoclopramide 5 mg	Biocraft Labs
BL 92	Saulron 50 mg	Bristol Labs
BL 93	Salutensin-Demi 10 mg	Bristol Labs
BL/93	Metoclopramide 10 mg	Biocraft Labs
BL 100	Videx 100 mg	Bristol-Myers
BL/130	Albuterol 2 mg	Biocraft Labs

Imprint	Ingredient/Brand Name	Manufacturer
BL/131	Albuterol 4 mg	Biocraft Labs
BL/132	Metaproterenol 10 mg	Biocraft Labs
BL/133	Metaproterenol 20 mg	Biocraft Labs
BL 136	Cephalexin 250 mg	Biocraft Labs
BL 137	Cephalexin 500 mg	Biocraft Labs
BL/141	Baclofen 10 mg	Biocraft Labs
BL/142	Baclofen 20 mg	Biocraft Labs
BL 150	Videx 150 mg	Bristol-Myers
BL/170	Amoxicillin Veterinary 50 mg	Biocraft Labs
BL/171	Amoxicillin Veterinary 100 mg	Biocraft Labs
BL/172	Amoxicillin Veterinary 200 mg	Biocraft Labs
BL/173	Amoxicillin Veterinary 400 mg	Biocraft Labs
BL 207	Corgard 40 mg	Bristol-Myers
BL 208	Corgard 120 mg	Bristol-Myers
BL/222	Amoxicillin 250 mg	Biocraft Labs
BL 232	Corgard 20 mg	Bristol-Myers
BL 241	Corgard 80 mg	Bristol-Myers
BL 246	Corgard 160 mg	Bristol-Myers
BL 283	Corzide 40 mg/5 mg	Bristol-Myers
BL 284	Corzide 80 mg/5 mg	Bristol-Myers
BL 512	Quibron-T 300 mg	Bristol Labs
BL 519	Quibron-T/SR 300 mg	Bristol Labs
Blaine	Magnesium Oxide 400 mg	Blaine Co.
BLAINE 0054	Magnesium Oxide 140 mg	Blaine Co.
BL B3	CONTROLLED - No Photo - Codeine 30 mg, Acetaminophen - DEA Schedule III	Bristol-Myers
BL C1	Ultracef 1000 mg	Bristol Labs
BL E1	Bristamycin 250 mg	Bristol-Myers
BL L1	Lysodren 500 mg	Bristol-Myers
BL N1	Naldecon 20 mg/5 mg/7.5 mg/2.5 mg	Bristol Labs
BL N2	Naldegesic 15 mg/325 mg	Bristol Labs
BL S1	Salutensin 50 mg/0.125 mg	Bristol Labs
BL S2	Saluron 50 mg	Bristol Labs
BL S3	Hydroflumethiazide 25 mg, Reserpine 125 mg	Bristol Labs
BL V1	Betapen-VK 250 mg	Bristol Labs
BL V2	Betapen-VK 500 mg	Bristol Labs
BM [logo]	Caffeine	Unknown
BMP 112	Dasin 3 mg/130 mg/100 mg/15 mg/8 mg/0.13 mg	Beecham Labs
BMP 121	Livitamin	Beecham Labs
BMP 122	Livitamin with Intrinsic Factor	Beecham Labs
BMP 123	Livitamin	Beecham Labs
BMP 125	Menest 0.3 mg	Beecham Labs
BMP 126	Menest 0.625 mg	Beecham Labs
BMP 127	Menest 1.25 mg	Beecham Labs
BMP 128	Menest 2.5 mg	Beecham Labs
BMP 132	Quinidine Sulfate	Beecham Labs
BMP 135	Semets 3 mg	Beecham Labs
BMP 140	Totacillin 250 mg	Beecham Labs
BMP 141	Totacillin 500 mg	Beecham Labs
BMP 143	Bactocill 250 mg	Beecham Labs
BMP 144	Bactocill 500 mg	Beecham Labs
BMP 145	Daricon 10 mg	Beecham Labs
BMP 148	Amoxil 250 mg	Beecham Labs
BMP 149	Amoxil 500 mg	Beecham Labs
BMP 156	Tigan 100 mg	Beecham Labs
BMP 157	Tigan 250 mg	Beecham Labs

Imprint	Ingredient/Brand Name	Manufacturer
BMP 165	Dycill 250 mg	Beecham Labs
BMP 166	Dycill 500 mg	Beecham Labs
BMP 169	Cloxapen 250 mg	Beecham Labs
BMP 170	Cloxapen 500 mg	Beecham Labs
BMP 182 NUCOFED	CONTROLLED - SEE PAGE 220	
BMP 185	Beepen-VK 250 mg	Beecham Labs
BMP 186	Beepen-VK 500 mg	Beecham Labs
BMP 188	CONTROLLED - SEE PAGE 204	
BMP 192	Metoclopramide 10 mg	Beecham Labs
BMP 207	CONTROLLED - SEE PAGE 198	
BMS 0814	Doxycycline 100 mg	Bristol-Myers
BMS 5040	Atenolol 50 mg	Bristol-Myers
BMS 5240	Atenolol 100 mg	Bristol-Myers
BMS 5250	Diltiazem 30 mg	Bristol-Myers
BMS 5550	Diltiazem 60 mg	Bristol-Myers
BMS 5770	Diltiazem 90 mg	Bristol-Myers
BMS 5850	Diltiazem 120 mg	Bristol-Myers
BMS 7720	Cefzil 250 mg	Bristol-Myers
BMS 7721	Cefzil 500 mg	Bristol-Myers
BNP 247	Caffeine, Ephedrine, Phenylpropanolamine	Unknown
BNR 157	Dexafed 150 mg/25 mg/50 mg	Russ Pharm
bock 460	Pseudoephedrine 60 mg, Guaifenesin 400 mg	Bock Pharm
BOCK BOCK	Poly-Histine-D 50 mg/16 mg/16 mg/16 mg	Bock Pharm
BOCK BOCK	Poly-Histine-D 25 mg/8 mg/8 mg/8 mg	Bock Pharm
bock/HS 33	Hemaspan 110 mg, 200 mg, 20 mg	Bock Pharm
bock PN 90	Vitamins, Minerals	Bock Pharm
bock/Z LA	Zephrex-LA 120 mg/600 mg	Bock Pharm
Bolar 0084	Phenytoin 100 mg	Bolar Pharm
BOLAR 227	Triamterene 50 mg, Hydrochlorothiazide 25 mg	Bolar Pharm
Bolar 277	Triamterene 50 mg, Hydrochlorothiazide 25 mg	Bolar Pharm
BOLAR KV KCl-10	Potassium Chloride 750 mg	Bolar Pharm
BOLAR NTS 5	Nitroglycerin Patch 5 mg	Bolar Pharm
BOLAR NTS15	Nitroglycerin Patch 15 mg	Bolar Pharm
BOLT	Caffeine 200 mg	D & E Pharm.
BONINE/201	Bonine 25 mg	Pfizer Labs
BOOTS 0051	Lopurin 100 mg	Boots Labs
BOOTS 0052	Lopurin 300 mg	Boots Labs
Boots 31 Ru-Tus 11 31	Ru-Tus II 75 mg/12 mg	Cord Labs
BOOTS [logo] 90	Guaifenesin 600 mg, Pseudoephedrine 120 mg	Boots Labs
bp 0001	Thioridazine 10 mg	Bolar Pharm
bp 0003	Brompheniramine 12 mg	Bolar Pharm
bp 0004	Primidone 250 mg	Bolar Pharm
bp 0005	Methocarbamol 500 mg	Bolar Pharm
bp 0006	Methocarbamol 750 mg	Bolar Pharm
bp 0007	Trihexyphenidyl 2 mg	Bolar Pharm
bp 0010	Dipyridamole 25 mg	Bolar Pharm
bp 0011	Furosemide 12.5 mg	Bolar Pharm
bp 0013	Chlorothiazide 500 mg	Bolar Pharm
bp 0016	Cyclandelate 200 mg	Bolar Pharm
bp 0017	Pentaerythritol Tetranitrate 80 mg	Bolar Pharm
bp 0020	Pseudoephedrine 60 mg	Bolar Pharm
bp 0024	Trihexphenidyl 5 mg	Bolar Pharm
bp 0026	Isosorbide Dinitrate 40 mg	Bolar Pharm
bp 0027	Theophylline, Guaifenesin	Bolar Pharm
bp 0028	Imipramine 20 mg	Bolar Pharm
bp 0029	Tripolidine, Pseudoephedrine	Bolar Pharm

Imprint	Ingredient/Brand Name	Manufacturer
bp 0031	Thioridazine 15 mg	Bolar Pharm
bp 0032	Dexamethasone 0.75 mg	Bolar Pharm
bp 0033	Chlorthalidone 25 mg	Bolar Pharm
bp 0034	Chlorthalidone 50 mg	Bolar Pharm
bp 0035	Chlorthalidone 100 mg	Bolar Pharm
bp 0036	Chlorothiazide 250 mg	Bolar Pharm
bp 0037	Orphenadrine 100 mg	Bolar Pharm
bp 0039	Imipramine 10 mg	Bolar Pharm
bp 0040	Imipramine 50 mg	Bolar Pharm
bp 0041	Ergoloid Mesylates 1 mg	Bolar Pharm
bp 0042	Acetazolamide 250 mg	Bolar Pharm
bp 0044	Warfarin 2.5 mg	Bolar Pharm
bp 0045	Warfarin 5 mg	Bolar Pharm
bp 0046	Warfarin 7.5 mg	Bolar Pharm
bp 0047	Warfarin 10 mg	Bolar Pharm
bp 0049	Isosorbide Dinitrate 20 mg	Bolar Pharm
bp 0050	Warfarin 2 mg	Bolar Pharm
bp 0052	Ergoloid Mesylates 0.5 mg	Bolar Pharm
bp 0055	Cyclandelate 400 mg	Bolar Pharm
bp 0056	Reserpine 0.125 mg, Chlorothiazide 250 mg	Bolar Pharm
bp 0058	Hydrochlorothiazide 100 mg	Bolar Pharm
bp 0059	Sulfasalazine 500 mg	Bolar Pharm
bp 0060	Liothyronine 0.025 mg	Bolar Pharm
bp 0062	Methyclothiazide 2.5 mg	Bolar Pharm
bp 0063	Methyclothiazide 5 mg	Bolar Pharm
bp 0064	Hydralazine 100 mg, Hydrochlorothiazide 50 mg	Bolar Pharm
bp 0065	Hydralazine 25 mg, Hydrochlorothiazide 25 mg	Bolar Pharm
bp 0066	Hydralazine 50 mg, Hydrochlorothiazide 50 mg	Bolar Pharm
bp 0069	Ergoloid Mesylates 1 mg	Bolar Pharm
bp 0072	Hydroflumethiazide 50 mg	Bolar Pharm
bp 0073	Bethanechol 5 mg	Bolar Pharm
bp 0074	Bethanechol 10 mg	Bolar Pharm
bp 0075	Bethanechol 25 mg	Bolar Pharm
bp 0076	Oxtriphylline 100 mg	Bolar Pharm
bp 0077	Oxtriphylline 200 mg	Bolar Pharm
bp 0078	Cyproheptadine 4 mg	Bolar Pharm
bp 0082	Chlormezanone 200 mg	Bolar Pharm
bp 0083	Hydralazine 25 mg, Hydrochlorothiazide 15 mg	Bolar Pharm
bp 0084	Phenytoin 100 mg	Bolar Pharm
bp 0087	Sulfamethoxazole 500 mg	Bolar Pharm
bp 0088	Primidone 250 mg	Bolar Pharm
bp 0090	Isosorbide Dinitrate 5 mg	Bolar Pharm
bp 0091	Chlorzoxazone 250 mg, Acetaminophen 300 mg	Bolar Pharm
bp 0093	Prochlorperazine 10 mg	Bolar Pharm
bp 0094	Carisoprodol 350 mg	Bolar Pharm
bp 0096	Anisotropine 50 mg	Bolar Pharm
bp 0098	Sulfamethoxazole 1000 mg	Bolar Pharm
bp 095	Carisoprodol 200 mg, Aspirin 325 mg	Bolar Pharm
bp 0100	Hydroxyzine 25 mg	Bolar Pharm
bp 0101	Hydroxyzine 50 mg	Bolar Pharm
bp 0103	Hydroxyzine 10 mg	Bolar Pharm
bp 0104	Hydroxyzine 25 mg	Bolar Pharm
bp 0105	Hydroxyzine 50 mg	Bolar Pharm
bp 0106	Hydroxyzine 100 mg	Bolar Pharm
bp 0110	Isosorbide Dinitrate 2.5 mg	Bolar Pharm
bp 0111	Prochlorperazine 5 mg	Bolar Pharm

Imprint	Ingredient/Brand Name	Manufacturer
bp 0112	Prochlorperazine 25 mg	Bolar Pharm
bp 0118	Thioridazine 25 mg	Bolar Pharm
bp 0119	Thioridazine 50 mg	Bolar Pharm
bp 0120	Thioridazine 100 mg	Bolar Pharm
bp 0121	Thioridazine 150 mg	Bolar Pharm
bp 0122	Thioridazine 200 mg	Bolar Pharm
bp 0127	Reserpine 0.125 mg, Hydroflumethiazide 25 mg	Bolar Pharm
bp 0128	Reserpine 0.125 mg, Hydroflumethiazide 50 mg	Bolar Pharm
bp 0129	Spironolactone 25 mg, Hydrochlorothiazide 25 mg	Bolar Pharm
bp 0131	Sulfasalazine 500 mg	Bolar Pharm
bp 0132	Reserpine 0.125 mg, Chlorothiazide 500 mg	Bolar Pharm
bp 0133	Allopurinol 100 mg	Bolar Pharm
bp 0134	Allopurinol 300 mg	Bolar Pharm
bp 0135	Guanethidine 10 mg	Bolar Pharm
bp 0136	Guanethidine 25 mg	Bolar Pharm
bp 0144	Carisoprodol 200 mg, Aspirin 325 mg	Bolar Pharm
bp 0152	Procainamide 250 mg	Bolar Pharm
bp 0153	Procainamide 500 mg	Bolar Pharm
bp 0154	Procainamide 750 mg	Bolar Pharm
bp 0157	Deserpidine 0.25 mg, Methyclothiazide 5 mg	Bolar Pharm
bp 0158	Deserpidine 0.25 mg, Methyclothiazide 5 mg	Bolar Pharm
bp 0167	Chlorpropamide 100 mg	Bolar Pharm
bp 0168	Chlorpropamide 250 mg	Bolar Pharm
bp 0187	Procainamide 1000 mg	Bolar Pharm
bp 0211	Maprotiline 25 mg	Bolar Pharm
bp 0212	Maprotiline 50 mg	Bolar Pharm
bp 0213	Maprotiline 75 mg	Bolar Pharm
bp/1	Thioridazine 10 mg	Bolar Pharm
bp 6	Methocarbamol 750 mg	Bolar Pharm
bp 13	Chlorthiazide 500 mg	Bolar Pharm
bp 22	Decongestabs 10 mg/40 mg/15 mg /5 mg	Bolar Pharm
bp 28	Imipramine 25 mg	Bolar Pharm
bp/31	Thioridazine 15 mg	Bolar Pharm
bp 32	Dexamethasone 0.75 mg	Bolar Pharm
bp 33	Chlorthalidone 25 mg	Bolar Pharm
bp 34	Chlorthalidone 50 mg	Bolar Pharm
bp 35	Chlorthalidone 100 mg	Bolar Pharm
bp 39	Imipramine 10 mg	Bolar Pharm
bp 40	Imipramine 50 mg	Bolar Pharm
bp 41	Ergoloid Mesylates 1 mg	Bolar Pharm
bp 42	Acetazolamide 250 mg	Bolar Pharm
bp 44	Warfarin Sodium 2.5 mg	Bolar Pharm
bp 46	Warfarin Sodium 7.5 mg	Bolar Pharm
bp 47	Warfarin Sodium 10 mg	Bolar Pharm
bp 50	Warfarin Sodium 2 mg	Bolar Pharm
bp 56	Chlothiazide 250 mg, Reserpine 0.125 mg	Bolar Pharm
bp 60	Liothyronine Sodium 25 mcg	Bolar Pharm
bp 61	Sodium Liothyronine 0.050 mg	Bolar Pharm
bp 62	Methyclothiazide 2.5 mg	Bolar Pharm
bp 63	Methyclothiazide 5 mg	Bolar Pharm
bp 64	Hydralazine 100 mg, Hydrochlorthiazide 50 mg	Bolar Pharm
bp 72	Hydroflumethiazide 50 mg	Bolar Pharm
bp 76	Oxtriphylline 100 mg	Bolar Pharm
bp 77	Oxtriphylline 200 mg	Bolar Pharm
bp 78	Cyproheptadine 4 mg	Bolar Pharm
bp 79	Clonidine 0.1 mg	Bolar Pharm

Imprint	Ingredient/Brand Name	Manufacturer
bp 80	Clonidine 0.2 mg	Bolar Pharm
bp 81	Clonidine 0.3 mg	Bolar Pharm
bp 87	Sulfamethoxazole 500 mg	Bolar Pharm
bp/93	Prochlorperazine 10 mg	Bolar Pharm
bp 100	Hydroxyzine Pamoate 25 mg	Bolar Pharm
bp 101	Hydroxyzine Pamoate 50 mg	Bolar Pharm
bp 102	Hydroxyzine 100 mg	Bolar Pharm
bp/111	Prochlorperazine 5 mg	Bolar Pharm
bp/112	Prochlorperazine 25 mg	Bolar Pharm
bp 117	Trifluoperazine 5 mg	Bolar Pharm
bp/118	Thioridazine 25 mg	Bolar Pharm
bp/119	Thioridazine 50 mg	Bolar Pharm
bp/120	Thioridazine 100 mg	Bolar Pharm
bp/121	Thioridazine 150 mg	Bolar Pharm
bp/122	Thioridazine 200 mg	Bolar Pharm
bp 123	Propranolol 10 mg	Bolar Pharm
bp 124	Propranolol 20 mg	Bolar Pharm
bp 125	Propranolol 40 mg	Bolar Pharm
bp 126	Propranolol 80 mg	Bolar Pharm
bp 132	Chlorothiazide 500 mg, Reserpine 0.125 mg	Bolar Pharm
bp 140	Chlorthalidone 25 mg	Bolar Pharm
bp 141	Chlorthalidone 50 mg	Bolar Pharm
bp 143	Trimethobenzamide 250 mg	Bolar Pharm
bp 145	Indomethacin 25 mg	Bolar Pharm
bp 146	Indomethacin 50 mg	Bolar Pharm
bp 148	Oxyphenbutazone 100 mg	Bolar Pharm
bp 151	Trifluoperazine 10 mg	Bolar Pharm
bp/152	Procainamide 250 mg	Bolar Pharm
bp/153	Procainamide 500 mg	Bolar Pharm
bp/154	Procainamide 750 mg	Bolar Pharm
bp 163	Fluphenazine 1 mg	Bolar Pharm
bp 164	Fluphenazine 2.5 mg	Bolar Pharm
bp 165	Fluphenazine 5 mg	Bolar Pharm
bp 166	Fluphenazine 10 mg	Bolar Pharm
bp 168	Chlorpropamide 250 mg	Bolar Pharm
bp 171	Trifluoperazine 1 mg	Bolar Pharm
bp 172	Trifluoperazine 2 mg	Bolar Pharm
bp 173	Benztropine Mesylate 0.5 mg	Bolar Pharm
bp 174	Benztropine Mesylate 1 mg	Bolar Pharm
bp 175	Benztropine Mesylate 2 mg	Bolar Pharm
bp 187	Procainamide 1000 mg	Bolar Pharm
bp 211	Maprotiline 25 mg	Bolar Pharm
bp 212	Maprotiline 50 mg	Bolar Pharm
bp 213	Maprotiline 75 mg	Bolar Pharm
bp 227	Triamterene 50 mg, Hydrochlorothiazide 25 mg	Bolar Pharm
BP 956	CONTROLLED - SEE PAGE 199	
BP 958	CONTROLLED - SEE PAGE 212	
BP 996	CONTROLLED - SEE PAGE 204	
bp 1007	Trazodone 50 mg	Bolar Pharm
bp 1008	Trazodone 100 mg	Bolar Pharm
bp 1015	Nitrofurantoin 50 mg	Bolar Pharm
bp 1016	Nitrofurantoin 100 mg	Bolar Pharm
bp 1027	Amantadine 100 mg	Bolar Pharm
bp 2005	Disopyramide 100 mg	Bolar Pharm
bp 2006	Disopyramide 150 mg	Bolar Pharm
bp 2013	Chlorpheniramine 4 mg	Bolar Pharm

Imprint	Ingredient/Brand Name	Manufacturer
bp 2014	Methyldopa 125 mg	Bolar Pharm
bp 2015	Methyldopa 250 mg	Bolar Pharm
bp 2016	Methyldopa 500 mg	Bolar Pharm
bp 2017	Brompheniramine 4 mg	Bolar Pharm
bp 2023	Dicyclomine 10 mg	Bolar Pharm
bp 2024	Meclpfenamate 50 mg	Bolar Pharm
bp 2025	Meclofenamate 100 mg	Bolar Pharm
bp 2026	Dicyclomine 20 mg	Bolar Pharm
bp 2027	Metoclopramide 10 mg	Bolar Pharm
bp 2036	Methyldopa 250 mg, Hydrochlorothiazide 15 mg	Bolar Pharm
bp 2037	Methyldopa 250 mg, Hydrochlorothiazide 25 mg	Bolar Pharm
bp 2038	Methyldopa 500 mg, Hydrochlorothiazide 30 mg	Bolar Pharm
bp 2039	Methyldopa 500 mg, Hydrochlorothiazide 50 mg	Bolar Pharm
bp 2042	Verapamil 80 mg	Bolar Pharm
bp 2043	Verapamil 120 mg	Bolar Pharm
bp 2047	Reserpine 0.125 mg, Hydrochlorothiazide 25 mg	Bolar Pharm
bp 2048	Reserpine 0.125 mg, Hydrochlorothiazide 50 mg	Bolar Pharm
bp 2049	Hydrochlorothiazide, Reserpine, Hydralazine	Bolar Pharm
bp 2051	Isosorbide Dinitrate 5 mg	Bolar Pharm
bp 2052	Isosorbide Dinitrate 10 mg	Bolar Pharm
bp 2053	Perphenazine 2 mg, Amitriptyline 25 mg	Bolar Pharm
bp 2054	Perphenazine 4 mg, Amitriptyline 25 mg	Bolar Pharm
bp 2055	Methocarbamol 500 mg	Bolar Pharm
bp 2055	Perphenazine 2 mg, Amitriptyline 50 mg	Bolar Pharm
bp 2056	Perphenazine 2 mg, Amitriptyline 10 mg	Bolar Pharm
bp 2057	Perphenazine 4 mg, Amitriptyline 10 mg	Bolar Pharm
bp 2059	Nitrofurantoin 100 mg	Bolar Pharm
bp 2060	Propranolol 60 mg	Bolar Pharm
bp 2061	Nitrofurantoin 100 mg	Bolar Pharm
bp 2064	Pentaerythritol Tetranitrate 10 mg	Bolar Pharm
bp 2066	Lithium Carbonate 300 mg	Bolar Pharm
bp 2067	Pentaerythritol Tetranitrate 20 mg	Bolar Pharm
bp 2068	Tolazamide 100 mg	Bolar Pharm
bp 2069	Tolazamide 250 mg	Bolar Pharm
bp 2070	Tolazamide 500 mg	Bolar Pharm
bp 2074	Probenecid 500 mg, Colchicine 0.5 mg	Bolar Pharm
bp 2075	Nitrofurantoin 50 mg	Bolar Pharm
bp 2076	Procainamide 250 mg	Bolar Pharm
bp 2078	Procainamide 500 mg	Bolar Pharm
bp 2079	Propantheline 15 mg	Bolar Pharm
bp 2080	Nitrofurantoin 100 mg	Bolar Pharm
bp 2088	Primidone 250 mg	Bolar Pharm
bp 2092	Reserpine 0.1 mg, Trichlormethiazide 4 mg	Bolar Pharm
bp 2093	Hydrochlorothiazide 25 mg	Bolar Pharm
bp 2094	Hydrochlorothiazide	Bolar Pharm
bp 2118	Disopyramide Phosphate 100 mg	Bolar Pharm
bp 2119	Disopyramide Phosphate 150 mg	Bolar Pharm
bp 2126	Potassium Chloride 750 mg	Bolar Pharm
bp 2130	Tripelennamine 50 mg	Bolar Pharm
bp 2135	Propoxyphene 65 mg	Bolar Pharm
bp 2150	Isoniazid 100 mg	Bolar Pharm
bp 2155	Isoniazid 300 mg	Bolar Pharm
bp 2200	Folic Acid 1 mg	Bolar Pharm
bp 3000	Quinidine 324 mg	Bolar Pharm
bp 3020	Trichlormethiazide 4 mg	Bolar Pharm
bp 4111	Pyrilamine 25 mg	Bolar Pharm

Imprint	Ingredient/Brand Name	Manufacturer
bp 4112	Brompheniramine 8 mg	Bolar Pharm
bp 5000	Spironolactone 25 mg	Bolar Pharm
bp 5010	Bethanechol 50 mg	Bolar Pharm
bp 9000	Quinine 260 mg	Bolar Pharm
BPM 189	Amoxicillin 125 mg, Clavulanate Potassium 31.25 mg	Beecham
BPM 190	Amoxicillin 250 mg, Clavulanate Potassium 62.5 mg	Beecham
BRA200	Calcium Acetate 667 mg	Braintree Labs
BREON 100	Bronkodyl 100 mg	Breon Labs
BREON 200	Bronkodyl 200 mg	Breon Labs
BREON/T 100	Trancopal 100 mg	Winthrop-Breon
BREON/T 200	Trancopal 200 mg	Winthrop-Breon
BRICANYL 2 1/2	Bricanyl 2.5 mg	Merrell Dow
BRICANYL 5	Bricanyl 5 mg	Merrell Dow
BRISTOL 515	Quibron 300 mg	Bristol Labs
BRISTOL 516	Quibron150 mg	Bristol Labs
BRISTOL 518	Quibron Plus 150 mg	Bristol-Myers
BRISTOL 732 ENKAID 25mg	Enkaid 25 mg	Bristol Labs
BRISTOL 734 ENKAID 35mg	Enkaid 35 mg	Bristol Labs
BRISTOL 735 ENKAID 50mg	Enkaid 50 mg	Bristol Labs
BRISTOL 3030	CeeNU 10 mg	Bristol-Myers Prod
BRISTOL 3031	CeeNU 40 mg	Bristol-Myers Prod
BRISTOL 3032	CeeNU 100 mg	Bristol-Myers Prod
BRISTOL 3091	VePesid 50 mg	Bristol-Myers Prod
BRISTOL 3506	Kantrex 500 mg	Bristol-Myers Prod
BRISTOL 7271	Ultracef 500 mg	Bristol Labs
BRISTOL 7278	Polymox 250 mg	Bristol Labs
BRISTOL 7279	Polymox 500 mg	Bristol Labs
BRISTOL 7375	Cefanex 250 mg	Bristol-Myers
BRISTOL 7376	Cefanex 500 mg	Bristol-Myers
BRISTOL 7496	Tegopen 500 mg	Bristol Labs
BRISTOL 7658	Dynapen 500 mg	Bristol Labs
BRISTOL 7892	Dynapen 125 mg	Bristol Labs
BRISTOL 7893	Dynapen 250 mg	Bristol Labs
BRISTOL 7935	Tegopen 250 mg	Bristol Labs
BRISTOL 7977	Prostaphlin 250 mg	Bristol Labs
BRISTOL 7982	Prostaphlin 500 mg	Bristol Labs
BRISTOL 7992	Polycillin 250 mg	Bristol Labs
BRISTOL 7993	Polycillin 500 mg	Bristol Labs
BRONTEX	CONTROLLED - SEE PAGE 226	
BT 10-845	Caffeine, Ephedrine, Phenylpropanolamine	Unknown
BT 10-984	Caffeine, Ephedrine, Phenylpropanolamine	Unknown
BT 18-845	Caffeine, Ephedrine, Phenylpropanolamine	Unknown
BT 18-894	Caffeine, Ephedrine, Phenylpropanolamine	Unknown
BT 72	Caffeine, Ephedrine, Phenylpropanolamine	Unknown
BTP L14	Caffeine, Ephedrine, Phenylpropanolamine	Unknown
BTP L17	Caffeine, Ephedrine, Phenylpropanolamine	Unknown
BTP L19	Caffeine, Ephedrine, Phenylpropanolamine	Unknown
BUCET	Bucet 50 mg/650 mg	UAD Labs
Bufferin Nite Time	Bufferin AF Nite Time	Bristol-Myers
BUMEX 0.5/ROCHE	Bumex 0.5 mg	Roche Labs
BUMEX 1/ROCHE	Bumex 1 mg	Roche Labs
BUMEX 2/ROCHE	Bumex 2 mg	Roche Labs
BUTAZOLIDIN 100MG GEIGY 44	Butazolidin 100 mg	Geigy Pharm
BWP 147	Caffeine, Ephedrine, Phenylpropanolamine	Unknown
C	Propagest	Carnrick Labs
C	Cod Liver Oil	Schering Corp

Imprint	Ingredient/Brand Name	Manufacturer
C	Coorectol Laxative Tablets	Schering Corp
C	Cascara Sagrada Extract 50 mg, Phenolphthalein 32.4 mg	Mentholatum
C[in flask]	Quinaglute 324 mg	Berlex Labs
C 1	Rauwolfia Serpentine 50 mg, Bendroflumethiazide 4 mg	Econolab
C 1	Pseudoephedrine 60 mg, Triprolidine 2.5 mg	K.C. Pharm
C-2	Docusate Sodium 50 mg	Chase
C2C	Lanoxicaps 0.2 mg	Burroughs Wellcome
C5	CONTROLLED - SEE PAGE 220	
C 7	Chlorthalidone 25 mg	Lederle Labs
C10	CONTROLLED - SEE PAGE 223	
C 15	Chlorthalidone 50 mg	Lederle Labs
C25	CONTROLLED - SEE PAGE 220	
C-26	Docusate Calcium 240 mg	Chase
C-27	Docusate Sodium 100 mg	Chase
C 29	Docusate Sodium 250 mg	Chase
C-35	Docusate Calcium 60 mg, Phenolphthalein 65 mg	Chase
C 35/15	Leucovorin 15 mg	Lederle Labs
C 37	Chlorpropamide 100 mg	Lederle Labs
C 38	Chlorpropamide 250 mg	Lederle Labs
C-39	Docusate Sodium 100 mg, Casantranol 30 mg	Chase
C 64	Cephalexin 250 mg	Lederle Labs
C 65	Cephalexin 500 mg	Lederle Labs
C 67/LL	Chlordiazepoxide 5 mg, Amitriptyline 12.5 mg	Lederle Labs
C 68/LL	Chlordiazepoxide 10 mg, Amitriptyline 25 mg	Lederle Labs
C 69/LL	CONTROLLED - SEE PAGE 210	
C 86 62	Skelaxin 400 mg	Carnrick Labs
C71	Atenolol 100 mg, Chlorthalidone 25 mg	IPR
C 71/LL	CONTROLLED - SEE PAGE 191	
C-85	Nighttime Cold Medicine	Hall Labs
C90	Atenolol 100 mg	IPR
C 111	Clofibrate 500 mg	Pharm Basics
C-122	Amantadine 100 mg	Parm Basics
C 127	Caffeine, Ephedrine, Phenylpropanolamine	Unknown
C 133	Valproic Acid 250 mg	Pharm Basics
C 135	Doxylamine Succinate 25 mg	Granutec
C177	Brompheniramine 12 mg, Phenylpropanolamine 75 mg	Granutec
C229	Brompheril 12-Hour Cold & Allergy Medication	Granutec
C 275/PF	Cardioquin 275 mg	Purdue Frederick
C 360-LL	Vitamins	Lederle
C771	Aspirin 325 mg	Upsher-Smith
C 875	Caffeine, Ephedrine, Phenylpropanolamine	Unknown
C 3148	Clofibrate 500 mg	Chase Pharm
C3227	Nifedipine 10 mg	Chase Pharm
C3453	Nifedipine 20 mg	Chase Pharm
C 8625	Sinulin 37.5 mg/2 mg/325 mg/250 mg/0.75 mg	Carnrick Labs
C 8647	CONTROLLED - SEE PAGE 221	
C 8650	Phrenilin 50 mg/325 mg	Carnrick Labs
C 8651	Phenylpropanolamine 25 mg	Carnrick Labs
C 8652	Phenindamine Tartrate 25 mg	Carnrick Labs
C 8656	Phrenlin Forte 50 mg/650 mg	Carnrick Labs
C 8657	CONTROLLED - SEE PAGE 219	
C 8658	Caffeine, Ephedrine, Phenylpropanolamine	Unknown
C 8666	Acetaminophen 650 mg, Chlorpheniramine 4 mg Phenylpropanolamine 25 mg	Carnrick
C 8671	Salsalate 500 mg	Carnrick
C 8672	Salsalate 750 mg	Carnrick

Imprint	Ingredient/Brand Name	Manufacturer
C 8673	Phenylpropanolamine 75 mg, Guaifenesin 400 mg	Carnrick
C 8704	Caffeine, Ephedrine, Phenylpropanolamine	Unknown
C 8858	Caffeine, Ephedrine, Phenylpropanolamine	Unknown
C 86120	Midrin 65 mg/100 mg/325 mg	Carnrick Labs
C 86204	Nolamine 4 mg/24 mg/50 mg	Carnrick Labs
CAFERGOT	Cafergot 1 mg/100 mg	Sandoz Pharm
CAFERGOT/78-34	Cafergot 1 mg/100 mg	Sandoz Pharm
CAFERGOT/S	Cafergot 1 mg/100 mg	Sandoz Pharm
Caffedrine	Caffeine	Unknown
CALAN 40	Calan 40 mg	Searle Pharm
CALAN 80	Calan 80 mg	Searle Pharm
CALAN 120	Calan 120 mg	Searle Pharm
CALAN SR 120	Caland SR 120 mg	Searle Pharm
CALAN/SR 240	Calan 240 mg	Searle Pharm
C ALLEREST	Childrens Chewable Allerest	CIBA
CAMA 500/	Cama 500 mg/150 mg/150 mg	Sandoz
C AMEN	Amen 10 mg	Carnrick Labs
Capoten 12.5mg	Capoten 12.5 mg	Bristol-Myers
Capoten 25mg	Capoten 25 mg	Bristol-Myers
Capoten 50mg	Capoten 50 mg	Bristol-Myers
Capoten 100mg	Capoten 100 mg	Bristol-Myers
Capozide 25/15	Capozide 25 mg/15 mg	Bristol-Myers
Capozide 25/25	Capozide 25 mg/25 mg	Bristol-Myers
Capozide 50/15	Capozide 50 mg/15 mg	Bristol-Myers
Capozide 50/25	Capozide 50 mg/25 mg	Bristol-Myers
CARACO 872	Nifedipine 10 mg	Caraco Pharm
CARAFATE/1712	Carafate 1000 mg	Marion Labs
Cardene 20mg Syntex 2437	Cardene 20 mg	Syntex
Cardene 30mg Syntex 2438	Cardene 30 mg	Syntex
Cardene SR 30mg Syntex 2440	Cardene SR 30 mg	Syntex
Cardene SR 45mg Syntex 2441	Cardene SR 45 mg	Syntex
Cardene SR 60mg Syntex 2442	Cardene SR 60 mg	Syntex
CARDILATE X7A	Cardilate 10 mg	Burroughs Wellcome
CARDIZEM/90 mg	Cardizem 90 mg	Marion Labs
CARDIZEM/120 mg	Cardizem 120 mg	Marion Labs
CARDIZEM CD 120 mg	Cardizem CD 120 mg	Marion Labs
CARDIZEM SR 60 mg	Cardizem 60 mg	Marion Labs
CARDIZEM SR 90 mg	Cardizem 90 mg	Marion Labs
CARDIZEM SR 120 mg	Cardizem 120 mg	Marion Labs
C C	Phenylpropanolamine 75 mg	CIBA
CC	Benzocaine 5 mg	Proctor & Gamble
CC/SCHERING	Chlor-Trimeton 8 mg	Schering Corp
C-C[in box] 0147	CONTROLLED - SEE PAGE 214, 218, 218	
C-C[in box] 18.75	CONTROLLED - SEE PAGE 222	
C-C[in box] 37.5	CONTROLLED - SEE PAGE 214, 218, 220, 223, 223, 224	
C-C[in box] 37.5P	Phenylpropanolamine 37.5 mg	Camall Corp
C-C[in box] 75P	Phenylpropanolamine 75 mg	Camall Corp
C-C[in box] 101	Meclizine 25 mg	Camall Corp
C-C[in box] 102	CONTROLLED - SEE PAGE 212	
C-C[in box] 105	CONTROLLED - SEE PAGE 193, 207, 213	
C-C[in box] 107	CONTROLLED - SEE PAGE 205	
C-C[in box] 108	Hydrochlorothiazide 50 mg	Camall Corp
C-C[in box] 109	CONTROLLED - SEE PAGE 194	
C-C[in box] 116	Hydrochlorothiazide 25 mg	Camall Corp
C-C[in box] 123	Hydrochlorothiazide 50 mg	Camall Corp
C-C[in box] 124	Hydralazine 25 mg, Hydrochlorothiazide 15 mg, Reserpine 0.1 mg	Cama

Imprint	Ingredient/Brand Name	Manufacturer
C-C[in box] 125	Hydrochlorothiazide 50 mg, Reserpine 0.125 mg	Camall Corp
C-C[in box] 135	CONTROLLED - SEE PAGE 199, 211	
C-C[in box] 136	CONTROLLED - No Photo - Phentermine HCl 8 mg - DEA Schedule IV	Camall Corp
C-C[in box] 137	Meclizine 12.5 mg	Camall Corp
C-C[in box] 143	Trichlormethiazide 4 mg	Camall Corp
C-C[in box] 227	Thyroid 3 grains	Camall Corp
C-C[in box] 232	CONTROLLED - SEE PAGE 199, 206	
C-C[in box] 236	Cyproheptadine 4 mg	Camall Corp
C-C[in box] 238	Potassium Gluconate 500 mg	Camall Corp
C-C[in box] 242	Thyroid 1/2 grain	Camall Corp
C-C[in box] 243	Thyroid 1 grain	Camall Corp
C-C[in box] 244	Thyroid 2 grains	Camall Corp
C-C[in box] 245	Chromium Picolinate 200 mcg	Camall Corp
C-C[in box] 250	Vitamins	Camall Corp
C-C[in box] 255	Hydralazine 10 mg	Camall Corp
C-C[in box] 256	Hydralazine 25 mg	Camall Corp
C-C[in box] 257	Hydralazine 50 mg	Camall Corp
C-C[in box] 258	Hydralazine 100 mg	Camall Corp
C-C[in box] 270	Phenylpropanolamine 37.5 mg	Camall Corp
C-C[in box] 424	Benzocaine 3 mg	Camall Corp
C-C[in box] 425	Benzocaine 3 mg	Camall Corp
C.E.G.	Correctol Stool Softener	Schering Corp
Central	Vitamins	Central Pharm
Central	Guaifenesin 200 mg	Central Pharm
Central	Chlorpheniramine maleate 2 mg, Pseudoephedrine 30 mg, Acetaminophen 325 mg	Central Pharm
CENTRAL/1 0	Vitamins	Central Pharm
Central/20	Iron 150 mg	Central Pharm
Central/21	CONTROLLED - No Photo - Hydrocodone Bitartrate 5 mg, Aspirin 500 mg - Mottled pink tablet - DEA Schedule III	Central Pharm
Central 40	Chlorpheniramine Maleate 8 mg, Pseudoephedrine 120 mg	Central
Central 44	Vitamins	Central Pharm
CENTRAL 60/4	Chlorpheniramine Maleate 4 mg, Pseudoephedrine 60 mg	Central
Central/100mg	Theoclear-100 100 mg	Central Pharm
Central 130 mg	Theophylline 130 mg	Central Pharm
Central 260mg	Theophylline 260 mg	Central Pharm
Central 500 mg	Salsalate 500 mg	Central Pharm
Central/500 5	CONTROLLED - SEE PAGE 201	
Central 750 mg	Salsalate 750 mg	Central Pharm
CENTRAL 2200	Vitamins/Minerals	Central Pharm
Centrax P-D 552	CONTROLLED - SEE PAGE 217	
Centrax P-D 553	CONTROLLED - SEE PAGE 217	
Centrax P-D 554	CONTROLLED - SEE PAGE 214	
CFL	Phenolphthalein 90 mg	Leiner Health
CHOOZ	Chooz Antacid Gum	Schering Corp
Ciba	Slow FE 160 mg	Ciba Pharm
CIBA/7	CONTROLLED - SEE PAGE 205	
CIBA/13	Serpasil 0.1 mg/25 mg	Ciba Pharm
CIBA 16	CONTROLLED - SEE PAGE 189	
CIBA/22	Esidrix 25 mg	Ciba Pharm
CIBA/23	Priscoline 25 mg	Ciba Pharm
CIBA 24	Cytadren 250 mg	Ciba Pharm
CIBA/26	Ludiomil 50 mg	Ciba Pharm
CIBA/33	Pyribenzamine 50 mg	Ciba Pharm
CIBA/35	Serpasil 0.1 mg	Ciba Pharm

Imprint	Ingredient/Brand Name	Manufacturer
CIBA/36	Serpasil 0.25 mg	Ciba Pharm
CIBA/37	Apresoline 10 mg	Ciba Pharm
CIBA/39	Apresoline 25 mg	Ciba Pharm
CIBA/40	Serpasil 0.1 mg/25 mg	Ciba Pharm
CIBA 41	Anturane 100 mg	Ciba Pharm
CIBA/46	Esidrix 50 mg	Ciba Pharm
CIBA/47	Esimil 10 mg/25 mg	Ciba Pharm
CIBA 48	PBA-SR 100 mg	Ciba Pharm
CIBA/49	Ismelin 10 mg	Ciba Pharm
CIBA/50	Priscoline 80 mg	Ciba Pharm
CIBA/53	Serpasil 1 mg	Ciba Pharm
CIBA 65	Lithobid 300 mg	Ciba Pharm
CIBA/71	Ser-Ap-Es	Ciba Pharm
CIBA/73	Apresoline 50 mg	Ciba Pharm
CIBA/97	Serpasil-Esidrix 0.1 mg/50 mg	Ciba Pharm
CIBA/101	Apresoline 100 mg	Ciba Pharm
CIBA/103	Ismelin 25 mg	Ciba Pharm
CIBA/104	Serpasil-Apresoline 0.2 mg/50 mg	Ciba Pharm
CIBA/110	Ludiomil 25 mg	Ciba Pharm
CIBA/129	Apresoline-Esidrix 25 mg/15 mg	Ciba Pharm
CIBA/130	Metopirone 250 mg	Ciba Pharm
CIBA/135	Ludiomil 75 mg	Ciba Pharm
CIBA/135	Metopirone 75 mg	Ciba Pharm
CIBA 139	Apresazide 25 mg/25 mg	Ciba Pharm
CIBA 149	Apresazide 50 mg/50 mg	Ciba Pharm
CIBA/152	Regitine 50 mg	Ciba Pharm
CIBA 154	Rimactane 300 mg	Ciba Pharm
CIBA/157	Pyribenzamine 100 mg	Ciba Pharm
CIBA 159	Apresazide 100 mg/50 mg	Ciba Pharm
CIBA 165	Slow-K 600 mg	Ciba Pharm
CIBA 168	Anturane 200 mg	Ciba Pharm
CIBA/192	Esidrix 100 mg	Ciba Pharm
CIBA NR	Ferrous Sulfate 60 mg	Ciba Pharm
CL/001	Peritrate 20 mg	Warner Chilcott
CL/004	Peritrate SA 80 mg	Warner Chilcott
CL 007	Peritrate 10 mg	Warner Chilcott
CL 008	Peritrate 40 mg	Warner Chilcott
CLARITIN 10/458	loratadine 10 mg	Schering Corp.
CLEOCIN	Cleocin 75 mg	Upjohn Comp
CLEOCIN 150mg	Cleocin 150 mg	Upjohn Comp
CLOMID 50	Clomid 50 mg	Merrell Dow
Cognex 10	Tacrine HCl 10 mg	Parke-Davis
Cognex 20	Tacrine HCl 20 mg	Parke-Davis
Cognes 30	Tacrine HCl 30 mg	Parke-Davis
Cognex 40	Tacrine HCl 40 mg	Parke-Davis
COLD AS + ALLERGY	Aspirin 500 mg, Chlopheniramine Maleate 2 mg, Phenylpropanolamine 24.08 mg, Dextromethorphan 10 mg	Miles
COLE 2658	Niac 300 mg	Cole Pharmacal Co
COMHIST	Comhist 2 mg/25 mg/10 mg	Norwich Eaton Pharm
COMHIST LA	Comhist LA 4 mg/50 mg/20 mg	Norwich Eaton Pharm
COMPOZ	Diphenhydramine 50 mg	Medtech Labs
COMTREX	Comtrex Multi-Sympton Cold Releiver	Bristol-Myers
Comtrex A/S	Comtrex-A/S 500 mg/30 mg/2 mg	Bristol-Meyers Prod
COMTREX DAY	Comtrex Non-Drowsy Liqui-Gels	Bristol-Myers
COMTREX LG	Comtrex Multi-Symptom Cold Releiver Liqui-Gels	Bristol-Myers
Comtrex ND	Comtrex Non-Drowsy Liqui-Gel	Bristol-Myers

Imprint	Ingredient/Brand Name	Manufacturer
Contac Contac	Phenylpropanolamine 75 mg, Chlorpheniramine 8 mg	SmithKline
CONTAC MENJ	Contac 8 mg/75 mg	Menley & James Labs
CONTROL CONTROL	Phenylpropanolamine 75 mg	Thompson Medical
Cooper 0123	Elixophyllin 250 mg	Cooper Labs
Cooper 0129	Elixophyllin 125 mg	Cooper Labs
COOPER 184	Deconamine 60 mg/4 mg	Berlex Labs
COPE	Aspirin 421 mg, Caffeine 32 mg,	Mentholatum Co.
COPLEY 111	Vitamins	Copley Pharm
COPLEY 113	Phenylephrine 25 mg, Chlorpheniramine 8 mg, Pyrilamine 25 mg	Copley
COPLEY 114	Procainamide 750 mg	Copley Pharm
COPLEY 123	Sodium Fluoride 0.5 mg	Copley Pharm
COPLEY 126	Vitamins	Copley Pharm
COPLEY 131	Sodium Fluoride 1 mg	Copley Pharm
COPLEY 143	Salsalate 500 mg	Copley Pharm
COPLEY 144	Salsalate 750 mg	Copley Pharm
COPLEY 146	Naproxen 250 mg	Copley Pharm
COPLEY 150	Naproxen 150 mg	Copley Pharm
COPLEY 151	Vitamins	Copley Pharm
COPLEY 152	Vitamins, Minerals	Copley Pharm
COPLEY 158	Vitamins	Copley Pharm
COPLEY 159	Florvite + Iron	Copley Pharm
COPLEY 166	Vitamins, Fluoride	Copley Pharm
COPLEY 169	Folic Acid 1 mg	Copley Pharm
COPLEY 176	Vitamins	Copley Pharm
COPLEY 182	Piroxicam 10 mg	Copley Pharm
COPLEY 188	Procainamide 500 mg	Copley Pharm
COPLEY 192	Vitamins	Copley Pharm
COPLEY 195	Piroxicam 20 mg	Copley Pharm
COPLEY 197	Vitamins	Copley Pharm
COPLEY 206	Amitriptyline 10 mg	Copley Pharm
COPLEY 207	Amitriptyline 25 mg	Copley Pharm
COPLEY 208	Amitriptyline 50 mg	Copley Pharm
COPLEY 209	Amitriptyline 75 mg	Copley Pharm
COPLEY 210	Amitriptyline 100 mg	Copley Pharm
COPLEY 211	Amitriptyline 150 mg	Copley Pharm
COPLEY 225	Potassium Chloride 600 mg	Copley Pharm
COPLEY 411	Methazolamide 25 mg	Copley Pharm
COPLEY 424	Methazolamide 50 mg	Copley Pharm
COPLEY 443	Naproxen 375 mg	Copley Pharm
COPLEY 447	Iodinated Glycerol 30 mg	Copley Pharm
COPLEY 457	Magnesium Gluconate	Copley Pharm
COPLEY 631	Diltiazem HCL 30 mg	Copley Pharm
COPLEY 662	Diltiazem HCL 60 mg	Copley Pharm
COPLEY 691	Diltiazem HCL 90 mg	Copley Pharm
COPLEY 720	Diltiazem HCL 120 mg	Copley Pharm
CORICIDIN SINUS	Sinus Headache Caplets	Schering Corp
CORRECTOL	Laxative Caplets	Schering Corp
Cortef 5	Cortef 5 mg	Upjohn
Cortef 10	Cortef 10 mg	Upjohn
Cortef 20	Cortef 20 mg	Upjohn
COTRIM/93 93	Cotrim 400 mg/80 mg	Lemmon Pharm
COTRIM DS/93 93	Cotrim-DS 800 mg/160 mg	Lemmon Pharm
Coumadin 1	Coumadin 1 mg	DuPont Pharm
COUMADIN 2	Coumadin 2 mg	DuPont Pharm
COUMADIN 2 1/2	Coumadin 2.5 mg	DuPont Pharm
COUMADIN 5	Coumadin 5 mg	DuPont Pharm

Imprint	Ingredient/Brand Name	Manufacturer
COUMADIN 7 1/2	Coumadin 7.5 mg	DuPont Pharm
COUMADIN 10	Coumadin 10 mg	DuPont Pharm
CP250	Nortriptyline Hydrochloride 10 mg	Creighton Corp.
CP251	Nortriptyline Hydrochloride 25 mg	Creighton Corp
CP252	Nortriptyline Hydrochloride 50 mg	Creighton Corp
CP253	Nortriptyline Hydrochloride 75 mg	Creighton Corp
CPC 464	Ferrous Fumarate 115 mg, Vitamins	H.L. Moore
CPC 836	Diphenhydramine 25 mg	H.L. Moore
CPI	Pseudoephedrine 60 mg, Triprolidine 2.5 mg	Century Pharm
CPW[in diamond] 18-704	Caffeine, Ephedrine, Phenylpropanolamine	Unknown
CPW[in diamond] 18-789	Caffeine, Ephedrine, Phenylpropanolamine	Unknown
CPW[in diamond] 18-858	Caffeine, Ephedrine, Phenylpropanolamine	Unknown
CPW[in diamond] 18-985	Caffeine, Ephedrine, Phenylpropanolamine	Unknown
CPW[in diamond] 50-888	Caffeine, Ephedrine, Phenylpropanolamine	Unknown
CPW[in diamond] 172	Caffeine, Ephedrine, Phenylpropanolamine	Unknown
CPW[in diamond] RJS	Caffeine, Ephedrine, Phenylpropanolamine	Unknown
C RJB	Caffeine, Ephedrine, Phenylpropanolamine	Unknown
CS	Zaditen 1 mg	Sandoz Pharm
CS-11 SILVER	Vitamins	Lederle Labs
CS 12	Caffeine, Ephedrine, Phenylpropanolamine	Unknown
CS 16	Caffeine, Ephedrine, Phenylpropanolamine	Unknown
CT 937	Calcium Lactate 10 grains	Freshlabs
CTM SINUS	Chlor-Trimeton Allergy Tablets	Schering Corp
CY	Cyklokapron 500 mg	Pharmacia
Cx	Day & Night Comtrex Allergy Sinus Treatment	Bristol-Myers
Cx-D	Day & Night Comtrex Allergy Sinus Treatment	Bristol-Myers
d	Dristan Cold Multi-Symptom	Whitehall Robins
D	Chlorpheniramine Maleate .5 mg, Phenylpropanolamine 6.25 mg	Sandoz
D4	DayQuil 4 Hour Allergy Relief	Proctor & Gamble
D 31 [diamond logo]	CONTROLLED - SEE PAGE 207	
D 33	Docusate 250 mg	Lederle Labs
D 35/W	CONTROLLED - SEE PAGE 187	
D 37/W	CONTROLLED - SEE PAGE 192	
D 41	Doxycycline 100 mg	Lederle Labs
D 51/LL	CONTROLLED - SEE PAGE 190	
D 52/LL	CONTROLLED - SEE PAGE 203	
D 53/LL	CONTROLLED - SEE PAGE 212	
d[in box] 810	Caffeine, Ephedrine, Phenylpropanolamine	Unknown
d[in box] 812	Caffeine, Ephedrine, Phenylpropanolamine	Unknown
d[in box] 814	Caffeine, Ephedrine, Phenylpropanolamine	Unknown
d[in box] 816	Caffeine, Ephedrine, Phenylpropanolamine	Unknown
Dallergy-D Laser 175	Pseudoephedrine 120 mg, Chlorpheniramine 12 mg	Laser
DALMANE 15 ROCHE	CONTROLLED - SEE PAGE 221	
DALMANE 30 ROCHE	CONTROLLED - SEE PAGE 221	
DAN 526	Isoniazid 300 mg	Danbury Pharm
DAN 944	Colchicine 0.6 mg	Danbury Pharm
DAN 5003	Diphenhydramine 50 mg	Danbury Pharm
DAN 5026	Procainamide 250 mg	Danbury Pharm
DAN 5028	Quinine Sulfate 5 grains	Danbury Pharm
DAN 5052	Prednisone 5 mg	Danbury Pharm
DAN 5058	Tripelennamine 50 mg	Danbury Pharm
DAN 5059	Prednisolone 5 mg	Danbury Pharm
DAN 5162	Tetracycline 250 mg	Danbury Pharm
DAN 5216	Folic Acid 1 mg	Danbury Pharm
DAN 5307	Promethazine 25 mg	Danbury Pharm
DAN 5319	Promethazine 50 mg	Danbury Pharm

Imprint	Ingredient/Brand Name	Manufacturer
DAN 5321	Primidone 250 mg	Danbury Pharm
DAN 5325	Colchicine 0.5 mg,Probenecid 500 mg	Danbury Pharm
DAN 5333	Procainamide 500 mg	Danbury Pharm
DAN 5335	Trihexyphenidyl 2 mg	Danbury Pharm
DAN 5337	Trihexyphenidyl 5 mg	Danbury Pharm
DAN 5345	Hydrochlorothiazide 50 mg	Danbury Pharm
DAN 5347	Probenecid 500 mg	Danbury Pharm
DAN 5350	Procainamide 375 mg	Danbury Pharm
DAN 5361 0.75	Dexamethasone 0.75 mg	Danbury Pharm
DAN 5368	Disulfiram 500 mg	Danbury Pharm
DAN 5369	Bethanechol 10 mg	Danbury Pharm
DAN 5373	Isosorbide Dinitrate 10 mg	Danbury Pharm
DAN 5374	Isosorbide Dinitrate 5 mg	Danbury Pharm
DAN 5376	Disulfiram 250 mg	Danbury Pharm
DAN 5381	Methocarbamol 500 mg	Danbury Pharm
DAN 5382	Methocarbamol 750 mg	Danbury Pharm
DAN 5385	Isosorbide Dinitrate 5 mg	Danbury Pharm
DAN 5387	Isosorbide Dinitrate 2.5 mg	Danbury Pharm
DAN 5388	Triamcinolone 4 mg	Danbury Pharm
DAN 5402	Bethanechol 25 mg	Danbury Pharm
DAN 5406	Hydrochlorothiazide 25 mg, Reserpine 0.125 mg	Danbury Pharm
DAN 5407	Hydrochlorothiazide 50 mg, Reserpine 0.125 mg	Danbury Pharm
DAN 5428	HCTZ 15 mg, Reserpine 0.1 mg,Hydralazine 25 mg	Danbury Pharm
DAN 5430	Acetazolamide 250 mg	Danbury Pharm
DAN 5438	Quinidine Sulfate 200 mg	Danbury Pharm
DAN 5440	Doxycycline 100 mg	Danbury Pharm
DAN 5442	Prednisone 10 mg	Danbury Pharm
DAN 5443	Prednisone 20 mg	Danbury Pharm
DAN 5444	Chlorothiazide 250 mg	Danbury Pharm
DAN 5449 0.25	Dexamethasone 0.25 mg	Danbury Pharm
DAN 5450 0.50	Dexamethasone 0.5 mg	Danbury Pharm
DAN 5451 1.5	Dexamethasone 1.5 mg	Danbury Pharm
DAN 5454	Quinidine Sulfate 300 mg	Danbury Pharm
DAN 5479	Erythromycin 250 mg	Danbury Pharm
DAN 5496	Spironolactone 25 mg, Hydrochlorothiazide 25 mg	Danbury Pharm
DAN 5501	Ergoloid Mesylates 1 mg	Danbury Pharm
DAN 5502	Ergoloid Mesylates 0.5 mg	Danbury Pharm
DAN 5504	Ergoloid Mesylates 1 mg	Danbury Pharm
DAN 5507	Chlorthalidone 25 mg	Danbury Pharm
DAN 5508	Tolbutamide 500 mg	Danbury Pharm
DAN 5513	Carisoprodol 350 mg	Danbury Pharm
DAN 5515	Bethanechol 50 mg	Danbury Pharm
DAN 5516	Quinine Sulfate 260 mg	Danbury Pharm
DAN 5518	Chlorthalidone 50 mg	Danbury Pharm
DAN 5520	Tetracycline 500 mg	Danbury Pharm
DAN 5522	Hydroxyzine 10 mg	Danbury Pharm
DAN 5523	Hydroxyzine 25 mg	Danbury Pharm
DAN 5535	Doxycycline 50 mg	Danbury Pharm
DAN 5538	Quinidine 324 mg	Danbury Pharm
DAN 5540	Metronidazole 250 mg	Danbury Pharm
DAN 5542/25	Thioridazine 25 mg	Danbury Pharm
DAN 5543	Allopurinol 100 mg	Danbury Pharm
DAN 5544	Allopurinol 300 mg	Danbury Pharm
DAN 5546	Sulfamethoxazole 400 mg, Trimethoprim 80 mg	Danbury Pharm
DAN 5547	Sulfamethoxazole 800 mg, Trimethoprim 160 mg	Danbury Pharm
DAN 5549	Chloroquine Phosphate 500 mg	Danbury Pharm

Imprint	Ingredient/Brand Name	Manufacturer
DAN 5552	Metronidazole 500 mg	Danbury Pharm
DAN 5553	Doxycycline 100 mg	Danbury Pharm
DAN 5554/10	Propranolol 10 mg	Danbury Pharm
DAN 5555/20	Propranolol 20 mg	Danbury Pharm
DAN 5556/40	Propranolol 40 mg	Danbury Pharm
DAN 5557/80	Propranolol 80 mg	Danbury Pharm
DAN 5560	Disopyramide 100 mg	Danbury Pharm
DAN 5561	Disopyramide 150 mg	Danbury Pharm
DAN 5562	Procainamide 250 mg	Danbury Pharm
DAN 5563	Procainamide 500 mg	Danbury Pharm
DAN 5564	Procainamide 750 mg	Danbury Pharm
DAN 5565	Hydroxyzine 50 mg	Danbury Pharm
DAN 5566/10	Thioridazine 10 mg	Danbury Pharm
DAN 5568/50	Thioridazine 50 mg	Danbury Pharm
DAN 5569	Thioridazine 100 mg	Danbury Pharm
DAN 5571	Trimethoprim 100 mg	Danbury Pharm
DAN 5572	Thioridazine 15 mg	Danbury Pharm
DAN 5575	Furosemide 40 mg	Danbury Pharm
DAN 5576	Furosemide 20 mg	Danbury Pharm
DAN 5579	Chlorpropamide 100 mg	Danbury Pharm
DAN 5580	Thioridazine 150 mg	Danbury Pharm
DAN 5581	Thioridazine 200 mg	Danbury Pharm
DAN 5582	Tolazamide 250 mg	Danbury Pharm
DAN 5585	Ibuprofen 200 mg	Danbury Pharm
DAN 5587	Methyldopa 500 mg	Danbury Pharm
DAN 5588	Methyldopa 250 mg	Danbury Pharm
DAN 5589	Metoclopramide 10 mg	Danbury Pharm
DAN 5590	Tolazamide 500 mg	Danbury Pharm
DAN 5591	Tolazamide 100 mg	Danbury Pharm
DAN 5592	Thiothixene 2 mg	Danbury Pharm
DAN 5593	Thiothixene 1 mg	Danbury Pharm
DAN 5594	Thiothixene 10 mg	Danbury Pharm
DAN 5595	Thiothixene 5 mg	Danbury Pharm
DAN 5597	Acetohexamide 500 mg	Danbury Pharm
DAN 5598	Acetohexamide 250 mg	Danbury Pharm
DAN 5599	Trazodone 100 mg	Danbury Pharm
DAN 5600	Trazodone 50 mg	Danbury Pharm
DAN 5601	Verapamil 80 mg	Danbury Pharm
DAN 5602	Verapamil 120 mg	Danbury Pharm
DAN 5603/2	Haloperidol 2 mg	Danbury Pharm
DAN 5604/1	Haloperidol 1 mg	Danbury Pharm
DAN 5605/0.5	Haloperidol 0.5 mg	Danbury Pharm
DAN 5606/5	Haloperidol 5 mg	Danbury Pharm
DAN 5607/15	Methyldopa 250 mg, Hydrochlorothiazide 15 mg	Danbury Pharm
DAN 5608/25	Methyldopa 250 mg, Hydrochlorothiazide 25 mg	Danbury Pharm
DAN 5609/0.1	Clonidine 0.1 mg	Danbury Pharm
DAN 5610/50	Methyldopa 500 mg, Hydrochlorothiazide 50 mg	Danbury Pharm
DAN 5611/30	Methyldopa 500 mg, Hydrochlorothiazide 30 mg	Danbury Pharm
DAN 5612/0.2	Clonidine 0.2 mg	Danbury Pharm
DAN 5613/0.3	Clonidine 0.3 mg	Danbury Pharm
DAN 5614	CONTROLLED - SEE PAGE 219	
DAN 5615	CONTROLLED - SEE PAGE 217	
DAN 5616	CONTROLLED - SEE PAGE 228	
DAN 5617	CONTROLLED - SEE PAGE 213	
DAN 5618	CONTROLLED - SEE PAGE 228	
DAN 5619/5	CONTROLLED - SEE PAGE 205	

Imprint	Ingredient/Brand Name	Manufacturer
DAN 5620/10	CONTROLLED - SEE PAGE 209	
DAN 5621/2	CONTROLLED - SEE PAGE 192	
DAN 5622/2	CONTROLLED - SEE PAGE 188	
DAN 5624/1	CONTROLLED - SEE PAGE 185	
DAN 5625/0.5	CONTROLLED - SEE PAGE 184	
DAN 5629	Doxepin 10 mg	Danbury Pharm
DAN 5630	Doxepin 25 mg	Danbury Pharm
DAN 5631	Doxepin 50 mg	Danbury Pharm
DAN 5632	Doxepin 75 mg	Danbury Pharm
DAN 5633	Doxepin 100 mg	Danbury Pharm
DAN 5636	Meclofenamate 50 mg	Danbury Pharm
DAN 5637	Meclofenamate 100 mg	Danbury Pharm
DAN 5642/2.5	Minoxidil 2.5 mg	Danbury Pharm
DAN 5643/10	Minoxidil 10 mg	Danbury Pharm
DAN 5658	Cyclobenzaprine 10 mg	Danbury Pharm
DAN 5659	Furosemide 80 mg	Danbury Pharm
DAN 5660	Sulindac 200 mg	Danbury Pharm
DAN 5661	Sulindac 150 mg	Danbury Pharm
DAN 5662	Nalidixic Acid 1 gm	Danbury Pharm
DAN 5677	Nalidixic Acid 500 mg	Danbury Pharm
DAN 5682	Triamterene 75 mg, Hydrochlorothiazide 50 mg	Danbury Pharm
DAN 5693	Prazosin 5 mg	Danbury Pharm
DAN 5694	Minocycline 50 mg	Danbury Pharm
DAN 5695	Minocycline 100 mg	Danbury Pharm
DAN 5696	Prazosin 2 mg	Danbury Pharm
DAN 5697	Prazosin 1 mg	Danbury Pharm
DAN 5704	Fenoprofen Calcium 600 mg	Danbury Pharm
DAN 5706/500	Chlorzoxazone 500 mg	Danbury Pharm
DAN 5708	Clindamycin 150 mg	Danbury Pharm
DAN 5710/2	Albuterol Sulfate 2 mg	Danbury Pharm
DAN 5711/4	Albuterol Sulfate 4 mg	Danbury Pharm
DAN 5713/25	Amoxapine 25 mg	Danbury Pharm
DAN 5714/50	Amoxapine 50 mg	Danbury Pharm
DAN 5715/100	Amoxapine 100 mg	Danbury Pharm
DAN 5716/150	Amoxapine 150 mg	Danbury Pharm
DAN 5721	Fenoprofen Calcium 300 mg	Danbury Pharm
DAN 5724/10	Metaproterenol Sulfate 10 mg	Danbury Pharm
DAN 5725/20	Metaproterenol Sulfate 20 mg	Danbury Pharm
DAN 5726	Hydroxyzine Pamoate 25 mg	Danbury Pharm
DAN 5730/10	Baclofen 10 mg	Danbury Pharm
DAN 5731/20	Baclofen 20 mg	Danbury Pharm
DAN 5736 5	Timolol Maleate 5 mg	Danbury Pharm
DAN 5737 10	Timolol Maleate 10 mg	Danbury Pharm
DAN 5738/20	Timolol Maleate 20 mg	Danbury Pharm
DAN 5777 50	Atenolol 50 mg	Danbury Pharm
DAN 5778 100	Atenolol 100 mg	Danbury Pharm
DAN 5782	Atenolol 50 mg, Chlorthalidone 25 mg	Danbury Pharm
DAN 5783	Atenolol 100 mg, Chlorthalidone 25 mg	Danbury Pharm
DARAPRIM A3A	Pyrimethamine 25 mg	Burroughs Wellcome
D&E 25-25	Caffeine	D&E Pharm
D&E 85-25	Caffeine	D&E Pharm
D&E 127	Caffeine	D&E Pharm
D&E 160	Caffeine	D&E Pharm
D&E 190	Caffeine	D&E Pharm
D&E 200	Caffeine	D&E Pharm
D&E 225	Caffeine	D&E Pharm

Imprint	Ingredient/Brand Name	Manufacturer
D&E 260	Caffeine	D&E Pharm
D&E 290	Caffeine	D&E Pharm
D&E 500	Caffeine	D&E Pharm
D&E M E	Caffeine	D&E Pharm
D&E WNM	Caffeine	D&E Pharm
Danocrine Winthrop D05	Danocrine 200 mg	Winthrop
DARVOCET-N 100/Lilly	CONTROLLED - SEE PAGE 208	
DATRIL	Datril 500 mg	Bristol-Meyers Prod
Day	Pseudoephedrine 30 mg, Dextromethorphan 10 mg, Acetaminophen 250 mg, Guaifenesin 100 mg	Granutec
DayQuil	Vicks DayQuil Liquicaps	Proctor & Gamble
Day time	Caffeine, Ephedrine, Phenylpropanolamine	Unknown
D-C/M	CONTROLLED - No Photo - Hydrocodone 5 mg, Acetaminophen 500 mg - White, pink mottle tablet - DEA Schedule III	Mason Pharm
d d	Phenylpropanolamine 75 mg	Thompson Medical
D E	Caffeine	D&E Pharm
DELO 156	Acetaminophen, Salicylamide	Unknown
DELO F80	Methapyrilene	Unknown
DELO L19	Ephedrine	Unknown
Deltasone 2.5	Deltasone 2.5 mg	Upjohn Comp
DELTASONE 5	Deltasone 5 mg	Upjohn Comp
DELTASONE 10	Deltasone 10 mg	Upjohn Comp
DELTASONE 20	Deltasone 20 mg	Upjohn Comp
Deltasone 500	Deltasone 500 mg	Upjohn Comp
Desyrel MJ 775	Desyrel 50 mg	Bristol-Myers
Desyrel MJ 776	Desyrel 100 mg	Bristol-Myers
Desyrel MJ 778	Desyrel 150 mg	Bristol-Myers
DEX	Caffeine, Ephedrine, Phenylpropanolamine	Unknown
Dexatrim Vitamin	Dexatrim Plus Vitamins	Thompson Medical
DEX L10	Caffeine, Ephedrine, Phenylpropanolamine	Unknown
DEX L10	Phenylpropanolamine	Unknown
Dexatrim	Dexatrim	Thompson Medical
DF [logo]	Hytrin 1 mg	Abbott Labs
DH [logo]	Hytrin 2 mg	Abbott Labs
DI [logo]	Hytrin 10 mg	Abbott Labs
Dia β	DiaBeta 5 mg	Hoechst-Roussel
DIALOSE	Docusate Sodium 100 mg	Johnson & Johnson
DIALOSE PLUS	Docusate Sodium 100 mg, Phenolphthalein 65 mg	Johnson & Johnson
Diamox 125 D1LL	Diamox 125 mg	Lederle Labs
DIAMOX 250 D2LL	Diamox 250 mg	Lederle Labs
DIAMOX 500	Diamox 250 mg	Lederle Labs
DIAMOX D3	Diamox Sequels 500 mg	Lederle Labs
DIAR AID	Activated Attapulgite 750 mg	Thompson Medical
Diasorb	Activated Nonfibrous Attapulgite 750 mg	Columbia Labs
DIDREX 25	CONTROLLED - No Photo - Benzphetamine 25 mg - Yellow, round tablet - DEA Schedule III	Upjohn
DIDREX 50	CONTROLLED - SEE PAGE 203	
DI-GEL	Di-Gel Antacid Tablets	Schering Corp
Dilacor XR 180 mg 0251	Dilacor XR 180 mg	Rorer
Dilacor XR 240 mg 0252	Dilacor XR 240 mg	Rorer
DIMETAPP AHR	Brompheniramine 12 mg, Phenylpropanolamine 75 mg	Whitehall Robins
DIMETAPP SINUS	Ibuprofen 200 mg, Pseudoephedrine 30 mg	Whitehall Robins
DIMACOL	Dimacol Cold & Cough	Whitehall Robins
DIPENTUM 250 mg	Olsalazine Sodium 250 mg	Pharmacia
DISALCID/3M	Disalcid 500 mg	3M
DISALCID 750/3M	Disalcid 750 mg	3M

Imprint	Ingredient/Brand Name	Manufacturer
DISALCID TM/3M	Disalcid	3M
DISTA 3055	Cinobac 250 mg	Dista Prod
DISTA 3056	Cinobac 500 mg	Dista Prod
DISTA 3122	Co-Pyronil 2 2 mg/30 mg	Dista Prod
DISTA 3123	Co-Pyronil 2 4 mg/60 mg	Dista Prod
DISTA C03	Ilotycin 250 mg	Dista Prod
DISTA C19	Mi-Cebrin	Dista Prod
DISTA C20	Mi-Cebrin T	Dista Prod
DISTA C22	Becotin-T	Dista Prod
DISTA F01	Trinsicon 240 mg/0.0075 mg/110 mg/0.5 mg/75 mg	Dista Prod
DISTA F62	Becotin	Dista Prod
DISTA F77	Becotin with Vitamin C	Dista Prod
DISTA F91	Co-Pyronil 15 mg/25 mg/12.5 mg	Dista Prod
DISTA F93	Co-Pyronil 7.5 mg/12.5 mg/6.25 mg	Dista Prod
DISTA H07	Ilosone 125 mg	Dista Prod
DISTA H09	Ilosone 250 mg	Dista Prod
DISTA H69	Keflex 250 mg	Dista Prod
DISTA H71	Keflex 500 mg	Dista Prod
DISTA H74	Ethinamate 500 mg	Dista Prod
DISTA H76	Nalfon 200	Dista Prod
DISTA H77	Nalfon 300 mg	Dista Prod
DISTA U05	Ilosone 125 mg	Dista Prod
DISTA U25	Ilosone 250 mg	Dista Prod
DISTA U26	Ilosone 500 mg	Dista Prod
DISTA U59	Nalfon 600 mg	Dista Prod
DISTA U60	Keflex 1000 mg	Dista Prod
DIUCARDIN 50	Diucardin 50 mg	Ayerst Labs
DI [logo]	Hytrin 10 mg	Abbott Labs
DJ [logo]	Hytrin 5 mg	Abbott Labs
DOAN'S	Magnesium Salicylate 325 mg	CIBA
DOAN'S PM	Magnesium Salicylate 500 mg, Diphenhydramine 25 mg	CIBA
DOONER 351	Slo-Phyllin 100 mg	Dooner Labs
DOONER 352	Slo-Phyllin 200 mg	Dooner Labs
DORAL/7.5	CONTROLLED - SEE PAGE 204	
DORAL/15	CONTROLLED - SEE PAGE 204	
DORSEY/10	Metaprel 10 mg	Dorsey Labs
DORSEY/20	Metaprel 20 mg	Dorsey Labs
Dorsey 43-27	Triaminic Juvelets 25 mg/12.5 mg/12.5 mg	Dorsey Labs
DORSEY TRIAMINIC	Triaminic 12.5 mg/2 mg	Dorsey Labs
DORSEY TRIAMINIC 12	Triaminic-12 75 mg/12 mg	Dorsey Labs
Dorsey TRIAMINIC TR	Triaminic TR 50 mg/25 mg/25 mg	Dorsey Labs
DORSEY TRIAMINICOL	Traminicol 12.5 mg/2 mg/10 mg	Dorsey Labs
DORYX	Doryx 100 mg	Parke-Davis
DOW[in diamond] 31	Lorelco 250 mg	Merrell Dow Pharm
DOW[in diamond] 51	Lorelco 250 mg	Merrell Dow Pharm
DOW[in diamond] 80	Lorelco	Merrell Dow Pharm
DOW[in diamond] 104	Novafed 120 mg	Merrell Dow Pharm
DOW[in diamond] 106	Novafed A 120 mg/8 mg	Merrell Dow Pharm
DOW[in diamond] 508	Rifadin 300 mg	Merrell Dow Pharm
DOW[in diamond] 509	Rifamate 300 mg/150 mg	Merrell Dow Pharm
DOW[in diamond] 510	Rifadin 150 mg	Merrell Dow Pharm
Doxidan	Doxidan 60 mg/50 mg	Hoechst-Roussel Pharm
DOXY/93	Doxy-Lemmon 100 mg	Lemmon Pharm
dp 01	Clonidine 0.1 mg	Duramed Pharm
dp 02	Clonidine 0.2 mg	Duramed Pharm
dp 03	Clonidine 0.3 mg	Duramed Pharm

Imprint	Ingredient/Brand Name	Manufacturer
dp 082/TUSSIGON	CONTROLLED - SEE PAGE 209	
dp 10	Propranolol 10 mg	Duramed Pharm
dp 11	Trifluoperazine 1 mg	Duramed Pharm
dp 12	Trifluoperazine 2 mg	Duramed Pharm
dp 12-1/2	Levothyroxine Sodium 0.0125 mg	Daniels Pharm
dp 13	Trifluoperazine 5 mg	Duramed Pharm
dp 14	Trifluoperazine 10 mg	Duramed Pharm
dp 20	Propranolol 20 mg	Duramed Pharm
dp 25	Dipridamole 25 mg	Duramed Pharm
dp 25/LEVOXINE	Levoxine 0.025 mg	Daniels Pharm
dp 30	Duramed 0.3 mg	Duramed Pharm
dp 31	Estrogens 0.625 mg	Duramed Pharm
dp 32	Estrogens 1.25 mg	Duramed Pharm
dp 34	Estrogens 2.5 mg	Duramed Pharm
dp 40	Propranolol 40 mg	Duramed Pharm
dp 50	Dipyridamole 50 mg	Duramed Pharm
dp 50	Levothyroxine Sodium 0.05 mg	Daniels Pharm
dp 60	Propranolol 60 mg	Duramed Pharm
dp 75	Levoxine 0.075 mg	Daniels Pharm
dp 75	Dipyridamole 75 mg	Duramed Pharm
DP 75/LEVOXINE	Levoxine 0.075 mg	Daniels Pharm
dp 80	Propranolol 80 mg	Duramed Pharm
dp 90	Propranolol 90 mg	Duramed Pharm
DP 100/LEVOXINE	Levoxine 0.1 mg	Daniels Pharm
dp 112	Levothyroxine Sodium 0.112 mg	Duramed Pharm
dp 125/LEVOXINE	Lovoxine 0.125 mg	Daniels Pharm
dp 150/LEVOXINE	Levoxine 0.15 mg	Daniels Pharm
dp 175/LEVOXINE	Levoxine 0.175 mg	Daniels Pharm
dp 200/LEVOXINE	Levoxine 0.2 mg	Daniels Pharm
dp 215	Chlorzoxazone 250 mg, Acetaminophen 300 mg	Duramed Pharm
dp 223	Aminophylline 100 mg	Duramed Pharm
dp 224	Aminophylline 200 mg	Duramed Pharm
dp 225	Haloperidol 0.5 mg	Duramed Pharm
dp 226	Haloperidol 1 mg	Duramed Pharm
dp 227	Haloperidol 2 mg	Duramed Pharm
dp 228	Haloperidol 5 mg	Duramed Pharm
dp 229	Haloperidol 10 mg	Duramed Pharm
dp 230	Haloperidol 20 mg	Duramed Pharm
dp 241	Choline Magnesium Trisalate 500 mg	Duramed Pharm
dp 242	Choline Magnesium Trisalate 750 mg	Duramed Pharm
dp 246	Cyproheptadine 4 mg	Duramed Pharm
dp 249	Iodoquinol 650 mg	Duramed Pharm
dp 251	Chlorpropamide 250 mg	Duramed Pharm
dp 252	Chlorpropamide 100 mg	Duramed Pharm
dp 255	Dipyridamole 25 mg	Duramed Pharm
dp 257	Dipyridamole 50 mg	Duramed Pharm
dp 258	Dipyridamole 75 mg	Duramed Pharm
dp 265	Hydroxyzine 25 mg	Duramed Pharm
dp 266	Hydroxyzine 50 mg	Duramed Pharm
dp 267	Hydroxyzine 100 mg	Duramed Pharm
dp 274	Isoniazid 100 mg	Duramed Pharm
dp 275	Indomethacin 25 mg	Duramed Pharm
dp 276	Indomethacin 50 mg	Duramed Pharm
dp 277	Isoniazid 300 mg	Duramed Pharm
dp 293	Phenylephrine 5 mg, Phenylpropanolamine 45 mg, Guaifenesin 200 mg	Duramed Pharm

Imprint	Ingredient/Brand Name	Manufacturer
dp 294	Phenylpropanolamine 75 mg, Guaifenesin 400 mg	Duramed Pharm
dp 295	Phenylpropanolamine 75 mg, Guaifenesin 400 mg	Duramed Pharm
dp 296	Salsalate 500 mg	Duramed Pharm
dp 297	Salsalate 750 mg	Duramed Pharm
dp 298	Salsalate 500 mg	Duramed Pharm
dp 299	Salsalate 750 mg	Duramed Pharm
dp 300/LEVOXINE	Levoxine 0.3 mg	Daniels Pharm
dp 301	Methylprednisolone 4 mg	Duramed Pharm
dp 305	Papverine 150 mg	Duramed Pharm
dp 311	Prednisone 5 mg	Duramed Pharm
dp 312	Prednisone 10 mg	Duramed Pharm
dp 313	Prednisone 20 mg	Duramed Pharm
dp 314	Prochlorperazine 5 mg	Duramed Pharm
dp 315	Prochlorperazine 10 mg	Duramed Pharm
dp 316	Prochlorperazine 25 mg	Duramed Pharm
dp 325	Tolazamide 100 mg	Duramed Pharm
dp 326	Tolazamide 250 mg	Duramed Pharm
dp 327	Tolazamide 500 mg	Duramed Pharm
dp 332	Propranolol 40 mg, Hydrochlorothiazide 25 mg	Duramed Pharm
dp 333	Propranolol 80 mg, Hydrochlorothiazide 25 mg	Duramed Pharm
dp 364	Isometheptene Mucate 65 mg, Dichloralphenazone 100 mg Acetaminophen 325 mg	Duramed Pharm
dp 371	Methyldopa 250 mg	Duramed Pharm
dp 372	Methyldopa 500 mg	Duramed Pharm
dp 401	Pseudoephedrine 120 mg, Guaifenesin 600 mg	Duramed Pharm
dp 651	CONTROLLED - SEE PAGE 218	
dp 661	CONTROLLED - SEE PAGE 213	
DPI/2	CONTROLLED - No Photo - Acetaminophen 300 mg, Codeine 15 mg - Tablet - DEA Schedule III	Duramed Pharm
DPI/3	CONTROLLED - No Photo - Acetaminophen 300 mg, Codeine 30 mg - Tablet - DEA Schedule III	Duramed Pharm
DPI/4	CONTROLLED - No Photo - Acetaminophen 300 mg, Codeine 60 mg - Tablet - DEA Schedule III	Duramed Pharm
DPI 125	Estropipate 1.5 mg	Duramed Pharm
DPI 625	Estropipate .75 mg	Duramed Pharm
DPI 644	CONTROLLED - No Photo - Oxycodone 5 mg, Acetaminophen 500 mg - Tablet - DEA Schedule II	Duramed Pharm
dp/LEVOXINE	Levoxine 0.05 mg	Daniels Pharm
D-P/M	CONTROLLED - SEE PAGE 207	
DQ SC	DayQuil Sinus Pressure & Congestion Relief	Proctor & Gamble
DQ SP	DayQuil Sinus Pressure & Pain Relief	
Dristan	Dristan 12.5 mg/2 mg/325 mg/16 mg	Whitehall Labs
Dristan AF	Dristan AF 2 mg/5 mg/325 mg/16 mg	Whitehall Labs
Dristan Allergy	Pseudoephedrine 60 mg, Brompheniramine 4 mg	Whitehall Robins
Dristan Cold ND	Dristan Cold No-Drowsiness	Whitehall Robins
Dristan Sinus	Ibuprofen 200 mg, Pseudoephedrine 30 mg	Whitehall Labs
DRIXORAL/AMN	Allergy Tablets	Schering Corp
DUADACIN 0722	Acetaminophen 325 mg, Phenylpropanolamine 12.5 mg, Chlorpheniramine 2 mg	Kenwood Labs
DUNHALL 0409	Pseudoephedrine 120 mg, Chlorpheniramine 12 mg	Dunhall
DUNHALL 0805	Doxycycline Hyclate 100 mg	Dunhall
DUNHALL 2811	Acetaminophen 325 mg, Butalbital 50 mg	Dunhall
DUNHALL 2819 [logo]	CONTROLLED - SEE PAGE 222	
DUNHALL 2829	Cophene-X	Dunhall
DuPont/0072	Moban 5 mg	DuPont Pharm
DuPont/0073	Moban 10 mg	DuPont Pharm

Imprint	Ingredient/Brand Name	Manufacturer
DuPont/0074	Moban 25 mg	DuPont Pharm
DuPont/0076	Moban 50 mg	DuPont Pharm
DuPont/0077	Moban 100 mg	DuPont Pharm
DuPont MOBAN 5	Moban 5 mg	DuPont Pharm
DuPont MOBAN 10	Moban 10 mg	DuPont Pharm
DuPont MOBAN 25	Moban 25 mg	DuPont Pharm
DuPont MOBAN 50	Moban 50 mg	DuPont Pharm
DuPont MOBAN 100	Moban 100 mg	DuPont Pharm
DuPont/SYMMETREL	Symmetrel 100 mg	DuPont Pharm
DuPont/TREXAN	Trexan 50 mg	DuPont Pharm
DuPont VALPIN	Valpin 50 mg	DuPont Pharm
DuPont ZYDONE	CONTROLLED - SEE PAGE 214	
DURA 009	Guaifenesin 600 mg	Dura Pharm
Dura-Vent	Dura-Vent 75 mg/400 mg	Dura Pharm
Dura-Vent A	Dura-Vent A 75 mg/10 mg	Dura Pharm
DX	Ephedrine	Unknown
DYFLEX 400	Dyflex 400	Lemmon Pharm
DYFLEX-G	Dyflex-G 200 mg/200 mg	Econo Med Pharm
DynaCirc 2.5	DynaCirc 2.5 mg	Sandoz
DynaCirc 5	DynaCirc 5 mg	Sandoz
DYRENIUM 100 SKF	Dyrenium 100 mg	Smith, Kline & French
DYRENIUM 50 SKF	Dyrenium 50 mg	Smith, Kline & French
E	Excedrin 250 mg/250 mg/65 mg	Bristol-Meyers Prod
E 3	Ergoloid Mesylates 1 mg	Lederle Labs
E 12	Ferrous Sulfate 325 mg	Eon Labs
E 14	Chlorpheniramine maleate 4 mg	Eon Labs
E26	Docusate Calcium 240 mg	Chase
E27	Docusate Sodium 100 mg	Chase
E29	Docusate Sodium 250 mg	Chase
E 648	Diphenhydramine 25 mg	Eon Labs
E 649	Diphenhydramine 509 mg	Eon Labs
E 1303	Quinine Sulfate 325 mg	Eon Labs
E 5000	CONTROLLED - SEE PAGE 228	
E 5385	Ferrous Sulfate SR 250 mg	Eon Labs
E 8875	Caffeine, Ephedrine, Phenylprpanolamine	Unknown
EA [logo]	Erythromycin 500 mg	Abbott Labs
Eaton 007	Macrodantin 25 mg	Eaton Labs
Eaton 008	Macrodantin 50 mg	Eaton Labs
Eaton 009	Macrodantin 100 mg	Eaton Labs
Eaton 030	Dantrium 25 mg	Norwich Eaton Pharm
Eaton 033	Dantrium 100 mg	Norwich Eaton Pharm
Eaton 036	Furadantin 50 mg	Norwich Eaton Pharm
Eaton 037	Furadantin 100 mg	Norwich Eaton Pharm
Eaton 045	Duvoid 10 mg	Norwich Eaton Pharm
Eaton 046	Duvoid 25 mg	Norwich Eaton Pharm
Eaton 047	Duvoid 50 mg	Norwich Eaton Pharm
Eaton 072	Furoxone 100 mg	Norwich Eaton Pharm
EB [logo]	Erythromycin 250 mg	Abbott Labs
EC [logo]	Ery-Tab 250 mg	Abbott Labs
ECR 0131	CONTROLLED - SEE PAGE 225	
ECR 0141	CONTROLLED - SEE PAGE 226	
ED [logo]	Ery-Tab 500 mg	Abbott Labs
EE [logo]	EES 400	Abbott Labs
EF [logo]	EES 200	Abbott Labs
EH [logo]	Ery-Tab 333 mg	Abbott Labs
EK [logo]	Erythromycin 500 mg	Abbott Labs

Imprint	Ingredient/Brand Name	Manufacturer
EL 040	Guaifenesin 600 mg	Econolab
EL 090	Dextromethorphan Hydrobromide 30 mg, Guaifenesin 600 mg	Econolab
EL 140	Pseudoephedrine 60 mg, Guaifenesin 600 mg	Econolab
EL 222	Brompheniramine Maleate 6 mg, Pseudoephedrine 60 mg	Econolab
EL 320	Lipase 8,000 units, Protease 30,000 units, Amylase 30,000 units	Econola
EL 323	Lipase 4,000 units, Amylase 20,000 units, Protease 25,000 units	Econola
EL 444	Trimethobenzamide 250 mg	Econolab
EL 514	Aspirin 800 mg	Econolab
EL 522	Dyphylline 200 mg, Guaifenesin 200 mg	Econolab
EL 525	Pentobarbital Sodium30 mg, Belladonna Alkaloids 125 mg Ergotamine Tartrate 1.0 mg	Econolab
EL 717	Hyoscyamine Sulfate .125 mg	Econolab
EL 740	Chlorpheniramine maleate 8 mg, Pseudoephedrine 120 mg	Econolab
EL 860	Pseudoephedrine 120 mg, Guaifenesin 250 mg	Econolab
EL 870	Pseudoephedrine 60 mg, Guaifenesin 300 mg	Econolab
EL 880	Lipase 10,000 units, Amylase 33,200 units, Protease 37,500 units	Econol
ELDER	Trisoralen 5 mg	Burroughs Wellcome
ELDER 600	Oxsoralen 10 mg	Burroughs Wellcome
ELLO[in box] 35-866	Caffeine, Ephedrine, Phenylpropanolamine	Unknown
EM	Dyflex-200	Econo Med Pharm
EMCYT KP 132	Emcyt 140 mg	Pharmacia
EMCYT ROCHE	Emcyt 140 mg	Roche Labs
EMPIRIN 2	CONTROLLED - SEE PAGE 198	
EMPIRIN 3	CONTROLLED - SEE PAGE 198	
EMPIRIN 4	CONTROLLED - SEE PAGE 198	
ENDEP 10 ROCHE	Endep 10 mg	Roche Labs
ENDEP 25 ROCHE	Endep 25 mg	Roche Labs
ENDEP 50 ROCHE	Endep 50 mg	Roche Labs
ENDEP 75 ROCHE	Endep 75 mg	Roche Labs
ENDEP 100 ROCHE	Endep 100 mg	Roche Labs
ENDEP 150 ROCHE	Endep 150 mg	Roche Labs
Endo/0072	Moban 5 mg	Endo Labs
Endo/0073	Moban 10 mg	Endo Labs
Endo/0074	Moban 25 mg	Endo Labs
Endo 051	Promethazine	Endo Labs
Endo 132	Percogesic 30 mg/325 mg	Endo Labs
Endo 173/7 1/2	Coumadin 7.5 mg	Endo Labs
Endo 602	CONTROLLED - No Photo - Oxycodone 5 mg, Acetaminophen 325 mg - White, riound tablet - DEA Schedule II	Endo Labs
Endo 610	CONTROLLED - No Photo - Oxycodone Hydrochloride 4.5 mg, Oxycodone Terephthalate 0.38 mg, Aspirin 325 mg - Yellow, round tablet - DEA Schedule II	Endo Labs
ENDURON [logo]	Enduron	Abbott Labs
ENTEX	Entex 5 mg/45 mg/200 mg	Norwich Eaton Pharm
ENTEX LA	Entex LA 400 mg/75 mg	Norwich Eaton Pharm
EPITOL/93 93	Epitol 200 mg	Lemmon Pharm
ER [logo]	Erythromycin 250 mg	Abbott Labs
ERVA 5.4	Yohimbine HCl 5.4 mg	Royce
Eryc	Eryc 250 mg	Parke-Davis
ES [logo]	Erythrocin 250 mg	Abbott Labs
ES BUFFERIN	ES Bufferin 500 mg	Bristol-Myers Prod
ESB	Extra Strength Bufferin 500 mg	Bristol-Myers Prod
E/Searle	Enovid-E 2.5 mg/0.1 mg	Searle Pharm
ESKALITH SKF	Eskalith 300 mg	Smith, Kline & French
ESLC	Quinine Sulfate 162.5 mg	P.L. Developments
Espo	Phenolphthalein 97.2 mg	Combe

Imprint	Ingredient/Brand Name	Manufacturer
ET [logo]	Erythrocin 500 mg	Abbott Labs
Ethavex	Ethavex-100 100 mg	Econo Med
ETHEX/001	Potassium Chloride 750 mg	Ethex
ETHEX/002	Disopyramide Phosphate 150 mg	Ethex
ETHEX/003	Disopyramide Phosphate 100 mg	Ethex
ETHEX/004	Nitroglycerin 2.5 mg	Ethex
ETHEX/005	Nitroglycerin 6.5 mg	Ethex
ETHEX/006	Nitroglycerin 9 mg	Ethex
ETHEX 205	Guaifenesin 600 mg	Ethex
ETHEX 208	Guaifenesin 600 mg	Ethex
ETHEX 212	Prenatal MR 90	Ethex
ETHEX 213	Guaifenesin 600 mg	Ethex
ETHEX 214	Guaifenesin 600 mg	Ethex
EV201	Bacmin	Marnel
EVAC-U-GEN	Yellow Phenolphthalein 97.2 mg	Walker Corp.
EVERETT	Pavatym 150 mg	Everett Labs
EVERETT 0072	Vitafol	Everett Labs
EVERETT 0201	Strovite Plus	Everett Labs
EVERETT 162	Repan 50 mg	Everett Labs
EVERETT 166	Repan CF	Everett Labs
EX-1B	Ibuprofen 200 mg	Bristol-Myers
EXCEDRIN	Excedrin 250 mg/250 mg/65 mg	Bristol-Meyers Prod
Excedrin PM	Acetaminophen 500 mg, Diphenhydramine 38 mg	Bristol-Myers
EX-LAX	Phenolphthalein 135 mg	Sandoz
EXTRA STRENGTH SINE-AID	Sine-Aid 500 mg/30 mg	McNeil Pharm
EZ [logo]	Erythromycin 200 mg	Abbott Labs
F 04	Cycloserine 250 mg	Eli Lilly
F 11	Furosemide 20 mg	Lederle Labs
F 12	Furosemide 40 mg	Lederle Labs
F 13	Furosemide 80 mg	Lederle Labs
F16	Principen with Probenecid	Bristol-Myers
F 25	Ephedrine 50 mg	Eli Lilly
F 39	Quinidine Sulfate 200 mg	Eli Lilly
F 66	Doxylamine	Unknown
F 66/LL	Fibercon 625 mg	Lederle Labs
F 74	Vitamins	Eli Liily
F 96	Vitamins	Eli Lilly
F-9031	Caffeine	Unknown
FAM	Feen-A-Mint Laxative	Schering Corp
F CIBA	Calcium Polycarbophil	CIBA
Fe	Ferrous Gluconate 300 mg	Upsher-Smith
Feen-A-Mint	Feen-A-Mint Laxative	Schering Corp
Feverall 80 mg	Acetaminophen 80 mg	Upsher-Smith
Feverall 160 mg	Acetaminophen 160 mg	Upsher-Smith
F [in triangle] Jr	Anhydrous Theophyilline 130 mg	Fleming
F [in triangle] Jr	Guaifenesin 125 mg, Pseudoephedrine 60 mg	Fleming
F [in triangle] Jr	Chlorpheniramine 4 mg, Phenylephrine 10 mg, Methscopolamine 1.25 mg	Fleming
F [in triangle] Sr	Anhydrous Theophylline 260 mg	Fleming
F [in triangle] Sr	Guaifenesin 250 mg, Pseudoephedrine 120 mg	Fleming
F [in triangle] Sr	Chlorpheniramine 8 mg, Phenylephrine 20 mg, Methscopolamine 2.50 mg	Fleming
FAST LENE	Caffeine, Phenylpropanolamine	Unknown
FC 2	Ergomar 2 mg	Fisons Corp
FC 1125	Vitron-C-Plus 400 mg/250 mg	Fisons Corp
FC [logo]	Temafloxacin 400 mg	Abbott Labs

Imprint	Ingredient/Brand Name	Manufacturer
FELDENE PFIZER 322	Feldene 10 mg	Pfizer Labs
FELDENE PFIZER 323	Feldene 20 mg	Pfizer Labs
Feosol	Feosol 159 mg	SmithKline
FIORICET CODEINE	CONTROLLED - SEE PAGE 228	
Fioricet [logo]	Fioricet 50 mg/325 mg/40 mg	Sandoz Pharm
FIORINAL 78-103	CONTROLLED - SEE PAGE 220	
FIORINAL/SANDOZ	CONTROLLED - SEE PAGE 196	
FISONS 670	Intal 20 mg	Fisons Corp
FL	Pseudoephedrine 120 mg, Chlorpheniramine Maleate 8 mg	Ferndale
FL 0496	Phenylephrine 25 mg, Chlorpheniramine 8 mg, Pyrilamine 25 mg	Econolab
FL 1033	Belladonna, Phenobarbital, Ergotamine	Ferndale
FLAGYL 250	Flagyl 250 mg	Searle Pharm
FLAGYL/500	Flagyl 500 mg	Searle Pharm
FLINT 1	Choloxin 1 mg	Flint Labs
FLINT 2	Choloxin 2 mg	Flint Labs
FLINT 4	Choloxin 4 mg	Flint Labs
FLINT 6	Choloxin 6 mg	Flint Labs
FLINT 25	Synthroid 0.025 mg	Flint Labs
FLINT 50	Synthroid 0.05 mg	Flint Labs
FLINT 75	Synthroid 0.075 mg	Flint Labs
FLINT 88	Synthroid 0.088 mg	Flint Labs
FLINT 100	Synthroid 0.1 mg	Flint Labs
FLINT 112	Synthroid 0.112 mg	Flint Labs
FLINT 125	Synthroid 0.125 mg	Flint Labs
FLINT 150	Synthroid 0.15 mg	Flint Labs
FLINT 175	Synthroid 0.175 mg	Flint Labs
FLINT 200	Synthroid 0.2 mg	Flint Labs
FLINT 300	Synthroid 0.3 mg	Flint Labs
FLT	Bisacodyl 5 mg	C.B. Fleet
FOREST 100	Theophylline 100 mg	Forest Pharm
FOREST 150	Guaifenesin 200 mg	Forest Pharm
FOREST 200	Theophylline 200 mg	Forest Pharm
FOREST 245	Aminoacetic Acid 150 mg, Calcium Carbonate 300 mg	Forest Pharm
FOREST 251	Sulfamethoxazole 500 mg	Forest Pharm
FOREST 295	Potassium Iodide 135 mg, Niacinamide 25 mg	Forest Pharm
FOREST 300	Theophylline 300 mg	Forest Pharm
FOREST 346	Rauwolfia Serpentina 50 mg	Forest Pharm
FOREST 355	Pedameth 200 mg	Forest Pharm
FOREST 372	Feostat 100 mg	Forest Pharm
FOREST 452	Tetracycline HCl 250 mg	Forest Pharm
FOREST 536	Rauwolfia Serpentina 100 mg	Forest Pharm
FOREST 591	Dextromethorphan Hydrobromide 15 mg, Guaifenesin 100 mg	Forest
FOREST 610	CONTROLLED - SEE PAGE 224	
FOREST 610A	CONTROLLED - SEE PAGE 228	
FOREST 621	Hyoscamine Sulfate 0.125 mg	Forest Pharm
FOREST 624	Phenylpropanolamine 25 mg, Chlorpheniramine 4 mg, Acetaminophen 325 mg	Forest Pharm
FOREST 627	Phenylpropanolamine 37.5 mg, Chlorpheniramine 4 mg	Forest Pharm
FOREST 628	Dehist 8 mg/75 mg	Forest Pharm
FOREST 630	Acetaminophen 325 mg, Caffeine 40 mg, Butalbital 50 mg	Forest Pharm
FOREST 642	Theophylline 100 mg	Forest Pharm
FOREST 643	Theophylline 200 mg	Forest Pharm
FOREST 646	Theophylline 125 mg	Forest Pharm
FOREST 647	Theophylline 250 mg	Forest Pharm
FOREST 678	Butalbital 50 mg, Acetaminophen 500 mg, Caffeine 40 mg	Forest Pharm

Imprint	Ingredient/Brand Name	Manufacturer
FOREST 707	Sucrose and Starch	Forest Pharm
FOREST 708	Sucrose and Starch	Forest Pharm
FOREST 709	Sucrose and Starch	Forest Pharm
FOREST 1054	Racemethionine 200 mg	Forest Pharm
F P	Caffeine, Ephedrine	Unknown
FP [in diamond] 12463	Caffeine, Phenylpropanolamine	Unknown
FS [logo]	Temafloxacin Hydrochloride 600 mg	Abbott Labs
FULVICIN/352	Fulvicin 330 mg	Schering Corp
FULVICIN/654	Fulvicin 165 mg	Schering Corp
G00	Phenolphthalein 65 mg, Docusate Sodium 100 mg	G & W Labs
G01	Phenolphthalein 90 mg	G & W Labs
G-026	Piroxicam 10 mg	Par
G-027	Piroxicam 20 mg	Par
G-0104	Phenylpropanolamine 75 mg, Caramiphen Edisylate 40 mg	Pioneer
G 0506	Seragen 0.1 mg/25 mg/15 mg	Reid-Provident Labs
G1-LL	Vitamin Supplement	Lederle
G10C 2/879	CONTROLLED - SEE PAGE 195	
G11C 3/879	CONTROLLED - SEE PAGE 195	
G12C 4/879	CONTROLLED - SEE PAGE 194	
G20C 879	CONTROLLED - SEE PAGE 197	
G 30 30	Caffeine, Ephedrine	Unknown
G 41 879	Aminophylline 100 mg	Halsey Drug
G85C 879/2	CONTROLLED - SEE PAGE 198	
G86C 879/3	CONTROLLED - SEE PAGE 197	
G87C 879/4	CONTROLLED - SEE PAGE 198	
G88C 879	CONTROLLED - SEE PAGE 185 or 186	
G122C 879	CONTROLLED - SEE PAGE 211	
G 180 879	Chlorpheniramine 4 mg	Halsey Drug
G 283	Diphenhydramine 25 mg	Granutec
G 284	Diphenhydramine 25 mg, Pseudoephedrine 60 mg	Granutec
G292 Cold Cap	Phenylpropanolamine 75 mg, Chlorpheniramine 8 mg	Granutec
G 297	CONTROLLED - SEE PAGE 217	
G 302 879	Diphenhydramine 25 mg	Halsey Drug
G 303 879	Diphenhydramine 50 mg	Halsey Drug
G 324	CONTROLLED - SEE PAGE 216	
G 368 879	Folic Acid 1 mg	Halsey Drug
G383	Liquitussin Cold & Cough Liquigels	Granutec
G385	Liquitussin Severe Congestion Liquigels	Granutec
G 406 879	Hydrochlorothiazide 25 mg	Halsey Drug
G 407 879	Hydrochlorothiazide 50 mg	Halsey Drug
G468C 879	CONTROLLED - SEE PAGE 192	
G469C 879	CONTROLLED - SEE PAGE 193	
G 545 879	Prednisolone 5 mg	Halsey Drug
G 549 879	Prednisone 20 mg	Halsey Drug
G 587 879	Rauwolfia Serpentina 100 mg	Halsey Drug
G-600	Guaifenesin 600 mg	Trinity
G650C 879	CONTROLLED - SEE PAGE 206	
G 1063	Amitriptyline	Unknown
G 1140	Amitriptyline 150 mg	MD Pharm
G 1157	Spironolactone 25 mg	Bolar Pharm
G 1189 500	Chlorzoxazone 500 mg	Goldline
G 1481	Allopurinol 100 mg	Boots Labs
G 1482	Allopurinol 300 mg	Boots Labs
G 3717	CONTROLLED - SEE PAGE 227	
G 3718	CONTROLLED - SEE PAGE 227	
G 3719	CONTROLLED - SEE PAGE 227	

Imprint	Ingredient/Brand Name	Manufacturer
G 3720	CONTROLLED - SEE PAGE 227	
G 3721	CONTROLLED - SEE PAGE 227	
G 3722	CONTROLLED - SEE PAGE 225	
G 3723	Flurbiprofen 50 mg	Greenstone
G 3724	Flurbiprofen 100 mg	Greenstone
G 3725	Glyburide 1.25 mg	Greenstone
G 3726	Glyburide 2.5 mg	Greenstone
G 3727	Glyburide 5 mg	Greenstone
G 3740	Medroxyprogesterone Acetate 2.5 mg	Greenstone
G 3741	Medroxyprogesterone Acetate 5 mg	Greenstone
G 3742	Medroxyprogesterone Acetate 10 mg	Greenstone
G Antacid 3	Calcium Carbonate 311 mg, Magnesium Carbonate 232 mg	Granutec
GANTANOL-DS	Gantanol-DS 1000 mg	Roche Labs
GAS-X	Simethicone 125 mg	Sandoz
GAVISCON 1172 2/MARION	Gaviscon 160 mg/40 mg	Marion Labs
GAVISCON 1175/MARION	Gaviscon 80 mg/20 mg	Marion Labs
GBN/10	Baclofen 10 mg	Genpharm
GBN/20	Baclofen 20 mg	Genpharm
Geigy 02	Butazolidin 100 mg/100 mg/150 mg	Geigy Pharm
Geigy 11	Tofranil 25 mg	Geigy Pharm
Geigy/14	Butazolidin 100 mg	Geigy Pharm
Geigy 20	Tofranil-PM 75 mg	Geigy Pharm
Geigy 21	Tofranil 10 mg	Geigy Pharm
Geigy 22	Tofranil-PM 150 mg	Geigy Pharm
Geigy 23	Loiresal 10 mg	Geigy Pharm
GEIGY 27	Tegretol 200 mg	Geigy Pharm
Geigy/32	Tofranil 10 mg	Geigy Pharm
Geigy/33	Lioresal 20 mg	Geigy Pharm
GEIGY/35	Lopressor HCT 50 mg/25 mg	Geigy Pharm
Geigy 40	Tofranil-PM 100 mg	Geigy Pharm
Geigy/42	Constant-T 200 mg	Geigy Pharm
GEIGY 43	PBZ 50 mg	Geigy Pharm
GEIGY 44	Butazolidin 100 mg	Geigy Pharm
Geigy 45	Tofranil-PM 125 mg	Geigy Pharm
Geigy 47	Tegretol 100 mg	Geigy Pharm
GEIGY 48	PBZ-SR 100 mg	Geigy Pharm
GEIGY/51 51	Lopressor 50 mg	Geigy Pharm
GEIGY 52	Tegretol 100 mg	Geigy Pharm
GEIGY/53	Lopressor HCT 100 mg/25 mg	Geigy Pharm
Geigy/57	Constant-T 300 mg	Geigy Pharm
Geigy 67	Tegretol 200 mg	Geigy Pharm
GEIGY/71 71	Lopressor 100 mg	Geigy Pharm
Geigy 72	Brethine 2.5 mg	Geigy Pharm
GEIGY/73	Lopressor HCT 100 mg/50 mg	Geigy Pharm
Geigy 74	Tofranil 50 mg	Geigy Pharm
Geigy 105	Brethine 5 mg	Geigy Pharm
GEIGY/108	Lamprene 50 mg	Geigy Pharm
GEIGY/109	Lamprene 100 mg	Geigy Pharm
GEIGY 111	PBZ 25 mg	Geigy Pharm
GEIGY 117	PBZ 50 mg	Geigy Pharm
Geigy/136	Tofranil 50 mg	Geigy Pharm
Geigy/140	Tofranil 25 mg	Geigy Pharm
GEIGY 146	Ten-K 750 mg	Geigy Pharm
GEIGY DK	Clomipramine 10 mg	Geigy Pharm
GEIGY FH	Clomipramine 25 mg	Geigy Pharm
GEIGY FP	Phenylbutazone 100 mg	Geigy Pharm

Imprint	Ingredient/Brand Name	Manufacturer
GEIGY GM	Clofazimine 100 mg	Geigy Pharm
GEIGY LP	Clomipramine Hydrochlortide	Geigy Pharm
GG 1	Isosorbide Dinitrate 2.5 mg	Geneva
GG 2	Isosorbide Dinitrate 5 mg	Geneva
GG 4	CONTROLLED - SEE PAGE 186	
GG 8	Nylidrin 6 mg	Geneva
GG 11	Chlorthalidone 25 mg	Geneva
GG 12	Medroxyprogesterone 10 mg	Geneva
GG 13	Chlorthalidone 50 mg	Geneva
GG 14	Prednisolone 5 mg	Geneva
GG 15	Nylidrin 12 mg	Geneva
GG 18	Perphenazine 2 mg	Geneva
GG 21	Furosemide 20 mg	Geneva Pharm
GG 22	Pseudoephedrine 60 mg	Geneva
GG 24	Theophylline 130 mg, Ephedrine 25 mg, Hydroxyzine 10 mg	Geneva
GG 25	Trifed 2.5 mg/60 mg	Geneva
GG 26	Isosorbide Dinitrate 10 mg	Geneva
GG 27	Hydrochlorothiazide 50 mg	Geneva
GG 28	Hydrochlorothiazide 25 mg	Geneva
GG 30	Thioridazine 10 mg	Geneva
GG 31/15	Thioridazine 15 mg	Geneva
GG 31 25	Thioridazine 50 mg	Geneva
GG 32/25	Thioridazine 25 mg	Geneva
GG 33/50	Thioridazine 50 mg	Geneva
GG 34/100	Thioridazine 100 mg	Geneva
GG 35	Thioridazine 150 mg	Geneva
GG 36	Thioridazine 200 mg	Geneva
GG 37	Hydroxyzine 10 mg	Geneva
GG 38	Hydroxyzine HCL 25 mg	Geneva
GG 39	Hydroxyzine 50 mg	Geneva
GG 40	Amitriptyline 10 mg	Geneva
GG 41	Imipramine 10 mg	Geneva
GG 42	Imipramine 50 mg	Geneva
GG 44	Amitriptyline 25 mg	Geneva
GG 45	Dipyridamole 50 mg	Geneva
GG 47	Imipramine 25 mg	Geneva
GG 48	Pseudoephedrine 30 mg	Geneva
GG 49	Dipyridamole 25 mg	Geneva
GG 51/1	Trifluoperazine 1 mg	Geneva
GG 52	l-Thyroxin 0.1 mg	Geneva
GG 53/2	Trifluoperazine 2 mg	Geneva
GG 54	l-Thyroxin 0.2 mg	Geneva
GG 55/5	Trifluoperazine HCL 5 mg	Geneva
GG 56	Disopyramide Phosphate 100 mg	Geneva
GG 57	Disopyramide Phosphate 150 mg	Geneva
GG 58/10	Trifluoperazine HCL 10 mg	Geneva
GG 59	Allopurinol 100 mg	Geneva
GG 60	Allopurinol 300 mg	Geneva
GG 61	Chlorpropamide 100 mg	Geneva
GG 62	Sodium Fluoride 2.2 mg	Geneva
GG 63	Desipramine HCL 10 mg	Geneva
GG 64	Desipramine HCL 25 mg	Geneva
GG 65	Desipramine HCL 50 mg	Geneva
GG 66	CONTROLLED - SEE PAGE 193	
GG 67	CONTROLLED - SEE PAGE 203	
GG 68	CONTROLLED - SEE PAGE 211	

Imprint	Ingredient/Brand Name	Manufacturer
GG 71	Propranolol 10 mg	Geneva
GG 72	Propranolol 20 mg	Geneva
GG 73	Propranolol 40 mg	Geneva
GG 74	Propranolol 60 mg	Geneva
GG 75	Propranolol 80 mg	Geneva
GG 76	l-Thyroxin 0.3 mg	Geneva
GG 77	l-Thyroxin 0.15 mg	Geneva
GG 78	Methazolamide 25 mg	Geneva
GG 79	Prednisone 5 mg	Geneva
GG 80	Furosemide 80 mg	Geneva
GG 81	Clonidine 0.1 mg	Geneva
GG 82	Clonidine 0.2 mg	Geneva
GG 83	Clonidine 0.3 mg	Geneva
GG 84	Timolol Maleate 5 mg	Geneva
GG 85	Spironolactone 25 mg	Geneva
GG 89	Amoxapine 25 mg	Geneva
GG 90	Amoxapine 50 mg	Geneva
GG 92	CONTROLLED - SEE PAGE 189	
GG 93	CONTROLLED - SEE PAGE 193	
GG 94	Albuterol 2 mg	Geneva
GG 95	Spironolactone 25 mg, Hydrochlorothiazide 25 mg	Geneva
GG 97	Fluphenazine HCL 1 mg	Geneva
GG 100	CONTROLLED - SEE PAGE 201	
GG 101	Methocarbamol 750 mg	Geneva
GG 103	Metronidazole 250 mg	Geneva
GG 104	Methyldopa 125 mg	Geneva
GG 105	Haloperidol 0.5 mg	Geneva
GG 107	Perphenazine 4 mg	Geneva
GG 108	Perphenazine 8 mg	Geneva
GG 109	Perphenazine 16 mg	Geneva
GG 110	Chlorzoxazone 250 mg, Acetaminophen 300 mg	Geneva
GG 111	Methyldopa 250 mg	Geneva
GG 112	CONTROLLED - SEE PAGE 208	
GG 113	Metoclopramide 10 mg	Geneva
GG 114	Ergoloid Mesylates 1 mg	Geneva
GG 115	Ergoloid Mesylates 1 mg	Geneva
GG 116	Ergoloid Mesylates 0.5 mg	Geneva
GG 118	Phenylephrine 10 mg, Phenylpropanolamine 40 mg, Phenyltoloxamine 15 mg, Chloropheniramine 5 mg	Geneva
GG 119	CONTROLLED - SEE PAGE 196	
GG 121/4	CONTROLLED - SEE PAGE 195	
GG 122	Sulfasalazine 500 mg	Geneva
GG 123	Haloperidol 1 mg	Geneva
GG 124	Haloperidol 2 mg	Geneva
GG 125	Haloperidol 5 mg	Geneva
GG 126	Haloperidol 10 mg	Geneva
GG 127	Quinine Sulfate 260 mg	Geneva
GG 130	Aminophylline 100 mg	Geneva
GG 132	Verapamil 80 mg	Geneva
GG 133	Verapamil 120 mg	Geneva
GG 134	Haloperidol 20 mg	Geneva
GG 141	Meclizine 12.5 mg	Geneva
GG 142	Tolbutamide 500 mg	Geneva
GG 144	Chlorpropamide 250 mg	Geneva
GG 145	Dimenhydrinate 50 mg	Geneva
GG 150	CONTROLLED - SEE PAGE 196	

Imprint	Ingredient/Brand Name	Manufacturer
GG 151/3	CONTROLLED - SEE PAGE 198	
GG 153	Propranolol 40 mg, Hydrochlorothiazide 25 mg	Geneva
GG 154	Propranolol 80 mg, Hydrochlorothiazide 25 mg	Geneva
GG 155	Prednisone 20 mg	Geneva
GG 156	Prednisone 10 mg	Geneva
GG 157	Prednisone 50 mg	Geneva
GG 158	Sulfisoxazole 500 mg	Geneva
GG 159	Clemastine 1.34 mg	Geneva
GG 160	Clemastine 2.68 mg	Geneva
GG 161/4	CONTROLLED - SEE PAGE 198	
GG 162	CONTROLLED - SEE PAGE 227	
GG 163	CONTROLLED - SEE PAGE 227	
GG 165	Triamterene 37.5 mg, Hydrochlorothiazide 25 mg	Geneva
GG 166	Desipramine HCL 75 mg	Geneva
GG 167	Desipramine HCL 100 mg	Geneva
GG 168	Desipramine HCL 150 mg	Geneva
GG 172	Triamterene 75 mg, Hydrochlorothiazide 50 mg	Geneva
GG 174	Sulfamethoxazole 400 mg, Trimethoprim 80 mg	Geneva
GG 175	Sulfamethoxazole 800 mg, Trimethoprim 160 mg	Geneva
GG 180	Aminophylline 200 mg	Geneva
GG 181	Methazolamide 50 mg	Geneva
GG 182	Timolol Maleate 10 mg	Geneva
GG 183	Timolol Maleate 20 mg	Geneva
GG 184	Isoxsuprine 20 mg	Geneva
GG 185	CONTROLLED - SEE PAGE 198	
GG 190	Methocarbamol 500 mg	Geneva
GG 191	Amoxapine 100 mg	Geneva
GG 192	Amoxapine 150 mg	Geneva
GG 195	Metronidazole 500 mg	Geneva
GG 196	Chlorpheniramine 4 mg	Geneva
GG 197	Acetahexamide 250 mg	Geneva
GG 198	Acetohexamide 500 mg	Geneva
GG 199	Acetaminophen 325 mg	Geneva
GG 201	Furosemide 40 mg	Geneva
GG 213	Perphenazine 2 mg, Amitriptyline 10 mg	Geneva
GG 214	Perphenazine 2 mg, Amitriptyline 25 mg	Geneva
GG 215	Perphenazine 4 mg, Amitriptyline 10 mg	Geneva
GG 216	Perphenazine 4 mg, Amitriptyline 25 mg	Geneva
GG 217	Perphenazine 4 mg, Amitriptyline 50 mg	Geneva
GG 219	Methyldopa 250 mg, Hydrochlorothiazide 15 mg	Geneva
GG 220/3	CONTROLLED - SEE PAGE 195	
GG 224	Phenylpropanolamine 75 mg, Guaifenesin 400 mg	Geneva
GG 225	Promethazine 25 mg	Geneva
GG 227	Isosorbide Dinitrate 20 mg	Geneva
GG 229	Isosorbide Dinitrate 40 mg	Geneva
GG 234	Methylprednisolone 4 mg	Geneva
GG 235	Promethazine 50 mg	Geneva
GG 236	Sulindac 150 mg	Geneva
GG 237	Sulindac 200 mg	Geneva
GG 238	Glyburide 1.25 mg	Greenstone Labs
GG 239	Glyburide 2.5 mg	Greenstone Labs
GG 240	Glyburide 5.0 mg	Greenstone Labs
GG 242	Methyclothiazide 5 mg	Geneva
GG 243	Methyldopa 500 mg, Hydrochlorothiazide 30 mg	Geneva
GG 244	Methyclothiazide 2.5 mg	Geneva
GG 245	Minoxidil 10 mg	Geneva

Imprint	Ingredient/Brand Name	Manufacturer
GG 249	CONTROLLED - SEE PAGE 225	
GG 250	Quinidine Gluconate 324 mg	Geneva
GG 254	Fenoprofen Calcium 600 mg	Geneva
GG 255	Pseudoephedrine 120 mg, Dexbrompheniramine 6 mg	Geneva
GG 256	CONTROLLED - SEE PAGE 227	
GG 257	CONTROLLED - SEE PAGE 227	
GG 258	CONTROLLED - No Photo - Alprazolam 1.0 mg - Blue round tablet - DEA Schedule IV	Geneva
GG 259	Isosorbide Dinitrate 5 mg	Geneva
GG 261	Meclizine 25 mg	Geneva
GG 263	Atenolol 50 mg	Geneva
GG 264	Atenolol 100 mg	Geneva
GG 265	Methyldopa 250 mg, Hydrochlorothiazide 25 mg	Geneva
GG 270	Tolazamide 100 mg	Geneva
GG 271	Tolazamide 250 mg	Geneva
GG 272	Tolazamide 500 mg	Geneva
GG 274	Isoxsuprine 10 mg	Geneva
GG 284	Isoxsuprine 10 mg	Geneva
GG 285	Quinidine Sulfate 3 grains	Geneva
GG 286	Quinidine Sulfate 300 mg	Geneva
GG 288	Cyclobenzaprine 10 mg	Geneva
GG 289	Methyldopa 500 mg, Hydrochlorothiazide 50 mg	Geneva
GG 291	Ibuprofen 400 mg	Geneva
GG 292	Ibuprofen 600 mg	Geneva
GG 293	Ibuprofen 200 mg	Invamed Inc.
GG 294	Ibuprofen 800 mg	Geneva
GG 295	Albuterol 4 mg	Geneva
GG 405	Acetaminophen 500 mg	Geneva
GG 407/50	Chlorpromazine HCL 50 mg	Geneva
GG 411	Carisoprodol 350 mg	Geneva
GG 414	Metoprolol Tartrate 50 mg	Geneva
GG 415	Metoprolol Tartrate 100 mg	Geneva
GG 416	Hydralazine 50 mg	Geneva
GG 417	Naproxen Sodium 275 mg	Geneva
GG 418	Naproxen Sodium 550 mg	Geneva
GG 419	Trazodone 50 mg	Geneva
GG 420	Trazodone 100 mg	Geneva
GG 421	Chlorzoxazone 250 mg	Geneva
GG 422	Chlorzoxazone 500 mg	Geneva
GG 431	Amitriptyline 50 mg	Geneva
GG 432	Conjugated Estrogens 0.3 mg	Geneva
GG 433	Conjugated Estrogens 0.625 mg	Geneva
GG 434	Conjugated Estrogens 1.25 mg	Geneva
GG 435	Conjugated Estrogens 2.5 mg	Geneva
GG 436	Nystatin Oral 500,000 units	Eon Labs
GG 437/100	Chlorpromazine HCL100 mg	Geneva
GG438	Pindolol 5 mg	Geneva
GG 439	Pindolol 10 mg	Geneva
GG 441	Vitamins, Fluoride	Geneva
GG 444	Pseudoephedrine 120 mg, Dexbrompheniramine 6 mg	Geneva
GG 447	Phenylpropanolamine 75 mg, Brompheniramine Sulfate 12 mg	Geneva
GG 450	Amitriptyline 150 mg	Geneva
GG 451	Amitriptyline 75 mg	Geneva
GG 455/10	Chlorpromazine HCL 10 mg	Geneva
GG 457/200	Chlorpromazine HCL 200 mg	Geneva
GG 458	Acetaminophen 500 mg	Geneva

Imprint	Ingredient/Brand Name	Manufacturer
GG 459	Acetaminophen 325 mg	Geneva
GG 461	Amitriptyline 100 mg	Geneva
GG 464	Dipyridamole	Geneva
GG 471	Methyldopa 500 mg	Geneva
GG 472	Procainamide 250 mg	Geneva
GG 473	Procainamide 500 mg	Geneva
GG 474	Procainamide 750 mg	Geneva
GG 475	Hydralazine 10 mg	Geneva
GG 476/25	Chlorpromazine HCL 25 mg	Geneva
GG 477	Tamine 12 mg/75 mg	Geneva
GG 480	Vitamins, Zinc	Geneva
GG 481	Vitamins	Geneva
GG 485	Hydralazine 25 mg	Geneva
GG 487	Probenecid 500 mg, Colchicine 0.5 mg	Geneva
GG 488	Fluphenazine HCL 2..5 mg	Geneva
GG 489	Fluphenazine HCL 5 mg	Geneva
GG 490	Fluphenazine HCL 10 mg	Geneva
GG 500	Acetaminophen 500 mg	Geneva
GG 501	Nitroglycerin 6.5 mg	Geneva
GG 502	Resaid 75 mg/12 mg	Geneva
GG 503	Papaverine 150 mg	Geneva
GG 505	CONTROLLED - SEE PAGE 213	
GG 506	CONTROLLED - SEE PAGE 213	
GG 507	CONTROLLED - SEE PAGE 213	
GG 511	Nitroglycerin 2.5 mg	Geneva
GG 512	Nitroglycerin 9 mg	Geneva
GG 515	Quinine Sulfate 5 grains	Geneva
GG 517	Indomethacin 25 mg	Geneva
GG 518	Indomethacin 50 mg	Geneva
GG 524	Meclofenamate 50 mg	Geneva
GG 525	Meclofenamate 100 mg	Geneva
GG 527	Prednisone 50 mg	Geneva
GG 530	Loperamide 2 mg	Geneva
GG 531	CONTROLLED - SEE PAGE 220	
GG 532	CONTROLLED - SEE PAGE 213	
GG 533	Diphenhydramine 25 mg	Geneva
GG 535	Nitrofurantoin 50 mg	Geneva
GG 536	Nitrofurantoin 100 mg	Geneva
GG 538	Nitrofurantoin 25 mg	Geneva
GG 541	Diphenhydramine 50 mg	Geneva
GG 551	Procainamide 250 mg	Geneva
GG 552	Procainamide 375 mg	Geneva
GG 553	Procainamide 500 mg	Geneva
GG 554	Niacin 125 mg	Geneva
GG 555	Cephalexin 500 mg	Geneva
GG 556	Cephalexin 250 mg	Geneva
GG 558	Fenoprofen Calcium 200 mg	Geneva
GG 559	Fenoprofen Calcium 300 mg	Geneva
GG 564	Niacin 250 mg	Geneva
GG 565	Nortriptyline 10 mg	Geneva
GG 566	Nortriptyline 25 mg	Geneva
GG 567	Nortriptyline 50 mg	Geneva
GG 568	Nortriptyline 75 mg	Geneva
GG 570	Chlorpheniramine 8 mg	Geneva
GG 571	Clinoxide 2.5 mg/5 mg	Geneva
GG 572	Doxepin HCL 25 mg	Geneva

Imprint	Ingredient/Brand Name	Manufacturer
GG 573	Doxepin HCL 50 mg	Geneva
GG 574	Doxepin HCL 75 mg	Geneva
GG 576	Doxepin HCL 10 mg	Geneva
GG 577	Doxepin HCL 100 mg	Geneva
GG 580	Triamterene 50 mg, Hydrochlorothiazide 25 mg	Geneva
GG 581	CONTROLLED - SEE PAGE 222	
GG 582	Hydroxyzine Pamoate 25 mg	Geneva
GG 583	Hydroxyzine 50 mg	Geneva
GG 584	Hydroxyzine Pamoate 100 mg	Geneva
GG 589	Thiothixene 1 mg	Geneva
GG 590	Chlorpheniramine 12 mg	Geneva
GG 591	CONTROLLED - SEE PAGE 215	
GG 592	Prazosin 1 mg	Geneva
GG 593	Prazosin 2 mg	Geneva
GG 594	Prazosin 5 mg	Geneva
GG 596	Thiothixene 2 mg	Geneva
GG 597	Thiothixene 5 mg	Geneva
GG 598	Thiothixene 10 mg	Geneva
GG 606	Triamterene 37.5, Hydrochlorothiazide 25 mg	Penn Labs
GG724	Naproxen 250 mg	Geneva
GG725	Naproxen 375 mg	Geneva
GG726	Naproxen 500 mg	Geneva
GG 733	Salsalate 500 mg	Geneva
GG 734	Salsalate 750 mg	Geneva
GG 735	Flurbiprofen 50 mg	Greenstone Labs
GG 736	Flurbiprofen 100 mg	Greenstone Labs
GG 1343	Reserpine 0.1 mg, Hydralazine 25 mg, Hydrochlorothiazide 15 mg	Geneva
GG 9533	Mudrane GG-2 130 mg/100 mg	Geneva
GG L7	Atenolol 25 mg	Geneva
GL/535-11	ESGIC 50 mg/325 mg/40 mg	Forest Pharm
GL/535-12	ESGIC 50 mg/325 mg/40 mg	Forest Pharm
Glaxo 268	Theobid 260 mg	Glaxo Inc
Glaxo/281	Ethatab 100 mg	Glaxo Inc
Glaxo 295	Theobid JR 130 mg	Glaxo Inc
Glaxo 309	Histabid 75 mg/8 mg	Glaxo Inc
Glaxo 316	Vicon Forte	Glaxo Inc
Glaxo/371	Trandate HCT 100 mg/25 mg	Glaxo Inc
Glaxo/372	Trandate HCT 200 mg/25 mg	Glaxo Inc
Glaxo/373	Trandate HCT 300 mg/25 mg	Glaxo Inc
GLAXO/378	Ceftin 250 mg	Glaxo Inc
GLAXO/387	Ceftin 250 mg	Glaxo Inc
GLAXO/394	Ceftin 500 mg	Glaxo Inc
GLAXO/395	Ceftin 125 mg	Glaxo Inc
GLAXO AMESEC	Amesec 130 mg/25 mg	Glaxo Inc
GLAXO TRINSICON	Trinsicon	Glaxo Inc
GLAXO TRINSICON-M	Trinsicon-M	Glaxo Inc
Glaxo/VENTOLIN 2	Ventolin 2 mg	Glaxo Inc
Glaxo/VENTOLIN 4	Ventolin 4 mg	Glaxo Inc
Glaxo/ZANTAC 150	Zantac 150 mg	Glaxo Inc
Glaxo/ZANTAC 300	Zantac 300 mg	Glaxo Inc
GLUTOFAC	Vitamins	Kenwood Labs
GN	Sennosides 20 mg	Sandoz
Goody's	Acetaminophen 130 mg, Aspirin 260 mg, Caffeine 16 mg	DeWitt Corp
G/P 5	Pindolol 5 mg	Par
G/P 10	Pindolol 10 mg	Par

Imprint	Ingredient/Brand Name	Manufacturer
GRISACTIN 125	Grisactin 125 mg	Ayerst Labs
GRISACTIN 250	Grisactin 250 mg	Ayerst Labs
GRISACTIN/500	Grisactin 500 mg	Ayerst Labs
GRISACTIN ULTRA 125	Grisactin Ultra 125 mg	Ayerst Labs
GRISACTIN ULTRA 250	Grisactin Ultra 250 mg	Ayerst Labs
GRISACTIN ULTRA 330	Grisactin Ultra 330 mg	Ayerst Labs
GTN/10	Tamoxifen Citrate 10 mg	Genpharm
GTN/20	Tamoxifen Citrate 20 mg	Genpharm
GUAIMAX-D	Pseudoephedrine 120 mg, Guaifenesin 600 mg	Central Pharm
GW0402	Senna Gloycosides 8.6 mg	G & W Labs
H 09	Erythromycin 250 mg	Eli Lilly
H1	Acetaminophen 325 mg	Hall Labs
H2	Acetaminophen 500 mg	Hall Labs
H3	Acetaminophen 80 mg	Hall Labs
H4	Acetaminophen 250 mg, Aspirin 250 mg, Caffeine 65 mg	Hall Labs
H5	Calcium Carbonate 500 mg	Hall Labs
H7	Calcium Carbonate 750 mg	Hall Labs
H8	Acetaminophen 500 mg, Diphenhydramine 25 mg	Hall Labs
H9	Caffeine 100 mg	Hall Labs
H 10	Vitamins	Eli Lilly
H 17	Nortriptyline 10 mg	Eli Lilly
H 17	Hydroxyzine 10 mg	Lederle Labs
H 18	Hygroton 50 mg	USV Labs
H 18	Hydroxyzine 25 mg	Lederle Labs
H 19	Nortriptylline 25 mg	Eli Lilly
H 19	Hygroton 25 mg	USV Labs
H 20	Chlorthalidone 50 mg	Rorer
H 22	Chlorthalidone 25 mg	Rorer
H 69	Cephalexin 250 mg	Eli Lilly
H 71	Cephalexin 500 mg	Eli Lilly
H 72	Vitamins	Eli Lilly
H 74	Ethinamate 500 mg	Eli Lilly
H 76	Fenoprofen Calcium 200 mg	Eli Lilly
H 77	Fenoprofen Calcium 300 mg	Eli Lilly
H111	Hyoscyamine .15 mg	Econolab
H 124	Hydrochlorothiazide 50 mg	Heather Drug
H 174	levo-Thyroxine 0.1 mg	Heather Drug
H 175	levo-Thyroxine 0.2 mg	Heather Drug
H 187	Prednisolone 5 mg	Heather Drug
H 188	Papaverine 150 mg	Heather Drug
H 189	Prednisone 5 mg	Heather Drug
H 193	Methocarbamol 500 mg	Heather Drug
H 196	Methenamine 500 mg	Heather Drug
H 202	Sulfisoxazole 500 mg	Heather Drug
H 203	Tetracycline 500 mg	Heather Drug
H 209	Thyroid 1 grain	Heather Drug
H 212	Thyroid 2 grains	Heather Drug
H 214	Tetracycline 250 mg	Heather Drug
H 309	Thyroid 60 mg	Heather Drug
H 403	Sulfamethoxazole 500 mg	Heather Drug
H 501	Methocarbamol 750 mg	Heather Drug
H 503	Methenamine 1000 mg	Heather Drug
H 505	Prednisone 10 mg	Heather Drug
H 506	Prednisone 20 mg	Heather Drug
H 510	Methylprednisolone 4 mg	Heather Drug
H 513	Cortisone Acetate 25 mg	Heather Drug

Imprint	Ingredient/Brand Name	Manufacturer
H 527	Prednisone 50 mg	Heather Drug
H 531	Furosemide 40 mg	Heather Drug
H 532	Furosemide 20 mg	Heather Drug
H 534	Sulfamethoxazole 400 mg, Trimethoprim 80 mg	Heather Drug
H 535	Sulfamethoxazole 800 mg, Trimethoprim 160 mg	Heather Drug
H 538	Doxycycline 100 mg	Heather Drug
H 539	Doxycycline 100 mg	Heather Drug
H 540	Doxycycline 50 mg	Heather Drug
HALCION 0.125	CONTROLLED - SEE PAGE 199	
HALCION 0.25	CONTROLLED - SEE PAGE 211	
HALDOL 1/2	Haldol 0.5 mg	McNeil Pharm
HALDOL 1	Haldol 1 mg	McNeil Pharm
HALDOL 2	Haldol 2 mg	McNeil Pharm
HALDOL 5	Haldol 5 mg	McNeil Pharm
HALDOL 10	Haldol 10 mg	McNeil Pharm
HALDOL 20	Haldol 20 mg	McNeil Pharm
Halodrin 38	Halodrin 0.02 mg, 1 mg	Upjohn
HALOTESTIN 2	CONTROLLED - SEE PAGE 202	
HALOTESTIN 5	CONTROLLED - SEE PAGE 211	
HALOTESTIN 10	CONTROLLED - SEE PAGE 212	
Hauck 077	Chlorpheniramine 8 mg, Pseudoephedrine 100 mg	Unknown
HAUCK 258	CONTROLLED - SEE PAGE 200	
HD 0656	Chlordiazepoxide 5 mg, Clidiinium Bromide 2.5 mg	Halsey Drug Co
HD 4	CONTROLLED - No Photo - Meperidine HCl 50 mg - DEA Schedule II	Halsey Drug Co
HD 5	CONTROLLED - No Photo - Meperidine HCl 100 mg - DEA Schedule II	Halsey Drug Co
HD 125	Digoxin 0.125 mg	Halsey Drug Co
HD 157	Quinine Sulfate 325 mg	Halsey Drug Co
HD 250	Digoxin 0.25 mg	Halsey Drug Co
HD 405	Amitriptyline 10 mg	Halsey Drug Co
HD 406	Amitriptyline 25 mg	Halsey Drug Co
HD 407	Amitriptyline 50 mg	Halsey Drug Co
HD 408	Amitriptyline 75 mg	Halsey Drug Co
HD 409	Amitriptyline 100 mg	Halsey Drug Co
HD 467	Dipyridamole 75 mg	Halsey Drug Co
HD 479	Dipyridamole 50 mg	Halsey Drug Co
HD 494	Dipyridamole 25 mg	Halsey Drug Co
HD 503	Chlorpropamide 250 mg	Halsey Drug Co
HD 506	Metronidazole 250 mg	Halsey Drug Co
HD 507	Indomethacin 25 mg	Halsey Drug Co
HD 508	Indomethacin 50 mg	Halsey Drug Co
HD 512	CONTROLLED - No Photo - Oxycodone 5 mg, Acetaminophen 325 mg - DEA Schedule II	Halsey Drug Co
HD 522	Chlorpropamide 100 mg	Halsey Drug Co
HD 532	CONTROLLED - SEE PAGE 222	
HD 533	CONTROLLED - SEE PAGE 217	
HD 534	CONTROLLED - SEE PAGE 219	
HD 535	Hydralazine 10 mg	Halsey Drug Co
HD 536	Hydralazine 25 mg	Halsey Drug Co
HD 537	Hydralazine 50 mg	Halsey Drug Co
HD 538	Hydralazine 100 mg	Halsey Drug Co
HD 540	Metronidazole 500 mg	Halsey Drug Co
HD 543	Butalbital 50 mg, Acetaminophen 325 mg	Halsey Drug Co
HD 544/5	CONTROLLED - SEE PAGE 205	
HD 546/2	CONTROLLED - SEE PAGE 191	

Imprint	Ingredient/Brand Name	Manufacturer
HD 549/10	CONTROLLED - SEE PAGE 209	
HD 550	CONTROLLED - SEE PAGE 197	
HD 557	Ibuprofen 200 mg	Halsey Drug Co
HD 559	Ibuprofen 400 mg	Halsey Drug Co
HD 560	Ibuprofen 600 mg	Halsey Drug Co
HD 561	Metoclopramide 10 mg	Halsey Drug Co
HD 562	Brompheniramine 4 mg	Halsey Drug Co
HD 565/0.5	CONTROLLED - SEE PAGE 186	
HD 572/1	CONTROLLED - SEE PAGE 187	
HD 573/2	CONTROLLED - SEE PAGE 192	
HD 574	CONTROLLED - SEE PAGE 201	
HD 581	Acetaminophen 500 mg	Halsey Drug Co
HD 582	Quinidine 324 mg	Halsey Drug Co
HD 606	Methyldopa 125 mg	Halsey Drug Co
HD 607	Methyldopa 250 mg	Halsey Drug Co
HD 608	Methyldopa 500 mg	Halsey Drug Co
HD 715/2	CONTROLLED - SEE PAGE 187	
HD 717/4	CONTROLLED - SEE PAGE 188	
HD 724	Doxycycline Hyclate 50 mg	Halsey Drug Co
HD 725	Doxycycline 100 mg	Houba Inc.
HH [logo]	Depakene 250 mg	Abbott Labs
HLT 41	Trimeprazine Tartrate 2.5 mg	Forest
HLT 50	Trimeprazine Tartrate 5 mg	Forest
HOECHST 70	Festal	Hoechst-Roussel Pharm
HOECHST 71	Festalan	Hoechst-Roussel Pharm
HOECHST 72	Festal II	Hoechst-Roussel Pharm
HOECHST 73	Festalan 1 mg	Hoechst-Roussel Pharm
HOECHST/LASIX	Lasix 20 mg	Hoechst-Roussel Pharm
HOPE 742	Atropine Sulfate 0.4 mg	Hope Pharm
HORNER 200 mg	Ibuprofen 200 mg	Horner
HORNER 300 mg	Ibuprofen 300 mg	Horner
HORNER 400 mg	Ibuprofen 400 mg	Horner
hoyt	Luride	Colgate-Hoyt Labs
Hoyt 006	Luride 1 mg	Colgate-Hoyt Labs
Hoyt 007	Luride 1 mg	Colgate-Hoyt Labs
Hoyt 013	Luride 0.5 mg	Colgate-Hoyt Labs
Hoyt 014	Luride 0.5 mg	Colgate-Hoyt Labs
Hoyt 140	Sodium Fluoride 1 mg	Colgate-Hoyt Labs
Hoyt 141	Sodium Fluoride 1 mg	Colgate-Hoyt Labs
Hoyt 142	Sodium Fluoride 1 mg	Colgate-Hoyt Labs
Hoyt 186	Sodium Fluoride 0.25 mg	Colgate-Hoyt Labs
HPC 30	Caffeine, Pseudoephedrine	Unknown
HR	Ephedrine	Unkniwn
HR 200	Caffeine, Ephedrine, Phenylpropanolamine	Unknown
H.R J.S	Caffeine, Ephedrine	Unknown
HS ALLEREST	Allerest Headache Strength	CIBA
HTI/76	Thalitone 25 mg	Horus Theraputics
HTI/77	Thalitone 15 mg	Horus Theraputics
Hy	Hytuss 100 mg	Hyrex Pharm
HY 408	Trac 2X 0.06 mg/0.03 mg/120 mg/30 mg	Hyrex Pharm
HYCODAN/DuPont	CONTROLLED - SEE PAGE 190	
HYCOMINE/DuPont	CONTROLLED - SEE PAGE 207	
Hydrogesic [logo]	CONTROLLED - SEE PAGE 214	
HYDERGINE 0.5	Hydergine 0.5 mg	Sandoz Pharm
HYDERGINE 1	Hydergine 1 mg	Sandoz Pharm
HYDERGINE/78-77	Mydergine 1 mg	Sandoz Pharm

Imprint	Ingredient/Brand Name	Manufacturer
HYDERGINE LC 1mg	Hydergine 1 mg	Sandoz Pharm
HYLOREL 10	Hylorel 10 mg	Pennwalt Corp
HYLOREL 25	Hylorel 25 mg	Pennwalt Corp
HyPam 0093	Hydroxyzine 25 mg	Lemmmon Pharm
HyPam 0093	Hydroxyzine 50 mg	Lemmon Pharm
HY-PAM 331	Hydroxyzine	Unknown
Hyrex	Hytuss 2X 200 mg	Hyrex Pharm
I	Isorbid 5 mg	Ives Labs
I-2	Ibuprofen 200 mg	Perrigo
I 67	Carbinoxamine Maleate 8 mg, Pseudoephedrine 120 mg	Econolab
IA [logo]	Cartedol 2.5 mg	Abbott
IBU 400	Ibuprofen 400 mg	Boots Labs
IBU 600	Ibuprofen 600 mg	Boots Labs
IBU 800	Ibuprofen 800 mg	Boots Labs
IB2	Ibuprofen 200 mg	Par Pharm
IC	Carteolol 5 mg	Abbott
ICI/101	Tenormin 100 mg	ICI Pharm
ICI/105	Atenolol 50 mg	ICI Pharm
ICI/115	Tenoretic 50 mg/25 mg	ICI Pharm
ICI/117	Tenoretic 100 mg/25 mg	ICI Pharm
ICN 0901	CONTROLLED - SEE PAGE 216	
ICN 60	Pyridostigmine Bromide 60 mg	ICN Pharm
ICN 303	Trioxsalen 5 mg	ICN Pharm
ICN/499	CONTROLLED - SEE PAGE 203	
ICN 650	Methoxsalen 10 mg	ICN Pharm
ICN M180	Mestinon Timespan 15 mg	ICN Pharm
ICN PROSTIGMIN	Neostigmine Bromide 15 mg	ICN Pharm
I/Inderal 10	Inderal 10 mg	Ayerst Labs
I/INDERAL 20	Inderal 20 mg	Ayerst Labs
I/INDERAL 40	Inderal 40 mg	Ayerst Labs
I/INDERAL 60	Inderal 60 mg	Ayerst Labs
I/INDERAL 80	Inderal 80 mg	Ayerst Labs
I/INDERAL 90	Inderal 90 mg	Ayerst Labs
I/INDERIDE 40 25	Inderide 40 mg/25 mg	Ayerst Labs
I/INDERIDE 80 50	Inderide 80 mg/50 mg	Ayerst Labs
II [logo]	Phenurone 500 mg	Abbott Labs
IL 3549	Isosorbide Dinitrate 40 mg	Inwood Labs
IL 3575	Isosorbide Dinitrate 40 mg	Inwood Labs
IL 3577	Pentaerythritol Tetranitrate 80 mg	Inwood Labs
IL 3581	Theochron 300 mg	Inwood Labs
IL 3583	Theochron 200 mg	Inwood Labs
IL 3584	Theochron 100 mg	Inwood Labs
IL 3587	Carbamazepine 200 mg	Inwood Labs
IL 3607	Indomethacin 75 mg	Inwood Labs
IL 3609	Propranolol 60 mg	Inwood Labs
IL 3610	Propranolol 80 mg	Inwood Labs
IL 3611	Propranolol 120 mg	Inwood Labs
IL 3612	Propranolol 160 mg	Inwood Labs
IMDUR/60	Isosorbide Mononitrate 60 mg	Schering Corp.
IMODIUM AD 2MG	Loperamide HCl 2 mg	McNeil
IMU RAN 50	Azathioprine 50 mg	Burroughs Wellcom
INDERAL/10	Inderal 10 mg	Ayerst Labs
INDERAL/20	Inderal 20 mg	Ayerst Labs
INDERAL/40	Inderal 40 mg	Ayerst Labs
INDERAL 80	Inderal 80 mg	Ayerst Labs
INDERAL LA 60	Inderal LA 60 mg	Ayerst Labs

Imprint	Ingredient/Brand Name	Manufacturer
INDERAL LA 80	Inderal LA 80 mg	Ayerst Labs
INDERAL LA 120	Inderal LA 120 mg	Ayerst Labs
INDERAL LA 160	Inderal LA 160 mg	Ayerst Labs
INDERIDE 80 25/I	Inderide 80 mg/25 mg	Ayerst Labs
INDERIDE 80 50	Inderide LA 80 mg/50 mg	Ayerst Labs
INDERIDE 120 50	Inderide LA 120 mg/50 mg	Ayerst Labs
INDERIDE 160 50	Inderide LA 160 mg/50 mg	Ayerst Labs
INV 101	Aluminum Hydroxide 80 mg, Magnesium Trisilicate 20 mg	Invamed
INV 102	Aluminum Hydroxide 200 mg, Magnesium Hydroxide 200 mg, Simethicone 25 mg	Invamed Labs
INV 103	Simethicone 80 mg	Invamed Labs
INV 119	Aluminum Hydroxide 475 mg	Invamed Labs
INV 122	Aluminum Hydroxide 200 mg, Magnesium Hydroxide 200 mg, Simethicone 20 mg	Invamed Labs
INV 123	Simethicone 40 mg	Invamed Labs
INV 138	Aspirin 500 mg, Aluminum Hydroxide 150 mg, Magnesium Oxide 150 mg	Invamed Labs
INV 139	Aluminum Hydroxide 400 mg, Magnesium Oxide 400 mg, Simethicone 30 mg	Invamed Labs
INV 140	Aspirin 325 mg, Aluminum Hydroxide 75 mg, Magnesium Hydroxide 75 mg	Invamed Labs
INV 141	Aspirin 325 mg, Aluminum Hydroxide 75 mg, Magnesium Hydroxide 75 mg	Invamed Labs
INV 148	Aluminum Hydroxide 160 mg, Magnesium Trisilicate 105 mg	Invamed
INV 150	Bismuth Subsalicylate 262 mg	Invamed
INV 201	Procainamide 500 mg	Invamed Labs
INV 205	Methyldopa 250 mg, Hydrochlorothiazide 15	Invamed Labs
INV 206	Methyldopa 250 mg, Hydrochlorothiazide 25 mg	Invamed Labs
INV 207	Metoclopramide 10 mg	Invamed Labs
INV 208	Benztropine Mesylate 0.5 mg	Invamed Labs
INV 209	Benztropine Mesylate 1 mg	Invamed Labs
INV 210	Benztropine Mesylate 2 mg	Invamed Labs
INV 211	Amantadine 100 mg	Invamed Labs
INV 220	Aspirin 975 mg	Invamed Labs
INV 223	Ibuprofen 400 mg	Invamed Labs
INV 224	Ibuprofen 600 mg	Invamed Labs
INV 225	Ibuprofen 800 mg	Invamed Labs
INV 227	Metoclopramide 5 mg	Invamed Labs
INV 232	Sloprin 800 mg	Invamed Labs
INV 234	Phenylephrine 25 mg, Chlorpheniramine 8 mg, Pyrilamine 25 mg	Invamed Labs
INV 241	Tricosal 500 mg	Duramed Pharm
INV 242	Tricosal 750 mg	Duramed Pharm
INV 245	Quinine Sulfate 162.5 mg	Invamed labs
INV 252	Cyclobenzaprine 10 mg	Duramed Pharm
INV 256	Atenolol 50 mg	Duramed Pharm
INV 257	Atenolol 100 mg	Duramed Pharm
INV 259	Atenolol 25 mg	Duramed Pharm
INV 296	Salsalate 500 mg	Invamed Labs
INV 297	Salsalate 750 mg	Invamed Labs
IONAMIN 15	CONTROLLED - SEE PAGE 222	
IONAMIN 30	CONTROLLED - SEE PAGE 215	
IP 001	Acetaminophen 500 mg	Interpharm
IP 011	Acetaminophen 325 mg	Interpharm
IP 018	Acetaminophen 500 mg	Interpharm
IP 029	Aspirin 800 mg	Interpharm

Imprint	Ingredient/Brand Name	Manufacturer
IP 037	Chlorpheniramine Maleate 4 mg	Interpharm
IP 050	Acetaminophen 325 mg, Pseudoephedrine 30 mg	Interpharm
IP 064	Diphenhydramine 25 mg	Interpharm
IP 96	Phenylpropanolamine 75 mg, Guaifenesin 400 mg	Interpharm
IP 131/400	Ibuprofen 400 mg	Interpharm
IP 132/600	Ibuprofen 600 mg	Interpharm
IP/135	Ibuprofen 200 mg	Interpharm
IP 136	Isomethoptane Mucate 65 mg, Dichloralphenazone 100 mg, Acetaminophen 325 mg	Interpharm
IP 137/800	Ibuprofen 800 mg	Interpharm
IP 138/200	Ibuprofen 200 mg	Interpharm
IP 141	Acetaminophen 325 mg, Dichloralphenaxzone 100 mg, Isometheptene Mucate 65 mg	Interpharm
IP 175	Metoclopramide 10 mg	Interpharm
IP 221	Pseudoephedrine 60 mg	Interpharm
IP 251	Quinine Sulfate 260 mg	Interpharm
IP 274	Simethecone 80 mg	Interpharm
IP 276	Salsalate 500 mg	Interpharm
IP 277	Salsalate 750 mg	Interpharm
IP 288	Triprolidine 2.5 mg, Pseudoephedrine 60 mg	Interpharm
IRCON	Ferrous Fumarate 200 mg	Kenwood Labs
IRCON FA	Ferrous Fumarate 200 mg	Kenwood Labs
ISMO 20W	ISMO 20 mg	Wyeth-Ayerst
Isoclor	Pseudoephedrine 60 mg, Chlorpheniramine 4 mg	Fisons
ISOPTIN 80 KNOLL	Isoptin 80 mg	Knoll Pharm
ISOPTIN 120 KNOLL	Isoptin 120 mg	Knoll Pharm
ISOPTIN SR/[triangles]	Isoptin SR 240 mg	Key Pharm
ISOPTIN SR 180 mg	Isoptin SR 180 mg	Knoll Pharm
Ives	Isordil 10 mg	Ives Labs
Ives 4120	Cyclospasmol 100 mg	Ives Labs
Ives 4124	Cyclospasmol 200 mg	Ives Labs
Ives 4125	Isordil 40 mg	Ives Labs
Ives 4132	Surmontil 25 mg	Ives Labs
Ives 4133	Surmontil 50 mg	Ives Labs
Ives 4140	Isordil 40 mg	Ives Labs
Ives 4148	Cyclospasmol 400 mg	Ives Labs
Ives 4152	Isordil 5 mg	Ives Labs
Ives 4153	Isordil 10 mg	Ives Labs
Ives 4154	Isordil 20 mg	Ives Labs
Ives 4158	Surmontil 100 mg	Ives Labs
Ives 4159	Isordil 30 mg	Ives Labs
Ives 4164	Isordil 10 mg	Ives Labs
Ives 4177	Sectral 200 mg	Ives Labs
Ives 4179	Sectral 400 mg	Ives Labs
J 02	Atropine Sulfate 0.4 mg	Eli Lilly
J 13	Colchicine 0.6 mg	Eli Lilly
J 20	Quinidine Sulfate 200 mg	Eli Lilly
J 25	Thyroid 60 mg	Eli Lilly
J 26	Thyroid 120 mg	Eli Lilly
J 29	Thyroid 30 mg	Eli Lilly
J 36	Ergonovine Maleate 0.2 mg	Eli Lilly
J 52	Diethylstilbestrol 1 mg	Eli Lilly
J 54	Diethylstilbestrol 5 mg	Eli Lilly
J 60	Digitoxin 0.1 mg	Eli Lilly
J 61	Papaverine 30 mg	Eli Lilly
J 62	Papaverine 60 mg	Eli Lilly

Imprint	Ingredient/Brand Name	Manufacturer
J 69	Propylthiouracil 50 mg	Eli Lilly
J 75	Digitoxin 0.05 mg	Eli Lilly
J 75/BREON	Isoproterenol 10 mg	Winthrop
J 76	Digitoxin 0.15 mg	Eli Lilly
J 77/BREON	Isoproterenol 15 mg	Winthrop
J 94	Methimazole	Eli Lilly
J 95	Methimazole 10 mg	Eli Lilly
Jacobus 101	Dapsone 100 mg	Jacobus Pharm
Jacobus 102	Dapsone 25 mg	Jacobus Pharm
JANSSEN/AST 10	Astemizole 10 mg	Janssen Pharm
JANSSEN IMODIUM	Imodium 2 mg	Janssen Pharm
JANSSEN L50	Levamisole 50 mg	Janssen Pharm
JANSSEN NIZORAL	Nizoral 200 mg	Janssen Pharm
JANSSEN P10	Cisapride 10 mg	Janssen Pharm
JANSSEN P20	Cisapride 20 mg	Janssen Pharm
JANSSEN R1	Risperidone 1 mg	Janssen Pharm
JANSSEN R2	Risperidone 2 mg	Janssen Pharm
JANSSEN R3	Risperidone 3 mg	Janssen Pharm
JANSSEN R4	Risperidone 4 mg	Janssen Pharm
JANSSEN Sproanox 100	Itraconazole 100 mg	Janssen Pharm
JANSSEN VERMOX	Mebendazole 100 mg	Janssen Pharm
JMI 626	Thyroid 30 mg	Jones Medical
JMI 627	Thyroid 60 mg	Jones Medical
JMI 628	Thyroid 120 mg	Jones Medical
JMI 629	Thyroid 180 mg	Jones Medical
JMI 674	Thyroid 60 mg	Jones Medical
JMI 675	Thyroid 120 mg	Jones Medical
JMI 686	Thyroid 30 mg	Jones Medical
JMI 777	Thyroid 64.8 mg	Jones Medical
JMI 778	Thyroid 129.6 mg	Jones Medical
JMI 3094	Phenylpropanolamine 25 mg	JMI Canton
JMI 5052	Chlorpheniramine maleate 4 mg	JMI Canton
JMI/Duotrate 30mg	Duotrate 30 mg	Jones Medical
JMI/Duotrate 45mg	Duotrate 45 mg	Jones Medical
JMI T-Dry	Pseudoephedrine 120 mg, Chlorpheniramine 12 mg	Jones Medical
JSP/10 1321	Caffeine	Unknown
JSP/10 1323	Caffeine	Unknown
JSP 507	CONTROLLED - SEE PAGE 219	
JSP 513	Levothyroxine Sodium 25 mcg	Jerome Stevens
JSP 514	Levothyroxine Sodium 50 mcg	Jerome Stevens
JSP 515	Levothyroxine Sodium 75 mcg	Jerome Stevens
JSP 526	Bromophen 6 mg, Pseudoephedrine 60 mg	Jerome Stevens
JSP 527	Bromophen 12 mg, Pseudoephedrine 120 mg	Jerome Stevens
K 0659	Ergoloid Mesylate 1 mg	KV
K 0849	Papaverine HCl 150 mg	KV
K/1	CONTROLLED - SEE PAGE 211	
K/2	CONTROLLED - SEE PAGE 202	
K/3	CONTROLLED - SEE PAGE 206	
K/4	CONTROLLED - SEE PAGE 204	
K 8	Potassium Chloride 600 mg	Alra Labs
K 10	Potassium Chloride 750 mg	Alra Labs
K/60	CONTROLLED - No Photo - Codeine Sulfate - Tablet DEA Schedule II	Knoll Pharm
K-200	Caffeine, Ephedrine, Phenylpropanolamine	Unknown
K 634	Nitroglycerin 2.5 mg	KV
K 635	Nitroglycerin 6.5 mg	KV

Imprint	Ingredient/Brand Name	Manufacturer
K 898	Nitroglycerin 9 mg	KV
K-DUR 10	Potassium Chloride 750 mg	Key Pharm
K-DUR 20	Potassium Chloride 1500 mg	Key Pharm
K-Norm 10	K-Norm 10 750 mg	Fisons
KEFLEX 250 mg	Keflex 250 mg	Dista Prod
KEFLEX 500 mg	Keflex 500 mg	Dista Prod
KEMADRIN S3A	Kemadrin 5 mg	Burroughs Wellcome
Kerlone 10	Kerlone 10 mg	Searle
Kerlone 20β	Kerlone 20 mg	Searle
KL [logo]	Clarithromycin 500 mg	Abbott labs
KLONOPIN 0.5 ROCHE	CONTROLLED - SEE PAGE 203	
KLONOPIN 1 ROCHE	CONTROLLED - SEE PAGE 210	
KLONOPIN 2 ROCHE	CONTROLLED - SEE PAGE 190	
KLOR-CON 8	Klor-con 600 mg	Upsher-Smith Labs
KLOR-CON 10	Klor-con 750 mg	Upsher-Smith Labs
Klotrix MJ 770	Klotrix 10mEq	Bristol-Myers
KMP 25	Caffeine, Ephedrine, Phenylpropanolamine	Unknown
Knoll/120SR	Verapamil 120 mg	Knoll Pharm
KP 101	Sulfasalazine 500 mg	Kabi
KP 102	Sulfasalazine 500 mg	Kabi
KREMERS URBAN 053	Pseudoephedrine 65 mg, Chlorpheniramine Maleate 10 mg	Kremers
KREMERS URBAN 055	Pseudoephedrine 120 mg, Chlorpheniramine Maleate 8 mg	Kremers
KREMERS URBAN 475	Digestive enzyme supplement	Kremers Urban
KREMERS URBAN 505	Lactase Enzyme 250 mg	Kremers Urban
KREMERS URBAN 522	Digestive enzyme supplement	Kremers Urban
KREMERS URBAN 525	Digestive enzyme supplement	Kremers Urban
KREMERS URBAN 537	Hyoscamine Sulfate 0.375 mg	Kremers Urban
KT [logo]	Clarithromycin 250 mg	Abbott Labs
K-U	Levsin 0.125 mg	Rorer Pharm
KU 050	Pseudoephedrine 60 mg, Chlorpheniramine 4 mg	Schwarz Pharma
KU 1	Ergocalciferol 1.25 mg	Schwarz Pharma
KU 202	Belladonna Extract 15 mg, Phenobarbital 15 mg	Schwarz Pharma
KU 531	Hyoscamine Sulfate 0.125 mg	KU
KU 534	Hyoscyamine 0.125 mg, Phenobarbital 15 mg	Schwarz Pharma
L	Iodinated Glycerol 30 mg	LuChem
L010	Acetaminophen 325 mg	Leiner health
L011	Phenylpropanolamine 75 mg	Proctor & Gamble
L012	Aspirin 325 mg	Leiner health
L013	Acetaminophen 250 mg, Aspirin 250 mg, Caffeine 65 mg	Leiner Health
L014	Acetaminophen 500 mg	Leiner Health
L015	Pseudoephedrine60 mg, Tripolidine 2.5 mg	Leiner Health
L016	Acetaminophen 500 mg	Leiner Health
L017	Acetaminophen 80 mg	Leiner Health
L019	Aspirin 325 mg	Leiner Health
L021	Chlorpheniramine Maleate 4 mg	Leiner Health
L022	Acetaminophen 80 mg	Leiner Health
L023	Acetaminophen 80 mg	Leiner Health
L024	Tri-Buffered Aspirin325 mg	Leiner Health
L025	Calcium Carbonate 500 mg	Leiner Health
L026	Calcium Carbonate 500 mg	Leiner Health
L027	Calcium Carbonate 750 mg	Leiner Health
L029	Diuretic	Leiner Health
L030	Phenylpropanolamine 75 mg	Leiner Health
L031	Bismuth Subsalicylate 262 mg	Leiner Health
L032	Caffeine 200 mg	Leiner Health
L033	Dimenhydrinate 50 mg	Leiner Health

Imprint	Ingredient/Brand Name	Manufacturer
L034	Diphenhydramine 25 mg	Leiner Health
L035	Natural Laxative	Leiner Health
L036	Acetaminophen 500 mg, Diphenhydramine 25 mg	Leiner Health
L039	Aspirin 500 mg	Leiner Health
L040	Diphenhydramine 50 mg	Leiner Health
L042	Iron 50 mg, Docusate Sodium 100 mg	Leiner Health
L043	Acetaminophen 500 mg	Leiner Health
L044	Cold & Cough Caplets	Leiner Health
L045	Multiple Symptom Cold Caplets	Leiner Health
L046	Multiple Symptom Cold Caplets	Leiner Health
L047	Bismuth Subsalicylate 262 mg	Leiner Health
L049	Acetaminophen 160 mg	Leiner Health
L051	Aspirin 325 mg	Leiner Health
L052	Calcium Polycarbophil 625 mg	Leiner Health
L053	Meclizine HCl 25 mg	Leiner Health
L054	Sinus Tablets	Leiner Health
L055	Pseudoephedrine 30 mg, Acetaminophen 325 mg	Leiner Health
L056	Acetaminophen 500 mg	Leiner Health
L057	Dihydroxyaluminum Sodium Carbonate 300 mg	Leiner Health
L061	Phenylpropanolamine 18.7 mg, Chlorpheniramine Maleate 2 mg	Leiner
L074	Multi-Symptom Cold Tablet	Leiner Health
L077	Pseudoephedrine 30 mg, Acetaminophen 500 mg	Leiner Health
L079	Pseudoephedrine 30 mg, Acetaminophen 500 mg	Leiner Health
L080	Pseudoephedrine 30 mg, Acetaminophen 500 mg	Leiner Health
L081	Aspirin 500 mg	Leiner Health
L082	Aspirin 500 mg	Leiner Health
L083	Magnesium Hydroxide 311 mg	Leiner Health
L086	Pseudoephedrine 60 mg, Chlorpheniramine 4 mg	Leiner Health
L087	Dihydroxyaluminum Sodium Carbonate 334 mg	Leiner Health
L089	Pseodoephedrine 60 mg, Chlorpheniramine Maleate 4 mg	Leiner Health
L090	Pseudoephedrine 30 mg, Acetaminophen 500 mg	Leiner Health
L091	Magnesium Trisilicate 60 mg, Aluminum Hydroxide 80 mg	Leiner Health
L099	Acetaminophen 160 mg	Leiner Health
L-2	Loperamide 2 mg	Perrigo
L 9	Ledercillin VK 500 mg	Lederle Labs
L 10	Ledercillin VK 250 mg	Lederle Labs
L 11	Thyroid 3 grains	LuChem Pharm
L 33/3	CONTROLLED - SEE PAGE 199	
L 53/W	CONTROLLED - SEE PAGE 208	
L100	Acetaminophen 160 mg	Leiner Health
L101	Cold & Cough Caplet	Leiner Health
L102	Maximum Strength Allergy Sinus	Leiner Health
L105	Acetaminophen 500 mg, Pseudoephedrine 30 mg	Leiner Health
L110	Aspirin 81 mg	Leiner Health
L 110	Yohimbine 5.4 mg	LuChem Pharm
L111	Pseudoephedrine 30 mg, Chlorpheniramine Maleate 2 mg	Leiner Health
L126	Dextromethorphan 15 mg, Pseudoephedrine 30 mg, Acetaminophen 325 mg	Perrigo
L172	Acetaminophen 160 mg	Perrigo
L179	Calcium Carbonate 750 mg	Perrigo
L235	Dihydroxaluminum Sodium Carbonate 300 mg	Perrigo
L240	Yellow Phenolphthalein 90 mg	Perrigo
L403 325mg	Acetaminophen 325 mg	Perrigo
L405 500mg	Acetaminophen 500 mg	Perrigo
L406	Diphenhydramine 25 mg	Perrigo
L415	Aspirin 400 mg, Caffeine 32 mg	Perrigo

Imprint	Ingredient/Brand Name	Manufacturer
L419	Nite Cold Relief	Perrigo
L420	Complete Multi-Symptom Cold Reliever	Perrigo
L421	Aspirin 325 mg, Sodium Bicarb 1916 mg, Citric Acid 1000 mg	Perrigo
L427	Non-Aspirin Allergy Sinus Tablets	Perrigo
L429	Aspirin 325 mg	Perrigo
L430	Acetaminophen 250 mg, Caffeine 65 mg, Aspirin 250 mg	Perrigo
L432	Pseudoephedrine 30 mg	Perrigo
L434	Pseudoephedrine 60 mg, Tripolidine 2.5 mg	Perrigo
L438	Acetaminophen 500 mg, Pseudoephedrine 30 mg	Perrigo
L442	Docusate Sodium 100 mg, Yellow Phenolphthalein 65 mg	Perrigo
L447	Acetaminophen 500 mg, Pseudoephedrine 30 mg	Perrigo
L449	Acetaminophen 150 mg	Perrigo
L450	Pseudoephedrine 60 mg, Chlorpheniramine 4 mg	Perrigo
L459	Chlorpheniramine 4 mg, Phenylpropanolamine 25 mg	Perrigo
L462	Diphenhydramine 25 mg	Perrigo
L463	Chlorpheniramine maleate 4 mg	Perrigo
L465 PM	Acetaminophen 500 mg, Diphenhydramine 25 mg	Perrigo
L467	Aspirin 81 mg	Perrigo
L469	Bismuth Subsalicylate 262 mg	Perrigo
L470	Acetaminophen 500 mg	Perrigo
L478	Calcium Carbonate 500 mg	Perrigo
L479	Diphenhydramine 25 mg	Perrigo
L480	Maximum Strentgh Sinus Caplets	Perrigo
L481	Acetaminophen 80 mg	Perrigo
L482	Phenylpropanolamine 75 mg, Chlorpheniramine 8 mg	Perrigo
L484	Acetaminophen 500 mg	Perrigo
L485	Calcium Carbonate 500 mg	Perrigo
L486	Docusate Sodium 100 mg	Perrigo
L492	Acetaminophen 80 mg	Perrigo
L494	Effervescent Cold Relief	Perrigo
L496	Brompheniramine maleate 4 mg, Phenylpropanolamine	Perrigo
L501	Severe Cold Caplets	Perrigo
L524	Pseudoephedrine 30 mg, Acetaminophen 325 mg	Perrigo
L596	Severe Cold Tablets	Perrigo
L 609	Decongestant Antihistamine Combination	LuChem Pharm
L642	Aspirin 325 mg	Perrigo
L643	Acetaminophen 500 mg, Pseudoephedrine 30 mg	Perrigo
L/670	Quinine Sulfate 260 mg	LuChem Pharm
L-685	Thyroid 0.5 grain	LuChem Pharm
L-686	Thyroid 1 grain	LuChem Pharm
L-687	Thyroid 2 grains	LuChem Pharm
L 816	Chlorpheniramine 8 mg, Pseudoephedrine 12 mg	LuChem Pharm
LactAid	LactAid	Lactaid Inc
LA CTM D	Chlor-Trimeton 120 mg/8 mg	Schering Corp
LAN 1231	Primidone 250 mg	Lannett
LANOXIN T9A	Lanoxin 0.5 mg	Burroughs Wellcome
LANOXIN X3A	Lanoxin 0.25 mg	Burroughs Wellcome
LANOXIN Y3B	Lanoxin 0.125 mg	Burroughs Wellcome
LAROBEC ROCHE	Larobec	Roche Labs
LARODOPA 100 ROCHE	Larodopa 100 mg	Roche Labs
LARODOPA 250 ROCHE	Larodopa 250 mg	Roche Labs
LARODOPA 500 ROCHE	Larodopa 500 mg	Roche Labs
LASER 0169	Pseudoephedrine 120 mg, Guaifenesin 250 mg	Laser
LASER 0174	Pseudoephedrine 60 mg, Guaifenesin 200 mg	Laser
LASER 173	Lactocal-F	Laser
LASIX 40	Lasix 40 mg	Hoechst-Roussel Pharm

Imprint	Ingredient/Brand Name	Manufacturer
LASIX 80	Lasix 80 mg	Hoechst-Roussel Pharm
L/Aspirin	Aspirin 325 mg	Cumberlad Swan
LaxCaps	Phillips LaxCaps 90 mg/83 mg	Glenbrook Labs
LBQ	BQ Cold Tablets 325 mg/12.5 mg/2 mg	Bristol-Meyers Prod
LC 738	Propranolol 10 mg	Chelsea Labs
LC 739	Propranolol 20 mg	Chelsea Labs
LC 740	Propranolol 40 mg	Chelsea Labs
LC 741	Propranolol 80 mg	Chelsea Labs
LC/770	Phenytoin 100 mg	Rugby Labs
LE [logo]	Trimethadione 150 mg	Abbott Labs
Lederle 250 A31	Ampicillin Trihydrate 250 mg	Lederle Labs
Lederle A 3 250	Achromycin V 250 mg	Lederle Labs
Lederle A 5 500	Achromycin V 500 mg	Lederle Labs
Lederle A20	Acetaminophen 500 mg	Lederle Labs
Lederle A31	Ampicillin 250 mg	Lederle Labs
Lederle A32	Ampicillin 500 mg	Lederle Labs
Lederle A33	Amoxicillin 250 mg	Lederle Labs
Lederle A34	Amoxicillin 500 mg	Lederle Labs
Lederle C17	Chlorpheniramine maleate 8 mg	Lederle Labs
Lederle C18	Chlorpheniramine maleate 12 mg	Lederle Labs
Lederle C56	CONTROLLED - SEE PAGE 222	
Lederle C57	CONTROLLED - SEE PAGE 217	
Lederle C61	Cephradine 250 mg	Lederle Labs
Lederle C62	Cephradine 500 mg	Lederle Labs
Lederle C64	Cephalexin 250 mg	Lederle Labs
Lederle C65	Cephalexin 500 mg	Lederle Labs
Lederle D3	Acetazolamide 500 mg	Lederle Labs
Lederle D16	Dicloxacillin Sodium 250 mg	Lederle Labs
Lederle D17	Dictoxacillin Sodium 500 mg	Lederle Labs
Lederle D22	Doxycycline 50 mg	Lederle Labs
Lederle D23	Dicyclomine 10 mg	Lederle Labs
Lederle D25	Doxycycline 100 mg	Lederle Labs
Lederle D36	CONTROLLED - SEE PAGE 216	
Lederle D43	Disopyramide 150 mg	Lederle Labs
Lederle D47	Doxepin 25 mg	Lederle Labs
Lederle D48	Doxepin 50 mg	Lederle Labs
Lederle D49	Doxepin 75 mg	Lederle Labs
Lederle D50	Doxepin 10 mg	Lederle Labs
Lederle D54	Doxepin 100 mg	Lederle Labs
Lederle D55	Doxepin 150 mg	Lederle Labs
Lederle D62	Disopyramide 100 mg	Lederle Labs
Lederle E 5	Erythromycin 500 mg	Lederle Labs
Lederle F 2	Ferro-Sequels	Lederle Labs
LEDERLE I19	Indomethacin 25 mg	Lederle Labs
LEDERLE I20	Indomethacin 50 mg	Lederle Labs
Lederle L 1	Loxitane 5 mg	Lederle Labs
Lederle L 2	Loxitane 10 mg	Lederle Labs
Lederle L 3	Loxitane 25 mg	Lederle Labs
Lederle L 4	Loxitane 50 mg	Lederle Labs
Lederle LL C81	Cephalexin 250 mg	Lederle Labs
Lederle LL C82	Cephalexin 500 mg	Lederle Labs
Lederle M 2	Minocin 50 mg	Lederle Labs
Lederle M 4	Minocin 100 mg	Lederle Labs
Lederle M41	Meclofenamate Sodium 50 mg	Lederle Labs
Lederle M42	Meclofenamate Sodium 100 mg	Lederle Labs
Lederle M45	Minocycline 50 mg	Lederle Labs

Imprint	Ingredient/Brand Name	Manufacturer
Lederle M 46	Minocycline 100 mg	Lederle Labs
Lederle N20	Nitroglycerin 2.5 mg	Lederle Labs
Lederle N21	Nitroglycerin 6.5 mg	Lederle Labs
Lederle N22	Nitroglycerin 9 mg	Lederle Labs
Lederle P11	Papaverine 150 mg	Lederle Labs
Lederle P29	Procainamide 250 mg	Lederle Labs
Lederle P30	Procainamide 375 mg	Lederle Labs
Lederle P31	Procainamide 500 mg	Lederle Labs
Lederle P69	Prazosin HCl 1 mg	Lederle Labs
Lederle P70	Prazosin HCl 2 mg	Lederle Labs
Lederle P71	Prazosin HCl 5 mg	Lederle Labs
Lederle Q15	Quinine Sulfate 325 mg	Lederle Labs
Lederle S5	Vitamins/Minerals	Lederle Lab
Lederle V7	Verelan 180 mg	Lederle Lab
Lederle V8 Verelan 120 mg	Verelan 120 mg	Lederle Lab
Lederle V9	Verelan 240 mg	Lederle Lab
Legatrin	Quinine Sulfate 162.5 mg	Columbia Labs
LEMMON/30	Neothylline 200 mg	Lemmon Pharm
LEMMON/37	Neothylline 300 mg	Lemmon Pharm
LEMMON 110	Acetaminophen 300 mg, Salicylamide 300 mg, Phenylpropanolamine 6 mg, Chlorpheniramine 4 mg	Lemmon Pharm
LEMMON/128 128	Neothylline-GG 200 mg/200 mg	Lemmon Pharm
LEMMON/ORAP 2	Pimozide 2 mg	Lemmon Pharm
LEVO-DROMORAN/ROCHE	CONTROLLED - SEE PAGE 186	
LF [logo]	Panwarfin 10 mg	Abbott Labs
LH	Levothroid 0.125 mg	USV Labs
LH 524	Chlorpheniramine 4 mg, Phenyltoloxamine 20 mg, Phenylephrine 50 mg	Econolab
LIBRITABS 5/ROCHE	CONTROLLED - SEE PAGE 211	
LIBRITABS 10/ROCHE	CONTROLLED - SEE PAGE 211	
LIBRITABS 25/ROCHE	CONTROLLED - SEE PAGE 211	
LIBRIUM 5 ROCHE	CONTROLLED - SEE PAGE 221	
LIBRIUM 10 ROCHE	CONTROLLED - SEE PAGE 223	
LIBRIUM 25 ROCHE	CONTROLLED - SEE PAGE 220	
Lilly 3061	Ceclor 250 mg	Eli Lilly & Co
Lilly 3062	Ceclor 500 mg	Eli Lilly & Co
Lilly 3111 DARVON COMP.65	CONTROLLED - SEE PAGE 222	
Lilly 4131	Pergolide Mesylate 0.05 mg	Eli Lilly & Co
Lilly 4133	Pergolide Mesylate 0.25 mg	Eli Lilly & Co
Lilly 4135	Pergolide Mesylate 1 mg	Eli Lilly & Co
Lilly A01	Ammonium Chloride 486 mg	Eli Lilly & Co
Lilly A02	Ferrous Sulfate 324 mg	Eli Lilly & Co
Lilly A04	Pancreatin 1000 mg	Eli Lilly & Co
Lilly A05	Potassium Chloride 300 mg	Eli Lilly & Co
Lilly A06	Potassium Iodide 300 mg	Eli Lilly & Co
Lilly A09	Sodium Chloride 1004 mg	Eli Lilly & Co
Lilly A10	Sodium Salicylate 324 mg	Eli Lilly & Co
Lilly A11	Sodium Salicylate 648 mg	Eli Lilly & Co
Lilly A12	Ammonium Chloride 972 mg	Eli Lilly & Co
Lilly A14	Thyroid 30 mg	Eli Lilly & Co
Lilly A15	Thyroid 60 mg	Eli Lilly & Co
Lilly A16	Thyroid 120 mg	Eli Lilly & Co
Lilly A17	Thyroid 200 mg	Eli Lilly & Co
Lilly A19	Diethylstilbestrol 0.1 mg	Eli Lilly & Co
Lilly A20	Diethylstilbestrol 0.25 mg	Eli Lilly & Co
Lilly A21	Diethylstilbestrol 0.5 mg	Eli Lilly & Co

Imprint	Ingredient/Brand Name	Manufacturer
Lilly A22	Diethylstilbestrol 1 mg	Eli Lilly & Co
Lilly A25	A.S.A. 324 mg	Eli Lilly & Co
Lilly A26	Ox Bile Extract 324 mg	Eli Lilly & Co
Lilly A30	Aminosalicylic Acid 500 mg	Eli Lilly & Co
Lilly A31	Potassium Chloride 1000 mg	Eli Lilly & Co
Lilly A32	A.S.A. 648 mg	Eli Lilly & Co
Lilly A33	Diethylstilbestrol 5 mg	Eli Lilly & Co
Lilly A36	Ferrous Sulfate 324 mg	Eli Lilly & Co
Lilly C06	Cascara 324 mg	Eli Lilly & Co
Lilly C13	Ferrous Sulfate 324 mg	Eli Lilly & Co
Lilly C36	Quinine Sulfate 324 mg	Eli Lilly & Co
Lilly C47	Hepicebrin	Eli Lilly & Co
Lilly DARVOCET-N 50	CONTROLLED - SEE PAGE 208	
Lilly DARVON-N 100	CONTROLLED - SEE PAGE 204	
Lilly F04	Seromycin 250 mg	Eli Lilly & Co
Lilly F11	A.S.A. 324 mg	Eli Lilly & Co
Lilly F12	A.S.A. 324 mg	Eli Lilly & Co
Lilly F15	Lextron	Eli Lilly & Co
Lilly F16	Lextron Ferrous	Eli Lilly & Co
Lilly F24	Ephedrine 25 mg	Eli Lilly & Co
Lilly F25	Ephedrine 50 mg	Eli Lilly & Co
Lilly F26	Quinine Sulfate 130 mg	Eli Lilly & Co
Lilly F27	Quinine Sulfate 194 mg	Eli Lilly & Co
Lilly F29	Quinine Sulfate 324 mg	Eli Lilly & Co
Lilly F31	Acidulin 340 mg	Eli Lilly & Co
Lilly F39	Quinidine Sulfate 200 mg	Eli Lilly & Co
Lilly F40	CONTROLLED - SEE PAGE 216	
Lilly F41	Bilron 300 mg	Eli Lilly & Co
Lilly F42	CONTROLLED - SEE PAGE 215	
Lilly F44	Ferrous Gluconate 324 mg	Eli Lilly & Co
Lilly F54	Dicumarol 50 mg	Eli Lilly & Co
Lilly F61	Bilron 150 mg	Eli Lilly & Co
Lilly F65	CONTROLLED - SEE PAGE 219	
Lilly F66	CONTROLLED - SEE PAGE 219	
Lilly F71	Dicumarol 25 mg	Eli Lilly & Co
Lilly F96	Reticulex	Eli Lilly & Co
Lilly H02	CONTROLLED - SEE PAGE 215	
Lilly H03 DARVON	CONTROLLED - SEE PAGE 215	
Lilly H17	Aventyl 10 mg	Eli Lilly & Co
Lilly H19	Aventyl 25 mg	Eli Lilly & Co
Lilly H69	Keflex 250 mg	Eli Lilly & Co
Lilly H71	Keflex 500 mg	Eli Lilly & Co
Lilly J02	Atropine Sulfate 0.4 mg	Eli Lilly & Co
Lilly J03	Belladonna Extract 15 mg	Eli Lilly & Co
Lilly J10	CONTROLLED - SEE PAGE 185	
Lilly J11	CONTROLLED - SEE PAGE 185	
Lilly J13	Colchicine 0.6 mg	Eli Lilly & Co
Lilly J20	Quinidine Sulfate 200 mg	Eli Lilly & Co
Lilly J23	Soda Mint 324 mg	Eli Lilly & Co
Lilly J24	Sodium Bicarbonate 324 mg	Eli Lilly & Co
Lilly J25	Thyroid 60 mg	Eli Lilly & Co
Lilly J26	Thyroid 120 mg	Eli Lilly & Co
Lilly J29	Thyroid 30 mg	Eli Lilly & Co
Lilly J30	Thyroid 15 mg	Eli Lilly & Co
Lilly J31	CONTROLLED - SEE PAGE 187	
Lilly J32	CONTROLLED - SEE PAGE 187	

Imprint	Ingredient/Brand Name	Manufacturer
Lilly J33	CONTROLLED - SEE PAGE 190	
Lilly J36	Ergotrate Maleate 0.2 mg	Eli Lilly & Co
Lilly J37	CONTROLLED - SEE PAGE 187	
Lilly J41	Niacin 20 mg	Eli Lilly & Co
Lilly J42	Niacin 100 mg	Eli Lilly & Co
Lilly J43	Niacin 50 mg	Eli Lilly & Co
Lilly J45	Hexa-Betalin 25 mg	Eli Lilly & Co
Lilly J46	Niacinamide 50 mg	Eli Lilly & Co
Lilly J47	Riboflavin 5 mg	Eli Lilly & Co
Lilly J49	Diethylstilbestrol 0.1 mg	Eli Lilly & Co
Lilly J50	Diethylstilbestrol 0.25 mg	Eli Lilly & Co
Lilly J51	Diethylstilbestrol 0.5 mg	Eli Lilly & Co
Lilly J52	Diethylstilbestrol 1 mg	Eli Lilly & Co
Lilly J54	Diethylstilbestrol 5 mg	Eli Lilly & Co
Lilly J61	Papaverine 30 mg	Eli Lilly & Co
Lilly J62	Papaverine 60 mg	Eli Lilly & Co
Lilly J63	Riboflavid 10 mg	Eli Lilly & Co
Lilly J64	CONTROLLED - SEE PAGE 187	
Lilly J72	CONTROLLED - SEE PAGE 193	
Lilly J73	CONTROLLED - SEE PAGE 199	
Lilly J94	Tapazole 5 mg	Eli Lilly & Co
Lilly J95	Tapazole 10 mg	Eli Lilly & Co
Lilly S07	Diethylstilbestrol 0.1 mg	Eli Lilly & Co
Lilly S09	Diethylstilbestrol 0.5 mg	Eli Lilly & Co
Lilly S15	A.S.A. 324 mg	Eli Lilly & Co
Lilly S16	A.S.A. 648 mg	Eli Lilly & Co
Lilly T01	Zentron	Eli Lilly & Co
Lilly T05	A.S.A. 324 mg	Eli Lilly & Co
Lilly T06	A.S.A. 648 mg	Eli Lilly & Co
Lilly T13	Calcium Lactate 324 mg	Eli Lilly & Co
Lilly T14	Calcium Lactate 648 mg	Eli Lilly & Co
Lilly T20	Methenamine 500 mg	Eli Lilly & Co
Lilly T21	Methenamine 325 mg, Sodium Biphosphate 325 mg	Eli Lilly & Co
Lilly T23	Sodium Chloride 2250 mg	Eli Lilly & Co
Lilly T24	Sodium Chloride 1000 mg	Eli Lilly & Co
Lilly T26	Pancreatin 325 mg	Eli Lilly & Co
Lilly T29	Sodium Bicarbonate 648 mg	Eli Lilly & Co
Lilly T35	Calcium Carbonate 648 mg	Eli Lilly & Co
Lilly T36	Calcium Gluconate 1000 mg	Eli Lilly & Co
Lilly T39	Calcium Gluconate 486 mg	Eli Lilly & Co
Lilly T44	Clacium Gluconate 1000 mg, Vitamin D	Eli Lilly & Co
Lilly T45	Ascorbic Acid 100 mg	Eli Lilly & Co
Lilly T46	Sulfapyridine 500 mg	Eli Lilly & Co
Lilly T52	Thiamine 10 mg	Eli Lilly & Co
Lilly T53	Niacinamide 100 mg	Eli Lilly & Co
Lilly T54	Sulfadiazine 500 mg	Eli Lilly & Co
Lilly T55	Papaverine 100 mg	Eli Lilly & Co
Lilly T59	Thiamine 25 mg	Eli Lilly & Co
Lilly T60	Ascorbic Acid 250 mg	Eli Lilly & Co
Lilly T61	Calcium Phosphate 486 mg	Eli Lilly & Co
Lilly T62	Thiamine 50 mg	Eli Lilly & Co
Lilly T63	Thiamine 100 mg	Eli Lilly & Co
Lilly T67	Ascorbic Acid 500 mg	Eli Lilly & Co
Lilly T73	Papaverine 200 mg	Eli Lilly & Co
Lilly T93	Isoniazid 100 mg	Eli Lilly & Co
Lilly T96	Neomycin Sulfate 500 mg	Eli Lilly & Co

Imprint	Ingredient/Brand Name	Manufacturer
Lilly U03	Dymelor 250 mg	Eli Lilly & Co
Lilly U07	Dymelor 500 mg	Eli Lilly & Co
Lilly U23	Isoniazid 300 mg	Eli Lilly & Co
Lilly U53	CONTROLLED - SEE PAGE 204	
Lilly U56	Folic Acid 1 mg	Eli Lilly & Co
Lilly U60	Keflex 1000 mg	Eli Lilly & Co
LIMBITROL 10 25/ROCHE	CONTROLLED - SEE PAGE 193	
LIMBITROL DS/ROCHE	CONTROLLED - SEE PAGE 193	
LK	Levothroid 0.025 mg	USV Labs
LK [logo]	Deserpidine 0.25 mg	Abbott Labs
LL	Levothroid 0.05 mg	USV Labs
LL	Caltrate, Jr. 750 mg	Lederle Labs
LL [logo]	Oreticyl Forte 25 mg/0.25 mg	Abbott Labs
LL 5/C 33	Leucovorin Calcium 5 mg	Immunex
LL 10/C 12	Leocovorin Calcium 10 mg	Immunex
LL 15/C 35	Leucovorin Calcium 15 mg	Immunex
LL 53	Stresstabs & Zinc	Lederle Labs
LL A 1	Aristocort 1 mg	Lederle Labs
LL A 2	Aristocort 2 mg	Lederle Labs
LL A 4	Aristocort 4 mg	Lederle Labs
LL/A7	Atenolol 25 mg	Lederle Labs
LL A 8	Aristocort 8 mg	Lederle Labs
LL A 9	Artane 5 mg	Lederle Labs
LL A10	Amicar 500 mg	Lederle Labs
LL A11/ARTANE 2	Artane 2 mg	Lederle Labs
LL A12/ARTANE 5	Artane 5 mg	Lederle Labs
LL A13/25	Asendin 25 mg	Lederle Labs
LL A14	Amiloride 5 mg, Hydrochlorthiazide 50 mg	Lederle Labs
LL A15/50	Asendin 50 mg	Lederle Labs
LL A16	Aristocort 16 mg	Lederle Labs
LL A17/100	Asendin 100 mg	Lederle Labs
LL A18/150	Asendin 150 mg	Lederle Labs
LL A19	Acetaminophen 500 mg	Lederle Labs
LL A20	Acetaminophen 500 mg	Lederle Labs
LL A21	Acetaminophen 325 mg	Lederle Labs
LL A22	Acetaminophen 500 mg	Lederle Labs
LL A24	Amitriptyline 10 mg	Lederle Labs
LL A25	Amitriptyline 25 mg	Lederle Labs
LL A26	Amitriptyline 50 mg	Lederle Labs
LL A27	Amitriptyline 75 mg	Lederle Labs
LL A28	Amitriptyline 100 mg	Lederle Labs
LL A31	Ampicillin 250 mg	Lederle Labs
LL A32	Ampicillin 500 mg	Lederle Labs
LL A36	Ascorbic Acid 250 mg	Lederle Labs
LL A37	Ascorbic Acid 500 mg	Lederle Labs
LL A38	Ascorbic Acid 1000 mg	Lederle Labs
LL A39	Codeine 60 mg, Acetaminophen	Lederle Labs
LL A43	Allopurinol 100 mg	Lederle Labs
LL A44	Allopurinol 300 mg	Lederle Labs
LL A45	Albuterol Sulfate 2 mg	Lederle Labs
LL A46	Albuterol Sulfate 4 mg	Lederle Labs
LL A49	Atenolol 50 mg	Lederle Labs
LL A71	Atenolol 100 mg	Lederle Labs
LL B1	Zebeta 5 mg	Lederle Labs
LL B3	Zebeta 10 mg	Lederle Labs
LL B10	Benztropine Mesylate 1 mg	Lederle Labs

Imprint	Ingredient/Brand Name	Manufacturer
LL B11	Benztropine Mesylate 2 mg	Lederle Labs
LL C 1	Centrum	Lederle Labs
LL C 2	Centrum Jr.	Lederle Labs
LL C 7	Chlorthalidone 25 mg	Lederle Labs
LL C 13	Chlorthiazide 250 mg	Lederle Labs
LL C14	Chlorothiazide 500 mg	Lederle Labs
LL C15	Chlorthalidone 50 mg	Lederle Labs
LL C16	Chlorpheniramine 4 mg	Lederle Labs
LL C17	Chlorpheniramine 8 mg	Lederle Labs
LL C18	Chlorpheniramine 12 mg	Lederle Labs
LL C19	Chlorzoxazone 250 mg, Acetaminophen 300 mg	Lederle Labs
LL C22	Chlorpromazine 25 mg	Lederle Labs
LL C23	Chlorpromazine 50 mg	Lederle Labs
LL C24	Chlorpromazine 100 mg	Lederle Labs
LL C25	Chlorpromazine 200 mg	Lederle Labs
LL C30	Cloxacillin 250 mg	Lederle Labs
LL C31	Cloxacillin 500 mg	Lederle Labs
LL C33	Calcium Leucovorin 5 mg	Lederle Labs
LL C37	Chlorpropamide 100 mg	Lederle Labs
LL C38	Chlorpropamide 250 mg	Lederle Labs
LL C39	Centrum Jr + Extra C	Lederle Labs
LL C40	Caltrate 600+D	Lederle Labs
LL C42	Clonidine 0.1 mg	Lederle Labs
LL C43	Clonidine 0.2 mg	Lederle Labs
LL C44	Clonidine 0.3 mg	Lederle Labs
LL C45	Caltrate 600 + Iron	Lederle Labs
LL C61	Cephradine 250 mg	Lederle Labs
LL C62	Cephradine 500 mg	Lederle Labs
LL C66	Carbamazepine 200 mg	Lederle Labs
LL C600	Caltrate 1500 mg	Lederle Labs
LL D 1	Diamox 125 mg	Lederle Labs
LL D 2	Diamox 250 mg	Lederle Labs
LL D 3	Diamox Sequels 500 mg	Lederle Labs
LL D 9	Declomycin 150 mg	Lederle Labs
LL D11	Declomycin 150 mg	Lederle Labs
LL D12	Declomycin 300 mg	Lederle Labs
LL D16	Dicloxacillin 250 mg	Lederle Labs
LL D17	Dicloxacillin 500 mg	Lederle Labs
LL D22	Doxycycline 50 mg	Lederle Labs
LL D23	Dicyclomine 10 mg	Lederle Labs
LL D24	Dicyclomine 20 mg	Lederle Labs
LL D25	Doxycycline 100 mg	Lederle Labs
LL D27	Ergoloid Mesylates 0.5 mg	Lederle Labs
LL D28	Ergoloid Mesylates 1 mg	Lederle Labs
LL D32	Docusate 100 mg	Lederle Labs
LL D33	Docusate 250 mg	Lederle Labs
LL D34	Docusate 100 mg, Casanthranol 30 mg	Lederle Labs
LL D41	Doxycycline 100 mg	Lederle Labs
LL D43	Disopyramide 150 mg	Lederle Labs
LL D44	Dipyridamole 25 mg	Lederle Labs
LL D45	Dipyridamole 50 mg	Lederle Labs
LL D46	Dipyridamole 75 mg	Lederle Labs
LL D47	Doxepin 25 mg	Lederle Labs
LL D48	Doxepin 50 mg	Lederle Labs
LL D49	Doxepin 75 mg	Lederle Labs
LL D50	Doxepin 10 mg	Lederle Labs

Imprint	Ingredient/Brand Name	Manufacturer
LL D54	Doxepin 100 mg	Lederle Labs
LL D62	Disopyramide 100 mg	Lederle Labs
LL/D 71	Diltiazem 30 mg	Lederle Labs
LL/D 72	Diltiazem 60 mg	Lederle Labs
LL/D 75	Diltiazem 90 mg	Lederle Labs
LL E 2	Erythromycin 250 mg	Lederle Labs
LL E 3	Ergoloid Mesylates 1 mg	Lederle Labs
LL E 5	Erythromycin 500 mg	Lederle Labs
LL E10	Erythromycin Ethylsuccinate 400 mg	Lederle Labs
LL E 27	Ergoloid Mesylates 0.5 mg	Lederle Labs
LL E 28	Ergoloid Mesylates 1 mg	Lederle Labs
LL F 1	Folvite 1 mg	Lederle Labs
LL F 2	Ferro-Sequels	Lederle Labs
LL F 4	Filibon	Lederle Labs
LL F 5	Filibon F.A.	Lederle Labs
LL F 6	Filibon Forte	Lederle Labs
LL F 7	Vitamins/Minerals	Lederle Labs
LL F11	Furosemide 20 mg	Lederle Labs
LL F12	Furosemide 40 mg	Lederle Labs
LL F13	Furosemide 80 mg	Lederle Labs
LL F20	Ferrous Sulfate 300 mg	Lederle Labs
LL F21	Ferrous Gluconate 300 mg	Lederle Labs
LL/F 22	Fenoprofen Calcium 600 mg	Lederle Labs
LL F66	Calcium Polycarbophil 625 mg	Lederle Labs
LL G 1	Gevral	Lederle Labs
LL G 2	Gevral T	Lederle Labs
LL/G17	Gemfibrozil 600 mg	Lederle Labs
LL H 1	Hydromox 50 mg	Lederle Labs
LL H 2	Hydromox R 50/0.125 mg	Lederle Labs
LL H 5	Diethylcarbamazine Citrate 50 mg	Lederle Labs
LL H11	Hydralazine 25 mg	Lederle Labs
LL H12	Hydralazine 50 mg	Lederle Labs
LL H14	Hydrochlorothiazide 25 mg	Lederle Labs
LL H15	Hydrochlorothiazide 50 mg	Lederle Labs
LL H17	Hydroxyzine 10 mg	Lederle Labs
LL H18	Hydroxyzine 25 mg	Lederle Labs
LL H 21	Hydroxyzine 50 mg	Lederle Labs
LL H22	Reserpine 0.1 mg, Hydrochlorothiazide 15 mg, Hydralazine 25 mg	Lederle Labs
LL H25	Haloperidol 0.5 mg	Lederle Labs
LL H26	Haloperidol 1 mg	Lederle Labs
LL H 27	Haloperidol 2 mg	Lederle Labs
LL H28	Haloperidol 5 mg	Lederle Labs
LL H 29	Haloperidol 10 mg	Lederle Labs
LL I11	Imipramine 10 mg	Lederle Labs
LL I12	Imipramine 25 mg	Lederle Labs
LL I13	Imipramine 50 mg	Lederle Labs
LL I15	Isosorbide Dinitrate 5 mg	Lederle Labs
LL I16	Isosorbide Dinitrate 10 mg	Lederle Labs
LL I17	Isosorbide Dinitrate 2.5 mg	Lederle Labs
LL I18	Isosorbide Dinitrate 5 mg	Lederle Labs
LL I19	Indomethacin 25 mg	Lederle Labs
LL I20	Indomethacin 50 mg	Lederle Labs
LL I21	Isoxsuprine 10 mg	Lederle Labs
LL I22	Isoxsuprine 20 mg	Lederle Labs
LL I23	Isosorbide Dinitrate 40 mg	Lederle Labs

Imprint	Ingredient/Brand Name	Manufacturer
LL I24	Isosorbide Dinitrate 20 mg	Lederle Labs
LL I 27	Ibuprofen 200 mg	Lederla Labs
LL I28	Ibuprofen 400 mg	Lederle Labs
LL I29	Ibuprofen 600 mg	Lederle Labs
LL I 30	Ibuprofen 800 mg	Lederle Labs
LL L 6	Lederplex	Lederle Labs
LL L 9	Ledercillin VK 800,000 units	Lederle Labs
LL L10	Ledercillin VK 400,000 units	Lederle Labs
LL L11	Levothyroxine 0.1 mg	Lederle Labs
LL L12	Levothyroxine 0.2 mg	Lederle Labs
LL L13	Levothyroxine 0.3 mg	Lederle Labs
LL L15	Sequels 15 mg/12 mg/15 mg	Lederle Labs
LL L17	Levothyroxine 0.15 mg	Lederle Labs
LL M 1	Methotrexate 2.5 mg	Lederle Labs
LL M 3	Minocin 50 mg	Lederle Labs
LL M 5	Minocin 100 mg	Lederle Labs
LL M 6	Myambutol 100 mg	Lederle Labs
LL M 7	Myambutol 400 mg	Lederle Labs
LL M 8	Maxzide 75 mg/50 mg	Lederle Labs
LL M 8/MAXZIDE	Maxzide 75 mg/50 mg	Lederle Labs
LL M10	Materna	Lederle Labs
LL M12	Meclizine 12.5 mg	Lederle Labs
LL M13	Meclizine 25 mg	Lederle Labs
LL/M19	Methocarbamol 500 mg	Lederle Labs
LL/M20	Methocarbamol 750 mg	Lederle Labs
LL M21	Methyldopa 125 mg	Lederle Labs
LL/M22	Methyldopa 250 mg	Lederle Labs
LL/M23	Methyldopa 500 mg	Lederle Labs
LL M25	Methylclothiazide 5 mg	Lederle Labs
LL M26	Metronidazole 250 mg	Lederle Labs
LL M27	Metronidazole 500 mg	Lederle Labs
LL M28	Metoclopromide 10 mg	Lederle Labs
LL M35	Medroxyprogesterone 10 mg	Lederle Labs
LL M36	Methyldopa 250 mg, Hydrochlorothiazide 15mg	Lederle Labs
LL M37	Methyldopa 250 mg, Hydrochlorothiazide 25mg	Lederle Labs
LL N 1	Neptazane 50 mg	Lederle Labs
LL N 5	Nilstat	Lederle Labs
LL N 6	Nilstat	Lederle Labs
LL N10	Neomycin 500 mg	Lederle Labs
LL N20	Nitroglycerin 2.5 mg	Lederle Labs
LL N21	Nitroglycerin 6.5 mg	Lederle Labs
LL N22	Nitroglycerin 9 mg	Lederle Labs
LL N23	Nylidrin 6 mg	Lederle Labs
LL N24	Nylidrin 12 mg	Lederle Labs
LL O 4	Vitamins/Minerals	Lederle Labs
LL P 4	Pathilon 25 mg	Lederle Labs
LL P 7	Perihemin	Lederle Labs
LL P 8	Pronemia	Lederle Labs
LL P 9	Pronemia Hematinic	Lederle Labs
LL P11	Papavarine 150 mg	Lederle Labs
LL P13	Papaverine 100 mg	Lederle Labs
LL P17	Penicillin G	Lederle Labs
LL P24	Prednisone 5 mg	Lederle Labs
LL P25	Probenecid 500 mg	Lederle Labs
LL P26	Probenecid 500 mg, Colchicine 0.5 mg	Lederle Labs
LL P29	Procainamide 250 mg	Lederle Labs

Imprint	Ingredient/Brand Name	Manufacturer
LL P30	Procainamide 375 mg	Lederle Labs
LL P31	Procainamide 500 mg	Lederle Labs
LL P33	Propylthiouracil 50 mg	Lederle Labs
LL P34	Pseudoephedrine 60 mg	Lederle Labs
LL P35	Pseudoephedrine 30 mg	Lederle Labs
LL/P36	Pyrazinamide 500 mg	Lederle Labs
LL P37	Pyridoxine 25 mg	Lederle Labs
LL P38	Pyridoxine 50 mg	Lederle Labs
LL/P44	Propranolol 10 mg	Lederle Labs
LL/P45	Propranolol 20 mg	Lederle Labs
LL/P46	Propranolol 40 mg	Lederle Labs
LL/P47	Propranolol 80 mg	Lederle Labs
LL P48	Procainamide 250 mg	Lederle Labs
LL P49	Procainamide 500 mg	Lederle Labs
LL P50	Procainamide 750 mg	Lederle Labs
LL P53	Phenytoin 100 mg	Lederle Labs
LL P65	Propranolol 60 mg	Lederle Labs
LL P67	Propranolol 40 mg, Hydrochlorthiazide 25 mg	Lederle Labs
LL P68	Propranolol 80 mg, Hydrochlorthiazide 25 mg	Lederle Labs
LL P72	Perphenazine 2 mg, Amitriptyline 10 mg	Lederle Labs
LL P73	Perphenazine 2 mg, Amitriptyline 25 mg	Lederle Labs
LL P74	Perphenazine 4 mg, Amitriptyline 10 mg	Lederle Labs
LL P75	Perphenazine 4 mg, Amitriptyline 25 mg	Lederle Labs
LL P76	Perphenazine 4 mg, Amitriptyline 50 mg	Lederle Labs
LL/Q11	Quinidine 200 mg	Lederle Labs
LL Q13	Quinidine 324 mg	Lederle Labs
LL Q15	Quinine 325 mg	Lederle Labs
LL S 1	Stresstabs 600	Lederle Labs
LL S 2	Stresstabs 600 with Iron	Lederle Labs
LL S 3	Stresstabs 600 with Zinc	Lederle Labs
LL S 5	Stresscaps	Lederle Labs
LL S12	Spironolactone 25 mg, Hydrochlorothiazide 25 mg	Lederle Labs
LL S13	Spironolactone 25 mg	Lederle Labs
LL S14	Sulfalazine 500 mg	Lederle Labs
LL/S16	Sulindac 150 mg	Lederle Labs
LL/S17	Sulindac 200 mg	Lederle Labs
LL S22	Spartus	Lederle Labs
LL S23	Spartus + Iron	Lederle Labs
LL T 1	TriHemic 600	Lederle Labs
LL T10	Thioridazine 10 mg	Lederle Labs
LL T11	Thiamine 50 mg	Lederle Labs
LL T12	Thiamine 100 mg	Lederle Labs
LL T13	Trimethoprim 80 mg, Sulfamethoxazole 400 mg	Lederle Labs
LL T14	Thyroid 60 mg	Lederle Labs
LL T16	Trimethoprim 160 mg, Sulfamethoxazole 800 mg	Lederle Labs
LL T17	Tolbutamide 500 mg	Lederle Labs
LL T19	Tolazamide 100 mg	Lederle Labs
LL T20	Tolazamide 250 mg	Lederle Labs
LL T22	Tolazamide 500 mg	Lederle Labs
LL T23	Triprolidine 2.5 mg, Pseudoephedrine 60 mg	Lederle Labs
LL T25	Thioridazine 25 mg	Lederle Labs
LL T27	Thioridazine 50 mg	Lederle Labs
LL T28	Thioridazine 100 mg	Lederle Labs
LL T29	Trazodone 50 mg	Lederle Labs
LL T30	Trazodone 25 mg	Lederle Labs
LL T31-50/100	Trazodone 150 mg	Lederle Labs

Imprint	Ingredient/Brand Name	Manufacturer
LL T34	Theophylline 100 mg	Lederla Labs
LL T35	Theophylline 200 mg	Lederle Labs
LL T36	Theophylline 300 mg	Lederle Labs
LL U4	Aminophylline 100 mg	Lederle Labs
LL U5	Aminophylline 200 mg	Lederle Labs
LL U15	Ledercillin VK 500,000 units	Lederle Labs
LL V4	Verapamil 80 mg	Lederle Labs
LL V5	Verapamil 120 mg	Lederla Labs
LL V11	Vitamin A	Lederle Labs
LL V14	Vitamin C 250 mg	Lederle Labs
LL V15	Vitamin C 500 mg	Lederle Labs
LL V19	Vitamin E	Lederle Labs
LL V21	Vitamin E	Lederle Labs
LL V22	Vitamin E	Lederle Labs
LL V23	Vitamin E	Lederle Labs
LL V24	Vitamin E	Lederle Labs
LM	Levothroid 0.1 mg	USV Labs
LM [logo]	Panwarfin 2 mg	Abbott Labs
LN	Levothroid 0.15 mg	USV Labs
L/N 084-250	Cephalexin 250 mg	Novapharm
L/N 114-500	Cephalexin 250 mg	Novapharm
L/N 382	Clofibrate 500 mg	Novapharm
L/N 420-25	Indomethacin 25 mg	MP
L/N 439-50	Indomethacin 50 mg	MP
LN [logo]	Panwarfin 2.5 mg	Abbott Labs
LNK 25	Diphenhydramine 25 mg	Pioneer
LNK 50	Diphenhydramine 50 mg	Pioneer
LO [logo]	Panwarfin 5 mg	Abbott Labs
LONITEN 10	Loniten 10 mg	Upjohn Co
LORELCO 250	Lorelco 250 mg	Merrell Dow Pharm
Lotensin 5	Lotensin 5 mg	Ciba
Lotensin 10	Lotensin 10 mg	Ciba
Lotensin 20	Lotensin 20 mg	Ciba
Lotensin 40	Lotensin 40 mg	Ciba
LP 1 3/4	Levothroid 0.175 mg	USV Labs
LR	Levothroid 0.2 mg	USV Labs
LR [logo]	Panwarfin 7.5 mg	Abbott Labs
LS	Levothroid 0.3 mg	USV Labs
LS [logo]	Enduronyl 5 mg/0.25 mg	Abbott Labs
LT	Levothroid 0.075 mg	USV Labs
LT [logo]	Enduronyl Forte 5 mg/0.5 mg	Abbott Labs
LU [logo]	Ogen 0.75 mg	Abbott Labs
LuCHEM 5	CONTROLLED - SEE PAGE 200	
LUCHEM/7 43	Histatan 12 mg/8 mg/25 mg	LuChem Pharm
LuChem [logo] 110	Yohimbine 5.4 mg	LuChem Pharm
LuCHEM 649	Dexophed 6 mg/120 mg	LuChem Pharm
LuCHEM 663	CONTROLLED - SEE PAGE 224	
LuChem 741	Phenylpropanolamine 75 mg, Guaifenesin 400 mg	LeChem Pharm
LUCHEM 990	Quinine Sulfate 325 mg	LuChem Pharm
LUCHEM 992	Chlorpheniramine 12 mg	LuChem Pharm
LUCHEM 993	Chlorpheniramine 8 mg	LuChem Pharm
LV [logo]	Ogen 1.5 mg	Abbott Labs
LX [logo]	Ogen 3 mg	Abbott Labs
LY [logo]	Ogen 6 mg	Abbott Labs
M	Mylanta 600 mg	Johnson & Johnson
M	Aspirin 500 mg, Phenyltoloxamine Citrate	Whitehall Robins

Imprint	Ingredient/Brand Name	Manufacturer
M 1	Clonidine 0.1 mg, Chlorthalidone 15 mg	Mylan Pharm
M 1	Methenamine Mandelate 1 gram	Able Labs
M 2	Furosemide 20 mg	Mylan Pharm
M/4	Fluphenazine 1 mg	Mylan Pharm
M 5	Amitriptyline	Unknown
M/9	Fluphenazine 2.5 mg	Mylan Pharm
M 10	Propranolol 10 mg	Zenith Labs
M 11	Penicillin V 250 mg	Mylan Pharm
M 12	Penicillin V 500 mg	Mylan Pharm
M 12	Meclizine 12.5 mg	Lederle Labs
M 13	Meclizine 25 mg	Lederle Labs
M 13	Tolbutamide 500 mg	Mylan Pharm
M 14	Methotrexate 2.5 mg	Mylan Pharm
M 15	CONTROLLED - SEE PAGE 185	
M 15/PF	CONTROLLED - SEE PAGE 209	
M 19	Methocarbamol 500 mg	Lederle Labs
M 20	Methocarbamol 750 mg	Lederle Labs
M 20	Propranolol 20 mg	Zenith Labs
M 23	Diltiazem 30 mg	Mylan Pharm
M 25	Levothyroxine 0.025 mg	Duramed Pharm
M 26	Metronidazole 250 mg	Lederle Labs
M 27	Clonidine 0.2 mg, Chlorthalidone 15 mg	Mylan Pharm
M 27	Metronidazole 500 mg	Lederle Labs
M 28	Nadolol 20 mg	Mylan Pharm
M 29	Methyclothiazide 5 mg	Mylan Pharm
M 30	CONTROLLED - SEE PAGE 209	
M 30/PF	CONTROLLED - SEE PAGE 208	
M 31	Allopurinol 100 mg	Mylan Pharm
M 31/BREON	CONTROLLED - SEE PAGE 188	
M 32	Metoprolol Tartrate 50 mg	Mylan Pharm
M 32/BREON	CONTROLLED - SEE PAGE 191	
M 33	Chlorothiazide 250 mg, Reserpine 0.125 mg	Mylan Pharm
M 33/BREON	CONTROLLED - SEE PAGE 190	
M/35	Chlorthalidone 25 mg	Mylan Pharm
M 36	Amitriptyline 50 mg	Mylan Pharm
M 37	Amitriptyline 75 mg	Mylan Pharm
M 38	Amitriptyline 100 mg	Mylan Pharm
M 39	Amitriptyline 150 mg	Mylan Pharm
M 40	Propranolol 40 mg	Zentih Labs
M 40	CONTROLLED - SEE PAGE 202	
M 40/MATERNA	Materna	Lederle Labs
M 41	Spironolactone 25 mg, Hydrochlorothiazide 25 mg	Mylan Pharm
M 43	Chlorothiazide 500 mg, Reserpine 0.125 mg	Mylan Pharm
M 45	Diltiazem 60 mg	Mylan Pharm
M 47	Metoprolol Tartrate 100 mg	Mylan Pharm
M 50	Chlorothiazide 250 mg	Mylan Pharm
M 50	Milophene 50 mg	Milex
M 50	Levothyroxine 0.050 mg	Duramed Pharm
M 50 Levo	L-Thyroxin 0.050 mg	Mova Pharm
M 51	Amitriptyline 25 mg	Mylan Pharm
M 52	Pindolol 5 mg	Mylan Pharm
M/53	Cimetidine 200 mg	Mylan Pharm
M 54/10	Thioridazine 10 mg	Mylan Pharm
M 55	Timolol Maleate 5 mg	Mylan Pharm
M 58/25	Thioridazine 25 mg	Mylan Pharm
M 59/50	Thioridazine 50 mg	Mylan Pharm

Imprint	Ingredient/Brand Name	Manufacturer
M/60	Maprotiline 25 mg	Mylan Pharm
M 60/PF	CONTROLLED - SEE PAGE 203	
M 61/100	Thioridazine 100 mg	Mylan Pharm
M 63	Atenolol 50 mg, Chlorthalidone 25 mg	Mylan Pharm
M 64	Atenolol 100 mg, Chlorthalidone 25 mg	Mylan Pharm
M 70	CONTROLLED - SEE PAGE 202	
M 71	Allopurinol 300 mg	Mylan Pharm
M 71E	Caffeine, Ephedrine	Unknown
M 72	Clonidine 0.3 mg, Chlorthalidone 15 mg	Mylan Pharm
M/74	Fluphenazine 5 mg	Mylan Pharm
M 75	Chlorthalidone 50 mg	Mylan Pharm
M 75	Levothyroxine 0.075 mg	Duramed Pharm
M 77	Amitriptyline 10 mg	Mylan Pharm
M 80	Propranolol 80 mg	Zenith Labs
M/87	Maprotiline 50 mg	Mylan Pharm
M/92	Maprotiline 75 mg	Mylan Pharm
M 95	Penicillin V Potassium 250 mg	Mylan Pharm
M/97	Fluphenazine 10 mg	Mylan Pharm
M 98	Penicillin V Potassium 500 mg	Mylan Pharm
M 100	Levothyroxine 100 mg	Duramed Pharm
M 125	Levothyroxine 0.125 mg	Duramed Pharm
M 125 Levo	L-Thyroxin 0.125 mg	Mova Pharm
M 127	Pindolol 10 mg	Mylan Pharm
M 132	Nadolol 80 mg	Mylan Pharm
M 135	Diltiazem 90 mg	Mylan Pharm
M 150	Levothyroxine 0.150 mg	Duramed Pharm
M 150 Levo	L-Thyroxin 0.15 mg	Mova Pharm
M 171	Nadolol 40 mg	Mylan Pharm
M 200	Levothyroxine 0.200 mg	Duramed Pharm
M 200 Levo	L-Thyroxin 0.2 mg	Mova Pharm
M 200/P F	CONTROLLED - SEE PAGE 226	
M 221	Timolol Maleate 10 mg	Mylan Pharm
M/231	Atenolol 50 mg	Mylan Pharm
M 255	Albuterol Sulfate 2 mg	Mylan Pharm
M 300	Levothyroxine 0.300 mg	Duramed Pharm
M 300 Levo	L-Thyroxin 0.3 mg	Mova Pharm
M/317	Cimetidine 300 mg	Mylan Pharm
M/372	Cimetidine 400 mg	Mylan Pharm
M 400	Erythromycin Ethylsuccinate 400 mg	Mylan Pharm
M 471	Fenoprofen 600 mg	Mylan Pharm
M 525	Diltiazem 120 mg	Mylan Pharm
M 541	Cimetidine 800 mg	Mylan Pharm
M 572	Albuterol Sulfate 4 mg	Mylan Pharm
M 577	Amiloride 5 mg, Hydrochlorothiazide 50 mg	Mylan Pharm
M 715	Timolol Maleate 20 mg	Mylan Pharm
M/751	Cyclobenzaprine 10 mg	Mylan Pharm
M/757	Atenolol 100 mg	Mylan Pharm
M3052	Docusate Sodium 100 mg	Upsher-Smith
M3055	Docusate Sodium 100 mg, Casanthranol 30 mg	Upsher-Smith
M3063	Docusate Sodium 250 mg	Upsher-Smith
Maalox Plus/RORER	Maalox Plus 200 mg/200 mg/25 mg	Rorer Pharm
Maalox TC	Maalox TC 600 mg/600 mg	Rorer Pharm
Macrodantin 0149 0007	Macrodantin 25 mg	Norwich Eaton Pharm
Macrodantin 100mg	Macrodantin 100 mg	Norwich Eaton Pharm
Macrodantin 50mg	Macrodantin 50 mg	Norwich Eaton Pharm
MAGNUM	Caffeine, Ephedrine, Phenylpropanolamine	Unknown

Imprint	Ingredient/Brand Name	Manufacturer
MAGNUM 357	Caffeine, Ephedrine, Phenylpropanolamine	Unknown
MAGNUM H.R.	Caffeine	Unknown
MAOLATE	Maolate 400 mg	Upjohn Co
MARAX/ROERIG 254	Marax 25 mg/130 mg/10 mg	Pfizer Pharm
MAREZINE T4A	Marezine 50 mg	Burroughs Wellcome
MARGESIC#3	CONTROLLED - SEE PAGE 226	
MARGESIC H	CONTROLLED - SEE PAGE 228	
Marion 90 mg	Diltiazem 90 mg	Marion Labs
Marion 120 mg	Diltiazem 120 mg	Marion Labs
MARION/1375	Ditropan 5 mg	Marion Labs
MARION 1525	Duotrate 30 mg	Marion Labs
MARION 1530	Duotrate 45	Marion Labs
MARION 1550	Nitro-Bid 2.5 mg	Marion Labs
MARION 1551	Nitro-Bid 6.5 mg	Marion Labs
MARION 1553	Nitro-Bid 9 mg	Marion Labs
MARION 1555	Papaverine HCl 150 mg	Marion Labs
MARION 1575	Nico-400	Marion Labs
MARION/1712	Carafate 1000 mg	Marion Labs
MARION/1771	Cardizem 30 mg	Marion Labs
MARION/1772	Cardizem 60 mg	Marion Labs
MARION OS-CAL 1650	OS-CAL 250	Marion Labs
MARION/PAVABID HP	Pavabid HP 300 mg	Marion Labs
Marnatal-F	Marnatal F	Marnel
Martec 972	Piroxicam 10 mg	Pharm Basics
Martec 973	Piroxicam 20 mg	Pharm Basics
MATERNA M10	Materna 1.60	Lederle Labs
MATULANE ROCHE	Matulane 50 mg	Roche Labs
MaxEPA	MaxEPA	Solgar Vitamin Co
Maxzide LLM8	Maxzide 75 mg, 50 mg	Lederle Labs
Maxzide LLM9	Maxzide-25 mg	Lederle Labs
Maximum SINE-AID	Acetaminophen 500 mg, Pseudoephedrine 30 mg	McNeil Consumer
MAXIMUM-STRENGTH/TYLENOL SINUS	Aceta 500 mg, Pseudoephedrine 30 mg	McNeil
Mayrand/Nu-Iron 150 0291	Iron 150 mg	Mayrand Pharm
MC/a	CONTROLLED - SEE PAGE 190	
MCG 210	Rhinolar-EX 75 mg/8 mg	McGregor Pharm
MCG 211	Rhinolar-EX 12 mg/75 mg/12 mg	McGregor Pharm
MCG 215	Rhindecon 75 mg	McGregor Pharm
MCG 219	Rhinolar 75 mg, 8 mg, 2.5 mg	McGregor
MCI 18-845	Caffeine, Ephedrine, Phenylpropanolamine	Unknown
McNess	Aspirin 400 mg, Caffeine 32 mg	Furst-McNess
McNEIL 200	Tolectin 200 200 mg	McNeil Pharm
McNEIL/TOLECTIN 200	Tolectin 200 mg	McNeil Pharm
MD 518	CONTROLLED - SEE PAGE 210	
MD 529	CONTROLLED - SEE PAGE 198	
MD 538	Amitriptyline 10 mg	MD Pharm
MD/538	Amitriptyline 10 mg	MD Pharm
MD 539	Amitriptyline 25 mg	MD Pharm
MD 540	Amitriptyline 50 mg	MD Pharm
MD 541	Amitriptyline 75 mg	MD Pharm
MD 542	Amitriptyline 100 mg	MD Pharm
MD 543	Amitriptyline 150 mg	MD Pharm
MD 547	Cyproheptadine 4 mg	MD Pharm
MD 562	CONTROLLED - SEE PAGE 189	
MD 711	Triprolidine 2.5 mg, Pseudoephedrine 60 mg	MD Pharm
MD[in box] R-902	Caffeine, Ephedrine, Phenylpropanolamine	Unknown
ME/a	CONTROLLED - SEE PAGE 202	

Imprint	Ingredient/Brand Name	Manufacturer
Meclomen 50 PD	Meclofenamate Sodium 50 mg	Parke-Davis
Meclomen 100 PD	Meclofenamate Sodium 100 mg	Parke-Davis
Medics	Butalbital, Acetaminophen	Unknown
MEDIPREN	Medipren 200 mg	McNeil Pharm
MEDROL 2	Medrol 2 mg	Upjohn Co
MEDROL 4	Medrol 4 mg	Upjohn Co
MEDROL 8	Medrol 8 mg	Upjohn Co
MEDROL 16	Medrol 16 mg	Upjohn Co
MEDROL 24	Medrol 24 mg	Upjohn Co
MEDROL 32	Medrol 32 mg	Upjohn Co
Megace 40	Megace 40 mg	Bristol-Myers
MELLARIL 25	Mellaril 25 mg	Sandoz Pharm
MELLARIL 50	Mellaril 50 mg	Sandoz Pharm
Mellaril/78-2	Mellaril 10 mg	Sandoz Pharm
Mellaril/78-3	Mellaril 25 mg	Sandoz Pharm
Mellaril/78-4	Mellaril 50 mg	Sandoz Pharm
Mellaril/78-5	Mellaril 100 mg	Sandoz Pharm
Mellaril/78-6	Mellaril 150 mg	Sandoz Pharm
Mellaril/78-7	Mellaril 200 mg	Sandoz Pharm
Mellaril/78-8	Mellaril 15 mg	Sandoz Pharm
MELLARIL 100	Mellaril 100 mg	Sandoz Pharm
MELLARIL 150	Mellaril 150 mg	Sandoz Pharm
MELLARIL 200	Mellaril 200 mg	Sandoz Pharm
MERRELL 11	Norpramin 75 mg	Merrell Dow Pharm
MERRELL 15	Norpramin 50 mg	Merrell Dow Pharm
MERRELL 19	Norpramin 75 mg	Merrell Dow Pharm
MERRELL 20	Norpramin 100 mg	Merrell Dow Pharm
MERRELL 21	Norpramin 150 mg	Merrell Dow Pharm
MERRELL 37	Cantil 25 mg	Merrell Dow Pharm
MERRELL 62	Metahydrin 2 mg	Merrell Dow Pharm
MERRELL 63	Metahydrin 4 mg	Merrell Dow Pharm
MERRELL 64	Metatensin 2/0.1 mg	Merrell Dow Pharm
MERRELL 65	Metatensin 4/0.1 mg	Merrell Dow Pharm
MERRELL 68-692	Tace 72 mg	Merrell-Nationsl Labs
MERRELL 120	Bentyl 10 mg	Merrell Dow Labs
MERRELL 123	Bentyl 20 mg	Merrell Dow Labs
MERRELL 277	Hiprex 1000 mg	Merrell Dow Pharm
MERRELL 547	Quinamm 260 mg	Merrell Dow Pharm
MERRELL 690	Tace 12 mg	Merrell Dow Pharm
MERRELL 691	Tace 25 mg	Merrell Dow Pharm
MERRELL 692	Tace 72 mg	Merrell Dow Pharm
MERRELL 725	Bricanyl 2.5 mg	Merrell Dow Pharm
MERRELL 750	Bricanyl 5 mg	Merrell Dow Pharm
MESTINON 60 ROCHE	Mestinon 60 mg	Roche Labs
MF/a	CONTROLLED - SEE PAGE 204	
MGI/705	Pilocarpine HCl 5 mg	MCI Pharma
MI 15/P F	CONTROLLED - SEE PAGE 189	
MI 30/P F	CONTROLLED - SEE PAGE 199	
MIA 093	Tanamine 25 mg/8 mg/25 mg	Mikart Inc
MIA 110	Butalbital, Acetaminophen, Caffeine	Mikart Inc
M/IB	Ibuprofen 200 mg	Par Pharmaceutical
MICRONASE 5	Micronase 5 mg	Upjohn Co
MICRONASE/U 1.25	Micronase 1.25 mg	Upjohn Co
MICRONASE/U 2.5	Micronase 2.5 mg	Upjohn Co
MICRONASE/U 5	Micronase 5 mg	Upjohn Co
MILES/093	Mycelex 100 mg	Miles Pharm

Imprint	Ingredient/Brand Name	Manufacturer
MILES 095	Mycelex 10 mg	Miles Pharm
MILES/097	Mycelex 500 mg	Miles Pharm
MILES 20	Nifedipine 20 mg	Miles Pharm
MILES 121	Decholin 250 mg	Miles Pharm
MILES 132	Stilphostrol 50 mg	Miles Pharm
MILES 411	Domeboro	Miles Pharm
MILES 512	Cipro 250 mg	Miles Pharm
MILES 513	Cipro 500 mg	Miles Pharm
MILES 514	Cipro 750 mg	Miles Pharm
MILES 521	Biltricide 600 mg	Miles Pharm
MILES 721	Niclocide 500 mg	Miles Pharm
Miles 811	Adalat 10 mg	Miles Pharm
Miles 821	Adalat 20 mg	Miles Pharm
MILES 855	Nimodipine 30 mg	Miles Pharm
MILES 951	Lithane 300 mg	Miles Pharm
MILES DT	Nifedipine 10 mg	Miles Pharm
MINIPRESS PFIZER 431	Minipress 1 mg	Pfizer Labs
MINIPRESS PFIZER 437	Minipress 2 mg	Pfizer Labs
MINIPRESS PFIZER 438	Minipress 5 mg	Pfizer Labs
MINIZIDE PFIZER 430	Minizide 1 mg/0.5 mg	Pfizer Labs
MINIZIDE PFIZER 432	Minizide 2 mg/0.5 mg	Pfizer Labs
MINIZIDE PFIZER 436	Minizide 5 mg/0.5 mg	Pfizer Labs
Mlr	Ferrous Sulfate 195 mg	Schering Corp
MJ	Colace 50 mg	Mead Johnson
MJ 021	Estrace 0.5 mg	Mead Johnson
MJ 5	Buspar 5 mg	Mead Johnson
MJ 10	Buspar 10 mg	Mead Johnson
MJ 10mEq KLOTRIX	Klotrix 750 mg	Mead Johnson
MJ/20	Megace 20 mg	Mead Johnson
MJ/40	Megace 40 mg	Mead Johnson
MJ 158	Monopril 10 mg	Mead Johnson
MJ 240	Sotolol	Mead Johnson
MJ 468	Vitamins 0.5 mg	Mead Johnson
MJ 474	Vitamins 1.0 mg	Mead Johnson
MJ 476	Vitamins 1.0 mg	Mead Johnson
MJ 477	Vitamins 1.0 mg	Mead Johnson
MJ 482	Vitamins 0.5 mg	Mead Johnson
MJ 487	Vitamins 0.25 mg	Mead Johnson
MJ 488	Vitamins 0.25 mg	Mead Johnson
MJ 500	Duricef 500 mg	Mead Johnson
MJ 503	Cytoxan 50 mg	Mead Johnson
MJ 504	Cytoxan 25 mg	Mead Johnson
MJ 512	Quibron-T 300 mg	Mead Johnson
MJ 515	Quibron-300 300 mg/180 mg	Mead Johnson
MJ 516	Quibron 150 mg/90 mg	Mead Johnson
MJ 518	Quibron Plus 150 mg/100 mg/25 mg/20 mg	Mead Johnson
MJ 519	Quibron-T SR 300 mg	Mead Johnson
MJ 538	Ovcon-50 1 mg/0.05 mg	Mead Johnson
MJ 543	Vasodilan 10 mg	Mead Johnson
MJ 544	Vasodilan 20 mg	Mead Johnson
MJ 555	Deapril-ST	Mead Johnson
MJ 583	Ovcon 35	Mead Johnson
MJ 584	Ovcon 50	Mead Johnson
MJ 595	Megace 20 mg	Mead Johnson
MJ 596	Megace 40 mg	Mead Johnson
MJ 609	Monopril 20 mg	Mead Johnson

Imprint	Ingredient/Brand Name	Manufacturer
MJ 702	Natalins	Mead Johnson
MJ 755	Estrace 1 mg	Mead Johnson
MJ 756	Estrace 2 mg	Mead Johnson
MJ 770	Klotrix	Mead Johnson
MJ 775	Desyrel 50 mg	Mead Johnson
MJ 776	Desyrel 100 mg	Mead Johnson
MJ 778	Desyrel Dividose 150 mg	Mead Johnson
MJ 784	Duricef 500 mg	Mead Johnson
MJ 785	Duricef 1000 mg	Mead Johnson
MJ 796	Desyrel 300 mg	Mead Johnson
MJ/850	Placebo	Mead Johnson
MJT	Methamphetamine	Unknown
MK/a	CONTROLLED - SEE PAGE 210	
MK[in oval] 140	Diphenhydramine	McKesson Labs
ML	Caffeine, Ephedrine, Phenylpropanolamine	Unknown
M M	Sucrets MS 3 mg	Beecham Products
M MARION/PAVABID HP	Pavabid HP 300 mg	Marion Labs
MMS 830	Proglycem 50 mg	Medical Market
MMS PBA	Proglycem 50 mg	Medical Market
MO L.E	Caffeine, Ephedrine, Phenylpropanolamine	Unknown
MOTRIN 300mg	Motrin 300 mg	Upjohn Co
MOTRIN 400mg	Motrin 400 mg	Upjohn Co
MOTRIN 600mg	Motrin 600 mg	Upjohn Co
MOTRIN 800mg	Motrin 800 mg	Upjohn Co
MP 0364	Sterapred DS 10 mg	Mayrand
MP 0384	Vitamins	Scherer
MP 3	Hydroxyzine 10 mg	Mutual Pharm
MP 4	Imipramine Hydrochloride 10 mg	Mutual Pharm
MP 6	CONTROLLED - SEE PAGE 184	
MP 7	Hydroxyzine 25 mg	Mutual Pharm
MP 8	Imipramine Hydrochloride 25 mg	Mutual Pharm
MP 10	Amitriptyline 10 mg	Mutual Pharm
MP 11	Dipyridamole 25 mg	Mutual Pharm
MP 12	Thioridazine 10 mg	Mutual Pharm
MP 13	Hydroxyzine 50 mg	Mutual Pharm
MP 14	Thioridazine 25 mg	Mutual Pharm
MP 15	Dipyridamole 50 mg	Mutual Pharm
MP 17	Thioridazine 50 mg	Mutual Pharm
MP 18	Dipyridamole 75 mg	Mutual Pharm
MP 20	Ergoloid Mesylates 1 mg	Mutual Pharm
MP 22	Hydralazine 10 mg	Mutual Pharm
MP 25	Amitriptyline 25 mg	Mutual Pharm
MP 26	Amitriptyline 50 mg	Mutual Pharm
MP 27	Amitriptyline 75 mg	Mutual Pharm
MP 28	Amitriptyline 100 mg	Mutual Pharm
MP 29	Amitriptyline 150 mg	Mutual Pharm
MP 30	Chlorthalidone 25 mg	Mutual Pharm
MP 35	Spironolactone 25 mg	Mutual Pharm
MP 37	Doxycycline 100 mg	Mutual Pharm
MP 39	CONTROLLED - SEE PAGE 185	
MP40	Spironolactone 25 mg, Hydrochlorothiazide 25 mg	Mutual Pharm
MP 43	Chlorthalidone 50 mg	Mutual Pharm
MP 44	Benztropine Mesylate 1 mg	Mutual Pharm
MP 45	Metronidazole 250 mg	Mutual Pharm
MP 46	Metronidazole 500 mg	Mutual Pharm
MP 47	Albuterol 2 mg	Mutual Pharm

Imprint	Ingredient/Brand Name	Manufacturer
MP 50	Tolmetin Sodium 200 mg	Mutual Pharm
MP 51	Prednisone 5 mg	Mutual Pharm
MP 52	Prednisone 10 mg	Mutual Pharm
MP 53	Prednisone 20 mg	Mutual Pharm
MP 55	Hydralazine 50 mg	Mutual Pharm
MP 58	Carisoprodol 350 mg	Mutual Pharm
MP 64	Hydralazine 25 mg	Mutual Pharm
MP 65	Acetazolamide 125 mg	Mutual Pharm
MP 66	Quinidine Gluconate 324 mg	Mutual Pharm
MP 68	Tolazamide 100 mg	Mutual Pharm
MP 69	Verapamil 80 mg	Mutual Pharm
MP 70	Tolazamide 250 mg	Mutual Pharm
MP 71	Allopurinol 100 mg	Mutual Pharm
MP 72	Tolazamide 500 mg	Mutual Pharm
MP 74	Chlorzoxazone 500 mg	Mutual Pharm
MP 76	Verapamil 120 mg	Mutual Pharm
MP 77	Ibuprofen 200 mg	Mutual Pharm
MP 79	Imipramine Hydrochloride 50 mg	Mutual Pharm
MP 80	Allopurinol 300 mg	Mutual Pharm
MP 81	Sulfamethoxazole 400 mg, Trimethoprim 80 mg	Mutual Pharm
MP 83	Nystattin 0.5 mg	Mutual Pharm
MP 85	Sulfamethoxazole 800 mg, Trimethoprim 160 mg	Mutual Pharm
MP 88	Albuterol 4 mg	Mutual Pharm
MP 91	Sulfasalazine 500 mg	Mutual Pharm
MP 93	Quinidine Sulfate 100 mg	Mutual Pharm
MP 94	Ibuprofen 300 mg	Mutual Pharm
MP 95	Ibuprofen 400 mg	Mutual Pharm
MP 96	CONTROLLED - SEE PAGE 191	
MP 98	Ibuprofen 600 mg	Mutual Pharm
MP 99/800	Ibuprofen 800 mg	Mutual Pharm
MP 108	Quinidine Sulfate 200 mg	Mutual Pharm
MP 111/2	CONTROLLED - SEE PAGE 194	
MP 112	Sulindac 150 mg	Mutual Pharm
MP 114	Trazodone 100 mg	Mutual Pharm
MP 116	Sulindac 200 mg	Mutual Pharm
MP 118	Trazodone 50 mg	Mutual Pharm
MP 122/3	CONTROLLED - SEE PAGE 195	
MP 124	Quinidine Sulfate 300 mg	Mutual Pharm
MP 127/4	CONTROLLED - SEE PAGE 194	
MP 135	Acetaminophen 325 mg	Mutual Pharm
MP 140	Acetaminophen 500 mg	Mutual Pharm
MP 141	Acetazolamide 250 mg	Mutual Pharm
MP 145	Acetaminophen 500 mg	Mutual Pharm
MP 146	Atenolol 50 mg	Mutual Pharm
MP 147	Atenolol 75 mg	Mutual Pharm
MP 151	Prednisone 5 mg	Mutual Pharm
MP 152	Atenolol 100 mg, Chlorthalidone 25 mg	Mutual Pharm
MP 153	Atenolol 50 mg, Chlorthalidone 25 mg	Mutual Pharm
MP 155	Quinine Sulfate 260 mg	Mutual Pharm
MP 160	Thioridazine 100 mg	Mutual Pharm
MP 167	Fenoprofen 600 mg	Mutual Pharm
MP 174	Salsalate 500 mg	Mutual Pharm
MP 177	Salsalate 750 mg	Mutual Pharm
MP 184	Metoprolol Tartrate 50 mg	Mutual Pharm
MP 185	Metoprolol Tartrate 100 mg	Mutual Pharm
MPC 600	Potassium Citrate 5mEq	Mission

Imprint	Ingredient/Brand Name	Manufacturer
M R	Sedapap-10 50 mg/650 mg	Mayrand Inc
M/R	Sterapred 5 mg	Mayrand
MR 0379	Guaifenesin 400 mg, Pseudoephedrine 120 mg	Mayrand
MR 0382	Guaifenesin 400 mg, Dextromethorphan 20 mg, Pseudoephedrine 60 mg	Mayrand
M/R 1278	Butalbital 50 mg, Acetaminophen 650 mg	Mayrand
M [star logo]	Methamphetamine, Fenproporex, Caffeine	Unknown
MSAP	Arthritis Pain Formula	Whitehall Robins
MSD 014 Vasotec	Vasotec 2.5 mg	Merck Sharp
MSD 19 Prinivil	Prinivil 5 mg	Merck Sharp
MSD 20	Decadron 0.25 mg	Merck Sharp
MSD 21	Cogentin 0.5 mg	Merck Sharp
MSD 23	Elavil 10 mg	Merck Sharp
MSD 25	Indocin 25 mg	Merck Sharp
MSD 26	Vivactil 5 mg	Merck Sharp
MSD 41	Dacadron 0.5 mg	Merck Sharp
MSD 42	HydroDIURIL 25 mg	Merck Sharp
MSD 43	Mephyton 5 mg	Merck Sharp
MSD 45	Elavil 25 mg	Merck Sharp
MSD 47	Vivactil 10 mg	Merck Sharp
MSD 49	Daranide 50 mg	Merck Sharp
MSD 50	Indocin 50 mg	Merck Sharp
MSD 52	Inversine 2.5 mg	Merck Sharp
MSD 53	Hydropres 25 mg/0.125 mg	Merck Sharp
MSD 59 Blocadren	Blocadren 5 mg	Merck Sharp
MSD 60	Cogentin 2 mg	Merck Sharp
MSD 62	Periactin 4 mg	Merck Sharp
MSD 63	Decadron 0.75 mg	Merck Sharp
MSD 65	Edecrin 25 mg	Merck Sharp
MSD 67	Timolide 10 mg/25 mg	Merck Sharp
MSD 72 Proscar	Proscar 5 mg	Merck Sharp
MSD 90	Edecrin 50 mg	Merck Sharp
MSD 92	Midamor 5 mg	Merck Sharp
MSD 95	Decadron 1.5 mg	Merck Sharp
MSD 97	Decadron 4 mg	Merck Sharp
MSD 102	Elavil 50 mg	Merck Sharp
MSD 105	HydroDIURIL 50 mg	Merck Sharp
MSD 106 Prinivil	Prinivil 10 mg	Merck Sharp
MSD 126	Cortone 5 mg	Merck Sharp
MSD 127	Hydropres 50 mg/0.125 mg	Merck Sharp
MSD 135	Aldomet 125 mg	Merck Sharp
MSD 136 Blocadren	Blocadren 10 mg	Merck Sharp
MSD 147	Decadron 6 mg	Merck Sharp
MSD 150	Indocin 50 mg	Merck Sharp
MSD 207 Prinivil	Prinivil 20 mg	Merck Sharp
MSD 214	Diuril 250 mg	Merck Sharp
MSD 219	Cortone Acetate 25 mg	Merck Sharp
MSD 230	Diupres-250 250 mg/0.125 mg	Merck Sharp
MSD 237 Prinivil	Prinivil 40 mg	Merck Sharp
MSD 401	Aldomet 250 mg	Merck Sharp
MSD 403	Urecholine 5 mg	Merck Sharp
MSD 405	Diupres-500 500 mg/0.125 mg	Merck Sharp
MSD 410	HydroDIURIL 100 mg	Merck Sharp
MSD 412	Urecholine 10 mg	Merck Sharp
MSD 423	Aldoril 250 mg/15 mg	Merck Sharp
MSD 430	Elavil 75 mg	Merck Sharp

Imprint	Ingredient/Brand Name	Manufacturer
MSD 432	Diuril 500 mg	Merck Sharp
MSD 435	Elavil 100 mg	Merck Sharp
MSD 437 Blocadren	Blocadren 20 mg	Merck Sharp
MSD 456	Aldoril 250 mg/25 mg	Merck Sharp
MSD 457	Urecholine 25 mg	Merck Sharp
MSD 460	Urecholine 50 mg	Merck Sharp
MSD 501	Benemid 500 mg	Merck Sharp
MSD 516	Aldomet 500 mg	Merck Sharp
MSD 517	Triavil 4 mg/50 mg	Merck Sharp
MSD 602	Cuprimine 250 mg	Merck Sharp
MSD 612	Aldoclor 250 mg/150	Merck Sharp
MSD 614	ColBENEMID 500 mg/0.5 mg	Merck Sharp
MSD 619	Hydrocortone 10 mg	Merck Sharp
MSD 625	Hydrocortone 20 mg	Merck Sharp
MSD 634	Aldoclor 250 mg/250 mg	Merck Sharp
MSD 647	Sinemet 10 mg/100 mg	Merck Sharp
MSD 650	Sinemet 25 mg/100 mg	Merck Sharp
MSD 654	Sinemet 25 mg/250 mg	Merck Sharp
MSD 672	Cuprimine 125 mg	Merck Sharp
MSD 673	Elavil 150 mg	Merck Sharp
MSD 675	Dolobid 250 mg	Merck Sharp
MSD 679 CUPRID	Cuprid 250 mg	Merck Sharp
MSD 690	Demser 250 mg	Merck Sharp
MSD 693	Indocin 75 mg	Merck Sharp
MSD 694	Aldoril 500 mg/30 mg	Merck Sharp
MSD 697	Dolobid 500 mg	Merck Sharp
MSD 705	Tonocard 400 mg	Merck Sharp
MSD 707	Tonocard 400 mg	Merck Sharp
MSD 709	Tonocard 600 mg	Merck Sharp
MSD 712 Vasotec	Vasotec 5 mg	Merck Sharp
MSD 713 Vasotec	Vasotec 10 mg	Merck Sharp
MSD 714 Vasotec	Vasotec 20 mg	Merck Sharp
MSD 720	Vaseretic 10 mg/25 mg	Merck Sharp
MSD 730	Lovastatin 10 mg	Merck Sharp
MSD 731	Mevacor 20 mg	Merck Sharp
MSD 732	Lovastatin 40 mg	Merck Sharp
MSD 907	Mintezol 500 mg	Merck Sharp
MSD 914	Triavil 2 mg/10 mg	Merck Sharp
MSD 917	Moduretic 5 mg/50 mg	Merck Sharp
MSD 921	Triavil 2 mg/25 mg	Merck Sharp
MSD 931	Flexeril 10 mg	Merck Sharp
MSD 934	Triavil 4 mg/10 mg	Merck Sharp
MSD 935	Aldoril 500 mg/50 mg	Merck Sharp
MSD 941	Clinoril 150 mg	Merck Sharp
MSD 942	Clinoril 200 mg	Merck Sharp
MSD 946	Triavil 4 mg/25 mg	Merck Sharp
MSD 963	Pepcid 20 mg	Merck Sharp
MSD 964	Pepcid 40 mg	Merck Sharp
MSM	Magnesium Salicylate Tetrahydrate 580 mg	Whitehall Robins
MURO 6/60 BROMFED-PD	Bromfed P-D 6 mg/12 mg	Muro Pharm
MURO 12/120 BROMFED	Bromfed 12 mg/120 mg	Muro Pharm
MURO 60/300 GUAIFED-PD	Guaifed-PD 60 mg/300 mg	Muro Pharm
MURO 120/250 GUAIFED	Guaifed 120 mg/250 mg	Muro Pharm
MURO 400/60	Pseudoephedrine 60 mg, Guaifenesin 400 mg	Muro Pharm
MURO 4060	Bromfed 4 mg/60 mg	Muro Pharm

Imprint	Ingredient/Brand Name	Manufacturer
MURRELL	Caffeine 175 mg, Ephedrine 25 mg, Phenylpropanolamine 50 mg	BT Products Inc
MUTUAL 100	Doxycycline 50 mg	Mutual Pharm
MUTUAL 101	Indomethacin 25 mg	Mutual Pharm
MUTUAL 102	Quinine Sulfate 5 gr	Mutual Pharm
MUTUAL 103	Diphenhydramine 25 mg	Mutual Pharm
MUTUAL 105	Doxycycline 100 mg	Mutual Pharm
MUTUAL 106	Indomethacin 50 mg	Mutual Pharm
MUTUAL 107	Diphenhydramine 50 mg	Mutual Pharm
MUTUAL 110	Acetaminophen 500 mg	Mutual Pharm
MUTUAL 165	Piroxicam 10 mg	Mutual Pharm
MUTUAL 166	Piroxicam 20 mg	Mutual Pharm
MUTUAL 179	Tolmetin Sodium 400 mg	Mutual Pharm
MWP [in diamond] 10-4929	Caffeine, Ephedrine, Phenylpropanolamine	Unknown
MYL GAS 40	Mylanta Gas 40 mg	Johnson & Johnson
MYL GAS 80	Mylanta Gas 80 mg	Johnson & Johnson
MYL GAS 125	Mylanta Gas 125 mg	Johnson & Johnson
MYLANTA	Mylanta	Johnson & Johnson
MYLANTA DS	Mylanta Double Strength	Johnson & Johnson
MYLANTA GELCAP	Mylanta	Johnson & Johnson
MYLAN/73	Perphenazine 4 mg, Amitriptyline 50 mg	Mylan Pharm
MYLAN 101	Tetracycline 250 mg	Mylan Pharm
MYLAN 102	Tetracycline 500 mg	Mylan Pharm
MYLAN 106/250	Erythromycin Stearate 250 mg	Mylan Pharm
MYLAN 107/500	Erythromycin Stearate 500 mg	Mylan Pharm
MYLAN 115	Ampicillin Trihydrate 250 mg	Mylan Pharm
MYLAN 116	Ampicillin Trihydrate 500 mg	Mylan Pharm
MYLAN 143	Indomethacin 25 mg	Mylan Pharm
MYLAN 145	Doxycycline 50 mg	Mylan Pharm
MYLAN 146/25	Spironolactone 25 mg	Mylan Pharm
MYLAN 147	Indomethacin 50 mg	Mylan Pharm
MYLAN 148	Doxycycline 100 mg	Mylan Pharm
MYLAN 152	Clonidine 0.1 mg	Mylan Pharm
MYLAN 156/500	Probenecid 500 mg	Mylan Pharm
MYLAN 162	Chlorothiazide 500 mg	Mylan Pharm
MYLAN 167/100	Doxycycline Hyclate 100 mg	Mylan Pharm
MYLAN 182/10	Propranolol 10 mg	Mylan Pharm
MYLAN 183/20	Propranolol 20 mg	Mylan Pharm
MYLAN 184/40	Propranolol 40 mg	Mylan Pharm
MYLAN 185 80	Propranolol 80 mg	Mylan Pharm
MYLAN 186	Clonidine 0.2 mg	Mylan Pharm
MYLAN 197/100	Chlorpropamide 100 mg	Mylan Pharm
MYLAN 199	Clonidine 0.3 mg	Mylan Pharm
MYLAN 204	Amoxicillin Trihydrate 250 mg	Mylan Pharm
MYLAN 205	Amoxicillin Trihydrate 500 mg	Mylan Pharm
MYLAN 210/250	Chlorpropamide 250 mg	Mylan Pharm
MYLAN 214	Haloperidol 2 mg	Mylan Pharm
MYLAN 216/40	Furosemide 40 mg	Mylan Pharm
MYLAN 217/250	Tolazamide 250 mg	Mylan Pharm
MYLAN 232/80	Furosemide 80 mg	Mylan Pharm
MYLAN 257	Haloperidol 1 mg	Mylan Pharm
MYLAN 271	CONTROLLED - SEE PAGE 190	
MYLAN 327	Haloperidol 5 mg	Mylan Pharm
MYLAN/330	Perphenazine 2 mg, Amitriptyline 10 mg	Mylan Pharm
MYLAN 345	CONTROLLED - SEE PAGE 203	
MYLAN 347	Propranolol 80 mg, Hydrochlorothiazide 25 mg	Mylan Pharm

Imprint	Ingredient/Brand Name	Manufacturer
MYLAN 351	Haloperidol 0.5 mg	Mylan Pharm
MYLAN/377	Naproxen 250 mg	Mylan Pharm
MYLAN/421	Methyldopa 500 mg	Mylan Pharm
MYLAN/427	Sulindac 150 mg	Mylan Pharm
MYLAN/442	Perphenazine 2 mg, Amitriptyline 25 mg	Mylan Pharm
MYLAN/451	Naproxen 500 mg	Mylan Pharm
MYLAN 457	CONTROLLED - SEE PAGE 190	
MYLAN 477	CONTROLLED - SEE PAGE 212	
MYLAN/507	Methyldopa 250 mg, Hydrochlorothiazide 15 mg	Mylan Pharm
MYLAN 512	Verapamil 80 mg	Mylan Pharm
MYLAN 531	Sulindac 200 mg	Mylan Pharm
MYLAN 551	Tolazamide 500 mg	Mylan Pharm
MYLAN/555	Naproxen 375 mg	Mylan Pharm
MYLAN/574	Perphenazine 4 mg, Amitriptyline 25 mg	Mylan Pharm
MYLAN/611	Methyldopa 250 mg	Mylan Pharm
MYLAN/711	Methyldopa 250 mg, Hydrochlorothiazide 25 mg	Mylan Pharm
MYLAN/727	Perphenazine 4 mg, Amitriptyline 10 mg	Mylan Pharm
MYLAN 731	Propranolol 40 mg, Hydrochlorothiazide 25 mg	Mylan Pharm
MYLAN 772	Verapamil 120 mg	Mylan Pharm
MYLAN 777	CONTROLLED - SEE PAGE 192	
MYLAN 1001	Thiothixene 1 mg	Mylan Pharm
MYLAN 1010	Piroxicam 10 mg	Mylan Pharm
MYLAN 1049	Doxepin 10 mg	Mylan Pharm
MYLAN 1101	Prazosin 1 mg	Mylan Pharm
MYLAN 1401	Ibuprofen 400 mg	Mylan Pharm
MYLAN 1410	Nortriptyline 10 mg	Mylan Pharm
MYLAN 1601	Ibuprofen 600 mg	Mylan Pharm
MYLAN 1801	Ibuprofen 800 mg	Mylan Pharm
MYLAN 2002	Thiothixene 2 mg	Mylan Pharm
MYLAN 2020	Piroxicam 20 mg	Mylan Pharm
MYLAN 2100	Loperamide HCl 2 mg	Mylan Pharm
MYLAN 2150	Meclofenamate Sodium 50 mg	Mylan Pharm
MYLAN 2302	Prazosin 2 mg	Mylan Pharm
MYLAN 2325	Nortriptyline 25 mg	Mylan Pharm
MYLAN 3000	Meclofenamate Sodium 100 mg	Mylan Pharm
MYLAN 3005	Thiothixene 5 mg	Mylan Pharm
MYLAN 3125	Doxepin 25 mg	Mylan Pharm
MYLAN 3205	Prazosin 5 mg	Mylan Pharm
MYLAN 3250	Nortriptyline 50 mg	Mylan Pharm
MYLAN 4010	CONTROLLED - SEE PAGE 215	
MYLAN 4175	Nortriptyline 75 mg	Mylan Pharm
MYLAN 4250	Doxepin 50 mg	Mylan Pharm
MYLAN 4415	CONTROLLED - SEE PAGE 218	
MYLAN 4430	CONTROLLED - SEE PAGE 217	
MYLAN 5010	Thiothixene 10 mg	Mylan Pharm
MYLAN 5050	CONTROLLED - SEE PAGE 214	
MYLAN 5200	Tolmetin Sodium 400 mg	Mylan Pharm
MYLAN 5375	Doxepin 75 mg	Mylan Pharm
MYLAN 6410	Doxepin 100 mg	Mylan Pharm
MYLAN A	CONTROLLED - SEE PAGE 225	
MYLAN A 1	CONTROLLED - SEE PAGE 225	
MYLAN A 3	CONTROLLED - SEE PAGE 225	
MYLAN A 4	CONTROLLED - SEE PAGE 225	
MYLAN G1	Glipizide 5 mg	Mylan Pharm
MYLAN G2	Glipizide 10 mg	Mylan Pharm
MYLERAN K2A	Myleran 2 mg	Burroughs Wellcome

Imprint	Ingredient/Brand Name	Manufacturer
MYSOLINE 50	Mysoline 50 mg	Ayerst Labs
n	Chlorophyllin Copper Complex 33.3 mg	JB Labs
N	Diphenhydramine 25 mg	Block Drug Co.
N 020/2	Loperamide 2 mg	Novapharm
N039/50	Atenolol 50 mg	Novapharm
N 084-250	Cephalexin 250 mg	Novapharm
N088/5	Pindolol 5 mg	Novapharm
N093/10	Pindolol 10 mg	Novapharm
N2	Neptazane 25 mg	Lederle Labs
N 21/W[in box]	NegGram 250 mg	Winthrop-Breon Labs
N 22/W[in box]	NegGram 500 mg	Winthrop-Breon Labs
N 23/W[in box]	NegGram 1000 mg	Winthrop-Breon Labs
N 114-500	Cephalexin 500 mg	Novapharm
N126	CONTROLLED - No Photo - Alprazolam .25 mg - White, round tablet - DEA Schedule IV	Novapharm
N127	CONTROLLED - No Photo - Alprazolam .50 mg - Orange, round tablet - DEA Schedule IV	Novapharm
N131	CONTROLLED - No photo - Alprazolam 1 mg - Blue, round tablet - DEA Schedule IV	Novapharm
N/171	Nifedipine 10 mg	Novapharm
N181/200	Cimetidine 200 mg	Novapharm
N192/300	Cimetidine 300 mg	Novapharm
N204/400	Cimetidine 400 mg	Novapharm
N235/800	Cimetidine 800 mg	Novapharm
N/325	Aspirin 325 mg	P & G Pharma
N401/100	Atenolol 100 mg	Novapharm
N 420-25	Indomethacin 25 mg	Novapharm
N 439-50	Indomethacin 50 mg	Novapharm
N/463	Methyldopa 125 mg	Novapharm
N/471	Methyldopa 250 mg	Novapharm
N480/2	Albuterol Sulfate 2 mg	Novapharm
N/498	Methyldopa 500 mg	Novapharm
N499/4	Albuterol Sulfate 4 mg	Novapharm
N517/250	Naproxen 250 mg	Novapharm
N518/375	Naproxen 375 mg	Novapharm
N520/500	Naproxen 500 mg	Novapharm
N531/275	Naproxen 275 mg	Novapharm
N533/550	Naproxen 550 mg	Novapharm
N582	Calcium Carbonate 500 mg	Nutrilite
N583	Aspirin Free Cold Formula	Nutrilite
N584	Aspirin Free Sinus Relief	Nutrilite
N585	Allergy Relief Tablets	Nutrilite
N586	Acetaminophen 500 mg	Nutrilite
N587	Extra Strength Antacid	Nutrilite
N588	Aspirin 325 mg	Nutrilite
N589	Ferrous Sulfate 325 mg	Nutrilite
N591	Acetaminophen 80 mg	Nutrilite
N617/1	Piroxicam 10 mg	Novapharm
N/634	Methyldopa 250 mg, Hydrochlorothiazide 15 mg	Novapharm
N/635	Methyldopa 500 mg, Hydrochlorothiazide 30 mg	Novapharm
N640/20	Piroxicam 20 mg	Novapharm
N/642	Methyldopa 250 mg, Hydrochlorothiazide 25 mg	Novapharm
N/643	Methyldopa 500 mg, Hydrochlorothiazide 50 mg	Novapharm
N 716-500	Amoxicillin 500 mg	Novapharm
N 724-250	Amoxicillin 250 mg	Novapharm
N 815/400	Tolmetin Sodium 400 mg	Novapharm

Imprint	Ingredient/Brand Name	Manufacturer
NAL FON	Nalfon 600 mg	Dista Prod
NAPROXEN/250	Naproxen 250 mg	Hamilton
NAPROXEN/375	Naproxen 375 mg	Hamilton
NAPROXEN/500	Naproxen 500 mg	Hamilton
NAV 2/Pfizer	Navane 2 mg	Pfizer Labs
NAV 10/Pfizer	Navane 10 mg	Pfizer Labs
N-BACK	Magnesium Salicylate Tetrahydrate 580 mg	Bristol-Myers
ND [logo]	Janimine 10 mg	Abbott Labs
NE	Nicolar 500 mg	Rorer
NE [logo]	Janimine 25 mg	Abbott Labs
NE[in box] 225	Caffeine, Ephedrine, Phenylpropanolamine	Unknown
NE[in box] 275	Caffeine, Ephedrine	Unknown
NE[in box] 325	Caffeine, Ephedrine, Phenylpropanolamine	Unknown
NE[in box] 785	Caffeine, Ephedrine	Unknown
N E 406	Didronel 400 mg	Norwich Eaton Pharm
nervine	Diphenhydramine 25 mg	Miles, Inc.
Neurontin 100mg	Gabapentin 100 mg	Parke-Davis
Neurontin 300mg	Gabapentin 300 mg	Parke-Davis
Neurontin 400mg	Gabapentin 400 mg	Parke-Davis
NF [logo]	Tral 25 mg	Abbott Labs
NHC 1	Acetaminophen 500 mg	JMI Canton
Niche/420	Magnesium L-lactate Dihydrate 84 mg	Schering Corp.
Night	Aceta 250 mg, Pseudoephedrine 30 mg, Dextromethorphan 10 mg, Doxylamine Succinate 6.25 mg	Granutec
NJ [logo]	Cefol	Abbott Labs
NK [logo]	Eutron 25 mg/5 mg	Abbott Labs
NL [logo]	Janimine 50 mg	Abbott Labs
NM [logo]	Ktab 750 mg	Abbott Labs
NM11	Ferrous Sulfate 65 mg	Pharmavite
NM12	Ferrous Fumarate 60 mg	Pharmavite
NM13	Ferrous Sulfate 50 mg	Pharmavite
NoDoz	No Doz 100 mg	Bristol-Myers
No Doz CHEW	Caffeine 100 mg	Bristol-Myers
NOLUDAR 300 ROCHE	CONTROLLED - SEE PAGE 222	
NOLVADEX 600	Nolvadex 10 mg	Stuart Pharm
NOLVADEX/[head logo]	Nolvadex 10 mg	ICI Pharma
NORGESIC 3M	Norgesic	3M
NORGESIC FORTE 3M	Norgesic Forte	3M
NORMOZIDE/227	Labetalol 200 mg, Hydrochlorothiazide 25 mg	Schering Corp
NORMOZIDE/235	Labetalol 100 mg, Hydrochlorothiazide 25 mg	Schering Corp
NORMOZIDE/391	Labetalol 300 mg, Hydrochlorothiazide 25 mg	Schering Corp
NORPACE 100mg	Norpace 100 mg	Searle Pharm
NORPACE 150mg	Norpace 150 mg	Searle Pharm
NORPRAMIN 25	Norpramin 25 mg	Merrell Dow Pharm
NORPRAMIN 50	Norpramin 50 mg	Merrell Dow Pharm
NORPRAMIN 75	Norpramin 75 mg	Merrell Dow Pharm
NORPRAMINE 100	Norpramin 100 mg	Merrell Dow Pharm
NORPRAMINE 150	Norpramin 150 mg	Merrell Dow Pharm
NORTRIPTYLINE DAN 10 mg	Nortriptyline HCl 10 mg	Danbury Pharm
NORTRIPTYLINE DAN 25 mg	Nortriptyline HCl 25 mg	Danbury Pharm
NORTRIPTYLINE DAN 50 mg	Nortriptyline HCl 50 mg	Danbury Pharm
NORTRIPTYLINE DAN 75 mg	Nortriptyline HCl 75 mg	Danbury Pharm
Norvasc 2.5	Norvasc 2.5 mg	Pfizer
Norvasc 5	Norvasc 5 mg	Pfizer
Norvasc 10	Norvasc 10 mg	Pfizer
Norwich	Aspirin 500 mg	P & G Pharma

Imprint	Ingredient/Brand Name	Manufacturer
Norwich 325	Aspirin 325 mg	P & G Pharma
Norwich 500	Aspirin 500 mg	P & G Pharma
NOVAFED	Novafed 120 mg	Merrell Dow Pharm
NOVAFED A	Novafed A 120 mg/8 mg	Merrell Dow Pharm
npi 100	Caffeine, Ephedrine, Phenylpropanolamine	Unknown
NPI 136	Diphenhydramine 50 mg	Newtron Pharm
NPI 137	Diphenhydramine 25 mg	Newtron Pharm
NPL 51081/424	Isocom 65 mg, 100 mg, 325 mg	Nutripharm Labs
NR [logo]	Depakote 250 mg	Abbott Labs
NS [logo]	Depakote 500 mg	Abbott Labs
NT [logo]	Depakote 125 mg	Abbott Labs
Numark	Lipotriad	Numark
NUPRIN	Ibuprofen 200 mg	Bristol-Myers
O	Primatene 130 mg/24 mg	Whitehall Labs
O 600	Acetaminophen 500 mg	Ohm Labs
O 622	Docusate Potassium 100 mg	Ohm Labs
O 624	Acetaminophen 325 mg, Pseudoephedrine 30 mg, Dextromethorphan 10 mg, Chlorpheniramine 2 mg	Ohm Labs
O 625	Docusate Potassium 100 mg, Casanthranol 30 mg	Ohm Labs
OC CC	Acetaminophen 500 mg	Otis Clapp
OHM 010	Acetaminophen 325 mg	Ohm Labs
OHM 011	Acetaminophen 500 mg	Ohm Labs
OHM 013	Chlorpheniramine 2 mg, Phenylpropanolamine 18.7 mg	Ohm Labs
OHM 015	Aspirin 400 mg, Caffeine 32 mg	Ohm Labs
OHM 020	Aspirin 325 mg	Ohm Labs
OHM 021	Buffered Aspirin 325 mg	Ohm Labs
OHM 022	Aspirin 500 mg	Ohm Labs
OHM 031	Calcium Lactate 650 mg	Ohm Labs
OHM 038	Acetaminophen 325 mg, Phenylpropanolamine 12.5 mg, Dextromethorphan Hydrobromide 15 mg	Ohm Labs
OHM 045	Phenylephrine 5 mg, Chlorpheniramine 2 mg, Aceta 325 mg	Ohm Labs
OHM 055	Aceta 250 mg, Aspirin 250 mg, Caffeine 65 mg	Ohm Labs
OHM 076	Pseudoephedrine 60 mg	Ohm Labs
OHM 078	Phenyltoloxamine 30 mg, Acetaminophen 325 mg	Ohm Labs
OHM 117	Senna Concentrate	Ohm Labs
OHM 135	Acetaminophen 325 mg, Pseudoephedrine 30 mg, Dextromethorphan 10 mg, Chlorpheniramine 2 mg	Ohm Labs
OHM 160	Triprolidine 2.5 mg, Pseudoephedrine 60 mg	Ohm Labs
OHM 311	Acetaminophen 500 mg	Ohm Labs
OHM 400	Ibuprofen 400 mg	Ohm Labs
OJF 295	Iodo-Niacin 135 mg/25 mg	Forest Pharm
OJF 355	Pedameth 200 mg	Chromalloy Pharm
OJF 372	Feostat 100 mg	Forest Pharm
OJF 415	CONTROLLED - SEE PAGE 210	
OJF 1043	Dehist 8 mg/75 mg	Forest Pharm
One A Day	One-A-Day Stressgard	Miles
OPW 714	Doxylamine, Salicylamide, Acetaminphen	Unknown
ORAP McNEIL	Orap 2 mg	McNeil Pharm
ORETIC	Oretic 25 mg	Abbott Labs
ORETIC	Oretic 50 mg	Abbott Labs
ORG	Jenest-28	Organon Pharm
ORG 07	Jenest-28	Organon Pharm
ORG 14	Jenest-28	Organon Pharm
ORG 472	Calderol 0.02 mg	Organon Pharm
ORG 474	Calderol 0.05 mg	Organon Pharm
Organon 381	Cotazym	Organon Pharm

Imprint	Ingredient/Brand Name	Manufacturer
Organon 386	Cotazym 430 mg	Organon Pharm
Organon 388	Cotazym-S	Organon Pharm
Organon 393	Zymase	Organon Pharm
Organon 542	Wigraine 1 mg/100 mg	Organon Pharm
Organon 790	Hexadrol 1.5 mg	Organon Pharm
Organon 791	Hexadrol 0.75 mg	Organon Pharm
Organon 792	Hexadrol 0.5 mg	Organon Pharm
Organon 798	Hexadrol 4 mg	Organon Pharm
ORINASE 250	Orinase 250 mg	Upjohn Co
ORNADE	Ornade 75 mg/12 mg	Smith, Kline & French
ORNEX ORNEX	Acetaminophen 325 mg, Pseudoephedrine 30 mg	Menley & James
ORNEX MAX ORNEX MAX	Acetaminophen 500 mg, Pseudoephedrine 30 mg	Menley & James
ORNEX SC ORNES SC	Aceta 500 mg, Pseudoephedrine 30 mg, Dextromethorphan 15 mg	Menley & Ja
Ortho 0.35	Norethindrone 0.35 mg	Ortho Pharm
ORTHO-1/2	Ortho-Novum 0.5 mg/0.1 mg	Ortho Pharm
Ortho 1	Ortho-Novum 1 mg/0.08 mg	Ortho Pharm
Ortho 2	Ortho-Novum 2 mg/0.1 mg	Ortho Pharm
Ortho 10	Ortho-Novum 10 mg/0.06 mg	Ortho Pharm
Ortho 75	Ortho-Novum 0.75 mg/0.035 mg	Ortho Pharm
Ortho 135	Ortho-Novum 1/35	Ortho Pharm
Ortho 150	Ortho-Novum 1 mg/0.05 mg	Ortho Pharm
ORTHO 211	Grifulvin V 250 mg	Ortho Pharm
ORTHO 214	Grifulvin V 100 mg	Ortho Pharm
Ortho 535	Ortho-Novum 0.5 mg/0.035 mg	Ortho Pharm
ORTHO 735	Norethindrone 0.75 mg, Ethinyl Estradiol 0.035 mg	Ortho Pharm
ORTHO 1000 IMODIUM	Imodium 2 mg	Ortho Pharm
Ortho 1570	Protostat 250 mg	Ortho Pharm
Ortho 1571	Protostat 500 mg	Ortho Pharm
OS-CAL	Os-Cal 500 1250 mg	Marion Labs
OTIS CLAPP	Acetaminopehn 325 mg	Otis Clapp
P	Panadol 80 mg	Glenbrook Labs
P[crescent]	Pemoline 50 mg	Unknown
P[triangle]	Pemoline 25 mg	Unknown
P & G/402	Didronel 200 mg	Procter & Gamble
P 010	Chloral Hydrate	Unknown
P 0102	Vitamin A 50,000 units	Pharmacaps Inc
P 0109	Vitamin A 50,000 units	Pharmacaps Inc
P 0140	Vitmain A 50,000 units	Pharmacaps Inc
P1	Ibuprofen 200 mg	Granutec
P/1 1	Sodium Fluoride 1 mg	Pharmics
P/2 2	Sodium Fluoride 2 mg	Pharmics
P 9	Imipramine 25 mg	Vitarine Pharm
P 15	CONTROLLED - SEE PAGE 185	
P 15/DAN	CONTROLLED - SEE PAGE 185	
P20	Pseudoephedrine 60 mg	Circa Pharm
P-21	Imipramine 50 mg	Eon
P 25	Hydrochlorothiazide 25 mg	Vitarine Pharm
P 30	CONTROLLED - SEE PAGE 186	
P 30/DAN	CONTROLLED - SEE PAGE 186	
P32	Reserpine 0.1 mg	Eon Labs
P35	Pseudoephedrine 30 mg	Circa Pharm
P 36	Pyrazinamide 500 mg	Lederle Labs
P42	Ibuprofen 200 mg	Granutec
P 53	Phenytoin 100 mg	Lederle Labs
P 60/DAN	CONTROLLED - SEE PAGE 189	
P 61/W[in box]	Plaquenil 200 mg	Winthrop-Breon Labs

Imprint	Ingredient/Brand Name	Manufacturer
P 66	Caffeine, Ephedrine, Phenylpropanolamine	Unknown
KP 101	Azulfidine 500 mg	Pharmacia Labs
KP 102	Azulfidine 500 mg	Pharmacia Labs
P 3900	Theophylline 150 g, Guaifenesin 90 mg	Pharmacaps Inc
P/9523	CONTROLLED - SEE PAGE 202	
P&G 402	Didronel 200 mg	Norwich Eaton Pharm
P-32	Reserpine 0.1 mg	Vitarine Pharm
P47	Acetaminophen 80 mg	Granutec
P75	Magnesium Salicylate 325 mg	Granutec
P-75	Caffeine, Ephedrine, Phenylpropanolamine	Unknown
P 100/DAN	CONTROLLED - SEE PAGE 191	
P112	Multi-Symptom Cold Caplet	Granutec
P115	Multiple Symptom Cold Relief Tablets	Granutec
P-135	Caffeine, Ephedrine, Phenylpropanolamine	Unknown
P141	Maximum Strength Allergy Sinus Caplets	Granutec
P174	Multi-Symptom Cold Caplet	Granutec
P-175	Caffeine, Ephedrine, Phenylpropanolamine	Unknown
P-200	Caffeine	Unknown
P211	Acetaminophen 500 mg, Pseudoephedrine 30 mg	Granutec
P225	Magnesium Salicylate 500 mg	Granutec
P262	Yellow Phenolphthalein 90 mg	Granutec
P337	Cold Tablets	Granutec
P422	Maximum Strength Cold Tablets	Granutec
P [logo] 25	Diphenhydramine 25 mg	Medtech Labs
P 2120	Valproic Acid 250 mg	Sidmak Labs
P 4600	Benzonatate 100 mg	Sidmak Labs
P[in box] 51580	Caffeine, Ephedrine, Phenylpropanolamine	Unknown
P[in box] 81580	Caffeine, Ephedrine, Phenylpropanolamine	Unknown
P[in box] 81598	Caffeine, Ephedrine, Phenylpropanolamine	Unknown
PAMPRIN	Pamprin 500 mg/25 mg/15 mg	Chattem Prod
PAN/2000	Pancrelipase	Jones
PANADOL 500	Panadol 500 mg	Glenbrook Labs
Pancrease McNEIL	Pancrease 4000/20,000/25,000 units	McNeil Pharm
par 001	Cyclandelate 200 mg	Par Pharm
par 002	Cyclandelate 400 mg	Par Pharm
PAR 006	Chlorzoxazone 250 mg, Acetaminphen 300 mg	Par Pharm
par 008	Pseudoephedrine 60 mg	Par Pharm
par 009	Isosorbide Dinitrate 30 mg	Par Pharm
par 010	Isosorbide Dinitrate 10 mg	Par Pharm
par 011	Brompheniramine 4 mg	Par Pharm
par 012	Hydroxyzine 10 mg	Par Pharm
par 013	Hydroxyzine 25 mg	Par Pharm
par 014	Hydroxyzine 50 mg	Par Pharm
par 015	Meclizine 50 mg	Par Pharm
par 016	Chlorzoxazone 250 mg	Par Pharm
par 018	Doxycycline Hyclate 50 mg	Par Pharm
par 019	Doxycycline Hyclate 100 mg	Par Pharm
PAR 020	Isosorbide Dinitrate 5 mg	Par Pharm
PAR 021	Isosorbide Dinitrate 10 mg	Par Pharm
PAR 022	Isosorbide Dinitrate 20 mg	Par Pharm
par 023	Isosorbide Dinitrate 2.5 mg	Par Pharm
par 024	Isosorbide Dinitrate 5 mg	Par Pharm
par 025	Isosorbide Dinitrate 40 mg	Par Pharm
par 027	Hydralazine 25 mg	Par Pharm
par 028	Hydralazine 50 mg	Par Pharm
par 029	Hydralazine 10 mg	Par Pharm

Imprint	Ingredient/Brand Name	Manufacturer
par 030	Par-Decon 10 mg/40 mg/15 mg/5 mg	Par Pharm
par 031	Dipyridamole 50 mg	Par Pharm
par 034	Meclizine 12.5 mg	Par Pharm
par 035	Meclizine 25 mg	Par Pharm
par 036	Methocarbamol 500 mg	Par Pharm
par 037	Methocarbamol 750 mg	Par Pharm
par 038	Trichlormethiazide 2 mg	Par Pharm
par 039	Trichlormethiazide 4 mg	Par Pharm
par 041	Vitamins, Folic Acid	Par Pharm
par 042	Dipyridamole 25 mg	Par Pharm
par 043	Cyproheptadine 4 mg	Par Pharm
par 045	Dexchlorpheniramine 4 mg	Par Pharm
par 046	Dexchlorpheniramine 6 mg	Par Pharm
par 048	Isoxsuprine 10 mg	Par Pharm
par 049	Isoxsuprine 20 mg	Par Pharm
par 050	Guanethindine Sulfate 10 mg	Par Pharm
par 051	Guanethindine Sulfate 25 mg	Par Pharm
par 052	Iron, Vitamins	Par Pharm
par 053	Vitamin B Complex, Folic Acid	Par Pharm
par 054	Imipramine 10 mg	Par Pharm
par 055	Imipramine 25 mg	Par Pharm
par 056	Imipramine 50 mg	Par Pharm
par 057	Iron, Vitamins, Folic Acid	Par Pharm
par 058	Vitamins, Fluoride 1 mg	Par Pharm
par 06	Dexchlorophenriramine 6 mg	Par Pharm
par 061	Fluphenazine 1 mg	Par Pharm
par 062	Fluphenazine 2.5 mg	Par Pharm
par 064	Fluphenazine 10 mg	Par Pharm
par 065	Dipyridamole 75 mg	Par Pharm
par 066	Doxylamine 25 mg	Par Pharm
par 067	Indomethacin 25 mg	Par Pharm
par 068	Indomethacin 50 mg	Par Pharm
par 069	Hydroxyzine 25 mg	Par Pharm
par 070	Hydroxyzine 50 mg	Par Pharm
par 071	Hydroxyzine 100 mg	Par Pharm
par 076	Fluphenazine 5 mg	Par Pharm
par 077	Chlorpropamide 100 mg	Par Pharm
par 078	Chlorpropamide 250 mg	Par Pharm
par 082	Chlorzoxazone 500 mg	Par Pharm
par 083	Dexamethasone 0.25 mg	Par Pharm
par 084	Dexamethasone 0.5 mg	Par Pharm
par 085	Dexamethasone 0.75 mg	Par Pharm
par 086	Dexamethasone 1.5 mg	Par Pharm
par 087	Dexamethasone 4 mg	Par Pharm
par 088	Methandroxtenolone 2.5 mg	Par Pharm
par 089	Methandroxtenolone 5 mg	Par Pharm
par 090	Clidinium Bromide 2.5 mg, Chlordiazepoxide 5 mg	Par Pharm
par 095	Metronidazole 250 mg	Par Pharm
par 096	Thioridazine 10 mg	Par Pharm
par 097	Thioridazine 15 mg	Par Pharm
par 098	Thioridazine 25 mg	Par Pharm
par 099	Thioridazine 50 mg	Par Pharm
par 4	Dexchlorpheniramine 4 mg	Par Pharm
PAR 6	Polargen 4 mg	Par Pharm
par/25	Dipyridamole 25 mg	Par Pharm
PAR/50	Dipyridamole 50 mg	Par Pharm

Imprint	Ingredient/Brand Name	Manufacturer
PAR 75	Dipyridamole 75 mg	Par Pharm
par 101	Thioridazine 100 mg	Par Pharm
par 102	Thioridazine 150 mg	Par Pharm
par 103	Thioridazine 200 mg	Par Pharm
par 104	Allopurinol 100 mg	Par Pharm
par 105	Allopurinol 300 mg	Par Pharm
par 106	Propranolol 10 mg	Par Pharm
par 107	Propranolol 20 mg	Par Pharm
par 108	Propranolol 40 mg	Par Pharm
par 109	Propranolol 80 mg	Par Pharm
par 110	Clonidine 0.1 mg	Par Pharm
par 111	Clonidine 0.2 mg	Par Pharm
par 112	Clonidine 0.3 mg	Par Pharm
par 113	Clonidine 0.1 mg, Chlorthalidone 15 mg	Par Pharm
par 114	Metronidazole 500 mg	Par Pharm
par 115	Clonidine 0.3 mg, Chlorthalidone 15 mg	Par Pharm
par 116	Clonidine 0.3 mg, Chlorthalidone 15 mg	Par Pharm
par 117	Amiloride 5 mg	Par Pharm
par 118	Propantheline 15 mg	Par Pharm
par 119	Nystatin 500,000 units	Par Pharm
par 121	Hydralazine 100 mg	Par Pharm
par 122	Tolazamide 100 mg	Par Pharm
par 123	Tolazamide 250 mg	Par Pharm
par 124	Tolazamide 500 mg	Par Pharm
par 125	Valproic Acid 250 mg	Par Pharm
par 127	Propranolol 60 mg	Par Pharm
par 128	Amiloride 5 mg, Hydrochlorothiazide 50 mg	Par Pharm
par 129	Dexamethasone 6 mg	Par Pharm
par 130	Metronidazole 250 mg	Par Pharm
par 131	Metronidazole 500 mg	Par Pharm
par 132	Metoclopramide 10 mg	Par Pharm
par 133	Amitriptyline 10 mg	Par Pharm
par 134	Amitriptyline 25 mg	Par Pharm
par 135	Amitriptyline 50 mg	Par Pharm
par 136	Amitriptyline 75 mg	Par Pharm
par 137	Amitriptyline 100 mg	Par Pharm
par 138	Amitriptyline 150 mg	Par Pharm
par 139	Sulfamethoprim 400 mg/80 mg	Par Pharm
Par 140	Sulfamethoxazole 800 mg, Trimethoprim 160 mg	Par Pharm
par 143	Hydra-zide 25 mg/25 mg	Par Pharm
par 144	Hydra-zide 50 mg/50 mg	Par Pharm
par 145	Hydra-zide 100 mg/50 mg	Par Pharm
par 147	Hydroflumethiazide 50 mg	Par Pharm
par 148	Hydroflumethiazide 50 mg, Reserpine 0.125 mg	Par Pharm
par 150	Methyldopa 125 mg	Par Pharm
par 151	Methyldopa 250 mg	Par Pharm
par 152	Methyldopa 500 mg	Par Pharm
par 153	Disulfiram 250 mg	Par Pharm
par 154	Disulfiram 500 mg	Par Pharm
par 155	Methylprednisolone 2 mg	Par Pharm
par 156	Methylprednisolone 4 mg	Par Pharm
par 157	Methylprednisolone 8 mg	Par Pharm
par 158	Methylprednisolone 16 mg	Par Pharm
par 159	Methylprednisolone 24 mg	Par Pharm
par 160	Methylprednisolone 32 mg	Par Pharm
par 161	Ibuprofen 300 mg	Par Pharm

Imprint	Ingredient/Brand Name	Manufacturer
par 162 /400	Ibuprofen 400 mg	Par Pharm
par 163 /600	Ibuprofen 600 mg	Par Pharm
par 164	Benztropine Mesylate 0.5 mg	Par Pharm
par 165	Benztropine Mesylate 1 mg	Par Pharm
par 166	Benztropine Mesylate 2 mg	Par Pharm
par 170	Sulfinpyrazone 100 mg	Par Pharm
par 171	Sulfinpyrazone 200 mg	Par Pharm
par 176	CONTROLLED - SEE PAGE 212	
par 177	Methyclothiazide 2.5 mg	Par Pharm
par 178	Methyclothiazide 5 mg	Par Pharm
par 181	Perphenazine 2 mg, Amitriptyline 25 mg	Par Pharm
par 182	Perphenazine 2 mg, Amitriptyline 25 mg	Par Pharm
par 183	Perphenazine 4 mg, Amitriptyline 10 mg	Par Pharm
par 184	Perphenazine 4 mg, Amitriptyline 25 mg	Par Pharm
par 185	Perphenazine 4 mg, amitriptyline 50 mg	Par Pharm
par 186	Methyldopa 250 mg, Hydrochlorothiazide 15 mg	Par Pharm
par 187	Methyldopa 250 mg, Hydrochlorothiazide 25 mg	Par Pharm
par 188	Methyldopa 500 mg, Hydrochlorothiazide 30 mg	Par Pharm
par 189	Methyldopa 500 mg, Hydrochlorothiazide 50 mg	Par Pharm
par 193	CONTROLLED - SEE PAGE 218	
par 194	CONTROLLED - SEE PAGE 217	
PAR 200	Ibuprofen 200 mg	Par Pharm
par 202	Methyldopa 150 mg, Chlorothiazide 250 mg	Par Pharm
par 203	Methyldopa 250 mg, Chlorothiazide 250 mg	Par Pharm
par 206	CONTROLLED - SEE PAGE 184	
par 207	CONTROLLED - SEE PAGE 188	
par 208	CONTROLLED - SEE PAGE 193	
par 213	Orphengesic 25 mg/30 mg/385 mg	Par Pharm
par 214	Orphengesic Forte 50 mg/60 mg/770 mg	Par Pharm
par 216/800	Ibuprofen 800 mg	Par Pharm
par 217	Doxepin 10 mg	Par Pharm
par 218	Doxepin 25 mg	Par Pharm
par 219	Doxepin 50 mg	Par Pharm
par 220	Doxepin 75 mg	Par Pharm
par 221	Doxepin 100 mg	Par Pharm
par 222	Doxepin 150 mg	Par Pharm
par 223	Haloperidol 0.5 mg	Par Pharm
par 224	Haloperidol 1 mg	Par Pharm
par 225	Haloperidol 2 mg	Par Pharm
par 226	Haloperidol 5 mg	Par Pharm
par 227	Haloperidol 10 mg	Par Pharm
par 228	Haloperidol 20 mg	Par Pharm
par 229	Metronidazole 250 mg	Par Pharm
par 230	Metronidazole 500 mg	Par Pharm
par 231	Ibuprofen 200 mg	Par Pharm
par 237	Leucovorin 5 mg	Par Pharm
par 238	Leucovorin 25 mg	Par Pharm
par 239	Propranolol 90 mg	Par Pharm
par 240	CONTROLLED - SEE PAGE 220	
par 241	CONTROLLED - SEE PAGE 213	
Par/246	Carisoprodol 200 mg, Aspirin 325 mg	Par Pharm
PAR 247	Salsalate 500 mg	Par Pharm
PAR 248	Salsalate 750 mg	Par Pharm
Par/249	Methocarbamol 400 mg, Aspirin 325 mg	Par Pharm
PAR 250	Cephalexin 250 mg	Par Pharm
par 255	Ibuprofen 200 mg	Par Pharm

Imprint	Ingredient/Brand Name	Manufacturer
par 256	Minoxidil 2.5 mg	Par Pharm
par 257	Minoxidil 10 mg	Par Pharm
Par/258	Metaproterenol Sulfate 20 mg	Par Pharm
Par/259	Metaproterenol Sulfate 20 mg	Par Pharm
PAR 263	Meclofenamate 50 mg	Par Pharm
PAR 264	Meclofenamate 100 mg	Par Pharm
par 275	Cephalexin 250 mg	Par Pharm
par 276	Cephalexin 500 mg	Par Pharm
par 277	Leucovorin 15 mg	Par Pharm
Par/279	Triamterene 75 mg, Hydrochlorothiazide 50 mg	Par Pharm
Par/286	Fenoprofen Calcium 600 mg	Par Pharm
Par/287	Fenoprofen Calcium 200 mg	Par Pharm
Par/288	Fenoprofen Calcium 300 mg	Par Pharm
Par/289	Megestrol Acetate 20 mg	Par Pharm
Par/290	Megestrol Acetate 40 mg	Par Pharm
Par 304	Divalproex Sodium 250 mg	Par Pharm
Par 305	Divalproex Sodium 500 mg	Par Pharm
Par/500	Cephalexin 500 mg	Par Pharm
PARAFLEX McNEIL	Paraflex 250 mg	McNeil Pharm
PARAFON FORTE McNEIL	Parafon Forte 250 mg/300 mg	McNeil Pharm
PARLODEL 2 1/2/78 17	Parlodel 2.5 mg	Sandoz Pharm
PARLODEL 2 1/2	Parlodel 2.5 mg	Sandoz Pharm
Parlodel 5 mg	Parlodel 5 mg	Sandoz Pharm
PARNATE SKF	Parnate 10 mg	Smith, Kline & French
PBA/SCHERING	Proglycem 50 mg	Schering Corp
PBB/SCHERING	Proglycem 100 mg	Schering Corp
PC21	Ferrous Gluconate 38 mg	Pharmavite
PC22	Ferrous Sulfate 65 mg	Pharmavite
PC23	Ferrous Fumarate 50 mg	Pharmavite
PC24	Ferrous Sulfate 50 mg	Pharmavite
PC25	Ferrous Fumarate 50 mg, Docusate Sodium 100 mg	Pharmavite
PCE [logo]	PCE 333 mg	Abbott Labs
P-D 001	Peritrate 20 mg	Parke-Davis
P-D 004	Peritrate SR 80 mg	Parke-Davis
P-D 007	Dilantin 50 mg	Parke-Davis
P-D 008	Peritrate 40 mg	Parke-Davis
P-D 013	Peritrate 10 mg	Parke-Davis
P-D 034	Gelusil 200 mg/200 mg/25 mg	Parke-Davis
P-D 037	Ferrous Sulfate 325 mg	Parke-Davis
P-D 043	Gelusil-II 400 mg/400 mg/25 mg	Parke-Davis
P-D 045	Gelusil-M 300 mg/200 mg/25 mg	Parke-Davis
P-D 070	Propranolol 10 mg	Parke-Davis
P-D 071	Propranolol 20 mg	Parke-Davis
P-D 072	Propranolol 40 mg	Parke-Davis
P-D 073	Propranolol 60 mg	Parke-Davis
P-D 074	Propranolol 80 mg	Parke-Davis
P-D 0260	Euthroid 30 mg	Parke-Davis
P-D 0261	Euthroid 60 mg	Parke-Davis
P-D 0262	Euthroid 120 mg	Parke-Davis
P-D 0263	Euthroid 180 mg	Parke-Davis
P-D 0557	Verapamil 80 mg	Parke-Davis
P-D 0573	Verapamil 120 mg	Parke-Davis
P-D 111	Ergostat 2 mg	Parke-Davis
P-D 121	Chlorthalidone 50 mg	Parke-Davis
P-D 123	Chlorthalidone 25 mg	Parke-Davis
PD 141/2	CONTROLLED - SEE PAGE 199	

Imprint	Ingredient/Brand Name	Manufacturer
PD 142	CONTROLLED - No Photo - Diazepam 5 mg - DEA Schedule IV	Parke-Davis
PD 143	CONTROLLED - No Photo - Diazepam 10 mg - DEA Schedule IV	Parke-Davis
P-D 166	Mandelamine 500 mg	Parke-Davis
P-D 167	Mandelamine 1000 mg	Parke-Davis
P-D 177	Sinubid 300 mg/100 mg/66 mg	Parke-Davis
P-D 180	Pyridium 100 mg	Parke-Davis
P-D 181	Pyridium 200 mg	Parke-Davis
P-D 182	Pyridium Plus 150 mg/0.3 mg/15 mg	Parke-Davis
P-D 200	Brondecon 200 mg/100 mg	Parke-Davis
P-D 202	Procan SR 250 mg	Parke-Davis
PD 204	Procan SR 500 mg	Parke-Davis
PD 205	Procan SR 750 mg	Parke-Davis
PD 207	Procan SR 1000 mg	Parke-Davis
P-D 210	Choledyl 100 mg	Parke-Davis
P-D 211	Choledyl 200 mg	Parke-Davis
P-D 212	Natafort	Parke-Davis
P-D 214	Choledyl 400 mg	Parke-Davis
P-D 221	Choledyl 600 mg	Parke-Davis
P-D 230	Tedral 8 mg, 130 mg, 24 mg	Parke-Davis
P-D 231	Tedral SA 180 mg, 48 mg, 25 mg	Parke-Davis
P-D 237	Zarontin 250 mg	Parke-Davis
P-D 238	Tedral-2 130/24/25 mg	Parke-Davis
P-D 247	D-S-S 100 mg	Parke-Davis
P-D 248	D-S-S Plus 100/30 mg	Parke-Davis
P-D 251	Proloid 1/2 grain	Parke-Davis
P-D 252	Proloid 1 grain	Parke-Davis
P-D 253	Proloid 1 1/2 grains	Parke-Davis
P-D 254	Proloid 3 grains	Parke-Davis
P-D 257	Proloid 2 grains	Parke-Davis
P-D 260	Euthroid-1/2 0.030 mg/0.0075 mg	Parke-Davis
P-D 261	Euthroid-1 0.060 mg/0.015 mg	Parke-Davis
P-D 262	Euthroid-2 0.12 mg/0.03 mg	Parke-Davis
P-D 263	Euthroid-3 0.18 mg/0.045 mg	Parke-Davis
P-D 268	Meclomen 50 mg	Parke-Davis
P-D 269	Meclomen 100 mg	Parke-Davis
PD 269	Meclomen 100 mg	Parke-Davis
P-D 270	Nardil 15 mg	Parke-Davis
P-D 272	Amitriptyline 10 mg	Parke-Davis
P-D 273	Amitriptyline 25 mg	Parke-Davis
P-D 274	Amitriptyline 50 mg	Parke-Davis
P-D 275	Amitriptyline 75 mg	Parke-Davis
P-D 276	CONTROLLED - SEE PAGE 210	
P-D 278	Amitriptyline 150 mg	Parke-Davis
P-D 282	Natafort	Parke-Davis
P-D 320	Parsidol 10 mg	Parke-Davis
P-D 321	Parsidol 50 mg	Parke-Davis
P-D 337	Eldec	Parke-Davis
P-D 362	Dilantin 100 mg	Parke-Davis
P-D 365	Dilantin 30 mg	Parke-Davis
P-D 373	Benadryl 50 mg	Parke-Davis
P-D 379	Chloromycetin 250 mg	Parke-Davis
P-D 389	Bromdiphenhydramine 25 mg	Parke-Davis
P-D 390	Natabec	Parke-Davis
P-D 393	Milontin 500 mg	Parke-Davis

Imprint	Ingredient/Brand Name	Manufacturer
P-D 398	Eldec	Parke-Davis
P-D 402	Ampicillin 250 mg	Parke-Davis
P-D 404	Ampicillin 500 mg	Parke-Davis
P-D 407	Tetracycline HCl 250 mg	Parke-Davis
P-D 420	Quinine Sulfate 325 mg	Parke-Davis
P-D 437	Estrovis 0.1 mg	Parke-Davis
P-D 440	Furosemide 20 mg	Parke-Davis
P-D 441	Furosemide 40 mg	Parke-Davis
P-D 442	Furosemide 80 mg	Parke-Davis
P-D 443	Clonidine HCl 0.1 mg	Parke-Davis
P-D 444	Clonidine HCl 0.2 mg	Parke-Davis
P-D 445	Clonidine 0.3 mg	Parke-Davis
P-D 447	Benadryl 25 mg/60 mg	Parke-Davis
P-D 471	Benadryl 25 mg	Parke-Davis
P-D 490	Easprin 975 mg	Parke-Davis
P-D 525	Celontin 300 mg	Parke-Davis
P-D 527 5	Accupril 5 mg	Parke-Davis
P-D 529	Humatin 250 mg	Parke-Davis
P-D 530 10	Quinapril HCl 10 mg	Parke-Davis
P-D 532 20	Quinapril HCl 20 mg	Parke-Davis
P-D 533	Calcium Lactate 325 mg	Parke-Davis
P-D 534	Natabec with Fluoride	Parke-Davis
P-D 535 40	Quinapril HCl 40 mg	Parke-Davis
P-D 537	Celontin 150 mg	Parke-Davis
P-D 540	Ponstel 250 mg	Parke-Davis
P-D 541	Natabec-FA	Parke-Davis
P-D 544	Geriplex-FS	Parke-Davis
P-D 547	Natabec	Parke-Davis
P-D 550	Thera-Complex H-P	Parke-Davis
P-D 557	Verapamil 80 mg	Parke-Davis
P-D 573	Verapamil 120 mg	Parke-Davis
P-D 604	Calcium Lactate 650 mg	Parke-Davis
P-D 606	Aspirin 325 mg	Parke-Davis
P-D 618	Norlestrin	Parke-Davis
P-D 622	Ferrous Fumarate 75 mg	Parke-Davis
P-D 627	Thyroid 1 grain	Parke-Davis
P-D 638	Tabron	Parke-Davis
P-D 648	Penicillin V Potassium 250 mg	Parke-Davis
P-D 663	Erythromycin 125 mg	Parke-Davis
P-D 669	Lopid 300 mg	Parke-Davis
P-D 672	Erythromycin Stearate 250 mg	Parke-Davis
P-D 673	Penapar VK 500 mg	Parke-Davis
P-D 674	Thyroid 1 grain	Parke-Davis
P-D 696	ERYC 250 mg	Parke-Davis
P-D 697	Tetracycline 500 mg	Parke-Davis
P-D 702	Hydrochlorothiazide 25 mg	Parke-Davis
P-D 710	Hydrochlorothiazide 50 mg	Parke-Davis
P-D 712	Spironolactone 25 mg, Hydrochlorothiazide 25 mg	Parke-Davis
P-D 713	Spironolactone 25 mg	Parke-Davis
P-D 730	Amoxicillin 250 mg	Parke-Davis
P-D 731	Amoxicillin 500 mg	Parke-Davis
P-D 813	Doxycycline 100 mg	Parke-Davis
P-D 829	Doxycycline 50 mg	Parke-Davis
P-D 830	Doxycycline 100 mg	Parke-Davis
P-D 840	Benadryl 25 mg	Parke-Davis
P-D 849	Quinidine Sulfate 200 mg	Parke-Davis

Imprint	Ingredient/Brand Name	Manufacturer
P-D 850	Duraquin 330 mg	Parke-Davis
P-D 865	Methyldopa 250 mg	Parke-Davis
P-D 866	Methyldopa 500 mg	Parke-Davis
P-D 882	Norethindrone 5 mg	Parke-Davis
P-D 887	Indomethacin 25 mg	Parke-Davis
P-D 888	Indomethacin 50 mg	Parke-Davis
P-D 901	Norlestrin 2.5 mg/0.05 mg	Parke-Davis
P-D 904	Norlestrin 1 mg/0.02 mg	Parke-Davis
P-D 906	Ascorbic Acid	Parke-Davis
P-D 915	Loestrin 1 mg/0.02 mg	Parke-Davis
P-D 916	Loestrin 1.5 mg/0.03 mg	Parke-Davis
P-D 918	Norlutate 5 mg	Parke-Davis
P-D 919	Erythromycin Stearate 500 mg	Parke-Davis
PD Eryc 125	Eryc 125	Parke-Davis
PDK	Caffeine, Ephedrine, Phenylpropanolamine	Unknown
PDK 10-1362	Caffeine, Ephedrine, Phenylpropanolamine	Unknown
PDK 20 20	Caffeine, Phaylpropanolamine	Unknown
PDK 30 30	Caffeine	Unknown
PD Meclomen	Meclomen 50 mg	Parke-Davis
PD Meclomen 100	Meclomen 100 mg	Parke-Davis
PediaCare/CC	Pediacare Cough-Cold Caplet	McNeil Consumer
Pepto-Bismol	Pepto Bismol Tablets	Proctor & Gamble
PEPTO DC/2 MG	Pepto Diarrhea Control Caplets	Procotr & Gamble
PERCOCET/DuPont	CONTROLLED - SEE PAGE 198	
PERCODAN/DuPont	CONTROLLED - SEE PAGE 206	
PERCODAN DEMI/DuPont	CONTROLLED - SEE PAGE 207	
PERCOGESIC	Acetaminophen 325 mg, Phenyltoloxamine 30 mg	Proctor & Gamble
PF/100	CONTROLLED - SEE PAGE 212	
PFI 049	Ibuprofen 600 mg	Private Formulations
PFIZER 015	Tetracyn 250 mg	Pfizer Labs
PFIZER 016	Tetracyn 500 mg	Pfizer Labs
PFIZER 072	Terramycin 125 mg	Pfizer Labs
PFIZER 073	Terramycin 250 mg	Pfizer Labs
PFIZER 084	Terramycin 250 mg	Pfizer Labs
PFIZER 088	Terrastatin 250 mg	Pfizer Labs
PFIZER 092	Urobiotic 250 mg/250 mg/50 mg	Pfizer Labs
PFIZER 094	Vibramycin 50 mg	Pfizer Labs
PFIZER 095	Vibramycin 100 mg	Pfizer Labs
PFIZER 099	Vibra-Tabs 100 mg	Pfizer Labs
PFIZER 105	Phenoxymethyl Penicillin	Pfizer Labs
PFIZER 166	Tetracyn 250 mg	Pfizer Labs
PFIZER 172	Tetracyn 500 mg	Pfizer Labs
PFIZER 175	Tetracyn 250 mg	Pfizer Labs
Pfizer 260 Procardia	Procardia 10 mg	Pfizer Labs
PFIZER 261 PROCARDIA 20	Procardia 20 mg	Pfizer Labs
PFIZER 305	Azithromycin 250 mg	Pfizer Labs
PFIZER 322	Feldene 10 mg	Pfizer Labs
PFIZER 323	Feldene 20 mg	Pfizer Labs
PFIZER 375	Renese 1 mg	Pfizer Labs
PFIZER 376	Renese 2 mg	Pfizer Labs
PFIZER 377	Renese 4 mg	Pfizer Labs
PFIZER 393	Diabinese 100 mg	Pfizer Labs
PFIZER 394	Diabinese 250 mg	Pfizer Labs
PFIZER 411	Glucotrol 5 mg	Pfizer Labs
PFIZER 412	Glucotrol 10 mg	Pfizer Labs
PFIZER 431 Minipress	Minipress 1 mg	Pfizer Labs

Imprint	Ingredient/Brand Name	Manufacturer
PFIZER 432	Minizide 2 mg/0.5 mg	Pfizer Labs
PFIZER 436	Minizide 5 mg/0.5 mg	Pfizer Labs
PFIZER 437 Minipress	Minipress 2 mg	Pfizer Labs
PFIZER 438 Minipress	Minipress 5 mg	Pfizer Labs
Pfizer/441	Moderil 0.25 mg	Pfizer Labs
Pfizer/442	Moderil 0.5 mg	Pfizer Labs
PFIZER 446	Renese-R 2 mg/0.25 mg	Pfizer Labs
PFIZER 534	Sinequan 10 mg	Pfizer Labs
PFIZER 535	Sinequan 25 mg	Pfizer Labs
PFIZER 536	Sinequan 50 mg	Pfizer Labs
PFIZER 537	Sinequan 150 mg	Pfizer Labs
PFIZER 538	Sinequan 100 mg	Pfizer Labs
PFIZER 539	Sinequan 75 mg	Pfizer Labs
PFIZER 541	Vistaril 25 mg	Pfizer Labs
PFIZER 542	Vistaril 50 mg	Pfizer Labs
PFIZER 543	Vistaril 100 mg	Pfizer Labs
PFIZER 641 VANSIL	Vansil 250 mg	Pfizer Labs
PF/M 200	CONTROLLED - SEE PAGE 226	
PF MSIR 15 THIS END UP	CONTROLLED - SEE PAGE 228	
PF MSIR 30 THIS END UP	CONTROLLED - SEE PAGE 228	
PF Nz	Thiethylperazine Maleate 10 mg	Purdue Frederick
PFT 500	Choline Magnesium Trisalicylate 500 mg	Purdue Frederick
PFT 1000	Choline Magnesium Trisalicylate 1000 mg	Purdue Frederick
PF/U 200	Uniphyl 200 mg	Purdue Frederick
PF/U 400	Uniphyl 400 mg	Purdue Frederick
P&G 402	Didronel 200 mg	Procter & Gamble
pharmics	Vitamins/Minerals	Pharmics
Pharmics/0025	CONTROLLED - No Photo - Hydrocodone Bitartrate 5 mg, Acetaminophen 500 mg - White, oblong tablet - DEA Schedule III	Pharmics, Inc.
Phazyme	Simthicone 60 mg	Block Drug Co.
Phazyme 95	Simethicone 95 mg	Block Drug Co.
Phazyme 125	Simethicone 125 mg	Block Drug Co.
PhosChol	PhosChol 900	Advanced Nutritional
PKD/SCHERING	Coricidin 2 mg/325 mg	Schering Corp
PLACIDYL 500	CONTROLLED - SEE PAGE 216	
PLEGINE 35	CONTROLLED - SEE PAGE 205	
Plendil MSD 451	Plendil 5 mg	Merck Sharp
Plendil MSD 452	Plendil 10 mg	Merck Sharp
P M	Amobarbital, Secobarbital	Unknown
PM	Excedrin PM 500 mg/38 mg	Bristol-Meyers Prod
POSTURE	Tribasic Calcium 1565.2 mg	Wyeth-Ayerst
POSTURE/600 Ayerst	Posture 600 mg	Ayerst Labs
POSTURE D	Tribasic Calcium 1565.2 mg, Vitamin D 125 IU	Wyeth-Ayerst
POTABA 51	Potaba 500 mg	Glenwood Inc
POTABA 54	Potaba 500 mg	Glenwood Inc
PP-040	Furosemide 40 mg	Eon Labs
PP-071	Chlorthalidone 50 mg	Eon Labs
PP-073	Chlorthalidone 100 mg	Eon Labs
PP-081	Folic Acid 1 mg	Eon Labs
PP 3	Dipyridamole 25 mg	Eon Labs
PP 8	Imipramine 10 mg	Eon Labs
PP 9	Imipramine 25 mg	Eon Labs
PP-12	Ferrous Sulfate 325 mg	Eon Labs
PP-13	Ferrous Sulfate 325 mg	Eon Labs
PP 14	Chlorpheniramine 4 mg	Eon Labs

Imprint	Ingredient/Brand Name	Manufacturer
PP-16	Triprolidine 2.5 mg, Pseudoephedrine 60 mg	Eon Labs
PP-17	Baclofen 10 mg	Eon Labs
PP-18	Baclofen 20 mg	Eon Labs
PP-19	Desipramine 25 mg	Eon Labs
PP-21	Imipramine 50 mg	Eon Labs
PP-25	Hydrochlorothiazide 25 mg	Eon Labs
PP 29	Desipramine 10 mg	Eon Labs
PP-32	Reserpine 0.1 mg	Eon Labs
PP-50	Hydrochlorothiazide 50 mg	Eon Labs
PP-53	Vitamins, Iron, Folic Acid	Eon Labs
PP 54	Triamterene 75 mg, Hydrochlorothiazide 50 mg	Eon Labs
PP 58	Hydroxyzine 50 mg	Eon Labs
PP 59	Hydroxyzine 25 mg	Eon Labs
PP 60	Hydroxyzine 10 mg	Eon Labs
PP 75	CONTROLLED - No Photo - Phendimetrazine Tartrate 35 mg - Pink/white/blue capsule - DEA Schedule III	Eon Labs
PP 84	Iodinated Glycerol 30 mg	Eon Labs
PP-111	Sulfamethoxazole 400 mg, Trimethoprim 80 mg	Eon Labs
PP-112	Sulfamethoxazole 800 mg, Trimethoprim 160 mg	Eon Labs
PP-125	Methylprednisolone 4 mg	Eon Labs
PP-134	Reserpine 0.25 mg	Eon Labs
PP 200	Rescaps-D SR 40 mg/75 mg	Bolar Pharm
PP 220	Atrosept Tablets	Eon Labs
PP-226	Chlorzoxazone 250 mg, Acetaminophen 300 mg	Vitarine Pharm
PP-250	Mefenamic Acid 250 mg	Vitarine Pharm
PP-256	Chlorpheniramine 12 mg, Phenylpropanolamine 75 mg	Vitarine Pharm
PP-257	Vitamins	Vitarine Pharm
PP-259	Vitamins	Eon
PP 345	Phenylpropanolamine 75 mg, Caramiphen Edisylate 40 mg	Vitarine
PP-511	Quinidine 200 mg	Vitarine Pharm
PP-512	Quinidine 300 mg	Vitarine Pharm
PP-530	Isoxsuprine 10 mg	Vitarine Pharm
PP-531	Isoxsuprine 20 mg	Vitarine Pharm
PP 535	Tolbutamide 500 mg	Vitarine Pharm
PP-536	Tolbutamide 500 mg	Vitarine Pharm
PP-551	Metronidazole 250 mg	Vitarine Pharm
PP-555	Metronidazole 500 mg	Vitarine Pharm
PP 585	Methocarbamol 500 mg	Vitarine Pharm
PP 587	Methocarbamol 750 mg	Vitarine Pharm
PP 613	Hydroxyzine Pamoate 25 mg	Vitarine Pharm
PP 615	Hydroxyzine Pamoate 50 mg	Vitarine Pharm
PP 617	Chlordiazepoxide 5 mg, Clindinium Bromide 2.5 mg	Vitarine Pharm
PP 635	CONTROLLED - No Photo - Phentermine 30 mg - Red/black capsule - DEA Schedule IV	Vitarine Pharm
PP 640	CONTROLLED - No Photo - Phentermine 30 mg - Black capsule - DEA Schedule IV	Vitarine Pharm
PP 647	CONTROLLED - SEE PAGE 214	
PP 648	Diphenhydramine 25 mg	Vitarine Pharm
PP 649	Diphenhydramine 50 mg	Vitarine Pharm
PP-670	Tetracycline 250 mg	Vitarine Pharm
PP 671	Tetracycline 500 mg	Vitarine Pharm
PP 698	Doxycycline Hyclate 50 mg	Vitarine Pharm
PP-699	Doxycycline 100 mg	Vitarine Pharm
PP-711	Salsalate 500 mg	Vitarine Pharm
PP-712	Salsalate 750 mg	Vitarine Pharm
PP-713	Orphenadrine 25 mg, Aspirin 385 mg, Caffeine 60 mg	Vitarine Pharm

Imprint	Ingredient/Brand Name	Manufacturer
PP-714	Orphenadrine 50 mg, Aspirin 770 mg, Caffeine 60 mg	Vitarine Pharm
PP 716	CONTROLLED - SEE PAGE 193	
PP 717	CONTROLLED - SEE PAGE 195	
PP 718	Indomethacin 25 mg	Vitarine Pharm
PP 719	Indomethacin 50 mg	Vitarine Pharm
PP 720	Indomethacin 75 mg	Vitarine Pharm
PP 721	Desipramine 50 mg	Vitarine Pharm
PP 722	Desipramine 75 mg	Vitarine Pharm
PP 723	Carisoprodol 350 mg	Vitarine Pharm
PP 725	Meclofenamate Sodium 50 mg	Vitarine Pharm
PP 726	Meclofenemate Sodium 100 mg	Vitarine Pharm
PP 736	Desipramine 100 mg	Vitarine Pharm
PP 737	Cephradine 250 mg	Vitarine Pharm
PP 738	Cephradine 500 mg	Vitarine Pharm
PP 739	Timipramine 25 mg	Vitarine Pharm
PP 740	Timipramine 50 mg	Vitarine Pharm
PP 741	Timipramine 100 mg	Vitarine Pharm
PP 743	Niacin 250 mg	Vitarine Pharm
PP 745	Phenylpropanolamine 75 mg, Guaifenesin 400 mg	Vitarine Pharm
PP 750	Nystatin 500,000 units	Vitarine Pharm
PP 754	Clindamycin 75 mg	Vitarine Pharm
PP 755	Clindamycin 150 mg	Vitarine Pharm
PP 756	Triamterene 50 mg, Hydrochlorothiazide 25 mg	Vitarine Pharm
PP 760	Desipramine 150 mg	Vitarine Pharm
PP 761	Salsalate 500 mg	Vitarine Pharm
PP 762	Salsalate 750 mg	Vitarine Pharm
PP-777	Nystatin 100,000 units	Vitarine Pharm
PP 856	Salsalate 500 mg	Vitarine Pharm
PP 857	Salsalate 750 mg	Vitarine Pharm
PP 882	CONTROLLED - No Photo - Phentermine 15 mg - Gray/yellow capsule - DEA Schedule IV	Vitarine Pharm
PP 968	Chlordiazepoxide 5 mg, Clidinium 2.5 mg	Vitarine Pharm
PP 970	Cephalexin 250 mg	Vitarine Pharm
PP 971	Cephalexin 500 mg	Vitarine Pharm
PP 985	Choline Magnesium Trisalicylate 500 mg	Vitarine Pharm
PP 986	Choline Magnesium Trisalicylate 750 mg	Vitarine Pharm
PP 987	Choline Magnesium Trisalicylate	Vitarine Pharm
PP 988	Choline Magnesium Trisalicylate	Vitarine Pharm
PP 995	Choline Magnesium 500 mg	Vitarine Pharm
PP 996	Choline Magnesium 750 mg	Vitarine Pharm
PP 997	Choline Magnesium 1000 mg	Vitarine Pharm
PP 998	Yohimbine 5.4 mg	Vitarine Pharm
PP-1217	Nitroglycerin 9 mg	Vitarine Pharm
PP-1235	Nitroglycerin 6.5 mg	Vitarine Pharm
PP 1303	Quinine Sulfate 325 mg	Vitarine Pharm
PP 1304	Chlorpheniramine Maleate 8 mg, Pseudoephedrine 120 mg	Vitarine
PP 2002	Caramiphen 40 mg, Phenylpropanolamine 75 mg	Par Pharm
PP 2007	Genabid 150 mg	Pioneer Pharm
PP 4001	Cyclandelate 200 mg	Pioneer Pharm
PP 4002	Cyclandelate 400 mg	Pioneer Pharm
PP 4005	Indomethacin 25 mg	Pioneer Pharm
PP 4006	Indomethacin 50 mg	Pioneer Pharm
PP 4008	Diphenhydramine 50 mg	Pioneer Pharm
PP 4009	Chlordiazepoxide 5 mg, Clidinium 2.5 mg	Pioneer Pharm
PP 4011	CONTROLLED - SEE PAGE 223	
PP 4012	CONTROLLED - SEE PAGE 219	

Imprint	Ingredient/Brand Name	Manufacturer
PP 4013	Diphenhydramine 25 mg	Pioneer Pharm
PP 4017	Dicyclomine 10 mg	Pioneer Pharm
PP-4350	Isoniazid 300 mg	Vitarine Pharm
PP-4354	Isoniazid 100 mg	Vitarine Pharm
PP 5000	CONTROLLED - SEE PAGE 218	
PP 5023	Vitamins	Vitarine Pharm
PP-5156	Papaverine 150 mg	Vitarine Pharm
PP-5174	Nitroglycerin 2.5 mg	Vitarine Pharm
PP-5380	Vitamins, Iron, Folic Acid	Vitarine Pharm
PP-5511	Chlorpheniramine 8 mg	Vitarine Pharm
PP-5512	Chlorpheniramine 12 mg	Vitarine Pharm
PP 6001	Ephedrine 25 mg, Hydroxyzine 10 mg, Theophylline 130 mg	Vitarine
PP 6004	Folic Acid 1 mg	Pioneer Pharm
PP 6012	Chlorzoxazone 250 mg	Vitarine Pharm
PP 6013	Dicyclomine 20 mg	Vitarine Pharm
PP 6015	Cyproheptadine 4 mg	Vitarione Pharm
PP 6017	Chlorzoxazone 250 mg, Acetaminophen 300 mg	Pioneer Pharm
PP 6018	Carisoprodol 350 mg	Vitarine Pharm
PP 6048	Chlorzoxazone 500 mg	Vitarine Pharm
PP 6062	Chlorthalidone 25 mg	Vitarine Pharm
PP 6063	Chlorthalidone 50 mg	Vitarine Pharm
PP 6026	Chlorpheniramine 4 mg	Pioneer Pharm
PP 6031	Brompheniramine 4 mg	Pioneer Pharm
PP 6036	Methocarbamol 500 mg	Pioneer Pharm
PP 6038	Methocarbamol 750 mg	Pioneer Pharm
PPL 54	Triamterene 75 mg, Hydrochlorthiazide 10 mg	Eon
PPP 207	Nadolol 40 mg	Bristol
PPP 208	Nadolol 120 mg	Bristol
PPP 232	Nadolol 20 mg	Bristol
PPP 241	Nadolol 80 mg	Bristol
PPP 246	Nadolol 160 mg	Bristol
PPP 283	Nadolol 40 mg, Bendroflumethiazide 5 mg	Bristol
PPP 284	Nadolol 80 mg, Bendroflumethiazide 5 mg	Bristol
Pre-H-Cal TEW	Pre-H-Cal	T.E. Williams
PREMARIN 0.3 868	Premarin 0.3 mg	Ayerst Labs
PREMARIN 0.625 867	Premarin 0.625 mg	Ayerst Labs
PREMARIN 0.9 864	Premarin 0.9 mg	Ayerst Labs
PREMARIN 1.25 866	Premarin 1.25 mg	Ayerst Labs
PREMARIN 2.5 865	Premarin 2.5 mg	Ayerst Labs
PREMSYN PMS	Premsyn PMS 500 mg/25 mg/15 mg	Chattem Prod
PRL 200	Chlorpromazine	Philips Roxane Labs
PROLOPRIM 09A	Proloprim 100 mg	Burroughs Wellcome
PROLOPRIM 200	Proloprim 200 mg	Burroughs Wellcome
PROPACET	CONTROLLED - SEE PAGE 201	
PROSED/DS	Prosed DS	Star Pharm
PROSTIGMIN	Prostigmin 15 mg	Roche Labs
PROVENTIL 2	Proventil 2 mg	Schering Corp
PROVENTIL 4	Proventil 4 mg	Schering Corp
PROVERA 2.5	Provera 2.5 mg	Upjohn Co
PROVERA 5.0	Provera 5 mg	Upjohn Co
PROVERA 10	Provera 10 mg	Upjohn Co
PS 51-198	Caffeine	Unknown
P/T 222	Acetaminophen 500 mg	Hall Labs
PURDUE	CONTROLLED - SEE PAGE 228	
PURINETHOL 04A	Purinethol 50 mg	Burroughs Wellcome
PYRROXATE	Pyrroxate 4 mg/25 mg/500 mg	Upjohn Co

Imprint	Ingredient/Brand Name	Manufacturer
Q	Quinalan 324 mg	Lannett
Q 11	Quinidine Sulfate 200 mg	Lederle Labs
Q 13	Quinidine Gluconate 324 mg	Lederle Labs
Q 184	Doxepin 10 mg	Quantum Pharm
Q 185	Doxepin 25 mg	Quantum Pharm
Q 186	Doxepin 50 mg	Quantum Pharm
Q 187	Doxepin 75 mg	Quantum Pharm
Q 215	Meclofenamate 50 mg	Quantum Pharm
Q 216	Meclofenamate 100 mg	Quantum Pharm
QPL 114	Nystatin 500,000 units	Quantum Pharm
QPL 114	Nystatin 500,000 units	Quantum Pharm
QPL 154	Phenazopyradine 100 mg	Quantum Pharm
QPL 155	Phenazopyradine 200 mg	Quantum Pharm
QPL 156/0.5	CONTROLLED - SEE PAGE 184	
QPL/186	Doxepin 50 mg	Quantum Pharm
QPL 217 Q	Metaclopramide 10 mg	Quantum Pharm
QPL-220 Q	Triamterene 75 mg, Hydrochlorothiazide 50 mg	Quantum Pharm
QPL/228 10	Minodyl 10 mg	Quantum Pharm
QPL 236 Q	Fenoprofen 200 mg	Quantum Pharm
QPL 237 Q	Fenoprofen 300 mg	Quantum Pharm
QPL 243	Minoxidil 2.5 mg	Quantum Pharm
QPL 245-Q	Oxybutynin Chloride 5 mg	Quantum Pharm
QPL-270/Q	Metoclopramide 5 mg	Quantum Pharm
QPL 273/Q	Timolol Maleate 5 mg	Quantum Pharm
QPL 274/Q	Timolol Maleate 2 mg	Quantum Pharm
QPL 275/Q	Timolol Maleate 20 mg	Quantum Pharm
Q/QPL 115	Benztropine Mesylate 2 mg	Quantum Pharm
Q/QPL 116	Benztropine Mesylate 0.5 mg	Quantum Pharm
Q/QPL 117	Benztropine Mesylate 1 mg	Quantum Pharm
Q/QPL 194	Haloperidol 0.5 mg	Quantum Pharm
Q/QPL 195	Haloperidol 1 mg	Quantum Pharm
Q/QPL 196	Haloperidol 2 mg	Quantum Pharm
Q/QPL 197	Haloperidol 5 mg	Quantum Pharm
Q/QPL 213	Trazodone 50 mg	Quantum Pharm
Q/QPL 214	Trazodone 100 mg	Quantum Pharm
Q/QPL 228	Minoxidil 10 mg	Quantum Pharm
Q/QPL 238	Fenoprofen 600 mg	Quantum Pharm
QUARZAN 2.5 ROCHE	Quarzan 2.5 mg	Roche Labs
QUARZAN 5.0 ROCHE	Quarzan 5 mg	Roche Labs
QUINIDEX AHR	Quinidex Extentab 300 mg	A.H. Robins Co.
QUINORA 300	Quinidine Sulfate 300 mg	Key Pharm
Q-VEL	Quinine Sulfate 64.8 mg	Ciba Consumer
R	Menthol 10 mg	A.H. Robins
R	Vi-Daylin	Ross Labs
R	Acetaminophen 325 mg	Trinity Technologies
R Logo/249	Methocarbamol 750 mg	Purepac
R [in diamond] 10-10 T I	Caffeine, Ephedrine, Phenylpropanolamine	Unknown
R [in triangle] 200	Papaverine 200 mg	Rucker Pharm
R 001/3	CONTROLLED - SEE PAGE 197	
R 003/4	CONTROLLED - SEE PAGE 195	
R 006	Butalbital 50 mg, Aspirin 200 mg, Phenacetin 130 mg	Purepac Pharm
R-021	CONTROLLED - SEE PAGE 219	
R-022	CONTROLLED - SEE PAGE 217	
R 039	CONTROLLED - SEE PAGE 225	
R-067	CONTROLLED - SEE PAGE 215	
R-069	CONTROLLED - SEE PAGE 216	

Imprint	Ingredient/Brand Name	Manufacturer
R-073	CONTROLLED - SEE PAGE 216	
R-076	CONTROLLED - SEE PAGE 220	
R-077	CONTROLLED - SEE PAGE 213	
R-082	CONTROLLED - SEE PAGE 215	
R 2	Isosorbide Dinitrate 2.5 mg	Rugby Labs
R 5	Isosorbide Dinitrate 5 mg	Rugby Labs
R7	Lozol 1.25 mg	Rorer
R 8	Lozol 2.5 mg	Rorer
R 10	Isoxsuprine 10 mg	Rugby Labs
R 11	Verapamil 40 mg	Rugby Labs
R 20	Isoxsuprine 20 mg	Rugby Labs
R 27	Propanolol 10 mg	Purepac Pharm
R 29	Propanolol 20 mg	Purepac Pharm
R 31	Amitriptyline 10 mg	Purepac Pharm
R 31	Regroton 50 mg/0.25 mg	USV Labs
R 32	Amitriptyline 25 mg	Purepac
R 32	Demi-Regroton 25 mg/0.125 mg	USV Labs
R 70	Dipyridamole 25 mg	Rugby Labs
R 101	Acetazolamide 250 mg	Purepac Pharm
R 102	Acetaminophen 500 mg	Purepac Pharm
R 102	Allopurinol 100 mg	Purepac Pharm
R 103	Allopurinol 300 mg	Purepac Pharm
R 103	Acetaminophen 325 mg	Purepac Pharm
R 105	Aminophylline 100 mg	Purepac Pharm
R 106	Acetaminophen 500 mg	Purepac Pharm
R 107	Aminophylline 200 mg	Purepac Pharm
R 111	Ibuprofen 800 mg	Purepac Pharm
R 112	Ampicillin 250 mg	Purepac Pharm
R 114	Ampicillin 500 mg	Purepac Pharm
R 117	Amoxicillin 250 mg	Purepac Pharm
R 119	Amoxicillin 500 mg	Purepac Pharm
R 121	Pramilet	Ross Labs
R 124	Ibuprofen 400 mg	Purepac Pharm
R 125	Ibuprofen 600 mg	Purepac Pharm
R 127	Clonidine 0.1 mg	Purepac Pharm
R 128	Clonidine 0.2 mg	Purepac Pharm
R 129	Clonidine 0.3 mg	Purepac Pharm
R 131	Amitriptyline 10 mg	Purepac Pharm
R 132	Amitriptyline 25 mg	Purepac Pharm
R 133	Amitriptyline 50 mg	Purepac Pharm
R 134	Amitriptyline 75 mg	Purepac Pharm
R 135	Amitriptyline 100 mg	Purepac Pharm
R 136	Benztropine Mesylate 1 mg	Purepac Pharm
R 138	Benztropine Mesylate 2 mg	Purepac Pharm
R 138	Aspirin 500 mg	Purepac Pharm
R 139	Bethanechol 25 mg	Purepac Pharm
R 140	Aspirin 400 mg, Caffeine 32.4 mg	Purepac Pharm
R 141	Aspirin 320 mg	Purepac Pharm
R 143	Carbamazepine 200 mg	Purepac Pharm
R 147	Chlorothiazide 250 mg	Purepac Pharm
R 147	Pramet	Ross Labs
R 148	Chlorthiazide 500 mg	Purepac Pharm
R 149	Carisoprodol 350 mg	Purepac Pharm
R 150	Chlordiazepoxide 5 mg, Clindinium Bromide 2.5 mg	Purepac Pharm
R 151	Disopyramide 100 mg	Purepac Pharm
R 152	Chlorpheniramine 8 mg	Purepac Pharm

Imprint	Ingredient/Brand Name	Manufacturer
R 153	Chlorpropamide 250 mg	Purepac Pharm
R 154	Colchicine 1 mg/100 grain	Rondex Labs
R 155	Chlorpropamide 100 mg	Purepac Pharm
R 156	Chlorpheniramine 12 mg	Purepac Pharm
R 157	Chlorthalidone 100 mg	Purepac Pharm
R 158	Cortisone 25 mg	Purepac Pharm
R 160	Chlorpromazine 10 mg	Purepac Pharm
R 161	Chlorthalidone 25 mg	Purepac Pharm
R 161	Chlorpromazine 25 mg	Purepac Pharm
R 163	Chlorthalidone 50 mg	Purepac Pharm
R 164	Chlorpromazine 50 mg	Purepac Pharm
R 165	Chlorzoxazone 250 mg, Acetaminphen 300 mg	Purepac Pharm
R 166	Chlorpromazine 100 mg	Purepac Pharm
R 167	Cyproheptadine 4 mg	Purepac Pharm
R 168	Chlorpromazine 200 mg	Purepac Pharm
R 169	Conjugated Estrogens 0.3 mg	Purepac Pharm
R 171	Conjugated Estrogens 2.5 mg	Purepac Pharm
R 172	Conjugated Estrogens 0.625 mg	Purepac Pharm
R 173	Cyclandelate 200 mg	Purepac Pharm
R 174	Conjugated Estrogens 1.25 mg	Purepac Pharm
R 175	Cyclandelate 400 mg	Purepac Pharm
R 176	Digitoxin 0.1 mg	Purepac Pharm
R 178	Digitoxin 0.2 mg	Purepac Pharm
R 179	Disopyramide 150 mg	Purepac Pharm
R 180	Dexamethasone 0.75 mg	Purepac Pharm
R 182	Digitoxin 0.25 mg	Purepac Pharm
R 183	Dipyridamole 50 mg	Purepac Pharm
R 184	Erythromycin Ethylsuccinate 400 mg	Purepac Pharm
R 185	Dipyridamole 75 mg	Purepac Pharm
R 186	Bisacodyl 5 mg	Purepac Pharm
R 187	Doxycyline 100 mg	Purepac Pharm
R 191	Diphenhydramine 25 mg	Purepac Pharm
R 192	Diphenhydramine 50 mg	Purepac Pharm
R 193	Dipyridamole 25 mg	Purepac Pharm
R 194	Doxycycline 50 mg	Purepac Pharm
R 195	Doxycycline 100 mg	Purepac Pharm
R 196	Hydralazine 25 mg, Hydrochlorothiazide	Purepac Pharm
R 197	Erthromycin Estolate 250 mg	Purepac Pharm
R 198	Hydralazine 50 mg, Hydrochlorothiazide	Purepac Pharm
R 199	Hydroxyzine 10 mg	Purepac Pharm
R 200	Ergoloid Mesylates 1 mg	Purepac Pharm
R 201	Ergonovine 0.2 mg	Rondex Labs
R 203	Hydroxyzine 25 mg	Purepac Pharm
R 204	Erythromycin 250 mg	Rondex Labs
R/205	Pediamycin 200 mg	Ross Labs
R 205	Calcium Lactate 650 mg	Purepac Pharm
R 206	Hydroxyzine 50 mg	Purepac Pharm
R 207	Furosemide 20 mg	Purepac Pharm
R 208	Furosemide 40 mg	Purepac Pharm
R 209	Furosemide 80 mg	Purepac Pharm
R 210	Folic Acid 1 mg	Rondex Labs
R 211	Ibuprofen 800 mg	Purepac Pharm
R 212	Hydrocortisone 10 mg	Rondex Labs
R 213	Cascara Sagrada 300 mg	Purepac Pharm
R 214	Hydrocortisone 20 mg	Purepac Pharm
R 219	Hydralazine 50 mg	Purepac Pharm

Imprint	Ingredient/Brand Name	Manufacturer
R 220	Hydralazine 50 mg	Purepac Pharm
R 221	Hydrochlorothiazide 25 mg	Purepac Pharm
R222	Hydrochlorothiazide 50 mg	Purepac Pharm
R 224	Hydrochlorothiazide 25 mg, Reserpine 0.125 mg	Purepac Pharm
R 225	Hydrochlorothiazide 50 mg, Reserpine 0.125 mg	Purepac Pharm
R 226	Hydroflumethiazide 50 mg, Reserpine 0.125 mg	Purepac Pharm
R 227	Hydrochlorothiazide, Reserpine, Hydralazine	Purepac Pharm
R 228	Isosorbide Dinitrate 20 mg	Purepac Pharm
R 231	Chlorpheniramine 4 mg	Purepac Pharm
R 231	Imipramine 10 mg	Purepac Pharm
R 232	Imipramine 25 mg	Purepac Pharm
R 233	Imipramine 50 mg	Purepac Pharm
R 234	Isosorbide Dinitrate 40 mg	Purepac Pharm
R 235	Isosorbide Dinitrate 5 mg	Purepac Pharm
R 236	Isoniazid 100 mg	Rondex Labs
R 237	Isosorbide Dinitrate 5 mg	Purepac Pharm
R 238	Isosorbide Dinitrate 10 mg	Purepac Pharm
R 239	Isosorbide Dinitrate 40 mg	Purepac Pharm
R 243	Isoxsuprine 10 mg	Purepac Pharm
R 244	Indomethacin 25 mg	Purepac Pharm
R 245	Isoxsuprine 20 mg	Purepac Pharm
R 246	Indomethacin 50 mg	Purepac Pharm
R 247	Methocarbamol 500 mg	Purepac Pharm
R 248	Methyltestosterone 10 mg	Rondex Labs
R 249	Methocarbamol 750 mg	Purepac Pharm
R 253	Methyldopa 250 mg	Purepac Pharm
R 254	Meclofenamate 50 mg	Purepac Pharm
R 255	Methyldopa 500 mg	Purepac Pharm
R 256	Meclofenamate 100 mg	Purepac Pharm
R 257	Hydroxyzine 25 mg	Purepac Pharm
R 258	Metronidazole 250 mg	Purepac Pharm
R 259	Hydroxyzine 50 mg	Purepac Pharm
R 260	Metronidazole 500 mg	Purepac Pharm
R 261	Methyldopa 250 mg, Hydrochlorothiazide 15 mg	Purepac Pharm
R 262	Nitrofurantoin 50 mg	Purepac Pharm
R 263	Methyldopa 250 mg, Hydrochlorothiazide 25 mg	Purepac Pharm
R 264	Nitrofurantoin 100 mg	Purepac Pharm
R 265	Methyldopa 500 mg, Hydrochlorothiazide 30 mg	Purepac Pharm
R 266	Nitroglycerin 2.5 mg	Purepac Pharm
R 267	Methyldopa 500 mg, Hydrochlorothiazide 50 mg	Purepac Pharm
R 268	Nitroglycerin 6.5 mg	Purepac Pharm
R 269	Metoclopramide 10 mg	Purepac Pharm
R 271	Doxusate Sodium 100 mg, Casanthranol 30 mg	Purepac Pharm
R 272	Methylclothiazide 5 mg	Purepac Pharm
R 273	Docusate Sodium 100 mg	Purepac Pharm
R 276	Reserpine 0.25 mg	Purepac Pharm
R 277	Nystatin 500,000 units	Purepac Pharm
R 278	Oxytetracycline 250 mg	Rondex Labs
R 280	Haloperidol 1 mg	Purepac Pharm
R 281	Haloperidol 2 mg	Purepac Pharm
R 282	Haloperidol 5 mg	Purepac Pharm
R 283	Erythromycin 500 mg	Purepac Pharm
R 285	Medroxyprogesterone 10 mg	Purepac Pharm
R 286	Haloperidol 10 mg	Purepac Pharm
R 287	Haloperidol 20 mg	Purepac Pharm
R 288	Papaverine 1-1/2 grains	Rondex Labs

Imprint	Ingredient/Brand Name	Manufacturer
R 289	Haloperidol 0.5 mg	Purepac Pharm
R 290	Methyclothiazide 5 mg, Deserpidine 0.025 mg	Purepac Pharm
R 291	Amantadine 100 mg	Purepac Pharm
R 292	Papaverine 150 mg	Rondex Labs
R 294	Phenazopyridine 200 mg	Purepac Pharm
R 295	Clofibrate 500 mg	Purepac Pharm
R 296	Penicillin G 200,000 units	Rondex Labs
R 297	Ferrous Sulfate 300 mg	Purepac Pharm
R 300	Ferrous Sulfate 300 mg	Purepac Pharm
R 300	Penicillin G 250,000 units	Rondex Labs
R 301	Perphenazine 2 mg, Amitriptyline 10 mg	Purepac Pharm
R 302	Perphenazine 2 mg, Amitriptyline 25 mg	Purepac Pharm
R 302	Phenazopyridine 200 mg	Purepac Pharm
R 303	Perphenazine 4 mg, Amitriptyline 10 mg	Purepac Pharm
R 304	Penicillin G 400,000 units	Rondex Labs
R 305	Perphenazine 4 mg, Amitriptyline 25 mg	Purepac Pharm
R 307	Perphenazine 4 mg, Amitriptyline 50 mg	Purepac Pharm
R 311	Pentaerythritol Tetranitrate 80 mg	Purepac Pharm
R 312	Pentaerythritol Tetranitrate 20 mg	Purepac Pharm
R 313	Chlorpheniramine 12 mg, Phenylpropanolamine 75 mg	Purepac Pharm
R 317	Fenoprofen Calcium 600 mg	Purepac Pharm
R 321	Propranolol 60 mg	Purepac Pharm
R 322	Penicillin V 125 mg	Rondex Labs
R 324	Penicillin V 250 mg	Rondex Labs
R 327	Propranolol 10 mg	Purepac Pharm
R 329	Propranolol 20 mg	Purepac Pharm
R 330	Penicillin VK 500 mg	Purepac Pharm
R 331	Propranolol 40 mg	Purepac Pharm
R 332	Prednisolone 5 mg	Rondex Labs
R 333	Propranolol 80 mg	Purepac Pharm
R 335	Procainamide 375 mg	Purepac Pharm
R/336	Prednisone 5 mg	Rondex Labs
R/337	Prednisone 20 mg	Purepac Pharm
R/338	Prednisone 10 mg	Purepac Pharm
R 341	Probenecid, Colchicine	Purepac Pharm
R 342	Procainamide 250 mg	Purepac Pharm
R 343	Probenecid 500 mg	Purepac Pharm
R 345	Dexbrompheniramine, Pseudoephedrine	Purepac Pharm
R 346	Procainamide 500 mg	Purepac Pharm
R 347	Prochlorperazine 10 mg, Isopropamide 5 mg	Purepac Pharm
R 348	Propylthiouracil 50 mg	Rondex Labs
R 356	Quinidine Sulfate 200 mg	Rondex Labs
R 357	Quinidine Gluconate 324 mg	Purepac Pharm
R 358	Propranolol 40 mg, Hydrochlorothiazide 25 mg	Rondex Labs
R 360	Propranolol 80 mg, Hydrochlorothiazide 25 mg	Rondex Labs
R 364	Brompheniramine 4 mg, Phenylpropanolamine 12.5 mg	Purepac Pharm
R 368	Rauwolfia Serpentina 50 mg	Rondex Labs
R 370	Rauwolfia Serpentian 100 mg	Rondex Labs
R 371	Procainamide 250 mg	Purepac Pharm
R 372	Procainamide 500 mg	Purepac Pharm
R 373	Procainamide 750 mg	Purepac Pharm
R 374	Reserpine 0.1 mg	Rondex Labs
R 376	Reserpine 0.25 mg	Rondex Labs
R 384	Phenytoin 100 mg	Purepac Pharm
R 385	Sulfamethoxazole 500 mg	Purepac Pharm
R 386	Sulfisoxazole 500 mg	Purepac Pharm

Imprint	Ingredient/Brand Name	Manufacturer
R 387	Phenylazopyridine 50 mg, Sulfisoxazole 500 mg	Purepac Pharm
R 388	Spironolactone 25 mg	Purepac Pharm
R 390	Spironolactone 25 mg, Hydrochlorothiazide 25 mg	Purepac Pharm
R 395	Sulfamethoxazole 800 mg, Trimethoprim 160 mg	Purepac Pharm
R 397	Doxepin HCl 75 mg	Purepac Pharm
R 398	Doxepin 100 mg	Purepac Pharm
R 399	Sulfasalazine 500 mg	Purepac Pharm
R 400	Doxepin 150 mg	Purepac Pharm
R 404	Tetracycline 250 mg	Rondex Labs
R 406	Tetracycline 500 mg	Rondex Labs
R 407	Sulfamethoxazole 400 mg, Trimethoprim 80 mg	Purepac Pharm
R 409	Cephalexin 250 mg	Purepac Pharm
R 411	Thioridazine 10 mg	Purepac Pharm
R 412	Tolazamide 100 mg	Purepac Pharm
R 413	Thioridazine 25 mg	Purepac Pharm
R 414	Tolazamide 250 mg	Purepac Pharm
R 415	Thioridazine 50 mg	Purepac Pharm
R 416	Tolazamide 500 mg	Purepac Pharm
R 417	Thioridazine 100 mg	Purepac Pharm
R 418	Cephalexin 500 mg	Purepac Pharm
R 419	Thioridazine 200 mg	Purepac Pharm
R 421	Theophylline 100 mg	Purepac Pharm
R 423	Theophylline 200 mg	Purepac Pharm
R 425	Theophylline 300 mg	Purepac Pharm
R 432	Thyroid 1/2 grain	Rondex Labs
R 434	Thyroid 1 grain	Rondex Labs
R 438	Thyroid 120 mg	Purepac Pharm
R 439	Trazodone 50 mg	Purepac Pharm
R 440	Tolbutamide 500 mg	Purepac Pharm
R 441	Trazodone 100 mg	Purepac Pharm
R 443	Dicloxacillin 250 mg	Purepac Pharm
R 444	Dicloxacillin 500 mg	Purepac Pharm
R 450	Meclizine 12.5 mg	Purepac Pharm
R 452	Meclizine 25 mg	Purepac Pharm
R 454	Triamcinolone 4 mg	Purepac Pharm
R 455	Valproic Acid 250 mg	Purepac Pharm
R 459	Trifluoperazine 2 mg	Purepac Pharm
R 461	Trifluoperazine 5 mg	Purepac Pharm
R 463	Trifluoperazine 10 mg	Purepac Pharm
R 473	Verapamil 80 mg	Purepac Pharm
R 475	Verapamil 120 mg	Purepac Pharm
R 480	Tolmetin Sodium 600 mg	Purepac Pharm
R 481	Cephradine 250 mg	Purepac Pharm
R 482	Cephradine 500 mg	Purepac Pharm
R 490	levo-Thyroxine 0.1 mg	Purepac Pharm
R 491	levo-Thyroxine 0.15 mg	Purepac Pharm
R 497	Nifedipine 10 mg	Purepac Pharm
R 500	Prazosin 1 mg	Purepac Pharm
R 501	Prazosin 2 mg	Purepac Pharm
R 502	Prazosin 5 mg	Purepac Pharm
R 503	Triamterene 50 mg, Hydrochlorothiazide 25 mg	Purepac Pharm
R 504	Pseudoephedrine 30 mg	Purepac Pharm
R 507	Quinine Sulfate 200 mg	Purepac Pharm
R 511	Quinine Sulfate 325 mg	Purepac Pharm
R 520	Tolmetin Sodium 400 mg	Purepac Pharm
R 521	Naproxen 250 mg	Purepac Pharm

Imprint	Ingredient/Brand Name	Manufacturer
R 522	Naproxen 375 mg	Purepac Pharm
R 523	Naproxen 500 mg	Purepac Pharm
R 526	Minoxidil 10 mg	Purepac Pharm
R 530	Nifedipine 20 mg	Purepac Pharm
R 534	Pindolol 5 mg	Purepac Pharm
R 535	Pindolol 10 mg	Purepac Pharm
R 538	Carbidopa 10 mg, Levodopa 100 mg	Purepac Pharm
R 539	Carbidopa 25 mg, Levodopa 100 mg	Purepac Pharm
R 540	Carbidopa 25 mg, Levodopa 250 mg	Purepac Pharm
R 553	Erythromycin 250 mg	Purepac Pharm
R 573	Soda Mint	Purepac Pharm
R 643	Triprolidine 2.5 mg, Pseudoephedrine 60 mg	Purepac Pharm
R 840	Niacin 500 mg	Purepac Pharm
R 1103	Acetaminophen 325 mg	Purepac Pharm
R 1507	Quinine Sulfate 200 mg	Purepac Pharm
R 1511	Quinine Sulfate 352 mg	Purepac Pharm
R 3487	CONTROLLED - SEE PAGE 221	
R 3488	CONTROLLED - SEE PAGE 223	
R 3489	CONTROLLED - SEE PAGE 220	
R 4374	CONTROLLED - SEE PAGE 228	
R 4382	CONTROLLED - SEE PAGE 228	
R 4429	Quinidine Sulfate 300 mg	Rugby Labs
R 4519	Vi-Daylin	Ross Labs
R 4520	Vi-Daylin Plus Iron	Ross Labs
R/5726	Rondec 4 mg/60 mg	Ross Labs
R/6240	Rondec-TR 8 mg/120 mg	Ross Labs
R 7621	Vi-Daylin F Plus Iron	Ross Labs
R 7626	Vi-Daylin F	Ross Labs
R&C	Caffeine, Ephedrine, Phenylpropanolamine	Unknown
RACHELLE 553	Tetracycline	Rachelle Labs
RAM	Brompheniramine	R.A. McNeil Co
RC 0920	Dilatrate-SR 40 mg	Reed & Carnrick
RC 22	Levatol 20 mg	Reed & Carnrick
RD [logo]	Dialume 500 mg	Armour Pharm
REGAL 1010	Ampicillin	Unknown
REGAL 1011	Ampicillin	Unknown
REGAL 1090	Erythromycin	Unknown
REGAL 1805	Amoxicillin	Unknown
REGLAN 5	Reglan 5 mg	A.H. Robins Co.
RESTORIL 7.5 mg FOR SLEEP	CONTROLLED - SEE PAGE 228	
RESTORIL 15 mg FOR SLEEP	CONTROLLED - SEE PAGE 222	
RESTORIL 30mg FOR SLEEP	CONTROLLED - SEE PAGE 219	
REXIGEN FORTE	CONTROLLED - SEE PAGE 224	
RHM 156	Caffeine 175 mg	Unknown
RIFADIN 150	Rifadin 150 mg	Merrell Dow Pharm
RIFADIN 300	Rifadin 300 mg	Merrell Dow Pharm
RINADE	Rinade 120 mg/8 mg	Econo Med Pharm
RIOPAN	Riopan 480 mg	Ayerst Labs
RIOPAN PLUS	Riopan Plus 480 mg/20 mg	Ayerst Labs
RIOPAN PLUS 2	Magaldrate 1080 mg, Simethacone 30 mg	Ayerst Labs
RJ8/8	Caffeine, Ephedrine, Phenylpropanolamine	Unknown
RL	CONTROLLED - SEE PAGE 213, 215, 218	
RL	Calcium Gluconate 650 mg	Richlyn Labs
RL 1400	Tetracycline	Unknown
ROBAXISAL AHR	Robaxisal 400 mg/325 mg	A.H. Robins Co.

Imprint	Ingredient/Brand Name	Manufacturer
Roberts 138/Dolacet	CONTROLLED - No Photo - Hydrocodone 5 mg, Acetaminophen 500 mg - Black/gray capsule - DEA Schedule III	Roberts Pharm
ROCALTROL 0.25/ROCHE	Rocaltrol 0.00025 mg	Roche Labs
ROCALTROL 0.5/ROCHE	Rocaltrol 0.0005 mg	Roche Labs
ROCHE 21	Trimethobenzamide 100 mg	Roche Labs
ROCHE 33	Mestinon 60 mg	Roche Labs
ROCHE 35	Prostigmin 15 mg	Roche Labs
ROCHE 37	Synkayvite 5 mg	Roche Labs
ROCHE 45	Taractan 10 mg	Roche Labs
ROCHE 46	Taractan 25 mg	Roche Labs
ROCHE 47	Taractan 50 mg	Roche Labs
ROCHE 49	Taractan 100 mg	Roche Labs
ROCHE 54	Larodopa 500 mg	Roche Labs
ROCHE 55	Larodopa 250 mg	Roche Labs
ROCHE 57	Larodopa 250 mg	Roche Labs
ROCHE 103	Larodopa 100 mg	Roche Labs
ROCHE 106	Endep 10 mg	Roche Labs
ROCHE 107	Endep 25 mg	Roche Labs
ROCHE 109	Endep 50 mg	Roche Labs
ROCHE 114	Endep 75 mg	Roche Labs
ROCHE 115	Solatene 30 mg	Roche Labs
ROCHE 116	Endep 100 mg	Roche Labs
ROCHE/143	Rocaltrol 0.00025 mg	Roche Labs
ROCHE/144	Rocaltrol 0.0005 mg	Roche Labs
ROCHE 150	Endep 150 mg	Roche Labs
ROCHE AZO GANTANOL	Azo Gantanol 500 mg/100 mg	Roche Labs
ROCHE AZO GANTRISIN	Azo Gantrisin 500 mg/50 mg	Roche Labs
Roche Bumex 0.5	Bumex 0.5 mg	Roche Labs
Roche Bumex 1	Bumex 1 mg	Roche Labs
Roche bumex 2	Bumex 2 mg	Roche Labs
ROCHE GANTANOL	Gantanol 500 mg	Roche Labs
ROCHE GANTRISIN	Gantrisin 500 mg	Roche Labs
ROCHE/LIMBITROL	CONTROLLED - SEE PAGE 210	
ROCHE MARPLAN	Marplan 10 mg	Roche Labs
ROCHE [hexagon logo]	Fansidar 500 mg/25 mg	Roche Labs
ROERIG 143	Carbenicillin Indanyl 382 mg	Pfizer Pharm
ROERIG 159	TAO 250 mg	Pfizer Pharm
ROERIG 212	Antivert 25 mg	Pfizer Pharm
ROERIG 504	Heptuna Plus	Pfizer Pharm
ROERIG 534	Sinequan 10 mg	Pfizer Pharm
ROERIG 535	Sinequan 25 mg	Pfizer Pharm
ROERIG 536	Sinequan 50 mg	Pfizer Pharm
ROERIG 537	Sinequan 150 mg	Pfizer Pharm
ROERIG 538	Sinequan 100 mg	Pfizer Pharm
ROERIG 539	Sinequan 75 mg	Pfizer Pharm
ROERIG 571	Navane 1 mg	Pfizer Pharm
ROERIG 572	Navane 2 mg	Pfizer Pharm
ROERIG 573	Navane 5 mg	Pfizer Pharm
ROERIG 574	Navane 10 mg	Pfizer Pharm
ROERIG 577	Navane 20 mg	Pfizer Pharm
RONDEX 278	Navane 250 mg	Rondex Labs
RORER/136	ES Ascriptin 500 mg/82.5 mg/82.5 mg	Rorer Pharm
RORER 143/3	CONTROLLED - SEE PAGE 197	
ROSES 10 VALM	Pyrilamine, Chlorpheniramine	Unknown
Rowell 1611	Norlac Rx Tablets	Solvay
ROWELL 7512	Lithium Carbonate 300 mg	Reid-Rowell Labs

Imprint	Ingredient/Brand Name	Manufacturer
ROWELL 7720	Chenix 250 mg	Reid-Rowell Labs
RP/57	CONTROLLED - SEE PAGE 205	
RPC 005	CONTROLLED - No Photo - Codeine 20 mg, Pseudoephedrine 60 mg - Green/clear capsule - DEA Schedule III	Roberts Pharm
RPC 62	CONTROLLED - SEE PAGE 224	
RPC 69	CONTROLLED - SEE PAGE 214	
RPC 141	CONTROLLED - SEE PAGE 226	
RPL 063	P-V Tussin 5 mg/25 mg/200 mg	Reid-Rowell Labs
RPL 1007	Curretab 10 mg	Reid-Rowell Labs
RPL 1014	Estratab 0.3 mg	Reid-Rowell Labs
RPL 1022	Estratab 0.625 mg	Reid-Rowell Labs
RPL 1024	Estratab 1.25 mg	Reid-Rowell Labs
RPL 1025	Estratab 2.5 mg	Reid-Rowell Labs
RPL 1039	Histalet Forte 10 mg/50 mg/25 mg/4 mg	Reid-Rowell Labs
RPL 1050	Histalet-X 120 mg/400 mg	Reid-Rowell Labs
RPL 1132	Unipress 0.1 mg/25 mg/15 mg	Reid-Rowell Labs
RPL 1146	Zenate	Reid-Rowell Labs
RPL 7025	Ru-Vert-M 25 mg	Reid-Rowell Labs
RPR 20	Hygroton 50 mg	Rorer
RPR 21	Hygroton 100 mg	Rorer
RPR 22	Hygroton 25 mg	Rorer
RR 1	Orasone 1 mg	Solvay
RR5	Prednisone 5 mg	Reid-Rowell Labs
RR10	Prednisone 10 mg	Reid-Rowell Labs
RR20	Prednisone 20 mg	Reid-Rowell Labs
RR50	Prednisone 50 mg	Reid-Rowell Labs
RR 440	Amantadine 100 mg	Reid-Rowell Labs
RR 586	CONTROLLED - SEE PAGE 212	
RR 1007	Medroxyprogesterone Acetate 10 mg	Reid-Rowell Labs
RR 1014	Estratab 0.3 mg	Reid-Rowell Labs
RR 1022	Estratab 0.625 mg	Reid-Rowell Labs
RR 1023	Estratab 0.625 mg, 2.5 mg	Reid-Rowell Labs
RR 1024	Estratab 1.25 mg	Reid-Rowell Labs
RR 1025	Estratab 2.5 mg	Reid-Rowell Labs
RR 1026	Estratab 1.25 mg, 2.5 mg	Reid-Rowell Labs
RR 1039	Histalet Forte 50 mg, 25 mg, 4 mg, 10 mg	Reid-Rowell Labs
RR 1132	Unipres 25 mg, 0.1 mg, 15 mg	Reid-Rowell Labs
RR 1146	Vitamins	Reid-Rowell Labs
RR 1216	Vitamins	Reid-Rowell Labs
RR 1218	Vitamins	Reid-Rowell Labs
RR 1611	Vitamins, Minerals	Reid-Rowell Labs
RR 3205	Dexamethasone 0.5 mg	Reid-Rowell Labs
RR 3210	Dexamethasone 0.75 mg	Reid-Rowell Labs
RR 3215	Dexamethasone 1.5 mg	Reid-Rowell Labs
RR 3220	Dexamethasone 4 mg	Reid-Rowell Labs
RR 4020	Quinidine Sulfate 300 mg	Reid-Rowell Labs
RR 4024	Quinidine Sulfate 100 mg	Reid-Rowell Labs
RR 4028	Quinidine Sulfate 200 mg	Reid-Rowell Labs
RR 4032	Quinidine Sulfate 300 mg	Reid-Rowell Labs
RR 4120	Valproic Acid 250 mg	Reid-Rowell Labs
RR 7025	Meclizine 20 mg	Reid-Rowell Labs
RR 7512	Lithium Carbonate 300 mg	Reid-Rowell Labs
RR 7516	Lithium Carbonate 300 mg	Reid-Rowell Labs
R-R 4140	Amantadine 100 mg	RP Scherer Labs
RUFEN 6	Rufen 600 mg	Boots Pharm
Rufen 8	Rufen 800 mg	Boots Pharm

Imprint	Ingredient/Brand Name	Manufacturer
RUFEN 400	Rufen 400 mg	Boots Pharm
RUGBY 0200	Doxycylcine 50 mg	Rugby Labs
RUGBY 0230	Doxycycline 100 mg	Rugby Labs
RUGBY 0250	Erythromycin 250 mg	Rugby Labs
RUGBY 0265	Erythromycin 500 mg	Rugby Labs
RUGBY 0340	Doxycycline 100 mg	Rugby Labs
RUGBY 0390	Doxycycline 50 mg	Rugby Labs
RUGBY 2	Isosorbide 2.5 mg	Rugby Labs
RUGBY 5	Isosorbide 5 mg	Rugby Labs
RUGBY 10	Isoxsuprine 10 mg	Rugby Labs
RUGBY 20	Isoxsuprine 20 mg	Rugby Labs
RUGBY 70	Dipyridamole 25 mg	Rugby Labs
RUGBY 1820	Tetracycline 250 mg	Rugby Labs
RUGBY 1830	Tetracycline 250 mg	Rugby Labs
RUGBY 1870	Tetracycline 500 mg	Rugby Labs
RUGBY 3018	Allerfrin	Rugby Labs
RUGBY 3023	Phenylpropanolamine 75 mg, Chlorpheniramine 12 mg	Rugby Labs
RUGBY 3024	Phenylpropanolamine 75 mg, Chlorpheniramine 12 mg	Rugby Labs
RUGBY 3027/100	Allopurinol 100 mg	Rugby Labs
RUGBY 3028/300	Allopurinol 300 mg	Rugby Labs
RUGBY 3046	Aminophylline 100 mg	Rugby Labs
RUGBY 3060	Aminophylline 200 mg	Rugby Labs
RUGBY 3071	Amitriptyline 10 mg	Rugby Labs
RUGBY 3072	Amitriptyline 25 mg	Rugby Labs
RUGBY 3073	Amitriptyline 50 mg	Rugby Labs
RUGBY 3074	Amitriptyline 75 mg	Rugby Labs
RUGBY 3075	Amitriptyline 100 mg	Rugby Labs
RUGBY 3076	Amitriptyline 150 mg	Rugby Labs
RUGBY 3077	Perphenazine 2 mg, Amitriptylline 10 mg	Rugby Labs
RUGBY 3078	Perphenazine 4 mg, Amitriptylline 10 mg	Rugby Labs
RUGBY 3082	Perphenazine 2 mg, Amitriptylline 25 mg	Rugby Labs
RUGBY 3083	Perphenazine 4 mg, Amitriptylline 25 mg	Rugby Labs
RUGBY 3084	Perphenazine 4 mg, Amitriptylline 50 mg	Rugby Labs
RUGBY 3125	Vancomycin 125 mg	Rugby Labs
RUGBY 3126	Vancomycin 250 mg	Rugby Labs
RUGBY 3364	Bethanechol 5 mg	Rugby Labs
RUGBY 3365	Bethanechol 10 mg	Rugby Labs
RUGBY 3367	Dicyclomine 10 mg	Rugby Labs
RUGBY 3369	Bethanechol 25 mg	Rugby Labs
RUGBY 3370	Benztropine Mesylate 0.5 mg	Rugby Labs
RUGBY 3371	Benztropine Mesylate 1 mg	Rugby Labs
RUGBY 3372	Benztropine Mesylate 2 mg	Rugby Labs
RUGBY 3377	Dicyclomine 20 mg	Rugby Labs
RUGBY 3392	Bromophen 12 mg/15 mg/15 mg	Rugby Labs
RUGBY 3397	Bromophen	Rugby Labs
RUGBY 3415	Carbamazepine 200 mg	Rugby Labs
RUGBY 3420	Chlordrine 120 mg/8 mg	Rugby Labs
RUGBY 3435	Carisoprodol 350 mg	Rugby Labs
RUGBY 3437	Carisoprodol 200 mg, Phenacetin 160 mg, Caffeine 32 mg	Rugby Labs
RUGBY/3444	Chlorzoxazone 500 mg	Rugby Labs
RUGBY 3450	Chlorofon-F 250 mg/300 mg	Rugby Labs
RUGBY 3454	Chlorpromazine 10 mg	Rugby Labs
RUGBY 3455	Chlorpromazine 25 mg	Rugby Labs
RUGBY 3456	Chlorpromazine 50 mg	Rugby Labs
RUGBY 3457	Chlorpromazine 100 mg	Rugby Labs
RUGBY 3458	Chlorpromazine 200 mg	Rugby Labs

Imprint	Ingredient/Brand Name	Manufacturer
RUGBY 3460	Chlorothiazide 250 mg	Rugby Labs
RUGBY 3461	Chlorothiazide 500 mg	Rugby Labs
RUGBY 3462	Chlorpropamide 100 mg	Rugby Labs
RUGBY 3465	Chlorpropamide 250 mg	Rugby Labs
RUGBY 3468	Chlorthalidone 50 mg	Rugby Labs
RUGBY 3469	Chlorthalidone 100 mg	Rugby Labs
RUGBY 3485	Chlorthalidone 25 mg	Rugby Labs
RUGBY 3494	Colchicine 0.6 mg	Rugby Labs
RUGBY 3515	Cyproheptadine 4 mg	Rugby Labs
RUGBY 3516	Estrogens 0.625 mg	Rugby Labs
RUGBY 3517	Estrogens 0.3 mg	Rugby Labs
RUGBY 3522	Estrogens 1.25 mg	Rugby Labs
RUGBY 3523	Clonidine 0.1 mg	Rugby Labs
RUGBY 3524	Clonidine 0.2 mg	Rugby Labs
RUGBY 3526	Clonidine 0.3 mg	Rugby Labs
RUGBY 3528	Estrogens 2.5 mg	Rugby Labs
RUGBY 3529	Cyclandelate 400 mg	Rugby Labs
RUGBY 3530	Cortisone 25 mg	Rugby Labs
RUGBY 3531	Cyclandelate 200 mg	Rugby Labs
RUGBY 3571	Dipyridamole 50 mg	Rugby Labs
RUGBY 3572	Dipyridamole 75 mg	Rugby Labs
RUGBY 3583	Dexamethasone 0.75 mg	Rugby Labs
RUGBY 3595	Disopyramide 100 mg	Rugby Labs
RUGBY 3596	Disopyramide 150 mg	Rugby Labs
RUGBY 3642	Papaverine 150 mg	Rugby Labs
RUGBY 3728	Doxepin 25 mg	Rugby Labs
RUGBY 3729	Doxepin 50 mg	Rugby Labs
RUGBY 3730	Doxepin 100 mg	Rugby Labs
RUGBY 3737	Doxepin 75 mg	Rugby Labs
RUGBY 3738	Doxepin 150 mg	Rugby Labs
RUGBY 3743	Dipyridamole 25 mg	Rugby Labs
RUGBY 3747	Dipyridamole 75 mg	Rugby Labs
RUGBY 3748	Dipyridamole 50 mg	Rugby Labs
RUGBY 3758	Dipyridamole 50 mg	Rugby Labs
RUGBY 3762	Diphenhydramine 50 mg	Rugby Labs
RUGBY 3764	Phenytoin 100 mg	Rugby Labs
RUGBY 3767	Disulfiram 250 mg	Rugby Labs
RUGBY 3768	Disulfiram 500 mg	Rugby Labs
RUGBY 3770	Trichlormethiazide 4 mg	Rugby Labs
RUGBY 3778	Ephedrine 50 mg	Rugby Labs
RUGBY 3780	Ephedrine 25 mg	Rugby Labs
RUGBY 3795	CONTROLLED - SEE PAGE 219	
RUGBY 3796	CONTROLLED - SEE PAGE 217	
RUGBY 3835	Furosemide 80 mg	Rugby Labs
RUGBY 3840	Furosemide 20 mg	Rugby Labs
RUGBY 3841	Furosemide 40 mg	Rugby Labs
RUGBY 3845	Folic Acid 1 mg	Rugby Labs
RUGBY 3851	Dihydroergocornine, Dihydroergocristine, Dihydroergocrytine	Rugby Labs
RUGBY 3854	Dihydroergocornine, Dihydroergocristine, Dihydroergocrytine	Rugby Labs
RUGBY 3857	Dihydroergocornine, Dihydroergocristine, Dihydroergocrytine	Rugby Labs
RUGBY 3859	Dihydroergocornine, Dihydroergocristine, Dihydroergocrytine	Rugby Labs
RUGBY 3862	Hydralazine 25 mg	Rugby Labs

Imprint	Ingredient/Brand Name	Manufacturer
RUGBY 3863	Hydralazine 50 mg	Rugby Labs
RUGBY 3871	Phenylpropanolamine 75 mg, Guaifenesin 400 mg	Rugby Labs
RUGBY 3874	Hydroxyzine 10 mg	Rugby Labs
RUGBY 3875	Hydroxyzine 25 mg	Rugby Labs
RUGBY 3876	Hydroxyzine 50 mg	Rugby Labs
RUGBY 3882	Hydroflumethiazide 50 mg	Rugby Labs
RUGBY 3892	Hydroxyzine 10 mg	Rugby Labs
RUGBY 3893	Hydroxyzine 25 mg	Rugby Labs
RUGBY 3894	Hydroxyzine 50 mg	Rugby Labs
RUGBY 3895	Hydroxyzine 100 mg	Rugby Labs
RUGBY 3897	Hydroxyzine 25 mg	Rugby Labs
RUGBY 3898	Hydroxyzine 50 mg	Rugby Labs
RUGBY 3900	Theophylline 150 mg, Guaifenesin 90 mg	Rugby Labs
RUGBY 3906	Hydrophed 10 mg/25 mg/130 mg	Rugby Labs
RUGBY 3911	Hydralazine 50 mg	Rugby Labs
RUGBY 3913	Hydrochlorothiazide	Rugby Labs
RUGBY 3915	Hydroserpine #1 25 mg/0.125 mg	Rugby Labs
RUGBY 3916	Hydrochlorthiazide 50 mg, Reserpine 0.125 mg	Rugby Labs
RUGBY 3917	Hydralazine 25 mg	Rugby Labs
RUGBY 3919	Hydrochlorothiazide 50 mg	Rugby Labs
RUGBY 3921	Hydrochlorothiazide 50 mg	Rugby Labs
RUGBY 3922	Hydrochlorothiazide 25 mg	Rugby Labs
RUGBY 3923	Hydrochlorothiazide 100 mg	Rugby Labs
RUGBY 3927	Isosorbide Dinitrate 20 mg	Rugby Labs
RUGBY 3929	Imipramine 10 mg	Rugby Labs
RUGBY 3930	Imipramine 25 mg	Rugby Labs
RUGBY 3931	Imipramine 50 mg	Rugby Labs
RUGBY 3935	Isoxsuprine 10 mg	Rugby Labs
RUGBY 3936	Isoxsuprine 20 mg	Rugby Labs
RUGBY 3938	Isosorbide Dinitrate 30 mg	Rugby Labs
RUGBY 3940	Isosorbide Dinitrate 40 mg	Rugby Labs
RUGBY 3941	Isoniazid 300 mg	Rugby Labs
RUGBY 3943	Isosorbide Dinitrate 10 mg	Rugby Labs
RUGBY 3947	Isosorbide Dinitrate 5 mg	Rugby Labs
RUGBY 3948	Isoniazide 100 mg	Rugby Labs
RUGBY 3950	Isosorbide Dinitrate 10 mg	Rugby Labs
RUGBY 3952	l-Thyroxine 0.1 mg	Rugby Labs
RUGBY 3953	l-Thyroxine 0.15 mg	Rugby Labs
RUGBY 3954	l-Thyroxine 0.2 mg	Rugby Labs
RUGBY 3958	l-Thyroxine 0.3 mg	Rugby Labs
RUGBY 3977	Ibuprofen 400 mg	Rugby Labs
RUGBY 3978	Ibuprofen 600 mg	Rugby Labs
RUGBY 3979	Ibuprofen 800 mg	Rugby Labs
RUGBY 3981	Indomethacin 25 mg	Rugby Labs
RUGBY 3982	Indomethacin 50 mg	Rugby Labs
RUGBY 3985	Meclizine 12.5 mg	Rugby Labs
RUGBY 3986	Meclizine 12.5 mg	Rugby Labs
RUGBY 3987	Meclizine 12.5 mg	Rugby Labs
RUGBY 3988	Meclizine 25 mg	Rugby Labs
RUGBY 3990	Meclizine 25 mg	Rugby Labs
RUGBY 3995	Medroxyprogesterone 10 mg	Rugby Labs
RUGBY 3996	Methyldopa 250 mg, Hydrochlorothiazide 15 mg	Rugby Labs
RUGBY 3997	Methyldopa 250 mg, Hydrochlorothiazide 25 mg	Rugby Labs
RUGBY 4002	Meclofenemate 50 mg	Rugby Labs
RUGBY 4003	Meclofenemate 100 mg	Rugby Labs
RUGBY 4010	Methyldopa 250 mg	Rugby Labs

Imprint	Ingredient/Brand Name	Manufacturer
RUGBY 4011	Methyldopa 500 mg	Rugby Labs
RUGBY 4012	Methyldopa 125 mg	Rugby Labs
RUGBY 4018	Metronidazole 250 mg	Rugby Labs
RUGBY 4019	Metronidazole 500 mg	Rugby Labs
RUGBY 4020	Methyldopa 125 mg	Rugby Labs
RUGBY 4021	Methyldopa 250 mg	Rugby Labs
RUGBY 4022	Propranolol 40 mg, Hydrochlorothiazide 25 mg	Rugby Labs
RUGBY 4023	Propranolol 80 mg, Hydrochlorothiazide 25 mg	Rugby Labs
RUGBY 4026	Methocarbamol 500 mg	Rugby Labs
RUGBY 4027	Methocarbamol 750 mg	Rugby Labs
RUGBY 4028	Methocarbamol 400 mg, Aspirin 325 mg	Rugby Labs
RUGBY 4032	Metronidazole 500 mg	Rugby Labs
RUGBY 4033	Metronidazole 250 mg	Rugby Labs
RUGBY 4036	Methylprednisolone 4 mg	Rugby Labs
RUGBY 4040	Methyclothiazide 2.5 mg	Rugby Labs
RUGBY 4041	Methyclothiazide 5 mg	Rugby Labs
RUGBY 4042	Metoclopramide 10 mg	Rugby Labs
RUGBY 4043	Minoxidil 10 mg	Rugby Labs
RUGBY 4081	Nitrofurantoin 50 mg	Rugby Labs
RUGBY 4082	Nitrofurantoin 100 mg	Rugby Labs
RUGBY 4083	Nitroglycerin 2.5 mg	Rugby Labs
RUGBY 4084	Nitroglycerin 6.5 mg	Rugby Labs
RUGBY 4090	Nitroglycerin 9 mg	Rugby Labs
RUGBY 4091	Nystatin	Rugby Labs
RUGBY 4094	Nystatin	Rugby Labs
RUGBY 4124	Papaverine 150 mg	Rugby Labs
RUGBY 4130	Pentaerythritol Tetranitrate 10 mg	Rugby Labs
RUGBY 4138	Pentaerythritol Tetranitrate 20 mg	Rugby Labs
RUGBY 4147	Perphenzine 8 mg	Rugby Labs
RUGBY 4235	CONTROLLED - SEE PAGE 228	
RUGBY 4290	Phenylpropanolamine 25 mg	Rugby Labs
RUGBY 4295	Phenylbutazone 100 mg	Rugby Labs
RUGBY 4299	Pheylbutazone 100 mg	Rugby Labs
RUGBY 4305	Phenylbutazone 100 mg	Rugby Labs
RUGBY 4307	Vitamins	Rugby Labs
RUGBY 4309	Propranolol 10 mg	Rugby Labs
RUGBY 4312	Vitamins	Rugby Labs
RUGBY 4313	Propranolol 20 mg	Rugby Labs
RUGBY 4314	Propranolol 40 mg	Rugby Labs
RUGBY 4316	Propranolol 80 mg	Rugby Labs
RUGBY 4324	Prednisone 5 mg	Rugby Labs
RUGBY 4325	Prednisone 10 mg	Rugby Labs
RUGBY 4326	Prednisone 20 mg	Rugby Labs
RUGBY 4328	Prednisone 50 mg	Rugby Labs
RUGBY 4335	Vitamins	Rugby Labs
RUGBY 4339	Vitamins	Rugby Labs
RUGBY 4340	Prednisolone 5 mg	Rugby Labs
RUGBY 4346	Prednisolone 5 mg	Rugby Labs
RUGBY 4352	Prednisolone 5 mg	Rugby Labs
RUGBY 4363	Folic Acid, Iron	Rugby Labs
RUGBY 4365	Probenecid 500 mg, Colchicine 0.5 mg	Rugby Labs
RUGBY 4366	Probenecid 500 mg	Rugby Labs
RUGBY 4367	Procainamide 250 mg	Rugby Labs
RUGBY 4368	Procainamide 500 mg	Rugby Labs
RUGBY 4369	Promethazine 50 mg	Rugby Labs
RUGBY 4377	Procainamide 375 mg	Rugby Labs

Imprint	Ingredient/Brand Name	Manufacturer
RUGBY 4378	Promethazine 12.5 mg	Rugby Labs
RUGBY 4379	Promethazine 25 mg	Rugby Labs
RUGBY 4384	Propylthiouracil 50 mg	Rugby Labs
RUGBY 4390	Pseudoephedrine 60 mg	Rugby Labs
RUGBY 4391	Pseudoephedrine 30 mg	Rugby Labs
RUGBY 4402	Propranolol 40 mg, Hydrochlorothiazide 25 mg	Rugby Labs
RUGBY 4403	Propranolol 80 mg, Hydrochlorothiazide 25 mg	Rugby Labs
RUGBY 4411	Pyrilamine 25 mg	Rugby Labs
RUGBY 4426	Quinine 260 mg	Rugby Labs
RUGBY 4432	Quinidine 200 mg	Rugby Labs
RUGBY 4433	Quinine 325 mg	Rugby Labs
RUGBY 4434	Quinidine 324 mg	Rugby Labs
RUGBY 4458	Reserpine 0.25 mg	Rugby Labs
RUGBY 4494	Nylidrin 6 mg	Rugby Labs
RUGBY 4495	Nylidrin 12 mg	Rugby Labs
RUGBY 4503	Vitamins, Folic Acid	Rugby Labs
RUGBY 4515	Thiothixene 2 mg	Rugby Labs
RUGBY 4516	Thiothixene 5 mg	Rugby Labs
RUGBY 4517	Thiothixene 10 mg	Rugby Labs
RUGBY 4547	Sodium Fluoride 2.2 mg	Rugby Labs
RUGBY 4548	Sodium Fluoride 2.2 mg	Rugby Labs
RUGBY 4549	Sodium Fluoride 2.2 mg	Rugby Labs
RUGBY 4575	Spironolactone 25 mg	Rugby Labs
RUGBY 4576	Spironoloactone 25 mg, Hydrochlorothiazide 25 mg	Rugby Labs
RUGBY 4617	Sulfasalazine 500 mg	Rugby Labs
RUGBY 4618	Sulfisoxazole 500 mg	Rugby Labs
RUGBY 4640	Thioridazine 15 mg	Rugby Labs
RUGBY 4641	Thioridazine 10 mg	Rugby Labs
RUGBY 4642	Thioridazine 25 mg	Rugby Labs
RUGBY 4643	Thioridazine 50 mg	Rugby Labs
RUGBY 4644	Thioridazine 100 mg	Rugby Labs
RUGBY 4648	Theophylline 130 mg, Ephedrine 24 mg, Phenobarbital 8 mg	Rugby
RUGBY 4649	Theophylline 250 mg	Rugby Labs
RUGBY 4657	Theophylline 250 mg	Rugby Labs
RUGBY 4668	Tolbutamide 500 mg	Rugby Labs
RUGBY 4687	Trazodone 50 mg	Rugby Labs
RUGBY 4688	Trazodone 100 mg	Rugby Labs
RUGBY 4692	Trimeth-Sulfa SS 400 mg, 80 mg	Rugby Labs
RUGBY 4693	Trimth-Sulfa DS 160 mg, 800 mg	Rugby Labs
RUGBY 4694	Thyroid 30 mg	Rugby Labs
RUGBY 4698	Thyroid 30 mg	Rugby Labs
RUGBY 4702	Thyroid 60 mg	Rugby Labs
RUGBY 4706	Thyroid 60 mg	Rugby Labs
RUGBY 4710	Thyroid 125 mg	Rugby Labs
RUGBY 4714	Thyroid 125 mg	Rugby Labs
RUGBY 4717	Triamcinolone 4 mg	Rugby Labs
RUGBY 4720	Tri Hydroserpine 0.1 mg/25 mg/15 mg	Rugby Labs
RUGBY 4721	Tri Hydroserpine 0.1 mg/25 mg/15 mg	Rugby Labs
RUGBY 4725	Phenylephrine 10 mg, Phenyltoloxamine 15 mg, Phenylpropanolamine 40 mg, Chloroptheniramine 5 mg	Rugby Labs
RUGBY 4736	Tripelennamine 50 mg	Rugby Labs
RUGBY 4738	Tolazamide 100 mg	Rugby Labs
RUGBY 4739	Tolazamide 250 mg	Rugby Labs
RUGBY 4741	Caramiphen 40 mg, Phenylpropanolamine 75 mg	Rugby Labs
RUGBY 4744	Tolazamide 500 mg	Rugby Labs
RUGBY 4759	Vitamins	Rugby Labs

Imprint	Ingredient/Brand Name	Manufacturer
RUGBY 4812	Verapamil 80 mg	Rugby Labs
RUGBY 4813	Verapamil 120 mg	Rugby Labs
RUGBY 4903	Chlorpromazine 10 mg	Rugby Labs
RUGBY 4906	Chlorpromazine 25 mg	Rugby Labs
RUGBY 4915	Chlorpromazine 50 mg	Rugby Labs
RUGBY 4916	Chlorpromazine 100 mg	Rugby Labs
RUGBY 4918	Chlorpromazine 200 mg	Rugby Labs
RUGBY 4926	Triamterene 50 mg, Hydrochlorothiazide 25 mg	Rugby Labs
RUS	Caffeine, Ephedrine, Phenylpropanolamine	Unknown
RUSS 316	Vitamins/Minerals	Russ
RVJ	Caffeine, Ephedrine, Phenylprpranolamine	Unknown
RW/1	CONTROLLED - No Photo - Hydromorphone 1 mg - Green, round tablet - DEA Schedule II	Richwood Pharm
RW/2	CONTROLLED - No Photo - Hydromorphone 2 mg - Orange, round tablet - DEA Schedule II	Richwood Pharm
RW/3	CONTROLLED - No Photo - Hydromorphone 3 mg - Pink, round tablet - DEA Schedule II	Richwood Pharm
RW/4	CONTROLLED - No Photo - Hydromorphone 4 mg - Yellow, round tablet - DEA Schedule II	Richwood Pharm
RW/81	Aspirin 81 mg	Richwood Pharm
RX 101	Caffeine	Unknown
RX 102	Caffeine	Unknown
RX 103	Caffeine	Unknown
S	Clomiphene Citrate 50 mg	Serono Labs
S/5	Selegiline Hydrochloride 5 mg	Somerset Pharm
S 13	Spironolactone 25 mg	Lederle Labs
S 14	Sulfasalazine	Lederle Labs
S 18-985	Caffeine, Ephedrine	Unknown
S 78-2	Mellaril 10 mg	Sandoz
S 78-8	Mellaril 15 mg	Sandoz
S 78-30	Belladonna Alkaloids 0.25 mg	Sandoz
S-103	Dura-Vent 8 mg, 20 mg, 2.5 mg	Dura
S 547	Trichlormethiazide 4 mg	Schering
S/730	Sorbitrate 30 mg	ICI Pharm
S/760	Sorbitrate 5 mg	Stuart Pharm
S/761	Sorbitrate 10 mg	ICI Pharm
S/770	Sorbitrate 5 mg	ICI Pharm
S/773	Sorbitrate 30 mg	ICI Pharm
S/774	Sorbitrate 40 mg	ICI Pharm
S/780	Sorbitrate 10 mg	ICI Pharm
S/810	Sorbitrate 5 mg	ICI Pharm
S/815	Sorbitrate 10 mg	ICI Pharm
S/820	Sorbitrate 20 mg	ICI Pharm
S 822	Trichlormethiazide 2 mg	Schering
S/853	Sorbitrate 2.5 mg	Stuart Pharm
S/861	Haloperidol 5 mg	Searle Pharm
S/880	Sorbitrate S.A. 40 mg	ICI Pharm
S-1929	Caffeine, Ephedrine	Unknown
S 4140	Amantadine 100 mg	Solvay
S 7720	Chenodiol 250 mg	Solvay
S [cross]/547	Trichlormethiazide 4 mg	Nagua
S[in diamond] 10-1323	Caffeine, Ephedrine, Phenylpropanolamine	Unknown
s[in triangle]/MEL 50	Thioridazine	Unknown
S AHG	Trichlormethiazide 2 mg	Schering
S AHH	Trichlormethiazide 4 mg	Schering
Sal-Fayne	Aspirin, Caffeine, Phenacetin	Unknown

Imprint	Ingredient/Brand Name	Manufacturer
SANDOZ	Triaminic Allergy Tablets	Sandoz Pharm
SANDOZ/78-38	Cedilanid 0.5 mg	Sandoz Pharm
SANDOZ/78-52	Mesantoin 100 mg	Sandoz Pharm
SANDOZ/78-54	Methergine 0.2 mg	Sandoz Pharm
SANDOZ/78-58	Sansert 2 mg	Sandoz Pharm
SANDOZ 78-78	Pamelor 50 mg	Sandoz Pharm
SANDOZ 78-79	Pamelor 75 mg	Sandoz Pharm
SANDOZ 78-86	Pamelor 25 mg	Sandoz Pharm
SANDOZ 78-87	Pamelor 25 mg	Sandoz Pharm
SCHEIN 0765/400	Ibuprofen 400 mg	Danbury Pharm
SCHEIN 0766/600	Ibuprofen 600 mg	Danbury Pharm
SCHEIN 2137/800	Ibuprofen 800 mg	Danbury Pharm
SCHERING/011	Betamethasone 0.6 mg	Schering Corp
SCHERING/070	Ethinyl Estradiol 0.05 mg	Schering Corp
SCHERING/077	Perphenazine 16 mg	Schering Corp
SCHERING 080	Chlorpheniramine Maleate 4 mg	Schering Corp
SCHERING/095	Dexchlorpheniramine Maleate 4 mg	Schering Corp
SCHERING/119	Perphenazine 4 mg, Amitriptylline 10 mg	Schering Corp
SCHERING/148	Dexchlorpheniramine Maleate 6 mg	Schering Corp
SCHERING/150	Ethinyl Estradiol 0.5 mg	Schering Corp
SCHERING 160	Carisoprodol 350 mg	Schering Corp
SCHERING/228	Griseofulvin 125 mg	Schering Corp
SCHERING 244/100	Labetalol 100 mg	Schering Corp
SCHERING 251	CONTROLLED - No Photo - Halazepam 20 mg - Orange tablet - DEA Schedule IV	Schering Corp
SCHERING/252	Albuterol Sulfate 2 mg	Schering Corp
SCHERING/287	Perphenazine 2 mg, Amitriptylline 10 mg	Schering Corp
SCHERING/298	Ethinyl Estradiol 0.02 mg	Schering Corp
SCHERING 311	CONTROLLED - No Photo - Methyltestosterone 10 mg - White tablet - DEA Schedule III	Schering Corp
SCHERING/313	Perphenazine 8 mg	Schering Corp
SCHERING/316	Fluphenazine 10 mg	Schering Corp
SCHERING 402	Theophylline 125 mg	Schering Corp
SCHERING 431	Albuterol Sulfate 2 mg	Schering Corp
SCHERING 438/300	Labetalol 300 mg	Schering Corp
SCHERING/442	Fluphenazinel 2.5 mg	Schering Corp
SCHERING/507	Griseofulvin 250 mg	Schering Corp
SCHERING 522	Chlorpheniramine 2 mg, Acetaminophen 325 mg	Schering Corp
SCHERING 538	CONTROLLED - No Photo - Halazepam 20 mg - White tablet - DEA Schedule IV	Schering Corp.
SCHERING/550	Fluphenazine 5 mg	Schering Corp
SCHERING 555	Pseudoephedrine 120 mg, Dexbrompheniramine 6 mg	Schering Corp
SCHERING/573	Albuterol Sulfate 4 mg	Schering Corp
SCHERING/598	Perphenazine 2 mg, Amitriptylline 25 mg	Schering Corp
SCHERING 703	Azatadine Maleate 1 mg, Pseudoephedrine 120 mg	Schering Corp
SCHERING/705	Perphenazine 2 mg	Schering Corp
SCHERING/720	Perphenazine 4 mg, Amitriptylline 25 mg	Schering Corp
SCHERING 752/200	Labetalol 200 mg	Schering Corp
SCHERING 753	Theophylline 250 mg	Schering Corp
SCHERING/795	Anisindione 50 mg	Schering Corp
SCHERING/820	Dexchlorpheniramine Maleate 2 mg	Schering Corp
SCHERING/843	Prednisone 1 mg	Schering Corp
SCHERING 861	Pseudoephedrine 60 mg	Schering Corp
SCHERING 871	Decongestant Tablets	Schering Corp
SCHERING 901	Chlorpheniramine 4 mg, Pseudoephedrine 60 mg	Schering Corp
SCHERING/940	Perphenazine 4 mg	Schering Corp

Imprint	Ingredient/Brand Name	Manufacturer
SCHERING/251	CONTROLLED - SEE PAGE 203	
SCHERING/970	CONTROLLED - SEE PAGE 207	
SCHERING ADH	Perphenazine 2 mg	Schering Corp
SCHERING ADJ	Perphenazine 8 mg	Schering Corp
SCHERING ADK	Perphenazine 4 mg	Schering Corp
SCHERING ADM	Perphenazine 16 mg	Schering Corp
SCHERING AGT	Dexchlorpheniramine Maleate 2 mg	Schering Corp
SCHERING AHR	Carisoprodol 350 mg	Schering Corp
SCHERING ANA	Perphenazine 2 mg, Amitriptylline 10 mg	Schering Corp
SCHERING ANB	Perphenazine 4 mg, Amitriptylline 10 mg	Schering Corp
SCHERING ANC	Perphenazine 2 mg, Amitriptylline 25 mg	Schering Corp
SCHERING ANE	Perphenazine 4 mg, Amitriptylline 25 mg	Schering Corp
SCHERING EM	Ethinyl Estradiol 0.05 mg	Schering Corp
SCHERING ER	Ethinyl Estradiol 0.02 mg	Schering Corp
SCHERING EP	Ethinyl Estradiol 0.5 mg	Schering Corp
SCHERING/WDR	Fluphenazine 2.5 mg	Schering Corp
SCHERING/WFF	Fluphenazine 5 mg	Schering Corp
SCHERING/WFG	Fluphenazine 10 mg	Schering Corp
SCHWARZ 532	Hyoscyamine Sulfate 0.125 mg	Schwarz Pharma
SCHWARZ 610/10	Isosorbide Mononitrate 10 mg	Schwarz Pharma
SCHWARZ 620/20	Isosorbide Mononitrate 20 mg	Schwarz Pharma
SCS 431	Norethindrone 1 mg, Mestranol 50 mcg	Searle Pharm
SEARLE 5/51	Enovid 5 mg	Searle Pharm
SEARLE/10 01	Aldactone 25 mg	Searle Pharm
SEARLE/10 11	Aldactazide 25 mg/25 mg	Searle Pharm
SEARLE 10/101	Enovid 10 mg	Searle Pharm
SEARLE/12 51	Aminophylline 200 mg	Searle Pharm
SEARLE/15 01	Banthine 50 mg	Searle Pharm
SEARLE/71	Demulen 1 mg/0.05 mg	Searle Pharm
SEARLE 101	Norethynodrel 10 mg, Mestranol 75 mg	Searle Pharm
SEARLE/131	Enovid-E 2.5 mg/0.1 mg	Searle Pharm
SEARLE/151	Demulen 1 mg/0.035 mg	Searle Pharm
SEARLE 201	Spironolactone 25 mg, Hydrochlorothiazide 25 mg	Searle Pharm
SEARLE 205	Spironolactone 25 mg	Searle Pharm
SEARLE 210	Spironolactone 100 mg	Searle Pharm
SEARLE 221	Norethindrone 1 mg, Ethinyl Estradiol 35 mcg	Searle Pharm
SEARLE 244	Spironolactone 50 mg, Hydrochlorothiazide 50 mg	Searle Pharm
SEARLE 401	Ethynodiol Diacetate 1 mg, Mestranol 0.1 mcg	Searle Pharm
SEARLE 431	Norethindrone 1 mg, Mestranol 50 mcg	Searle Pharm
SEARLE/501	Diulo 2.5 mg	Searle Pharm
SEARLE/511	Diulo 5 mg	Searle Pharm
SEARLE/521	Diulo 10 mg	Searle Pharm
SEARLE 531	Chlorthalidone 25 mg	Searle Pharm
SEARLE 541	Chlorthalidone 50 mg	Searle Pharm
SEARLE 571	Furosemide 20 mg	Searle Pharm
SEARLE 581	Furosemide 40 mg	Searle Pharm
SEARLE/601	Pro-Banthine 15 mg	Searle Pharm
SEARLE/611	Pro-Banthine 7.5 mg	Searle Pharm
SEARLE/651	Pro-Banthine 30 mg	Searle Pharm
SEARLE 831	Haloperidol 0.5 mg	Searle Pharm
SEARLE 841	Haloperidol 1 mg	Searle Pharm
SEARLE 851	Haloperidol 2 mg	Searle Pharm
SEARLE 861	Haloperidol 5 mg	Searle Pharm
SEARLE 871	Haloperidol 10 mg	Searle Pharm
SEARLE 881	Haloperidol 20 mg	Searle Pharm
SEARLE 1001	Aldactazide 25 mg/25 mg	Searle Pharm

Imprint	Ingredient/Brand Name	Manufacturer
Searle 1041 Aldactone 50	Aldactone 50 mg	Searle Pharm
SEARLE 1021	Aldactone 50 mg/50 mg	Searle Pharm
SEARLE 1031	Aldactone 100 mg	Searle Pharm
SEARLE 1041	Aldactone 50 mg	Searle Pharm
SEARLE/1231	Aminophylline 100 mg	Searle Pharm
SEARLE/1251	Aminophylline 200 mg	Searle Pharm
SEARLE 1451	Misoprostol 100 mcg	Searle Pharm
SEARLE 1461	Misoprostol 200 mcg	Searle Pharm
SEARLE/1501	Banthine 50 mg	Searle Pharm
SEARLE/1701	Dramamine 50 mg	Searle Pharm
SEARLE/1801	Flagyl 250 mg	Searle Pharm
SEARLE 1831	Flagyl 250 mg	Searle Pharm
SEARLE 2732	Norpace 100 mg	Searle Pharm
SEARLE 2742	Norpace 150 mg	Searle Pharm
SEARLE 2752	Norpace 100 mg	Searle Pharm
SEARLE 2762	Norpace 150 mg	Searle Pharm
SELDANE	Seldane 60 mg	Merrell Dow Pharm
SEP 18-904	Caffeine, Ephedrine, Phenylpropanolamine	Unknown
SEPTRA DS 02C	Septra DS 160 mg/800 mg	Burroughs
SEPTRA Y2B	Septra 80 mg/400 mg	Burroughs
SFC-3512	Docusate Calcium 60 mg, Phenolphthaline 65 mg	Chase
S F-C SANDOZ 78-107	CONTROLLED - SEE PAGE 219	
SIDMAK/375	Nystatin 100,000 units	Sidmak Labs
SINE-AID	Maximum Strength Sine-Aid	McNeil Consumer
SINUS AS + ALLERGY	Alka-Seltzer Plus Sinus Allergy	Miles
Sinus Excedrin	Sinus Excedrin Caplet	Bristol-Myers
SJ	Chewable Aspirin	Schering Corp
SK + K	Caffeine	Unknown
SKF 2	Trifluoperazine 2 mg	Smith, Kline
SKF 5	Trifluoperazine 5 mg	Smith, Kline
SKF 10	Chlorpromazine	Smith, Kline
SKF 25	Vontrol 25 mg	Smith, Kline
SKF 101	Ampicillin 250 mg	Smith, Kline
SKF 102	Ampicillin 500 mg	Smith, Kline
SKF 107	Ampicillin 125 mg	Smith, Kline
SKF 111	Penicillin G	Smith, Kline
SKF 112	Penicillin G	Smith, Kline
SKF 116	Penicillin V 250 mg	Smith, Kline
SKF 117	Penicillin V 500 mg	Smith, Kline
SKF 120	Amitriptyline 10 mg	Smith, Kline
SKF 121	Amitriptyline 25 mg	Smith, Kline
SKF 122	Digoxin 0.25 mg	Smith, Kline
SKF 123	Amitriptyline 50 mg	Smith, Kline
SKF 124	Amitriptyline 75 mg	Smith, Kline
SKF 126	Tetracycline 250 mg	Smith, Kline
SKF 127	Tetracycline 500 mg	Smith, Kline
SKF 129	Niacin 50 mg	Smith, Kline
SKF 130	Niacin 100 mg	Smith, Kline
SKF 131	Amitriptyline 100 mg	Smith, Kline
SKF 132	Amitriptyline 150 mg	Smith, Kline
SKF 169	Reserpine 0.25 mg	Smith, Kline
SKF 171	Quinidine 200 mg	Smith, Kline
SKF 173	Acetaminophen 650 mg	Smith, Kline
SKF 174	Acetaminophen 325 mg	Smith, Kline
SKF 193	Bisacodyl 5 mg	Smith, Kline
SKF 200	Chlorpromazine 200 mg	Smith, Kline

Imprint	Ingredient/Brand Name	Manufacturer
SKF 303	Diphenhydramine 25 mg	Smith, Kline
SKF 304	Diphenhydramine 50 mg	Smith, Kline
SKF 310	Propantheline Bromide 15 mg	Smith, Kline
SKF 339	Prednisone 5 mg	Smith, Kline
SKF 340	Furosemide 20 mg	Smith, Kline
SKF 341	Furosemide 40 mg	Smith, Kline
SKF 347	Doxycycline 50 mg	Smith, Kline
SKF 348	Doxycycline 100 mg	Smith, Kline
SKF 363	Hydrochlorothiazide 25 mg	Smith, Kline
SKF 364	Hydrochlorothiazide 50 mg	Smith, Kline
SKF 367	Erythromycin 250 mg	Smith, Kline
SKF 369	Erythromycin 500 mg	Smith, Kline
SKF 371	Thioridazine 10 mg	Smith, Kline
SKF 372	Thioridazine 25 mg	Smith, Kline
SKF 373	Thioridazine 50 mg	Smith, Kline
SKF 374	Dexamethazone 0.5 mg	Smith, Kline
SKF 375	Thioridazine 100 mg	Smith, Kline
SKF 376	Dexamethazone 0.75 mg	Smith, Kline
SKF 377	Dexamethazone 1.5 mg	Smith, Kline
SKF 379	Dipyridamole 25 mg	Smith, Kline
SKF 380	Dipyridamole 50 mg	Smith, Kline
SKF 381	Dipyridamole 75 mg	Smith, Kline
SKF 403	Triamcinolone 2 mg	Smith, Kline
SKF 404	Triamcinolone 4 mg	Smith, Kline
SKF 406	Triamcinolone 8 mg	Smith, Kline
SKF 409	Tolbutamide 500 mg	Smith, Kline
SKF 419	Chlorothiazide 250 mg	Smith, Kline
SKF 420	Chlorothiazide 500 mg	Smith, Kline
SKF 426	Metronidazole 250 mg	Smith, Kline
SKF 499	Probenecid 500 mg	Smith, Kline
SKF A70	Anspor 250 mg	Smith, Kline
SKF A71	Anspor 500 mg	Smith, Kline
SKF C44	Compazine 10 mg	Smith, Kline
SKF C46	Compazine 15 mg	Smith, Kline
SKF C47	Compazine 30 mg	Smith, Kline
SKF C49	Compazine 75 mg	Smith, Kline
SKF C60	Compazine 2.5 mg	Smith, Kline
SKF C61	Compazine 5 mg	Smith, Kline
SKF C62	Compazine 25 mg	Smith, Kline
SKF C66	Compazine 5 mg	Smith, Kline
SKF C67	Compazine 10 mg	Smith, Kline
SKF C69	Compazine 25 mg	Smith, Kline
SKF D14	Cytomel 0.005 mg	Smith, Kline
SKF D16	Cytomel 0.025 mg	Smith, Kline
SKF D17	Cytomel 0.05 mg	Smith, Kline
SKF D62	Darbid 5 mg	Smith, Kline
SKF Dyazide	Dyazide 50,25 mg	Smith, Kline
SKF E12	CONTROLLED - SEE PAGE 223	
SKF E13	CONTROLLED - SEE PAGE 223	
SKF E14	CONTROLLED - SEE PAGE 223	
SKF E19	CONTROLLED - SEE PAGE 203	
SKF E33	Dibenzyline 10 mg	Smith, Kline
SKF E90	Dyazide 50 mg/25 mg	Smith, Kline
SKF E93	Triamterene 50 mg, Hydrochlorthiazide 25 mg	Smith, Kline
SKF H06	Dyrenium 50 mg	Smith, Kline
SKF H07	Dyrenium 100 mg	Smith, Kline

Imprint	Ingredient/Brand Name	Manufacturer
SKF H10	Triamterene 100 mg	Smith, Kline
SKF H11	Triamterene 50 mg	Smith, Kline
SKF H24	Ecotrin 5 grain	Smith, Kline
SKF J07	Eskalith 300 mg	Smith, Kline
SKF J09	Eskalith 300 mg	Smith, Kline
SKF J10	Eskalith CR 450 mg	Smith, Kline
SKF K31	Feosol 250 mg	Smith, Kline
SKF K32	Feosol 325 mg	Smith, Kline
SKF K33	Feosol	Smith, Kline
SKF K77	Hispril 5 mg	Smith, Kline
SKF N17	Ornex 18 mg/325 mg	Smith, Kline
SKF N23	Ornade 8 mg/50 mg	Smith, Kline
SKF N30	Ornade 8 mg/75 mg	Smith, Kline
SKF N31	Phenylpropanolamine 75 mg, Chlorpheniramine 12 mg	Smith, Kline
SKF N71	Parnate 10 mg	Smith, Kline
SKF P90	Isopropamide Iodide 5 mg	Smith, Kline
SKF P91	Isopropamide Iodide 5 mg, Trifluoperazine 2 mg	Smith, Kline
SKF P92	Isopropamide Iodide 7.5 mg, Trifluoperazine 2 mg	Smith, Kline
SKF P93	Isopropamide Iodide 10 mg, Trifluoperazine 2 mg	Smith, Kline
SKF S03	Stelazine 1 mg	Smith, Kline
SKF S04	Stelazine 2 mg	Smith, Kline
SKF S06	Stelazine 5 mg	Smith, Kline
SKF S07	Stelazine 10 mg	Smith, Kline
SKF S72	Teldrin 8 mg	Smith, Kline
SKF S73	Teldrin 12 mg	Smith, Kline
SKF T01	Temaril 5 mg	Smith, Kline
SKF T03	Temaril 2.5 mg	Smith, Kline
SKF T12	Tagamet 200 mg	Smith, Kline
SKF T13	Tagamet 300 mg	Smith, Kline
SKF T63	Thorazine 30 mg	Smith, Kline
SKF T64	Thorazine 75 mg	Smith, Kline
SKF T66	Thorazine 150 mg	Smith, Kline
SKF T67	Thorazine 200 mg	Smith, Kline
SKF T69	Thorazine 300 mg	Smith, Kline
SKF T70	Thorazine 300 mg	Smith, Kline
SKF T71	Thorazine 100 mg	Smith, Kline
SKF T73	Thorazine 10 mg	Smith, Kline
SKF T74	Thorazine 25 mg	Smith, Kline
SKF T76	Thorazine 50 mg	Smith, Kline
SKF T77	Thorazine 100 mg	Smith, Kline
SKF T79	Thorazine 200 mg	Smith, Kline
SKF V24	Troph-Iron	Smith, Kline
SKF V43	Trophite	Smith, Kline
SKF V71	Tuss-Ornade 20 mg/8 mg/50 mg	Smith, Kline
SKF V90	Urispas 100 mg	Smith, Kline
SKF X42	Vontrol 25 mg	Smith, Kline
SL/07	Hydroxyzine 10 mg	Sidmak Labs
SL/08	Hydroxyzine 25 mg	Sidmak Labs
SL/11	Dipyridamole 25 mg	Sidmak Labs
SL/36	Desipramine 25 mg	Sidmak Labs
SL/66	Amitriptyline 10 mg	Sidmak Labs
SL/67	Amitriptyline 25 mg	Sidmak Labs
SL 236	Pseudoephedrine 300 mg	Sidmak Labs
SL 273	Chlorpropamide 250 mg	Sidmak Labs
SL 301	Nitroglycerin 2.5 mg	Sidmak Labs
SL 302	Nitroglycerin 6.5 mg	Sidmak Labs

Imprint	Ingredient/Brand Name	Manufacturer
SL 303	Nitroglycerin 9 mg	Sidmak Labs
SL 308	Nitroglycerin 9 mg	Sidmak Labs
SL/309	Hydroxyzine 50 mg	Sidmak Labs
SL/312	Dipyridamole 50 mg	Sidmak Labs
SL/313	Dipyridamole 75 mg	Sidmak Labs
SL 314	Cyproheptadine 4 mg	Sidmak Labs
SL 318	Papaverine 150 mg	Sidmak Labs
SL 320	Vitamins, Fluoride 1 mg, Folic Acid	Sidmak Labs
SL 321/10	Isoxsuprine 10 mg	Sidmak Labs
SL 322/20	Isoxsuprine 20 mg	Sidmak Labs
SL 323	Bethanechol Chloride 5 mg	Sidmak Labs
SL 324	Bethanechol Chloride 10 mg	Sidmak Labs
SL 325	Bethanechol Chloride 25 mg	Sidmak Labs
SL 326	Bethanechol Chloride 50 mg	Sidmak Labs
SL 327	Hydralazine 25 mg	Sidmak Labs
SL 328	Hydralazine 50 mg	Sidmak Labs
SL 329	Cyclandelate 200 mg	Sidmak Labs
SL 330	Cyclandelate 400 mg	Sidmak Labs
SL 331	Disulfiram 250 mg	Sidmak Labs
SL 332	Disulfiram 500 mg	Sidmak Labs
SL 333	Metronidazole 250 mg	Sidmak Labs
SL 334	Metronidazole 500 mg	Sidmak Labs
SL 335	Ethaverine 100 mg	Sidmak Labs
SL 336	Ethaverine 100 mg	Sidmak Labs
SL 337	Nylidrin 6 mg	Sidmak Labs
SL 338	Nylidrin 12 mg	Sidmak Labs
SL 339	Procainamide 250 mg	Sidmak Labs
SL 340	Procainamide 500 mg	Sidmak Labs
SL 341	Sulfamethoxazole 400 mg, Trimethoprim 80 mg	Sidmak Labs
SL 342	Sulfamethoxazole 800 mg, Trimethoprim 160 mg	Sidmak Labs
SL 343	Papaverine 300 mg	Sidmak Labs
SL 346	Isosorbide Dinitrate 10 mg	Sidmak Labs
SL 347	Isosorbide Dinitrate 5 mg	Sidmak Labs
SL 348	Isosorbide Dinitrate 10 mg	Sidmak Labs
SL 349	Isosorbide Dinitrate 20 mg	Sidmak Labs
SL 350	Isosorbide Dinitrate 30 mg	Sidmak Labs
SL 351	Isosorbide Dinitrate 40 mg	Sidmak Labs
SL 353	Meclizine 12.5 mg	Sidmak Labs
SL 354	Meclizine 25 mg	Sidmak Labs
SL 355	Meclizine 25 mg	Sidmak Labs
SL 359	Dexchlorpheniramine 2 mg	Sidmak Labs
SL 362	Chlorthalidone 25 mg	Sidmak Labs
SL 363	Chlorthalidone 50 mg	Sidmak Labs
SL 364	Chlorthalidone 100 mg	Sidmak Labs
SL/368	Amitriptyline 50 mg	Sidmak Labs
SL/369	Amitriptyline 75 mg	Sidmak Labs
SL/370	Amitriptyline 100 mg	Sidmak Labs
SL/371	Amitriptyline 150 mg	Sidmak Labs
SL 372	Chlorpropamide 100 mg	Sidmak Labs
SL 373	Chlorpropamide 250 mg	Sidmak Labs
SL 375	Nystatin 100,000 units	Sidmak Labs
SL 377	Doxycycline Hyclate 100 mg	Sidmak Labs
SL 381	Phenylpropanolamine 40 mg, Chlorpheniramine Maleate 5 mg, Phenylephrine 10 mg, Phenyltoloxamine Citrate 15 mg	Sidmak Labs
SL 383	Sidcon TD	Sidmak Labs
SL 384	Isosorbide Dinitrate 20 mg	Sidmak Labs

Imprint	Ingredient/Brand Name	Manufacturer
SL 385	Phenylpropanolamine 75 mg, Guaifenesin 400 mg	Sidmak Labs
SL 387	Ibuprofen 400 mg	Sidmak Labs
SL 388	Ibuprofen 600 mg	Sidmak Labs
SL 390	Salgesic 500 mg	Sidmak Labs
SL 391	Salgesic 750 mg	Sidmak Labs
SL 393	Benztropine Mesylate 0.5 mg	Sidmak Labs
SL 394	Benztropine Mesylate 1 mg	Sidmak Labs
SL 395	Benztropine Mesylate 2 mg	Sidmak Labs
SL 396	Procainamide 750 mg	Sidmak Labs
SL 397	Hydralazine 100 mg	Sidmak Labs
SL 398	Hydralazine 10 mg	Sidmak Labs
SL 404	Phenytoin 100 mg	Sidmak Labs
SL 406	Indomethacin 25 mg	Sidmak Labs
SL 407	Indomethacin 50 mg	Sidmak Labs
SL 410	Carbamazepine 200 mg	Sidmak Labs
SL 415	Griseofulvin 165 mg	Sidmak Labs
SL 416	Griseofulvin 330 mg	Sidmak Labs
SL 425	Aspirin 15 mg	Sidmak Labs
SL 427	Phenylephrine 5 mg, Phenylpropanolamine 45 mg, Glyceryl Guaiacolate 200 mg	Sidmak Labs
SL 430	Metoclopramide 10 mg	Sidmak Labs
SL 433	Trazodone 50 mg	Sidmak Labs
SL 434	Trazodone 100 mg	Sidmak Labs
SL/437	Desipramine 50 mg	Sidmak Labs
SL/438	Desipramine 75 mg	Sidmak Labs
SL 439	Desipramine 100 mg	Sidmak Labs
SL 440	Desipramine 150 mg	Sidmak Labs
SL 441	Trazodone 150 mg	Sidmak Labs
SL 451	Ibuprofen 800 mg	Sidmak Labs
SL 456	Oxybutynin 5 mg	Sidmak Labs
SL 458	Theophylline 300 mg	Sidmak Labs
SL 459	Theophylline 300 mg	Sidmak Labs
SL 460	Clonidine 0.1 mg	Sidmak Labs
SL 461	Clonidine 0.2 mg	Sidmak Labs
SL 462	Clonidine 0.3 mg	Sidmak Labs
SL 463	Clonidine 0.1 mg, Chlorthalidone 15 mg	Sidmak Labs
SL 464	Clonidine 0.2 mg, Chlorthalidone 15 mg	Sidmak Labs
SL 465	Clonidine 0.3 mg, Chlorthalidone 15 mg	Sidmak Labs
SL 467	Propranolol 10 mg	Sidmak Labs
SL 468	Propranolol 20 mg	Sidmak Labs
SL 469	Propranolol 40 mg	Sidmak Labs
SL 470	Propranolol 60 mg	Sidmak Labs
SL 471	Propranolol 80 mg	Sidmak Labs
SL 472	Propranolol 90 mg	Sidmak Labs
SL 473	Propranolol 40 mg, Hydrochlorothiazide 25 mg	Sidmak Labs
SL 474	Propranolol 80 mg, Hydrochlorothiazide 25 mg	Sidmak Labs
SL 475	Methyldopa 125 mg	Sidmak Labs
SL 476	Methyldopa 250 mg	Sidmak Labs
SL 477	Methyldopa 500 mg	Sidmak Labs
SL 478	Methyldopa 250 mg, Hydrochlorothiazide 15 mg	Sidmak Labs
SL 479	Methyldopa 250 mg, Hydrochlorothiazide 25 mg	Sidmak Labs
SL 480	Methyldopa 500 mg, Hydrochlorothiazide 30 mg	Sidmak Labs
SL 481	Methyldopa 500 mg, Hydrochlorothiazide 50 mg	Sidmak Labs
SL 482	Theophylline 200 mg	Sidmak Labs
SL 483	Theophylline 100 mg	Sidmak Labs
SL 484	Sulindac 150 mg	Sidmak Labs

Imprint	Ingredient/Brand Name	Manufacturer
SL 485	Sulindac 200 mg	Sidmak Labs
SL 486	Verapamil 80 mg	Sidmak Labs
SL 487	Verapamil 120 mg	Sidmak Labs
SL 491	Albuterol Sulfate 2 mg	Sidmak Labs
SL 492	Albuterol Sulfate 4 mg	Sidmak Labs
SL 493	Aspirin 800 mg	Sidmak Labs
SL 497	Fenoprofen Calcium 600 mg	Sidmak Labs
SL 505	Triamterene 75 mg, Hydrochlorothiazide 50 mg	Sidmak Labs
SL 514	Meclizine 50 mg	Sidmak Labs
SL 515	Hydroxyzine 100 mg	Sidmak Labs
SL 517	Metoclopramide 5 mg	Sidmak Labs
SL 518	Theophylline 450 mg	Sidmak Labs
SL 520	Phenylephrine 25 mg, Chlorpheniramine 8 mg, Pyrilamine 25 mg	Sidmak Labs
SL 522	Phenylpropanolamine 75 mg, Guaifenesin 400 mg	Sidmak Labs
SL 528	Choline Magnesium Trisalicylate 500 mg	Sidmak Labs
SL 529	Choline Magnesium Trisalicylate 750 mg	Sidmak Labs
SL 530	Choline Magnesium Trisalicylate 1000 mg	Sidmak Labs
SLEEPINAL	Diphenhydramine 50 mg	Sidmak Labs
Slow-K	Slow-K 8mEq	Summit
SMR 22	Caffeine, Ephedrine, Phenylpropanolamine	Unknown
SOFARIN 93/2	Sofarin 2 mg	Lemmon Pharm
SOFARIN 93/2 1/2	Sofarin 2.5 mg	Lemmon Pharm
SOFARIN 93/5	Sofarin 5 mg	Lemmon Pharm
SOLATENE ROCHE	Solatene 30 mg	Roche Labs
SOLVAY 1007	Medroxyprogesterone Acetate 10 mg	Solvay
SOLVAY 1014	Esterified Estrogens 0.3 mg	Solvay
SOLVAY 1022	Esterified Estrogens 0.625 mg	Solvay
SOLVAY 1023	Estratab 0.625 mg, 2.5 mg	Solvay
SOLVAY 1024	Esterified Estrogens 1.25 mg	Solvay
SOLVAY 1025	Esterified Estrogens 2.5 mg	Solvay
SOLVAY 1026	Estratab 1.25 mg, 2.5 mg	Solvay
SOLVAY 1039	Histalet Forte 50 mg, 25 mg, 4 mg, 10 mg	Solvay
SOLVAY 1050	Pseudoephedrine 120 mg, Guaifenesin 400 mg	Solvay
SOLVAY 1082	CONTROLLED - SEE PAGE 221	
SOLVAY 1132	Unipress 25 mg/0.1 mg/15 mg	Solvay
SOLVAY 1146	Vitamins	Solvay
SOLVAY 1200	Creon	Solvay
SOLVAY 1216	Vitamins	Solvay
SOLVAY 1225	Creon-25	Solvay
SOLVAY 1611	Vitamins/Minerals	Solvay
SOLVAY 2808	Prednisone 1 mg	Solvay
SOLVAY 2810	Prednisone 5 mg	Solvay
SOLVAY 2812	Prednisone 10 mg	Solvay
SOLVAY 2814	Prednisone 20 mg	Solvay
SOLVAY 2816	Prednisone 50 mg	Solvay
SOLVAY 3205	Dexamethasone 0.5 mg	Solvay
SOLVAY 3210	Dexamethasone 0.75 mg	Solvay
SOLVAY 3215	Dexamethasone 1.5 mg	Solvay
SOLVAY 3220	Dexamethasone 4 mg	Solvay
SOLVAY 4020	Quinidine Sulfate 300 mg	Solvay
SOLVAY 4028	Quinidine Sulfate 200 mg	Solvay
SOLVAY 4032	Quinidine Sulfate	Solvay
SOLVAY 4120	Valproic Acid 250 mg	Solvay
SOLVAY 7512	Lithium Carbonate 300 mg	Solvay
SOLVAY 7516	Lithium Carbonate 300 mg	Solvay

Imprint	Ingredient/Brand Name	Manufacturer
SP 006	Chlorzoxazone 250 mg, Acetaminophen 300 mg	Superpharm Corp
SP 01	Furosemide 40 mg	Superpharm Corp
SP 02	Furosemide	Superpharm Corp
SP 026	Methocarbamol 500 mg	Superpharm Corp
SP 027	Methocarbamol 750 mg	Superpharm Corp
SP 057	Tolazamide 250 mg	Superpharm Corp
SP 058	Tolazamide 500 mg	Superpharm Corp
SP 091	Allopurinol 100 mg	Superpharm Corp
SP 092	Allopurinol 300 mg	Superpharm Corp
SP 094	Chlorpropamide 100 mg	Superpharm Corp
SP 095	Chlorpropamide 250 mg	Superpharm Corp
SP 3	Clonidine 0.1 mg	Superpharm Corp
SP 4	Clonidine 0.2 mg	Superpharm Corp
SP 5	Clonidine 0.3 mg	Superpharm Corp
SP 14/2	CONTROLLED - SEE PAGE 192	
SP 20	Pseudoephedrine 60 mg	Superpharm Corp
SP 23	Chlorthalidone 25 mg	Superpharm Corp
SP 24	Chlorthalidone 50 mg	Superpharm Corp
SP 26	Methocarbamol 500 mg	Superpharm Corp
SP 27	Methocarbamol 750 mg	Superpharm Corp
SP 38	Hydralazine 25 mg, Hydrochlorothiazide 25 mg	Superpharm Corp
SP 39	Hydralazine 50 mg, Hydrochlorothiazide 50 mg	Superpharm Corp
SP 41	Cyproheptadine 4 mg	Superpharm Corp
SP 43	Dipyridamole 25 mg	Superpharm Corp
SP 44	Dipyridamole 50 mg	Superpharm Corp
SP 45	Dipyridamole 75 mg	Superpharm Corp
SP 47	CONTROLLED - SEE PAGE 201	
SP 49	Triprolidine 2.5 mg, Pseudoephedrine 60 mg	Superpharm Corp
SP 52	Isosorbide Dinitrate 5 mg	Superpharm Corp
SP 53	Isosorbide Dinitrate 10 mg	Superpharm Corp
SP 54	Isosorbide Dinitrate 20 mg	Superpharm Corp
SP 57	Tolazamide 250 mg	Superpharm Corp
SP 58	Tolazamide 500 mg	Superpharm Corp
SP 62/4	CONTROLLED - SEE PAGE 195	
SP 63/3	CONTROLLED - SEE PAGE 194	
SP 74	Chlordiazepoxide 5 mg, Clidinium 2.5 mg	Superpharm Corp
SP 78	Ergoloid Mesylates 1 mg	Superpharm Corp
SP 84	Quinine Sulfate 260 mg	Superpharm Corp
SP 89	Ergoloid Mesylates 1 mg	Superpharm Corp
SP 90	Ergoloid Mesylates 0.5 mg	Vitarine Pharm
SP 91	Allopurinol 100 mg	Superpharm Corp
SP 92	Allopurinol 300 mg	Superpharm Corp
SP 96	Metronidazole 250 mg	Superpharm Corp
SP 97	Metronidazole 500 mg	Superpharm Corp
SP 98	Chlorthalidone 100 mg	Superpharm Corp
SP 100	Doxycycline 100 mg	Superpharm Corp
SP 101	Doxycycline 50 mg	Superpharm Corp
SP 102	Doxycycline 100 mg	Superpharm Corp
SP 103	Hydralazine 10 mg	Superpharm Corp
SP 104	Hydralazine 25 mg	Superpharm Corp
SP 105	Hydralazine 50 mg	Superpharm Corp
SP 106	Hydroxyzine 10 mg	Superpharm Corp
SP 107	Hydroxyzine 107	Superpharm Corp
SP 108	Hydroxyzine 50 mg	Superpharm Corp
SP 109	Tetracycline 250 mg	Superpharm Corp
SP 110	Tetracycline 500 mg	Superpharm Corp

Imprint	Ingredient/Brand Name	Manufacturer
SP 111	Tolbutamide 500 mg	Superpharm Corp
SP 112	Amitriptyline 10 mg	Superpharm Corp
SP 113	Amitriptyline 25 mg	Superpharm Corp
SP 114	Amitriptyline 50 mg	Superpharm Corp
SP 115	Amitriptyline 75 mg	Superpharm Corp
SP 116	Amitritpyline 100 mg	Superpharm Corp
SP 118	Hydroxyzine 25 mg	Superpharm Corp
SP 119	Hydroxyzine 50 mg	Superpharm Corp
SP 120	Hydroxyzine 100 mg	Superpharm Corp
SP 121	Prednisolone 5 mg	Superpharm Corp
SP 122	Prednisone 5 mg	Superpharm Corp
SP 123	Prednisone 10 mg	Superpharm Corp
SP 124	Predisone 20 mg	Superpharm Corp
SP 129	Hydrochlorothiazide 25 mg	Superpharm Corp
SP 130	Hydrochlorothiazide 50 mg	Superpharm Corp
SP 131	Hydrochlorothiazide 100 mg	Superpharm Corp
SP 132	Quinidine Sulfate 200 mg	Superpharm Corp
SP 136	Thioridazine 10 mg	Superpharm Corp
SP 137	Thioridazine 25 mg	Superpharm Corp
SP 138	Thioridazine 50 mg	Superpharm Corp
SP 140	Quinidine Gluconate 324 mg	Superpharm Corp
SP 140	Quinidine Gluconate 324 mg	Superpharm Corp
SP 142	Diphenhydramine 25 mg	Superpharm Corp
SP 143	Diphenhydramine 50 mg	Superpharm Corp
SP 144	Meclizine 12.5 mg	Superpharm Corp
SP 145	Meclizine 25 mg	Superpharm Corp
SP 146	Sulfamethoxazole 400 mg, Trimethoprim 80 mg	Superpharm Corp
SP 147	Sulfamethoxazole 800 mg, Trimethoprim 160 mg	Superpharm Corp
SP 148	Sulfasalazine 500 mg	Superpharm Corp
SP 152	Indomethacin 25 mg	Superpharm Corp
SP 153	Indomethacin 50 mg	Superpharm Corp
SP 154	Spironolactone 25 mg, Hyrochlorothiazide 25 mg	Superpharm Corp
SP 161	Metoclopramide 10 mg	Superpharm Corp
SP 164	Disopyramide 100 mg	Superpharm Corp
SP 165	Disopyramide 150 mg	Superpharm Corp
SP 166	Spironolactone 25 mg	Superpharm Corp
SP 170	Ibuprofen 400 mg	Superpharm Corp
SP 171	Ibuprofen 600 mg	Superpharm Corp
SP 175	CONTROLLED - SEE PAGE 208	
SP 181	CONTROLLED - SEE PAGE 185	
SP 182	CONTROLLED - SEE PAGE 187	
SP 184	CONTROLLED - SEE PAGE 218	
SP 185	CONTROLLED - SEE PAGE 217	
SP 189	Propranolol 10 mg	Superpharm Corp
SP 190	Propranolol 20 mg	Superpharm Corp
SP 191	Propranolol 40 mg	Superpharm Corp
SP 192	Propranolol 80 mg	Superpharm Corp
SP 384	Isosorbide Dinitrate 20 mg	Sidmak Labs
SPECTROBID/035	Spectrobid 400 mg	Pfizer Pharm
SP'D 37.5	Caffeine, Ephedrine, Phenylpropanolamine	Unknown
SPF ALLEREST	Allerest Sinus Pain Formula	Ciba
SQU 698	Dirocide 200 mg, Diethylcarbamaczine 200 mg	Unknown
SQUIBB 28	Imipramine 25 mg	Squibb
SQUIBB 39	Imipramine 10 mg	Squibb
SQUIBB 40	Imipramine 40 mg	Squibb
SQUIBB 45	Desipramine 25 mg	Squibb

Imprint	Ingredient/Brand Name	Manufacturer
SQUIBB 63	Ergoloid Mesylates 1 mg	Squibb
SQUIBB 105	Sulindac 150 mg	Squibb
SQUIBB 107	Sulindac 200 mg	Squibb
SQUIBB 109	Vitamin A 25,000 IU	Squibb
SQUIBB 110	Vitamin A 50,000 IU	Squibb
SQUIBB 111	Vitamin A 1,000 IU	Squibb
SQUIBB 112	Vitamin C 250 mg	Squibb
SQUIBB 113	Velosef 250	Squibb
SQUIBB 114	Velosef 500	Squibb
SQUIBB 133	CONTROLLED - No Photo - Clorazepate Dipotassium 3.75 mg - Tablet - DEA Schedule IV	Squibb
SQUIBB 138	Sulfamethoxazole 400 mg, Trimethoprim 80 mg	Squibb
SQUIBB 139	Chlorpropamide 100 mg	Squibb
SQUIBB 147	Velosef 1 gm	Squibb
SQUIBB 152	Chlorpropamide 250 mg	Squibb
SQUIBB 154	Pravastatin Sodium 10 mg	Squibb
SQUIBB 157	CONTROLLED - No Photo - Clorazepate Dippotassium 7.5 mg - Tablet - DEA Schedule IV	Squibb
SQUIBB 158	Monopril 10 mg	Squibb
SQUIBB 159	CONTROLLED - No Photo - Oxazepam 30 mg - Capsule - DEA Schedule IV	Squibb
SQUIBB 160	Erythromycin Stearate 250 mg	Squibb
SQUIBB 161	Erythromycin Stearate 500 mg	Squibb
SQUIBB 162	Chlorthalidone 25 mg	Squibb
SQUIBB 163	CONTROLLED - No Photo - Clorazepate Dipotassium 15 mg - Tablet - DEA Schedule IV	Squibb
SQUIBB 164	Pentids 200,000 units	Squibb
SQUIBB 165	Pentids 400	Squibb
SQUIBB 167	Pentids 400	Squibb
SQUIBB 168	Pentids 800	Squibb
SQUIBB 170	Gestest	Squibb
SQUIBB 171	Sulfamethoxazole 800 mg, Trimethoprim 160 mg	Squibb
SQUIBB 178	Prvastatin Sodium 20 mg	Squibb
SQUIBB 180	Chlorthalidone 50 mg	Squibb
SQUIBB 181	Cephalexin 250 mg	Squibb
SQUIBB 184	Amnestrogen 0.625 mg	Squibb
SQUIBB 185	CONTROLLED - No Photo - Diazepam 2 mg - Tablet - DEA Schedule IV	Squibb
SQUIBB 187	Chlorthalidone 100 mg	Squibb
SQUIBB 188	Amnestrogen 1.25 mg	Squibb
SQUIBB 189	Amnestrogen 2.5 mg	Squibb
SQUIBB 192	Ascorbic Acid 50 mg	Squibb
SQUIBB 193	Perphenazine 2 mg, Amitriptyline 10 mg	Squibb
SQUIBB 194	Vitamin C 100 mg	Squibb
SQUIBB 195	Tolazamide 100 mg	Squibb
SQUIBB 196	Vitamin C 250 mg	Squibb
SQUIBB 197	Vitamin C 500 mg	Squibb
SQUIBB 201	Aspirin 324 mg	Squibb
SQUIBB 202	Dicloxacillin Sodium 250 mg	Squibb
SQUIBB 203	Dicloxacillin 500 mg	Squibb
SQUIBB 204	Vitamins	Squibb
SQUIBB 207	Corgard 40 mg	Squibb
SQUIBB 208	Corgard 120 mg	Squibb
SQUIBB 211	Cloxacillin Sodium 250 mg	Squibb
SQUIBB 212	Cloxacillin Sodium 500 mg	Squibb
SQUIBB 230	Trimox 250	Squibb

Imprint	Ingredient/Brand Name	Manufacturer
SQUIBB 231	Trimox 500	Squibb
SQUIBB 232	Corgard 20 mg	Squibb
SQUIBB 238	CONTROLLED - No Photo - Diazepam 5 mg - Tablet - DEA Schedule IV	Squibb
SQUIBB 239	Cephalexin 500 mg	Squibb
SQUIBB 241	Corgard 80 mg	Squibb
SQUIBB 243	Corgard 100 mg	Squibb
SQUIBB 245	CONTROLLED - No Photo - Diazepam 10 mg - Tablet DEA Schedule IV	
SQUIBB 246	Corgard 160 mg	Squibb
SQUIBB 259	Perphenazine 2 mg, Amitriptyline 25 mg	Squibb
SQUIBB 267	Perphenazine 4 mg, Amitriptyline 10 mg	Squibb
SQUIBB 271	Perphenazine 4 mg, Amitriptyline 25 mg	Squibb
SQUIBB 274	Trazodone 50 mg	Squibb
SQUIBB 275	Triamterene 50 mg. Hydrochlorothiazide 25 mg	Squibb
SQUIBB 277	Tolazamide 250 mg	Squibb
SQUIBB 279	Isosorbide Dinitrate 40 mg	Squibb
SQUIBB 280	Indomethacin 25 mg	Squibb
SQUIBB 283	Corizide 40 mg/5 mg	Squibb
SQUIBB 284	Corizide 80 mg/5 mg	Squibb
SQUIBB 286	Quinidine Gluconate 324 mg	Squibb
SQUIBB 288	Allopurinol 300 mg	Squibb
SQUIBB 289	Clonidine 0.1 mg	Squibb
SQUIBB 295	Indomethacin 50 mg	Squibb
SQUIBB 297	Engran	Squibb
SQUIBB 298	CONTROLLED - No Photo - Lorazepam 0.5 mg - Tablet - DEA Schedule IV	Squibb
SQUIBB 300	Prazosin 1 mg	Squibb
SQUIBB 307	Rautraux with K 50 mg/50 mg	Squibb
SQUIBB 325	Trifluoperazine 10 mg	Squibb
SQUIBB 327	Triamterene 50 mg, Hydrochlorothiazide 25 mg	Squibb
SQUIBB 338	Capozide 25 mg/15 mg	Squibb
SQUIBB 341	Theragran Z	Squibb
SQUIBB 348	Indomethacin 75 mg	Squibb
SQUIBB 349	Capozide 25 mg/25 mg	Squibb
SQUIBB 355	Valadol 325 mg	Squibb
SQUIBB 357	Valadol 120 mg	Squibb
SQUIBB 359	Furosemide 20 mg	Squibb
SQUIBB 360	Furosemide 40 mg	Squibb
SQUIBB 365	Trifluoperazine 1 mg	Squibb
SQUIBB 368	TrifluoperAzine 2 mg	Squibb
SQUIBB 371	Digitoxin 0.1 mg	Squibb
SQUIBB 384	Capozide 50 mg/15 mg	Squibb
SQUIBB 386	Carisoprodol 350 mg	Squibb
SQUIBB 390	Capozide 50 mg/25 mg	Squibb
SQUIBB 399	Trifluoperazine 5 mg	Squibb
SQUIBB 400	Prazosin 2 mg	Squibb
SQUIBB 408	CONTROLLED - No Photo - Lorazepam 1 mg - Tablet - DEA Schedule IV	Squibb
SQUIBB 429	Florinef 0.1 mg	Squibb
SQUIBB 430	Fungilin 100 mg	Squibb
SQUIBB 431	Pronestyl 250 mg	Squibb
SQUIBB 433	Methyldopa 500 mg	Squibb
SQUIBB 434	Pronestyl 375 mg	Squibb
SQUIBB 438	Pronestyl 500 mg	Squibb
SQUIBB 447	Methyldopa 250 mg	Squibb

Imprint	Ingredient/Brand Name	Manufacturer
SQUIBB 450	Capoten 12.5 mg	Squibb
SQUIBB 452	Capoten 25 mg	Squibb
SQUIBB 455	Oragrafin 500 mg	Squibb
SQUIBB 457	Mycostatin 100,000 units	Squibb
SQUIBB 476	Engram - HP	Squibb
SQUIBB 478	Engram - HP	Squibb
SQUIBB 482	Capoten 50 mg	Squibb
SQUIBB 485	Capoten 100 mg	Squibb
SQUIBB 487	CONTROLLED - No Photo - Lorazepam 2 mg - Tablet - DEA Schedule IV	Squibb
SQUIBB 488	Metronidazole 250 mg	Squibb
SQUIBB 500	Prazosin 5 mg	Squibb
SQUIBB 504	Kenacort 2 mg	Squibb
SQUIBB 505	Ipral Calcium	Squibb
SQUIBB 511	Kenacort 1 mg	Squibb
SQUIBB 512	Kenacort 4 mg	Squibb
SQUIBB 513	Trimethoprim 100	Squibb
SQUIBB 518	Kenacort 8 mg	Squibb
SQUIBB 520	Clonidine 0.2 mg	Squibb
SQUIBB 527	Theragran M	Squibb
SQUIBB 534	Clonidine 0.3 mg	Squibb
SQUIBB 535	Theragran Hematinic	Squibb
SQUIBB 537	Niacin 500 mg	Squibb
SQUIBB 538	Rautrax-N Modified	Squibb
SQUIBB 539	Rautrax-N	Squibb
SQUIBB 547	Liafon	Squibb
SQUIBB 549	Iron, Vitamin C	Squibb
SQUIBB 560	Disopyramide 100 mg	Squibb
SQUIBB 567	Disopyramide 150 mg	Squibb
SQUIBB 570	Novo-Basic	Squibb
SQUIBB 572	Metronidazole 500 mg	Squibb
SQUIBB 573	Ora--Testryl	Squibb
SQUIBB 574	CONTROLLED - No Photo - Oxazepam 10 mg - Capsule - DEA Schedule IV	Squibb
SQUIBB 580	Mycostatin 500,000 units	Squibb
SQUIBB 598	Neomycin Sulfate 0.5 mg	Squibb
SQUIBB 599	CONTROLLED - No Photo - Oxazepam 15 mg - Capsule - DEA Schedule IV	Squibb
SQUIBB 602	Naturetin with K 2.5 mg/500 mg	Squibb
SQUIBB 603	Tetracycline 500 mg	Squibb
SQUIBB 605	Naturetin-2.5	Squibb
SQUIBB 606	Naturetin-5	Squibb
SQUIBB 607	Rauwolfia 50 mg, Hydroflumethiazide 25 mg	Squibb
SQUIBB 608	Naturetin 5 mg/500 mg	Squibb
SQUIBB 609	Fosinopril Sodium 20 mg	Squibb
SQUIBB 610	Niacin 25 mg	Squibb
SQUIBB 611	Niacin 50 mg	Squibb
SQUIBB 612	Niacin 100 mg	Squibb
SQUIBB 615	CONTROLLED - No Photo - Propoxyphene HCl 65 mg - Capsule - DEA Schedule IV	Squibb
SQUIBB 616	Principin with Probenecid	Squibb
SQUIBB 618	Naturetin-10	Squibb
SQUIBB 619	CONTROLLED - No Photo - Propoxyphene HCl 65 mg - Capsule - DEA Schedule IV	Squibb
SQUIBB 622	Meclofenamate 50 mg	Squibb

Imprint	Ingredient/Brand Name	Manufacturer
SQUIBB 623	CONTROLLED - No Photo - Noctec 250 mg - Capsule - DEA Schedule IV	Squibb
SQUIBB 626	CONTROLLED - No Photo - Noctec 500 mg - Capsule - DEA Schedule IV	Squibb
SQUIBB 629	Meclofenamate 100 mg	Squibb
SQUIBB 630	Methyldopa 250 mg, Hydrochlorothiazide 15 mg	Squibb
SQUIBB 637	Isoniazide 100 mg	Squibb
SQUIBB 648	Veetids 500	Squibb
SQUIBB 649	Trigot 0.5 mg	Squibb
SQUIBB 650	Re-Covr 500 mg	Squibb
SQUIBB 652	Methyldopa 500 mg, Hydrochlorothiazide 30 mg	Squibb
SQUIBB 654	Trigot 1 mg	Squibb
SQUIBB 655	Tetracycline 250 mg	Squibb
SQUIBB 663	Tetracycline 250 mg	Squibb
SQUIBB 671	Methyldopa 500 mg, Hydrochlorothiazide 50 mg	Squibb
SQUIBB 674	Doxycycline Hyclate 50 mg	Squibb
SQUIBB 677	Mysteclin	Squibb
SQUIBB/684	Veetids 250	Squibb
SQUIBB 685	Rautrax	Squibb
SQUIBB 689	Teslac 250 mg	Squibb
SQUIBB 690	Teslac 50 mg	Squibb
SQUIBB 692	Tolbutamide 500 mg	Squibb
SQUIBB 693	Metoclopramide 10 mg	Squibb
SQUIBB 694	Hydrochlorothiazide 50 mg	Squibb
SQUIBB 708	Rubraferate	Squibb
SQUIBB 713	Raudixin 50 mg	Squibb
SQUIBB 718	CONTROLLED - No Photo - Chlordiazepoxide 5 mg - Capsule - DEA Schedule IV	Squibb
SQUIBB 723	Phenytoin 100 mg	Squibb
SQUIBB 725	CONTROLLED - No Photo - Propoxyphene and Acetaminophen - Tablet - DEA Schedule IV	Squibb
SQUIBB 726	Procainamide 250 mg	Squibb
SQUIBB 727	CONTROLLED - No Photo - Chlordiazepoxide 10 mg - Capsule - DEA Schedule IV	Squibb
SQUIBB 729	Propranolol 10 mg	Squibb
SQUIBB 731	Propranolol 20 mg	Squibb
SQUIBB 736	CONTROLLED - No Photo - Chlordiazepoxide 25 mg - Capsule - DEA Schedule IV	Squibb
SQUIBB 738	CONTROLLED - No Photo - Temazepam 15 mg - Capsule - DEA Schedule IV	Squibb
SQUIBB 742	Procainamide 500 mg	Squibb
SQUIBB 745	Propranolol 40 mg	Squibb
SQUIBB 747	CONTROLLED - No Photo - Temazepam 30 mg - Capsule - DEA Schedule IV	Squibb
SQUIBB 749	Cephalexin 250 mg	Squibb
SQUIBB 750	Propranolol 60 mg	Squibb
SQUIBB 756	Pronestyl 375 mg	Squibb
SQUIBB 757	Pronestyl 500 mg	Squibb
SQUIBB 758	Pronestyl 250 mg	Squibb
SQUIBB 763	Sumycin 500	Squibb
SQUIBB 765	Propranolol 80 mg	Squibb
SQUIBB 766	Rauwolfia 50 mg, Hydroflumethiazide 25 mg	Squibb
SQUIBB 767	Thioridazine 10 mg	Squibb
SQUIBB 769	Rauzide 50 mg/4 mg	Squibb
SQUIBB 775	Pronestyl-SR 500 mg	Squibb
SQUIBB 776	Raudixin 100 mg	Squibb

Imprint	Ingredient/Brand Name	Manufacturer
SQUIBB 777	Procainamide 750 mg	Squibb
SQUIBB 778	Rutorbin 60-300	Squibb
SQUIBB 779	Tetracycline 250 mg, Amphotericin 50 mg	Squibb
SQUIBB 783	Rutorbin 20-100	Squibb
SQUIBB 788	Allopurinol 300 mg	Squibb
SQUIBB 789	Rubrafolin	Squibb
SQUIBB 790	Thioridazine 15 mg	Squibb
SQUIBB 797	Serenium 100 mg	Squibb
SQUIBB 798	Thioridazine 25 mg	Squibb
SQUIBB 802	CONTROLLED - No Photo - Clorazepate Dipotassium 3.75 mg - Capsule - DEA Schedule IV	Squibb
SQUIBB 812	Doxycycline Hyclate 100 mg	Squibb
SQUIBB 823	Theragran	Squibb
SQUIBB 825	Theragran-M	Squibb
SQUIBB 829	Chlorothiazide 500 mg	Squibb
SQUIBB 830	Hydrea 500 mg	Squibb
SQUIBB 831	Vitamin E 200 IU	Squibb
SQUIBB 833	Steclin 250 mg	Squibb
SQUIBB 834	Vitamins/Minerals	Squibb
SQUIBB 838	CONTROLLED - No Photo - Clorazepate Dipotassium 7.5 mg - Capsule - DEA Schedule IV	Squibb
SQUIBB 842	Vitamins	Squibb
SQUIBB 845	Allopurinol 100 mg	Squibb
SQUIBB 849	Theragran-M	Squibb
SQUIBB 851	Triamterene 75 mg, Hydrochlorothiazide 50 mg	Squibb
SQUIBB 862	CONTROLLED - No Photo - Clorazepate Dipotassium 3.75 mg - Tablet - DEA Schedule IV	Squibb
SQUIBB 863	Prolixin 1 mg	Squibb
SQUIBB 864	Prolixin 2.5 mg	Squibb
SQUIBB 870	CONTROLLED - No Photo - Clorazepate Dipotassium 15 mg - Capsule - DEA Schedule IV	Squibb
SQUIBB 872	Comoxol 400 mg/80 mg	Squibb
SQUIBB 873	Comoxol 800 mg/160 mg	Squibb
SQUIBB 874	Cephalexin 500 mg	Squibb
SQUIBB 876	Trigesic 2 mg/3.5 mg/0.5 grains	Squibb
SQUIBB 877	Prolixin 5 mg	Squibb
SQUIBB 883	Tetracycline 250 mg	Squibb
SQUIBB 887	Terfonyl 0.5 gm	Squibb
SQUIBB 889	Vitamin C 100 units	Squibb
SQUIBB 905	Theragran Junior	Squibb
SQUIBB 915	Vitamin B-1 50 mg	Squibb
SQUIBB 916	Vitamin B-1 100 mg	Squibb
SQUIBB 917	Amitid 10 mg	Squibb
SQUIBB 918	Amitid 25 mg	Squibb
SQUIBB 921	Vesprin 10 mg	Squibb
SQUIBB 922	Vesprin 25 mg	Squibb
SQUIBB 923	Vesprin 50 mg	Squibb
SQUIBB 929	Fungizone Lozenger 10 mg	Squibb
SQUIBB 937	Theragran	Squibb
SQUIBB 938	Thioridazine 50 mg	Squibb
SQUIBB 940	Doxycycline Hyclate 100 mg	Squibb
SQUIBB 942	Amitid 50 mg	Squibb
SQUIBB 943	Amitid 75 mg	Squibb
SQUIBB 955	Amitid 100 mg	Squibb
SQUIBB 956	Prolixin 10 mg	Squibb
SQUIBB 963	Trazodone 100 mg	Squibb

Imprint	Ingredient/Brand Name	Manufacturer
SQUIBB 964	Thioridazine 100 mg	Squibb
SQUIBB 971	Principen 250 mg	Squibb
SQUIBB 974	Principen 500 mg	Squibb
SQUIBB 977	Tolserol 0.5 gm	Squibb
SQUIBB 1175	Loxapine Succinate 5 mg	Squibb
SQUIBB 1235	Loxapine Succinate 10 mg	Squibb
SQUIBB 1455	Loxapine Succinate 25 mg	Squibb
SQUIBB 1535	Loxapine Succinate 50 mg	Squibb
SQUIBB 2201	Cephalexin Suspension 125 mg/5 mg	Squibb
SQUIBB 2202	Cephalexin Suspension 250 mg/5 mg	Squibb
S/S	Sleep-Eze 25 mg/0.125 mg	Whitehall Labs
S S	Sucrets 2.4 mg	Beecham Products
S S	Sucrets 1.2 mg	Beecham Products
ST 22	Caffeine, Ephedrine, Phenylpropanolamine	Unknown
STUART 021	Stuartnatal	Stuart Pharm
STUART 071	Stuartnatal	Stuart Pharm
STUART 115	Tenoretic 50 mg/25 mg	Stuart Pharm
STUART 117	Tenoretic 100 mg/25 mg	Stuart Pharm
STUART 330	Dialose 100 mg/400 mg	Stuart Pharm
STUART 350	Dialose Plus 30 mg/100 mg/400 mg	Stuart Pharm
STUART 380	Kasof 240 mg	Stuart Pharm
STUART/450	Mylicon 40 mg	Stuart Pharm
STUART 455	Simethicone 125 mg	Stuart Pharm
STUART 470	Dialose 100 mg	Stuart Pharm
STUART 475	Dialose Plus 100 mg/30 mg	Stuart Pharm
STUART 620	Mylanta 200 mg/200 mg/20 mg	Stuart Pharm
STUART 650	Ferancee	Stuart Pharm
STUART 651	Aluminum 400 mg, Magnesium Hydroxide 400 mg, Simethicone 40 mg	Stuart Pharm
STUART/710	Mulvidren-F	Stuart Pharm
STUART/770	Sorbitrate 5 mg	Stuart Pharm
STUART/773	Sorbitrate 30 mg	Stuart Pharm
STUART/774	Sorbitrate 40 mg	Stuart Pharm
STUART/780	Sorbitrate 10 mg	Stuart Pharm
STUART 790	Sorbitrate 10 mg, Phenobarbital 15 mg	Stuart Pharm
STUART/810	Sorbitrate 5 mg	Stuart Pharm
STUART/815	Sorbitrate 10 mg	Stuart Pharm
STUART/820	Sorbitrate 20 mg	Stuart Pharm
STUART 850	Stuartnatal 1+1	Stuart Pharm
STUART 851	Mylanta-II 400 mg/400 mg/30 mg	Stuart Pharm
STUART 858	Mylicon-80	Stuart Pharm
STUART/864	Bucladin 50 mg	Stuart Pharm
STUART/880	Sorbitrate 40 mg	Stuart Pharm
SU	Pseudoephedrine 30 mg	Burroughs Wellcom
Wellcome SUDAFED 12 HOUR	Pseudoephedrine 120 mg	Burroughs Wellcom
SUDAFED 60	Sudafed 60 mg	Burroughs Wellcome
SUDAFED PLUS	Sudafed Plus 60 mg/4 mg	Burroughs Wellcome
SUDAFED SINUS	Sudafed 120 mg	Burroughs Wellcome
Sunkist	Vitamin C 500 mg	Ciba
Sunkist 250	Vitamin C 250 mg	Ciba
Sunkist 500	Vitamin C 500 mg	Ciba
Sunkist V	Multivitamin	Ciba
SUPHEDRINE	Cold & Cough Liquigels	Granutec
SuperEPA	SuperEPA 1200 600 mg	Advanced Nutritional
SURE CURE ii	Phenylpropanolamine	Unknown
Surfak	Surfak 240 mg	Hoechst-Roussel Pharm

Imprint	Ingredient/Brand Name	Manufacturer
SUSTAIRE/220	Sustaire 100 mg	Pfizer Labs
SUSTAIRE/221	Sustaire 300 mg	Pfizer Labs
SV[in box] 18-789	Caffeine, Ephedrine, Phenylpropanolamine	Unknown
SV[in box] 18-850	Caffeine, Ephedrine, Phenylpropanolamine	Unknown
SV[in box] 18-906	Caffeine, Ephedrine, Phenylpropanolamine	Unknown
SV[in box] 18-985	Caffeine, Ephedrine, Phenylpropanolamine	Unknown
SV[in box] 895	Caffeine, Ephedrine, Phenylpropanolamine	Unknown
SYNTEX/1	Norinyl 1 mg/0.05 mg	Syntex Labs
SYNTEX/2	Norinyl 2 mg/0.1 mg	Syntex Labs
SYNTEX/3	Norinyl 1 mg/0.08 mg	Syntex Labs
SYNTEX/110	Brevicon 0.5 mg/0.035 mg	Syntex Labs
SYNTEX/111	Norinyl 1 mg	Syntex Labs
SYNTEX/272	Naprosyn 250 mg	Syntex Labs
SYNTEX/273	Naprosyn 375 mg	Syntex Labs
SYNTEX/274	Anaprox 275 mg	Syntex Labs
SYNTEX/277	Naprosyn 500 mg	Syntex Labs
SYNTEX/2107	Nor-QD 0.35 mg	Syntex Labs
SYNTEX/2110	Brevicon 0.5 mg/0.035 mg	Syntex Labs
T	Tessalon 100 mg	DuPont Pharm
T 10	Thioridazine 10 mg	Lederle Labs
T 13	Sulfamethoxazole 400 mg, Trimethoprim 80 mg	Lederle Labs
T 16	Sulfamethoxazole 800 mg, Trimethoprim 160 mg	Lederle Labs
T 17	Tolbutamide 500 mg	Lederle Labs
T-20	Caffeine, Ephedrine, Phenylpropanolamine	Unknown
T 21/W[in box]	Talwin 50 mg	Winthrop Labs
T 25	Thioridazine 25 mg	Lederle Labs
T 27	Thioridazine 50 mg	Lederle Labs
T27/Winthrop	CONTROLLED - SEE PAGE 200	
T 28	Thioridazine 100 mg	Lederle Labs
T 31/W[in box]	Telepaque 500 mg	Winthrop-Breon Labs
T 37/Winthrop	CONTROLLED - SEE PAGE 211	
T 41	Phenazopyridine 100 mg	Trinity
T 46	Sulfapyridine 500 mg	Eli Lilly
T 51/W	CONTROLLED - SEE PAGE 206	
T 54	Sulfadiazine 500 mg	Eli Lilly
T 55	Papaverine 100 mg	Eli Lilly
T-57	Phenylephrine 22 mg, Phenylpropanolamine 50 mg, Chlorpheniramine 8 mg, Hyoscyamine .19 mg, Atropine .04 mg	Econolab
T 73	Papaverine 200 mg	Eli Lilly
T77	Carbinoxamine Maleate 4 mg, Pseudoephedrine 60 mg	Econolab
T 93	Isoniazide 100 mg	Eli Lilly
T 96	Neomycin Sulfate 500 mg	Eli Lilly
T 99	Paramethasone Acetate 1 mg	Eli Lilly
T 100/W[in box]	Trancopal 100 mg	Winthrop-Breon Labs
T107	Tenormin 25 mg	ICI Pharma
T 109	Carbamazepine 200 mg	Lemmon Pharm
T 142	Phenazopyridine 200 mg	Trinity
T 147	Phenazopyridine 200 mg	Trinity
T 200/W[in box]	Trancopal 200 mg	Winthrop-Breon Labs
T 204	Colchicine 0.6 mg	Trinity
T 500/PF	Trilisate 500 mg	Purdue Frederick Co
T 750/PF	Trilisate 750 mg	Purdue Frederick Co
T 1000/PF	Trilisate 1000 mg	Purdue Frederick Co
TABLOID BRAND	Empirin 325 mg	Burroughs Wellcome
TAGAMET 200 SKF	Tagamet 200 mg	Smith, Kline & French
TAGAMET 300 SKF	Tagamet 300 mg	Smith, Kline & French

Imprint	Ingredient/Brand Name	Manufacturer
TAGAMET 400 SKF	Tagamet 400 mg	Smith, Kline & French
TARACTAN 10	Taractan 10 mg	Roche Labs
TARACTAN 25	Taractan 25 mg	Roche Labs
TARACTAN 50	Taractan 50 mg	Roche Labs
TARACTAN 100	Taractan 100 mg	Roche Labs
TAVIST-1/78-75	Tavist-1 1.34 mg	Sandoz Pharm
TAVIST/4370	Tavist 2.68 mg	Dorsey Labs
TAVIST D/78-221	Clemastine Fumarate 1.34 mg, Phenylpropanolamine 75 mg	Sandoz
T/B	Aspirin 325 mg	Ohm Labs
TC/a	CONTROLLED - SEE PAGE 186	
TCL 001	Aspirin 325 mg	Time-Cap Labs
TCL 002	Aspirin 650 mg	Time-Cap Labs
TCL 003	Bisacodyl 5 mg	Time-Cap Labs
TCL-005	Aspirin 500 mg	Time-Cap Labs
TCL 011	Aspirin 325 mg	Time-Cap Labs
TCL 016	Pseudoephedrine 30 mg	Time-Cap Labs
TCL 020	Docusate Sodium 100 mg, Yellow Phenolphthalein 65 mg	Time-Cap La
TCL 024	Aspirin 165 mg	Time-Cap Labs
TCL 025	Aspirin 81 mg	Time-Cap Labs
TCL 031	Ferrous Fumarate 150 mg, Docusate Sodium 100 mg	Time-Cap Labs
TCL 032	Aspirin 325 mg	Time-Cap Labs
TCL 1221	Nitroglycerin 2.5 mg	Time-Cap Labs
TCL 1222	Nitroglycerin 6.5 mg	Time-Cap Labs
TCL 1223	Nitroglycerin 9 mg	Time-Cap Labs
TCM	Tylenol Cold Effervescent Tablet	McNeil
TE/a	CONTROLLED - SEE PAGE 189	
TEGISON 10 ROCHE	Tegison 10 mg	Roche Labs
TEGISON 25 ROCHE	Tegison 25 mg	Roche Labs
Tempra	Acetaminophen 80 mg	Mead Johnson
Tempra 160	Acetaminophen 160 mg	Mead Johnson
TEN-K	Ten-K 750 mg	Geigy Pharm
TENORMIN 101	Tenormin 100 mg	Stuart Pharm
TENORMIN 105	Tenormin 50 mg	Stuart Pharm
TENUATE 25	CONTROLLED - SEE PAGE 196	
TENUATE 75	CONTROLLED - SEE PAGE 201	
TEPANIL TEN-TAB/RIKER	CONTROLLED - SEE PAGE 197	
TEPANIL/RIKER	CONTROLLED - SEE PAGE 194	
TERRAMYCIN PFIZER 073	Terramycin 250 mg	Pfizer Labs
TEW T-DIET	CONTROLLED - SEE PAGE 217	
TEW T-GESIC	CONTROLLED - SEE PAGE 214	
TF	Armour Thyroid 120 mg	Rorer
TG	Armour Thyroid 180 mg	Rorer
TH	Armour Thyroid 240 mg	Rorer
TH/a	CONTROLLED - SEE PAGE 190	
THEO-DUR 100	Theophylline 100 mg	Key Pharm
THEO-DUR 200	Theophylline 200 mg	Key Pharm
THEO-DUR 300	Theophylline 300 mg	Key Pharm
Theolair 250 3M	Theolair 250 mg	3M
THIS END UP PF MSIR 15	CONTROLLED - SEE PAGE 228	
THIS END UP PF MSIR 30	CONTROLLED - SEE PAGE 228	
TI	Armour Thyroid 300 mg	Rorer
TI/a	CONTROLLED - SEE PAGE 203	
Ticlid 250	Ticlid 250 mg	Syntex
TIGAN 100mg	Tigan 100 mg	Beecham Labs
TIGAN 250mg	Tigan 250 mg	Beecham Labs
TJ	Armour Thyroid 90 mg	Rorer

Imprint	Ingredient/Brand Name	Manufacturer
TJ/a	CONTROLLED - SEE PAGE 204	
TK/a	CONTROLLED - SEE PAGE 204	
TM AKG	Caffeine, Ephedrine, Phenylpropanolamine	Unknown
TM AKS 18-789	Caffeine, Ephedrine, Phenylpropanolamine	Unknown
TOLECTIN	Tolectin DS 400 mg	McNeil Pharm
TOLECTIN 600 McNEIL	Tolectin 600	McNeil Pharm
TOLINASE 100	Tolinase 100 mg	Upjohn Co
TOLINASE 250	Tolinase 250 mg	Upjohn Co
TOLINASE 500	Tolinase 500 mg	Upjohn Co
Tolmetin/1	Tolmetin Sodium 200 mg	Duramed Pharm
Tolmetin 400 mg	Tolmetin Sodium 400 mg	Duramed Pharm
Tolmetin 600 mg	Tolmetin Sodium 600 mg	Duramed Pharm
TP 305	Colchicine 648 mcg	Towne, Paulsen
TP 352	Zinc Sulfate 220 mg	Towne, Paulsen
TP 403	Hydrochlorothiazide 100 mg	Towne, Paulsen
TP 404	Hydrochlorothiazide 25 mg	Towne, Paulsen
TP 405	Hydrochlorothiazide 50 mg	Towne, Paulsen
TP 601	Colchicine 540 mcg	Towne, Paulsen
TP 604	Cortisone Acetate 25 mg	Towne, Paulsen
TP 606	Hydrocortisone 20 mg	Rondex Labs
TP 608	Hydrocortisone 10 mg	Rondex Labs
TP 758	Acetaminophen 325 mg	Towne, Paulsen
TP 816	Chlorpheniramine Maleate 4 mg	Towne, Paulsen
TP 826	Diphenhydramine 25 mg	Towne, Paulsen
TP 827	Diphenhydramine 50 mg	Towne, Paulsen
TP 833	Diphenhydramine 25 mg	Towne, Paulsen
TP 865	Isoniazide 100 mg	Towne, Paulsen
TP 873	Folic Acid 1 mg	Towne, Paulsen
TP 900	Quinidine Sulfate 200 mg	Towne, Paulsen
TP 913	Prednisone 10 mg	Towne, Paulsen
TP 922	Prednisone 5 mg	Towne, Paulsen
TP 924	Prednisone 5 mg	Towne, Paulsen
TP 925	Prednisone 20 mg	Towne, Paulsen
TP 926	Prednisone 2.5 mg	Towne, Paulsen
TR50 3M	Tambocor 50 mg	3M
TR100 3M	Tambocor 100 mg	3M
TR 125/G	CONTROLLED - SEE PAGE 226	
TR 250/G	CONTROLLED - SEE PAGE 226	
TRANDATE 100 GLAXO	Trandate 100 mg	Glaxo Inc
TRANDATE 200 GLAXO	Trandate 200 mg	Glaxo Inc
TRANDATE 300 GLAXO	Trandate 300 mg	Glaxo Inc
TRANQUIN	Trandate	Unknown
TRAVIST/78-72	Tavist 2.68 mg	Sandoz Pharm
TRENTAL	Trental 400 mg	Hoechst-Roussel
TRI 10-10	Caffeine, Ephedrine, Phenylpropanolamine	Unknown
TRIAD	Triad 50 mg/325 mg/40 mg	UAD Labs
TRIAMINIC SANDOZ	Chlorpheniramine 2 mg, Phenylpropanolamine 12.5 mg	Sandoz
TRIAMINICIN/SANDOZ	Triaminicin 25 mg/4 mg/650 mg	Dorsey Labs
TRIMPEX 100	Trimpex 100 mg	Roche Labs
TRINALIN 703	Azatadine Maleate 1 mg, Pseudoephedrine 120 mg	Schering Labs
Trofan DS IGM	Trofan-DS	Upsher-Smith
TRUST 250	Ampicillin	Unknown
TTTT 124	Hydrochlorothiazide 50 mg	Heather Drug
TTTT 174	Levo-Thyroxine 0.1 mg	Heather Drug
TTTT 175	Levo-Thyroxine 0.2 mg	Heather Drug
TTTT 187	Prednisolone 5 mg	Heather Drug

Imprint	Ingredient/Brand Name	Manufacturer
TTTT 188	Papaverine 150 mg	Heather Drug
TTTT 189	Prednisolone 5 mg	Heather Drug
TTTT 193	Methocarbamol 500 mg	Heather Drug
TTTT 196	Methenamine 500 mg	Heather Drug
TTTT 202	Sulfixoxazole 500 mg	Heather Drug
TTTT 203	Tetracycline 500 mg	Heather Drug
TTTT 209	Thyroid 1 grain	Heather Drug
TTTT 212	Thyroid 2 grains	Heather Drug
TTTT 214	Tetracycline 250 mg	Heather Drug
TTTT 403	Sulfamethoxazole 500 mg	Heather Drug
TTTT 501	Methocarbamol 750 mg	Heather Drug
TTTT 503	Methenamine 1000 mg	Heather Drug
TTTT 505	Prednisone 10 mg	Heather Drug
TTTT 506	Prednisone 20 mg	Heather Drug
TTTT 510	Methylpredisolone 4 mg	Heather Drug
TTTT 513	Cortisone 25 mg	Heather Drug
TTTT 527	Prednisolone 50 mg	Heather Drug
TTTT 531	Furosemide 40 mg	Heather Drug
TTTT 532	Furosemide 20 mg	Heather Drug
TTTT 534	Sulfamethoxazole 400 mg, Trimethoprim 160 mg	Heather Drug
TTTT 535	Sulfamethoxazole 800 mg, Trimethoprim 160 mg	Heather Drug
TTTT 538	Doxycycline 100 mg	Heather Drug
TTTT 539	Doxycycline 100 mg	Heather Drug
TTTT 540	Doxycycline 50 mg	Heather Drug
TYLENOL	Tylenol 325 mg	McNeil Pharm
TYLENOL 2 CODEINE/McNEIL	CONTROLLED - SEE PAGE 194	
TYLENOL 3 CODEINE/McNEIL	CONTROLLED - SEE PAGE 194	
TYLENOL 4 CODEINE/McNEIL	CONTROLLED - SEE PAGE 194	
TYLENOL 80	Tylenol 80 mg	McNeil Pharm
Tylenol 160	Junior Strength Tylenol 160 mg	McNeil Pharm
Tylenol 500mg	Extra-Strength Tylenol 500 mg	McNeil Pharm
TYLENOL A/S	Maximum Strength Tylenol Allergy Sinus	McNeil
TYLENOL SINUS	Tylenol Sinus 500 mg/30 mg	McNeil Pharm
TYLOX McNEIL	CONTROLLED - SEE PAGE 216	
T[in box] 10-845	Caffeine, Ephedrine, Phenylpropanolamine	Unknown
T[in box] 18-845	Caffeine, Ephedrine	Unknown
T[in box] 18-984	Caffeine, Ephedrine, Phenylpropanolamine	Unknown
U 01	Paramethasone Acetate 2 mg	Eli Lilly
U 03	Acetohexamide 250 mg	Eli Lilly
U 05	Erythromycin Estolate 125 mg	Eli Lilly
U 07	Acetohexamide 500 mg	Eli Lilly
U 09	Cyclothiazide 2 mg	Eli Lilly
U 23	Isoniazid 300 mg	Eli Lilly
U 25	Erythromycin 250 mg	Eli Lilly
U 26	Erythromycin Estolate 500 mg	Eli Lilly
U 29	Reserpine 0.25 mg	Eli Lilly
U 56	Folic Acid 1 mg	Eli Lilly
U 60	Cephalexin 1 gram	Eli Lilly
U 121/2 1/2	Loniten 2.5 mg	Upjohn Comp
U 137/Loniten10	Loniten 10 mg	Upjohn Comp
U/412	Maolate 400 mg	Upjohn Comp
UAD 1120	CONTROLLED - SEE PAGE 216	
UAD 2304	CONTROLLED - SEE PAGE 222	
ULTRASE MT6	Pancreatic Enzyme	Scandipharm
ULTRASE MT12	Pancreatic Enzyme	Scandipharm
ULTRASE MT18	Pancreatic Enzyme	Scandipharm

Imprint	Ingredient/Brand Name	Manufacturer
ULTRASE MT20	Pancreatic Enzyme	Scandipharm
Unisom	Doxylamine Succinate 25 mg	Pfizer, Inc.
U U 201	Lorcet Plus 7.5 mg/650 mg	Mikart Inc
UPJOHN 15	Cortisone Acetate 5 mg	Upjohn Co
UPJOHN 19	CONTROLLED - SEE PAGE 211	
UPJOHN 23	Cortisone Acetate 10 mg	Upjohn Co
UPJOHN 32	Deltasone 2.5 mg	Upjohn Co
UPJOHN 34	Cortisone Acetate 25 mg	Upjohn Co
UPJOHN 45	Deltasone 5 mg	Upjohn Co
UPJOHN 49	Medrol 24 mg	Upjohn Co
UPJOHN 50	Provera 10 mg	Upjohn Co
UPJOHN 56	Medrol 4 mg	Upjohn Co
UPJOHN 70	Tolinase 100 mg	Upjohn Co
UPJOHN 72	Medrol 8 mg	Upjohn Co
UPJOHN 73	Medrol 16 mg	Upjohn Co
UPJOHN 100	Orinase 500 mg	Upjohn Co
UPJOHN 114	Tolinase 250 mg	Upjohn Co
UPJOHN 155	Medrol 24 mg	Upjohn Co
UPJOHN 165	Deltasone 20 mg	Upjohn Co
UPJOHN 176	Medrol 32 mg	Upjohn Co
UPJOHN 193	Deltasone 10 mg	Upjohn Co
UPJOHN 225	Cleocin 150 mg	Upjohn Co
UPJOHN 310	Panmycin 500 mg	Upjohn Co
UPJOHN 331	Cleocin 75 mg	Upjohn Co
UPJOHN 388	Deltasone 50 mg	Upjohn Co
UPJOHN 477	Tolinase 500 mg	Upjohn Co
UPJOHN 701	Orinase 250 mg	Upjohn Co
UPJOHN 782	Panmycin 250 mg	Upjohn Co
UPJOHN 949	Uracil Mustard 1 mg	Upjohn Co
UPR	Acetaminophen 650 mg, Diphenhydramine 50 mg	Pfizer, Inc.
UREX 3M	Urex	3M
URISPAS SKF	Urispas 100 mg	Smith, Kline & French
UROLENE BLUE	Methylene Blue 65 mg	Star Pharm
US 303	Iron 50 mg, Vitamin C 250 mg	U.S. Pharmaceutical
US 500	Salsalate 500 mg	Upsher Smith
US 750	Salsalate 750 mg	Upsher Smith
USB001	Altretamine 50 mg	US Bioscience
USL 8	Potassium 600 mg	Upsher Smith
USL 10	Potassium 750 mg	Upsher Smith
USL 80	Zinc Sulfate 220 mg	Upsher Smith
USV 2835	Nicobid 125 mg	USV Labs
USV 2840	Nicobid 250 mg	USV Labs
USV 2841	Nicobid 500 mg	USV Labs
USV [logo] LH	Levothyroxine Sodium 125 mcg	USV Labs
USV [logo] LK	Levothyroxine Sodium 25 mcg	USV Labs
USV [logo] LL	Levothyroxine Sodium 50 mcg	USV Labs
USV [logo] LM	Levothyroxine Sodium 100 mcg	USV Labs
USV [logo] LN	Levothyroxine Sodium 150 mcg	USV Labs
USV [logo] LP	Levothyroxine Sodium 17 mcg	USV Labs
USV [logo] LR	Levothyroxine Sodium 200 mcg	USV Labs
USV [logo] LS	Levothyroxine Sodium 300 mcg	USV Labs
USV [logo] LT	Levothyroxine Sodium 75 mcg	USV Labs
UVS [logo]	Mephentermine	Unknown
U-ZOOM	Caffeine, Ephedrine, Phenylpropanolamine	Unknown
V	Menthol 5.3 mg	Proctor & Gamble
V60	Bisacodyl 5 mg	Vintage Pharm

Imprint	Ingredient/Brand Name	Manufacturer
V 5380	Contrin 0.5 mg/75 mg/110 mg/240 mg	Vitarine Pharm
VA 72	Acetaminophen 325 mg	Vitech Corp.
VA 73	Acetaminophen 500 mg	Vitech Corp.
VA 735	Acetaminophen 500 mg	Vitech Corp.
VALRELEASE 15 ROCHE	CONTROLLED - SEE PAGE 221	
Vascor 200	Vascor 200 mg	McNeil
Vascor 300	Vascor 300 mg	McNeil
Vascor 400	Vascor 400 mg	McNeil
VC	Menthol 10 mg, Benzocaine 6 mg	Proctor Gamble
V V	Vivarin 200 mg	Beecham Products
VIBRA PFIZER 094	Vibramycin 50 mg	Pfizer Labs
VIBRA PFIZER 095	Vibarmycin 100 mg	Pfizer Labs
VICODIN	CONTROLLED - SEE PAGE 200	
VICODIN ES	CONTROLLED - SEE PAGE 200	
VIOKASE AHR	Viokase	A.H. Robins Co.
VIRILON 10 MG [logo]	CONTROLLED - SEE PAGE 224	
VISKEN 5/78-111	Visken 5 mg	Sandoz Pharm
Visken 5V	Visken 5 mg	Sandoz Pharm
VISKEN 10/78-73	Visken 10 mg	Sandoz Pharm
Visken 10V	Visken 10 mg	Sandoz Pharm
VISTARIL PFIZER 541	Vistrail 25 mg	Pfizer Labs
VISTARIL PFIZER 542	Vistaril 50 mg	Pfizer Labs
VISTARIL PFIZER 543	Vistaril 100 mg	Pfizer Labs
Vitron C	Ascorbic Acid 125 mg	Fisons
VL	Senna Leaf Powder 324 mg, Senna Extract Powder 64.8 mg	Major Phar
VL 536	Prednisone 5 mg	Vangard Labs
VL 1537	Spironolactone 25 mg, Hydrochlorothiazide 25 mg	Vangard Labs
Volmax 4	Albuterol Sulfate 4 mg	Muro Pharm
Volmax 8	Albuterol Sulfate 8 mg	Muro Pharm
VT 76	CONTROLLED - SEE PAGE 205	
VT 77	CONTROLLED - No Photo- Phendimetrazine Tartrate 35 mg - Pink capsule - DEA Schedule III	Vitarine Pharm
VT 1052	Theophylline 260 mg	Vitarine Pharm
W	Phenazopyridine 97.2 mg	KV Pharm
W028	Cloxacillin Sodium	Bristol-Myers
W038	Cloxacillin Sodium	Bristol-Myers
W048	Dicloxacillin Sodium 250 mg	Bristol-Myers
W058	Dicloxacillin Sodium 500 mg	Bristol-Myers
W080	CONTROLLED - No Photo - Hydrocodone Bitartrate 5 mg, Acetaminophen 500 mg - Tablet - DEA Schedule III	
W090	Verapamil 80 mg	Bristol-Myers
W-1	Isosorbide Dinitrate 2.5 mg	West-ward Inc.
W/2.5	Isordil 2.5 mg	Wyeth Labs
W-3	Isosorbide Dinitrate 5 mg	West-ward Inc.
W 4/Wyeth 73	Wytensin 4 mg	Wyeth Labs
W/5	Isordil 5 mg	Wyeth Labs
W 8/Wyeth 74	Wytensin 8 mg	Wyeth Labs
W 10	Isosorbide Dinitrate 10 mg	Wyeth Labs
W 16/92	Wytensin 16 mg	Wyeth Labs
W 49	Aluminum 180 mg, Magnesium Hydroxide 160 mg	Winthrop
W 53/W	CONTROLLED - SEE PAGE 206	
W100	Verapamil 120 mg	Bristol-Myers
W110	Cefadroxil 500 mg	Bristol-Myers
W111	Thiothixene 1 mg	Bristol-Myers
W112	Haloperidol 5 mg	Bristol-Myers

Imprint	Ingredient/Brand Name	Manufacturer
W114	CONTROLLED - No Photo - Flurazepam 15 mg - Capsule - DEA Schedule IV	Bristol-Myers
W116	Hydroxyzine 25 mg	Bristol-Myers
W117	Prednisone 10 mg	Bristol-Myers
W118	Isosorbide Dinitrate ER	Bristol-Myers
W119	Methocarbamol 750 mg	Bristol-Myers
W122	Hydroxyzine 10 mg	Bristol-Myers
W125	Thiothixene 2 mg	Bristol-Myers
W127	CONTROLLED - No Photo - Flurazepam 30 mg - Capsule - DEA Schedule IV	Bristol-Myers
W128	Thiothixene 2 mg	Bristol-Myers
W131	Thiothixene 5 mg	Bristol-Myers
W134	Lithium Carbonate 300 mg	Bristol-Myers
W135	Haloperidol 2 mg	Bristol-Myers
W136	Meclizine 12.5 mg	Bristol-Myers
W137	Thiothixene 10 mg	Bristol-Myers
W260	CONTROLLED - No Photo - Propoxyphene HCl 65 mg - Tablet - DEA Schedule IV	Bristol-Myers
W280	CONTROLLED - No Photo - Propoxyphene Napsylate 100 mg, Acetaminophen 650 mg - Tablet - DEA Schedule IV	Bristol-Myers
W290	CONTROLLED - No Photo - Propoxyphene HCl 65 mg, Acetaminophen 640 mg - Tablet - DEA Schedule IV	Bristol-Myers
W300	Prazosin 1 mg	Bristol-Myers
W310	Erythromycin Stearate 250 mg	Bristol-Myers
W330	Erythromycin Stearate 500 mg	Bristol-Myers
W-332	Vitamins	West-ward
W340	Nitrofurantoin 100 mg	Bristol-Myers
W350	Nitrofurantoin 50 mg	Bristol-Myers
W400	Prazosin 2 mg	Bristol-Myers
W410	Amitriptyline	Bristol-Myers
W/434	Phenergan-D 6.25 mg/60 mg	Wyeth Labs
W460	Desipramine 50 mg	Bristol-Myers
W470	Desipramine 75 mg	Bristol-Myers
W 480	Propylthiouracil 50 mg	Rondex
W500	Prazosin 5 mg	Bristol-Myers
W540	Dicyclomine HCl 10 mg	Bristol-Myers
W550	Dicyclomine HCl 20 mg	Bristol-Myers
W610	Meclizine HCl 25 mg	Bristol-Myers
W613 562	Thyroid 32.4 mg	Western Reasearch
W614 562	Thyroid 64.8 mg	Western Reasearch
W615 562	Thyroid 129.6 mg	Western Reasearch
W616 562	Thyroid 194.4 mg	Western Reasearch
W 641	Triphasil	Wyeth-Ayerst
W 642	Triphasil	Wyeth-Ayerst
W 643	Triphasil	Wyeth-Ayerst
W 650	Triphasil	Wyeth-Ayerst
W720	Haloperidol 1 mg	Bristol-Myers
W777	Amoxapine 100 mg	Bristol-Myers
W790	Hydrochlorothiazide 25 mg	Bristol-Myers
W 791	Albuterol Sulfate 4 mg	Bristol-Myers
W830	Haloperidol 20 mg	Bristol-Myers
W840	Nitroglycerin 5 mg	Bristol-Myers
W870	Prednisone 5 mg	Bristol-Myers
W888	Amoxapine 50 mg	Bristol-Myers
W 891	Albuterol Sulfate 2 mg	Bristol-Myers
W900	Hydrochlorothiazide 50 mg	Bristol-Myers

Imprint	Ingredient/Brand Name	Manufacturer
W921	Metoprolol Tartrate 50 mg	Bristol-Myers
W930	Nitroglycerin SR 5 mg	Bristol-Myers
W933	Metoprolol Tartrate 100 mg	Bristol-Myers
W940	Haloperidol 10 mg	Bristol-Myers
W950	Prednisone 20 mg	Bristol-Myers
W970	Hydroxyzine 50 mg	Bristol-Myers
W999	Amoxapine 25 mg	Bristol-Myers
W 1620	Griseofulvin 125 mg	BiCoastal Pharm
W 1621	Griseofulvin 250 mg	BiCoastal Pharm
W 1623	Griseofulvin 165 mg	BiCoastal Pharm
W 1624	Griseofulvin 330 mg	BiCoastal Pharm
W 2225	Hyoscamine 0.15 mg	Webcon
W 2260	Hyoscamine 0.375 mg	Webcon
W 7300	Tacaryl 3.6 mg	Westwood Pharm
W 7400	Tacaryl 8 mg	Westwood Pharm
W 7400	Methdilazine 8 mg	Westwood
WA77	Chloroquine Phosphate 500 mg	Winthrop
WA79	Chloroquine Phosphate 500 mg, Primaquine Phos 79 mg	Winthrop
WA82	Quinacrine 100 mg	Winthrop
W & L -118	Diphenhydramine 50 mg	Weeks & Leo
WALLACE 37-1301 400	CONTROLLED - SEE PAGE 219	
WALLACE 37 1601/600	CONTROLLED - SEE PAGE 200	
WALLACE 153	Aquatensen 5 mg	Wallace Labs
WALLACE 272	Diutensen 2 mg/2.5 mg	Wallace Labs
WALLACE 274	Diutensen-R 2.5 mg/0.1 mg	Wallace Labs
WALLACE 521	Diphylline 200 mg	Wallace Labs
WALLACE 541	Diphylline 200 mg, Guaifenesin 200 mg	Wallace Labs
WALLACE 713	Rynatan 25 mg/8 mg/25 mg	Wallace Labs
WALLACE 717	Rynatuss 60 mg/5 mg/10 mg/10 mg	Wallace Labs
WALLACE 731	Lufyllin-400	Wallace Labs
WALLACE 2001/37	Soma 350 mg	Wallace Labs
WALLACE 2103	Soma Compound 350 mg/325 mg	Wallace Labs
WALLACE 2403/SOMA CC	CONTROLLED - SEE PAGE 206	
WALLACE 4224/37	Organidin 30 mg	Wallace Labs
WATSON 300	Fumide 20 mg	Everett Labs
WATSON 301	Fumide 40 mg	Everett Labs
WATSON 302	Furosemide 80 mg	Watson Labs
Watson 305	Propranolol 10 mg	Watson Labs
Watson 306	Propranolol 20 mg	Watson Labs
Watson 307	Propranolol 40 mg	Watson Labs
Watson 308	Propranolol 80 mg	Watson Labs
Watson 311	Furosemide 20 mg	Watson Labs
Watson 312	Metoclopramide 10 mg	Watson Labs
Watson 343	Verapamil 80 mg	Watson Labs
Watson 344	Verapamil 80 mg	Watson Labs
Watson 345	Verapamil 120 mg	Watson Labs
Watson 346	Verapamil 120 mg	Watson Labs
Watson 348	Triamterene 75 mg, Hydrochlorothiazide 50 mg	Watson Labs
WATSON 349	CONTROLLED - SEE PAGE 201	
Watson 352	Propranolol 60 mg	Watson Labs
WATSON 363/3.75	CONTROLLED - SEE PAGE 210	
WATSON 364/7.5	CONTROLLED - SEE PAGE 202	
WATSON 365/15	CONTROLLED - SEE PAGE 207	
Watson 369/5 mg	Loxapine Succinate 5 mg	Watson Labs
Watson 370/10 mg	Loxapine Succinate 10 mg	Watson Labs
Watson 371/25 mg	Loxapine Succinate 25 mg	Watson Labs

Imprint	Ingredient/Brand Name	Manufacturer
Watson 372/50 mg	Loxapine Succinate 50 mg	Watson Labs
Watson 373	Maprotiline 25 mg	Watson Labs
Watson 374	Maprotiline 50 mg	Watson Labs
Watson 375	Maprotiline 75 mg	Watson Labs
Watson 379	Amoxapine 25 mg	Watson Labs
Watson 380	Amoxapine 50 mg	Watson Labs
Watson 381	Amoxapine 100 mg	Watson Labs
Watson 382	Amoxapine 150 mg	Watson Labs
WATSON 385	CONTROLLED - SEE PAGE 200	
WATSON 387	CONTROLLED - SEE PAGE 201	
Watson 404	Verapamil 40 mg	Watson Labs
Watson 414	Estropipate .75 mg	Watson Labs
Watson 416	Estropipate 3 mg	Watson Labs
Watson 417	Estropipate 6 mg	Watson Labs
Watson 418	Cyclobenzaprine HCl 10 mg	Watson Labs
Watson 424	Triamterene 37.5 mg, Hydrochlorothiazide 25 mg	Watson Labs
Watson 430	Carbidopa 10 mg, Levodopa 100 mg	Watson Labs
Watson 431	Carbidopa 25 mg, Levodopa 100 mg	Watson Labs
Watson 432	Carbidopa 25 mg, Levodopa 250 mg	Watson Labs
Watson 515	Estropipate 1.5 mg	Watson Labs
WBS [logo]	Disophrol 6 mg/120 mg	Schering Corp
WC 014	Propranolol 40 mg, Hydrochlorothiazide 25 mg	Warner Chilcott
WC 015	Propranolol 80 mg, Hydrochlorothiazide 25 mg	Warner Chilcott
WC 030	Methyldopa 250 mg, Hydrochlorothiazide 15 mg	Warner Chilcott
WC 031	Methyldopa 250 mg, Hydrochlorothiazide 25 mg	Warner Chilcott
WC 032	Methyldopa 500 mg, Hydrochlorothiazide 30 mg	Warner Chilcott
WC 033	Methyldopa 500 mg, Hydrochlorothiazide 50 mg	Warner Chilcott
WC 034	Gelusil 200 mg/200 mg/25 mg	Warner Chilcott
WC 037	Ferrous Sulfate 325 mg	Warner Chilcott
WC 043	Gelusil II 400 mg/400 mg/30 mg	Warner Chilcott
WC 070	Propranolol 10 mg	Warner Chilcott
WC 071	Propranolol 20 mg	Warner Chilcott
WC 072	Propranolol 40 mg	Warner Chilcott
WC 073	Propranolol 60 mg	Warner Chilcott
WC 074	Propranolol 80 mg	Warner Chilcott
WC 077	Fenoprofen 600 mg	Warner Chilcott
WC 078	Nifedipine 10 mg	Warner Chilcott
WC 079	Nifedipine 800 mg	Warner Chilcott
WC 081	Fenoprofen 300 mg	Warner Chilcott
WC 084	Gemfibrozil 600 mg	Warner Chilcott
WC 100	Sinubid 100 mg/66 mg/300 mg/300 mg	Warner Chilcott
WC 110	Sinutab 25 mg/22 mg/325 mg	Warner Chilcott
WC 118	Extra Strength Sinutab 25 mg/22 mg/500 mg	Warner Chilcott
WC 121	Chlorthalidone 50 mg	Warner Chilcott
WC 123	Chlorthalidone 25 mg	Warner Chilcott
WC 142/5	CONTROLLED - SEE PAGE 191	
WC 143/10	CONTROLLED - SEE PAGE 192	
WC 180	Pyridium 100 mg	Warner Chilcott
WC 181	Pyridium 200 mg	Warner Chilcott
WC 200	Oxtriphylline 200 mg, Guaifenesin 100 mg	Warner Chilcott
WC 210	Choledyl 100 mg	Warner Chilcott
WC 211	Choledyl 200 mg	Warner Chilcott
WC 242	Carbamazepine 100 mg	Warner Chilcott
WC 243	Carbamazepine 200 mg	Warner Chilcott
WC 247	D-S-S 100 mg	Warner Chilcott
WC 248	D-S-S PLUS 100 mg/30 mg	Warner Chilcott

Imprint	Ingredient/Brand Name	Manufacturer
WC 250	Proloid 1/4 grain	Warner Chilcott
WC 251	Proloid 1/2 grain	Warner Chilcott
WC 252	Proloid 1 grain	Warner Chilcott
WC 253	Proloid 1 1/2 grains	Warner Chilcott
WC 254	Proloid 3 grains	Warner Chilcott
WC 255	Proloid 5 grains	Warner Chilcott
WC 257	Proloid 2 grains	Warner Chilcott
WC 260	Euthroid 1/2 grain	Warner Chilcott
WC 261	Euthroid 1 grain	Warner Chilcott
WC 262	Euthroid 2 grains	Warner Chilcott
WC 263	Euthroid 3 grains	Warner Chilcott
WC/270	Nardil 15 mg	Warner Chilcott
WC 271	Amitriptyline 100 mg	Warner Chilcott
WC 272	Amitriptyline 10 mg	Warner Chilcott
WC 273	Amitriptyline 25 mg	Warner Chilcott
WC 274	Amitriptyline 50 mg	Warner Chilcott
WC 275	Amitriptyline 75 mg	Warner Chilcott
WC 278	Amitriptyline 150 mg	Warner Chilcott
WC 402	Ampicillin 250 mg	Warner Chilcott
WC 404	Ampicillin 500 mg	Warner Chilcott
WC 407	Tetracycline 250 mg	Warner Chilcott
WC 420	Quinine Sulfate 325 mg	Warner Chilcott
WC 432/1	CONTROLLED - SEE PAGE 189	
WC 433/2	CONTROLLED - SEE PAGE 191	
WC 440	Furosemide 20 mg	Warner Chilcott
WC 441	Furosemide 40 mg	Warner Chilcott
WC 442	Furosemide 80 mg	Warner Chilcott
WC 443	Clonidine 0.1 mg	Warner Chilcott
WC 444	Clonidine 0.2 mg	Warner Chilcott
WC 445	Clonidine 0.3 mg	Warner Chilcott
WC 451	CONTROLLED - SEE PAGE 210	
WC 452	CONTROLLED - SEE PAGE 202	
WC 453	CONTROLLED - SEE PAGE 207	
WC 515	Allopurinol 100 mg	Warner Chilcott
WC 516	Ibuprofen 400 mg	Warner Chilcott
WC 517	Allopurinol 300 mg	Warner Chilcott
WC 533	Calcium Lactate 325 mg	Warner Chilcott
WC 538	Cefadroxil 500 mg	Warner Chilcott
WC 548	Cephalexin 250 mg	Warner Chilcott
WC 549	Cephalexin 500 mg	Warner Chilcott
WC 551	CONTROLLED - SEE PAGE 205	
WC 557	Verapamil 80 mg	Warner Chilcott
WC 558	Disopyramide Phosphate 100 mg	Warner Chilcott
WC 573	Verapamil 120 mg	Warner Chilcott
WC 573	Verapamil 120 mg	Warner Chilcott
WC 575	Danozol 200 mg	Warner Chilcott
WC 577	Trazodone 50 mg	Warner Chilcott
WC 577	Verapamil 80 mg	Warner Chilcott
WC 578	Trazodone 100 mg	Warner Chilcott
WC 592	Thephylline 300 mg	Warner Chilcott
WC 594	Desipramine 25 mg	Warner Chilcott
WC 595	Desipramine 50 mg	Warner Chilcott
WC 596	Desipramine 75 mg	Warner Chilcott
WC 604	Calcium Lactate 650 mg	Warner Chilcott
WC 606	Aspirin 325 mg	Warner Chilcott
WC 607	CONTROLLED - SEE PAGE 190	

Imprint	Ingredient/Brand Name	Manufacturer
WC 611	Baclofen 10 mg	Warner Chilcott
WC 612	Baclofen 20 mg	Warner Chilcott
WC 615	Minocycline 50 mg	Warner Chilcott
WC 616	Minocycline 100 mg	Warner Chilcott
WC 617	Quinidine Gluconate 324 mg	Warner Chilcott
WC 621	Loxapine 5 mg	Warner Chilcott
WC 632	Loxapine 10 mg	Warner Chilcott
WC 634/2	CONTROLLED - SEE PAGE 196	
WC 635/3	CONTROLLED - SEE PAGE 196	
WC 637/4	CONTROLLED - SEE PAGE 196	
WC 640	Acetaminophen 325 mg	Warner Chilcott
WC 648	Penicillin V Potassium 250 mg	Warner Chilcott
WC 650	Loxapine 25 mg	Warner Chilcott
WC 651	Loxapine 50 mg	Warner Chilcott
WC 657	Theophylline 100 mg	Warner Chilcott
WC 659	Thephylline 200 mg	Warner Chilcott
WC 672	Erythromycin Stearate 250 mg	Warner Chilcott
WC 673	Penicillin V Potassium 500 mg	Warner Chilcott
WC 697	Tetracycline 500 mg	Warner Chilcott
WC 698	CONTROLLED - SEE PAGE 190	
WC 699	CONTROLLED - SEE PAGE 186	
WC 700	CONTROLLED - SEE PAGE 188	
WC 702	Hydrochlorothiazide 25 mg	Warner Chilcott
WC 710	Hydrochlorothiazide 50 mg	Warner Chilcott
WC 712	Spironolactone, Hydrochlorothiazide	Warner Chilcott
WC 713	Spironolactone 25 mg	Warner Chilcott
WC 716	Trazodone 150 mg	Warner Chilcott
WC 720	Disopyramide Phosphate 150 mg	Warner Chilcott
WC 724	Timolol Maleate 20 mg	Warner Chilcott
WC 728	Timolol Maleate 10 mg	Warner Chilcott
WC 729	Timolol Maleate 5 mg	Warner Chilcott
WC 730	Amoxicillin 250 mg	Warner Chilcott
WC 731	Amoxicillin 500 mg	Warner Chilcott
WC 773	Sulindac 150 mg	Warner Chilcott
WC 774	Sulindac 200 mg	Warner Chilcott
WC 790	Maprotiline 25 mg	Warner Chilcott
WC 791	Maprotiline 50 mg	Warner Chilcott
WC 795	Maprotiline 75 mg	Warner Chilcott
WC 796	Fluphenazine 1 mg	Warner Chilcott
WC 797	Fluphenazine 2.5 mg	Warner Chilcott
WC 798	Fluphenazine 5 mg	Warner Chilcott
WC 799	Fluphenazine 10 mg	Warner Chilcott
WC 808	Cephradine 250 mg	Warner Chilcott
WC 809	Cephradine 500 mg	Warner Chilcott
WC 813	Doxycycline 100 mg	Warner Chilcott
WC 829	Doxycycline 50 mg	Warner Chilcott
WC 830	Doxycycline 100 mg	Warner Chilcott
WC 832	Amiloride 5 mg, Hydrochlorothiazide 50 mg	Warner Chilcott
WC 833	Triamterine 75 mg, Hydrochlorothiazide 50 mg	Warner Chilcott
WC 834	Triamterene 50 mg, Hydrochlorothiazide 25 mg	Warner Chilcott
WC 843	Prazosin 1mg	Warner Chilcott
WC 844	Prazosin 2 mg	Warner Chilcott
WC 845	Prazosin 5 mg	Warner Chilcott
WC 849	Quinidine Sulfate 200 mg	Warner Chilcott
WC 850	Quinidine Gluconate 330 mg	Warner Chilcott
WC 853	Amantadine 100 mg	Warner Chilcott

Imprint	Ingredient/Brand Name	Manufacturer
WC 865	Methyldopa 250 mg	Warner Chilcott
WC 866	Methyldopa 500 mg	Warner Chilcott
WC 868	Hydralazine 25 mg, Hydrochlorothiazide 25 mg	Warner Chilcott
WC 871	Hydralazine 50 mg, Hydrochlorothiazide 50 mg	Warner Chilcott
WC 874	Medroxyprogesterone 10 mg	Warner Chilcott
WC 875	Indomethacin 75 mg	Warner Chilcott
WC 878	Metoclopramide 10 mg	Warner Chilcott
WC 887	Indomethacin 25 mg	Warner Chilcott
WC 888	Indomethacin 50 mg	Warner Chilcott
WC 914	Ibuprofen 800 mg	Warner Chilcott
WC 919	Erythromycin 500 mg	Warner Chilcott
WC 922	Ibuprofen 600 mg	Warner Chilcott
WC 929	Nelova 0.5/35E	Warner Chilcott
WC 929	Nelova 10/11	Warner Chilcott
WC 930	Nelova 1/35E	Warner Chilcott
WC 930	Nelova 10/11	Warner Chilcott
WC 937	Nelova 10/11	Warner Chilcott
WC 938	Cephalexin 250 mg	Warner Chilcott
WC 939	Cephalexin 500 mg	Warner Chilcott
WC 940	R-Tannate 25 mg/8 mg/25 mg	Warner Chilcott
WC 941	Norethindrone 0.5 mg, Ethinyl Estradiol 35 mcg	Warner Chilcott
WC 942	Norethindrone 1 mg, Mestranol 50 mcg	Warner Chilcott
WC 945	Dicloxacillin 250 mg	Warner Chilcott
WC 946	Dicloxacillin 500 mg	Warner Chilcott
WC 949	Cloxacillin 250 mg	Warner Chilcott
WC 950	Cloxacillin 500 mg	Warner Chilcott
WC 951	Potassium Chloride 600 mg	Warner Chilcott
WC 956	Albuterol Sulfate 2 mg	Warner Chilcott
WC 957	Albuterol Sulfate 4 mg	Warner Chilcott
WC 966	Thioridazine 10 mg	Warner Chilcott
WC 967	Thioridazine 25 mg	Warner Chilcott
WC 968	Thioridazine 50 mg	Warner Chilcott
WC 969	Thioridazine 100 mg	Warner Chilcott
WC 970	Thiothixene 1 mg	Warner Chilcott
WC 971	Thiothixene 2 mg	Warner Chilcott
WC 972	Thiothixene 5 mg	Warner Chilcott
WC 975	Thiothixene 10 mg	Warner Chilcott
WC 977	CONTROLLED - SEE PAGE 214	
WC 978	CONTROLLED - SEE PAGE 214	
WC 981	Haloperidol 0.5 mg	Warner Chilcott
WC 982	Haloperidol 1 mg	Warner Chilcott
WC 983	Haloperidol 2 mg	Warner Chilcott
WC 984	Haloperidol 5 mg	Warner Chilcott
WC 985	Clonidine 0.1 mg, Chlorthalidone 15 mg	Warner Chilcott
WC 986	Clonidine 0.2 mg, Chlorthalidone 15 mg	Warner Chilcott
WC 987	Clonidine 0.3 mg, Chlorthalidone 15 mg	Warner Chilcott
WC 988	CONTROLLED - SEE PAGE 221	
WC 989	CONTROLLED - SEE PAGE 221	
WD 92	Ergocalciferol 1.25 mg	Winthrop
WELLBUTRIN 75	Bupropion HCl 75 mg	Burroughs
WELLBUTRIN 100	Bupropion HCl 100 mg	Burroughs
WELLCOME U3B	Thioguanine 40 mg	Burroughs
Wellcome Y9C 100	Zidovudine 100 mg	Burroughs Wellcom
Wellcome Zovirax 200	Zovirax 200 mg	Burroughs
Wellcovorin 5	Wellcovorin 5 mg	Burroughs
Wellcovorin 25	Wellcovorin 25 mg	Burroughs

Imprint	Ingredient/Brand Name	Manufacturer
West-ward 001	Acetaminophen 500 mg	West-ward Inc.
West-ward 010	Allopurinol 100 mg	West-ward Inc.
West-ward 020	Aminophylline 100 mg	West-ward Inc.
West-ward 025	Aminophylline 200 mg	West-ward Inc.
West-ward 030	Vitamins, Minerals	West-ward Inc.
West-ward 045	Amitriptyline 10 mg	West-ward Inc.
West-ward 046	Amitriptyline 25 mg	West-ward Inc.
West-ward 047	Amitriptyline 50 mg	West-ward Inc.
West-ward 048	Amitriptyline 75 mg	West-ward Inc.
West-ward 049	Amitriptyline 100 mg	West-ward inc.
West-ward 050	Amitriptyline 150 mg	West-ward Inc.
West-ward 060	Ascorbic Acid 500 mg	West-ward Inc.
West-ward 062	Aspirin 325 mg	West-ward Inc.
West-ward 063	Ampicillin 500 mg	West-ward Inc.
West-ward 070	Vitamins	West-ward Inc.
West-ward 080	Ascorbic Acid 100 mg	West-ward Inc.
West-ward 085	Ascorbic Acid 250 mg	West-ward Inc.
West-ward 087	Chlorpromazine 100 mg	West-ward Inc.
West-ward 087	Vitamins	West-ward Inc.
West-ward 090	Ascorbic Acid 500 mg	West-ward Inc.
West-ward 090	Chlorpromazine 200 mg	West-ward Inc.
West-ward 095	Aspirin 325 mg	West-ward Inc.
West-ward 107	Dipyridamole 25 mg	West-ward Inc.
West-ward 109	Dipyridamole 50 mg	West-ward Inc.
West-ward 110	CONTROLLED - SEE PAGE 217	
West-ward 111	Dipyridamole 75 mg	West-ward Inc.
West-ward 113	Chlorpheniramine 8 mg	West-ward Inc.
West-ward 114	Chlorpheniramine 12 mg	West-ward Inc.
West-ward 115	Ferrous Gluconate 325 mg	West-ward Inc.
West-ward 126	Ferrous Sulfate 325 mg	West-ward Inc.
West-ward 130	Docusate Sodium 100 mg	West-ward Inc.
West-ward 130	Ferrous Sulfate 325 mg	West-ward Inc.
West-ward 133	Docusate Sodium 250 mg	West-ward Inc.
West-ward 134	Docusate Sodium 100 mg, Casanthranol 30 mg	West-ward Inc.
West-ward 135	Docusate Sodium, Danthron	West-ward Inc.
West-ward 136	Diphenhydramine 25 mg	West-ward Inc.
West-ward 137	Diphenhydramine 50 mg	West-ward Inc.
West-ward 140	Hyoscyamine 0.1037 mg, Atropine Sulfate 0.0194 mg, Hyoscine HBr 0.0065 mg, Phenobarbital 16.2 mg	West-ward Inc.
West-ward 141	Doxycycline 50 mg	West-ward Inc.
West-ward 142	Doxycycline 100 mg	West-ward Inc.
West-ward 143	Benztropine Mesylate 1 mg	West-ward Inc.
West-ward 144	Benztropine Mesylate 2 mg	West-ward Inc.
West-ward 145	Ephedrine Sulfate 25 mg	West-ward Inc.
West-ward 147	Imipramine 25 mg	West-ward Inc.
West-ward 150	Aspirin 325 mg	West-ward Inc.
West-ward 150	Imipramine 50 mg	West-ward Inc.
West-ward 153	Methyldopa 250 mg	West-ward Inc
West-ward 155	Methyldopa 500 mg	West-ward Inc
West-ward 165	Calcium Gluconate 650 mg	West-ward Inc.
West-ward 165	Vitamins	West-ward Inc.
West-ward 166	Vitamins	West-ward Inc.
West-ward 170	Calcium Gluconate 1000 mg	West-ward Inc.
West-ward 175	Calcium Lactate 325 mg	West-ward Inc.
West-ward 175	Vitamins	West-ward Inc.
West-ward 177	Linolenic Acid	West-ward Inc.

Imprint	Ingredient/Brand Name	Manufacturer
West-ward 180	Calcium Lactate 650 mg	West-ward Inc.
West-ward 181	Carbamazepine 200 mg	West-ward Inc.
West-ward 183	Chlorpropamide 100 mg	West-ward Inc.
West-ward 185	Chlorpropamide 250 mg	West-ward Inc.
West-ward 186	Clonidine 0.1 mg	West-ward Inc.
West-ward 187	Clonidine 0.2 mg	West-ward Inc.
West-ward 195	Chloroquine 250 mg	West-ward Inc.
West-ward 200	Chlorpheniramine 4 mg	West-ward Inc.
West-ward 201	Colchicine 0.6 mg	West-ward Inc.
West-ward 202	Cortisone Acetate 25 mg	West-ward Inc.
West-ward 205	Chlorpromazine 25 mg	West-ward Inc.
West-ward 207	Chlorpromazine 50 mg	West-ward Inc.
West-ward 209	Chlorothiazide 250 mg	West-ward Inc.
West-ward 210	Chlorothiazide 500 mg	West-ward Inc.
West-ward 217	Chlorothiazide 250 mg, Reserpine 0.125 mg	West-ward Inc.
West-ward 218	Chlorothiazide 500 mg, Reserpine 0.125 mg	West-ward Inc.
West-ward 227	Prazosin 1 mg	West-ward inc.
West-ward 228	Prazosin 2 mg	West-ward Inc.
West-ward 229	Prazosin 5 mg	West-ward Inc.
West-ward 235	CONTROLLED - SEE PAGE 215	
West-ward 239	Dimenhydrinate 50 mg	West-ward Inc.
West-ward 245	Niacin 50 mg	West-ward Inc.
West-ward 247	Ergoloid Mesylates 1 mg	West-ward Inc.
West-ward 248	Folic Acid 1 mg	West-ward Inc.
West-ward 249	Furosemide 20 mg	West-ward inc.
West-ward 253	Furosemide 80 mg	West-ward inc.
West-ward 254	Hydrocortisone 20 mg	West-ward Inc.
West-ward 256	Hydrochlorothiazide 25 mg	West-ward Inc.
West-ward 257	Hydrochlorothiazide 50 mg	West-ward Inc.
West-ward 258	Isoxsuprine 10 mg	West-ward Inc.
West-ward 259	Isoxsuprine 20 mg	West-ward Inc.
West-ward 260	Vitamin C 250 mg	West-ward Inc.
West-ward 261	Isoniazid 300 mg	West-ward Inc.
West-ward 265	Reserpine 0.125 mg, Hydrochlorothiazide 50 mg	West-ward
West-ward 269	Hydralazine 25 mg	West-ward Inc.
West-ward 271	Hydralazine 50 mg	West-ward Inc.
West-ward 275	Meclizine 12.5 mg	West-ward Inc.
West-ward 276	Meclizine 25 mg	West-ward Inc.
West-ward 279	Phenylpropanolamine 40 mg, Phenylephrine 40 mg, Chlorpheniramine Maleate 5 mg, Phenyltoloxamine 15 mg	West-ward
West-ward 290	Methocarbamol 500 mg	West-ward Inc.
West-ward 292	Methocarbamol 750 mg	West-ward Inc.
West-ward 295	Tetracycline 250 mg	West-ward Inc.
West-ward 295	Vitamins, Minerals	West-ward Inc.
West-ward 296	Thioridazine 10 mg	West-ward Inc.
West-ward 297	Thioridazine 15 mg	West-ward Inc.
West-ward 298	Thioridazine 25 mg	West-ward Inc.
West-ward 299	Thioridazine 50 mg	West-ward Inc.
West-ward 300	Ibuprofen 400 mg	West-ward Inc.
West-ward 302	Thioridazine 100 mg	West-ward Inc.
West-ward 303	Thioridazine 150 mg	West-ward Inc.
West-ward 304	Thioridazine 200 mg	West-ward inc.
West-ward 307	Trifluoperazine 1 mg	West-ward inc.
West-ward 309	Trifluoperazine 2 mg	West-ward Inc.
West-ward 311	Trifluoperazine 5 mg	West-ward inc.
West-ward 313	Trifluoperazine 10 mg	West-ward inc.

Imprint	Ingredient/Brand Name	Manufacturer
West-ward 320	Hydroxyzine Pamoate 25 mg	West-ward inc.
West-ward 325	Hydroxyzine Pamoate 50 mg	West-ward Inc.
West-ward 329	Triamterene 50 mg, Hydrochlorothiazide 25 mg	West-ward Inc.
West-ward 330	Vitamin E 200 units	West-ward Inc.
West-ward 332	Vitamins	West-ward Inc.
West-ward 333	Vitamin E 500 units	West-ward Inc.
West-ward 335	Vitamin E 100 units	West-ward Inc.
West-ward 336	Acetaminophen 325 mg	West-ward Inc.
West-ward 337	Vitamin E 200 units	West-ward Inc.
West-ward 338	Vitamin E 400 units	West-ward Inc.
West-ward 339	Acetaminophen 500 mg	West-ward Inc.
West-ward 339	Vitamin E 1000 units	West-ward Inc.
West-ward 340	Niacin 25 mg	West-ward Inc.
West-ward 350	Niacin 100 mg	West-ward Inc.
West-ward 352	Niacin 500 mg	West-ward Inc.
West-ward 352	Wheat Germ Oil 20 minims	West-ward Inc.
West-ward 365	Docusate Calcium 240 mg	West-ward Inc.
West-ward 366	Nitrofurantoin 50 mg	West-ward Inc.
West-ward 445	CONTROLLED - SEE PAGE 187	
West-ward 450	CONTROLLED - SEE PAGE 188	
West-ward 473	Prednisone 10 mg	West-ward Inc.
West-ward 475	Prednisone 5 mg	West-ward Inc.
West-ward 476	Prednisone 5 mg	West-ward Inc.
West-ward 477	Prednisone 20 mg	West-ward Inc.
West-ward 480	Propylthiouracil 50 mg	West-ward Inc.
West-ward 481	Prednisone 50 mg	West-ward Inc.
West-ward 485	Pseudoephedrine 60 mg	West-ward Inc.
West-ward 502	Propranolol 10 mg	West-ward Inc.
West-ward 503	Propranolol 20 mg	West-ward Inc.
West-ward 504	Propranolol 40 mg	West-ward Inc.
West-ward 505	Propranolol 60 mg	West-ward Inc.
West-ward 506	Propranolol 80 mg	West-ward Inc.
West-ward 508	Quinidine Gluconate 324 mg	West-ward inc.
West-ward 510	Quinidine Sulfate 200 mg	West-ward Inc.
West-ward 530	Reserpine 0.1 mg	West-ward inc.
West-ward 535	Reserpine 0.25 mg	West-ward Inc.
West-ward 625	Sulfamethoxazole 800 mg, Trimethoprim 160 mg	West-ward Inc.
West-ward 680	Sulfinpyrazone 100 mg	West-ward inc.
West-ward 683	Sulfisoxazole 500 mg	West-ward Inc.
West-ward 689	Theophylline Anhydrous 200 mg	West-ward inc.
West-ward 690	Theophylline Anhydrous 300 mg	West-ward Inc.
West-ward 695	Theophylline 118.2 mg, Ephedrine 24 mg, Phenobarbital 8 mg	West-ward Inc.
West-ward 715	Thiamine 50 mg	West-ward Inc.
West-ward 720	Thiamine 100 mg	West-ward Inc.
West-ward 750	Triamterene 75 mg, Hydrochlorothiazide 50 mg	West-ward Inc.
West-ward 757	Vitamin C 500 mg	West-ward Inc.
West-ward 765	Isosorbide Dinitrate 2.5 mg	West-ward Inc.
West-ward 767	Isosorbide Dinitrate 5 mg	West-ward Inc.
West-ward 769	Isosorbide Dinitrate 5 mg	West-ward Inc.
West-ward 771	Isosorbide Dinitrate 10 mg	West-ward Inc.
West-ward 772	Isosorbide Dinitrate 20 mg	West-ward Inc.
West-ward 785	CONTROLLED - SEE PAGE 196	
West-ward 900	Triprolidine 2.5 mg, Pseudoephedrine 60 mg	West-ward Inc.
West-ward 3136	Diphenhydramine 25 mg	West-ward Inc.
West-ward 3141	Doxycycline 50 mg	West-ward Inc.

Imprint	Ingredient/Brand Name	Manufacturer
West-ward 3142	Doxycycline 100 mg	West-ward Inc.
West-ward 3145	Ephedrine Sulfate 25 mg	West-ward Inc.
West-ward Flurazepam 15	CONTROLLED - SEE PAGE 218	
West-ward Flurazepam 30	CONTROLLED - SEE PAGE 217	
WE[in box] 40 40	Caffeine	Unknown
Whitby 316	Vicon Forte	Whitby
WHR 050	Fedahist 60 mg/4 mg	Rorer Pharm
WHR 50mg	Slo-bid 50 mg	Rorer Pharm
WHR 75 mg	Theophylline 75 mg	Rorer Pharm
WHR 100	Slo-bid 100 mg	Rorer Pharm
WHR 125	Theophylline 125 mg	Rorer Pharm
WHR 137	Ascriptin 325 mg/150 mg/150 mg	Rorer Pharm
WHR 171	Gemnisyn 325 mg/325 mg	Rorer Pharm
WHR 200	Slo-bid 200 mg	Rorer Pharm
WHR/260	Fermalox 200 mg/100 mg/100 mg	Rorer Pharm
WHR 300	Slo-bid 300 mg	Rorer Pharm
WHR 351	Slo-Phyllin 100 mg	Rorer Pharm
WHR 352	Slo-Phyllin 200 mg	Rorer Pharm
WHR 1053	Fedahist 65 mg/10 mg	Rorer Pharm
WHR 1354	Slo-Phyllin 60 mg	Rorer Pharm
WHR 1355	Slo-Phyllin 125 mg	Rorer Pharm
WHR 1356	Slo-Phyllin 250 mg	Rorer Pharm
WHR 2358	Slo-Phyllin-GG 150 mg/90 mg	Rorer Pharm
Winthrop D03 50mg	Danocrine 50 mg	Winthrop
Winthrop D04 100mg	Danocrine 100 mg	Winthrop
WL STIM CAP-1	Caffeine	Unknown
WM 87	Ambenonium 10 mg	Winthrop
WM-90 60 mg	Trilostane 60 mg	Winthrop
WM 91 30 mg	Trilostane 30 mg	Winthrop
WMH	Brompheniramine, Pseudoephedrine	Unknown
WmP 9525	CONTROLLED - SEE PAGE 223	
WmP 9531	Uro-Phosphate 300 mg/500 mg	Poythress Labs
W N21	Nalidixic Acid 250 mg	Winthrop
W N22	Nalidixic Acid 500 mg	Winthrop
W N23	Nalidixic Acid 1000 mg	Winthrop
WP 61	Hydrochloroquine 200 mg	Winthrop
WP 97	Primaquine Phosphate 26.3 mg	Winthrop
WPPh/152	Methyldopa 250 mg	West Point Pharma
WPPh/153	Methyldopa 250 mg, Hydrochlorothiazide 25 mg	West Point Pharma
WPPh/154	Sulindac 200 mg	West Point Pharma
WPPh/156	Cyclobenzaprine 10 mg	West Point Pharma
WPPh 157	Indomethacin 75 mg	West Point Pharma
WPPh 159	Indomethacine 50 mg	West Point Pharma
WPPh/162	Amiloride 5 mg, Hydrochlorothiazide 50 mg	West Point Pharma
WPPH/170	Sulindac 150 mg	West Point Pharma
WPPh 172	Indomethacine 25 mg	West Point Pharma
WPPh/174	Methyldopa 125 mg	West Point Pharma
WPPh/176	Methyldopa 500 mg	West Point Pharma
WPPh/179	Methyldopa 250 mg, Hydrochlorothiazide 15 mg	West Point Pharma
WPPh/192	Timolol Maleate 5 mg	West Point Pharma
WPPh/194	Timolol Maleate 10 mg	West Point Pharma
WPPh/195	Diflunisal 250 mg	West Point Pharma
WPPh/196	Diflunisal 500 mg	West Point Pharma
WPPh/240	Chlorothiazide 250 mg	West Ponit Pharma
WPPh/241	Hydrochlorothiazide 25 mg	West Point Pharma
WPPh/243	Hydrochlorothiazide 50 mg	West Point Pharma

Imprint	Ingredient/Brand Name	Manufacturer
WPPh/245	Chlorothiazide 500 mg	West Point Pharma
WT 31	Iopanoic Acid 500 mg	Winthrop
W-T 4111	Magnesium Salicylate 500 mg	Adria
wt wt 41 11/Magan	Magan	Warren-Teed
WW[in box]	Caffeine, Ephedrine, Phenylpropanolamine	Unknown
WW 3145	Ephedrine 25 mg	H.L. Moore
Wyeth-6 SERAX 15	CONTROLLED - SEE PAGE 221	
WYETH/10	Isordil 10 mg	Wyeth Labs
WYETH 13	Amphojel 600 mg	Wyeth Labs
WYETH 19	Phenergan 12.5 mg	Wyeth Labs
WYETH 27	Phenergan 25 mg	Wyeth Labs
WYETH 28	Sparine 50 mg	Wyeth Labs
WYETH 29	Sparine 25 mg	Wyeth Labs
Wyeth-51 SERAX 10	CONTROLLED - SEE PAGE 222	
Wyeth-52 SERAX 30	CONTROLLED - SEE PAGE 222	
WYETH 53	Omnipen 250 mg	Wyeth Labs
WYETH 56	Ovral 0.5 mg	Wyeth Labs
WYETH 57	Unipen 250 mg	Wyeth Labs
WYETH 58	Pen-Vee K 125 mg	Wyeth Labs
WYETH 59	Pen-Vee K 250 mg	Wyeth Labs
WYETH 62	Ovrette 0.075 mg	Wyeth Labs
WYETH 75	Nordette 0.15 mg/0.03 mg	Wyeth Labs
WYETH 78	LO/Ovral 0.3 mg/0.03 mg	Wyeth Labs
WYETH 81/A	CONTROLLED - SEE PAGE 189	
WYETH/85	CONTROLLED - SEE PAGE 212	
WYETH 91	CONTROLLED - SEE PAGE 206	
WYETH 119	Amphojel 300 mg	Wyeth Labs
WYETH 165	Bicillin 125 mg	Wyeth Labs
WYETH 200	Sparine 100 mg	Wyeth Labs
WYETH 202	Sparine 10 mg	Wyeth Labs
WYETH 227	Phenergan 50 mg	Wyeth Labs
WYETH 261	CONTROLLED - SEE PAGE 216	
WYETH 272	Penicillin G 250 mg	Wyeth Labs
WYETH 309	Omnipen 500 mg	Wyeth Labs
WYETH 313	Aspirin 300 mg	Wyeth Labs
WYETH 317/S 15	CONTROLLED - SEE PAGE 206	
WYETH 360	Pathocil 250 mg	Wyeth Labs
WYETH 389	Tetracycline 250 mg	Wyeth Labs
WYETH 390	Pen-Vee K 500 mg	Wyeth Labs
WYETH 434	Phenergan-D 6.25 mg/60 mg	Wyeth Labs
WYETH 445	Ovral	Wyeth Labs
WYETH 464	Unipen 500 mg	Wyeth Labs
WYETH 471	Tetracycline 500 mg	Wyeth Labs
WYETH 472	Basaljel	Wyeth Labs
WYETH 473	Basaljel	Wyeth Labs
WYETH 486	Nordette	Wyeth Labs
WYETH 559	Wymox 250 mg	Wyeth Labs
WYETH 560	Wymox 500 mg	Wyeth Labs
WYETH 576	Wyamycin S 250 mg	Wyeth Labs
WYETH 578	Wyamycin S 500 mg	Wyeth Labs
WYETH 593	Pathocil 500 mg	Wyeth Labs
WYETH 614	Cyclacillin 250 mg	Wyeth Labs
WYETH 615	Cyclacillin 500 mg	Wyeth Labs
WYETH 641	Triphasil 0.05 mg/0.03 mg	Wyeth Labs
WYETH 642	Triphasil 0.075 mg/0.04 mg	Wyeth Labs
WYETH 643	Triphasil 0.125 mg/0.03 mg	Wyeth Labs

Imprint	Ingredient/Brand Name	Manufacturer
WYETH 650	Triphasil	Wyeth Labs
WYETH 4124	Cyclospasmol 200 mg	Wyeth Labs
WYETH 4125	Isosorbide Dinitrate 40 mg	Wyeth Labs
WYETH 4130	Ethionamide 250 mg	Wyeth Labs
WYETH 4132	Surmontil 25 mg	Wyeth Labs
WYETH 4133	Surmontil 50 mg	Wyeth Labs
WYETH 4140	Isordil 40 mg	Wyeth Labs
WYETH 4148	Cyclospasmol 400 mg	Wyeth Labs
WYETH/4152	Isordil 40 mg	Wyeth Labs
WYETH 4152	Isordil 5 mg	Wyeth Labs
WYETH 4153	Isordil 10 mg	Wyeth Labs
WYETH 4154	Isordil 20 mg	Wyeth Labs
WYETH 4158	Surmontil 100 mg	Wyeth Labs
WYETH 4159	Isordil 30 mg	Wyeth Labs
WYETH 4177 SECTRAL 200	Sectral 200 mg	Wyeth Labs
WYETH 4179 SECTRAL 400	Sectral 400 mg	Wyeth Labs
WYETH 4181 ORUDIS 50	Orudis 50 mg	Wyeth Labs
WYETH 4187 ORUDIS 75	Orudis 75 mg	Wyeth Labs
WYETH 4188	Cordarone 200 mg	Wyeth Labs
WYETH 4191	CONTROLLED - SEE PAGE 219	
WYETH 4192	Isordil 40 mg	Wyeth Labs
W[in box] B 34	Bilopaque 750 mg	Winthrop-Breon
W[in box] M- 90	Modrastane 60 mg	Winthrop-Breon
W[in box] M- 91	Modrastane 30 mg	Winthrop-Breon
X/2	Theophylline 60 mg, Ephedrine 12.5 mg, Gauifenesin 100 mg	Whitehall
X 7300	Verapamil HCl 240 mg	Baker
XANAX 0.25	CONTROLLED - SEE PAGE 199	
XANAX 0.5	CONTROLLED - SEE PAGE 203	
XANAX 1.0	CONTROLLED - SEE PAGE 211	
XANAX/2	CONTROLLED - SEE PAGE 199	
YC	Thyrdar 15 mg	Forest
YD	Thyrdar 30 mg	Forest
YE	Thyrdar 60 mg	Forest
YF	Thyrdar 120 mg	Forest
YH	Thyrdar 180 mg	Forest
YODOXIN 92	Yodoxin 210 mg	Glenwood Inc
YODOXIN 93	Yodoxin 650 mg	Glenwood Inc
YUTOPAR	Yutopar 10 mg	Astra Pharm
Z 1	Trifluoperazine 1 mg	Zenith Labs
Z-1	Trifluoperazine 1 mg	Zenith Labs
Z 2	Trifluoperazine 2 mg	Zenith Labs
Z-2	Trifluoperazine 2 mg	Zenith Labs
Z-5	Trifluoperazine 5 mg	Zenith Labs
Z 5	Trifluoperazine 5 mg	Zenith Labs
Z 10	Trifluoperazine 10 mg	Zenith Labs
Z-10	Trifluoperazine 10 mg	Zenith Labs
Z 50/2130	Nitrofurantoin 50 mg	Zenith Labs
Z 2042	Estrogen 0.625 mg	Zenith Labs
Z 2045	Estrogen 1.25 mg	Zenith Labs
Z 2047	Colchicine 0.6 mg	Zenith Labs
Z 2052	Chlorpromazine 25 mg	Zenith Labs
Z 2053	Chlorpromazine 50 mg	Zenith Labs
Z 2055	Diphenhydramine 25 mg	Zenith Labs
Z 2056	Diphenhydramine 50 mg	Zenith Labs
Z 2057	Phenytoin 100 mg	Zenith Labs
Z 2058	Digoxin 0.25 mg	Zenith Labs

Imprint	Ingredient/Brand Name	Manufacturer
Z 2083	Hydrochlorothiazide 25 mg	Zenith Labs
Z 2089	Hydrochlorothiazide 50 mg	Zenith Labs
Z 2150	Isosorbide Dinitrate 5 mg	Zenith Labs
Z 2151	Isosorbide Dinitrate 10 mg	Zenith Labs
Z 2160	Estrogen 2.5 mg	Zenith Labs
Z 2161	Chlorpromazine 10 mg	Zenith Labs
Z 2168	Hydrochlorothiazide 50 mg, Reserpine 0.125 mg	Zenith Labs
Z 2169	Hydrochlorothiazide 25 mg, Reserpine 0.125 mg	Zenith Labs
Z 2173	Propylthiouracil 50 mg	Zenith Labs
Z 2180	Papaverine 150 mg	Zenih Labs
Z 2184	Quinine Sulfate 325 mg	Zenith Labs
Z 2186	CONTROLLED - SEE PAGE 215	
Z 2190	Probenecid 500 mg	Zenith Labs
Z 2191	Chlorpromazine 100 mg	Zenith Labs
Z 2192	Chlorpromazine 200 mg	Zenith Labs
Z 2193	Probenecid 500 mg, Colchicine 0.5 mg	Zenith Labs
Z 2198	Reserpine 0.1 mg	Zenith Labs
Z 2199	Reserpine 0.25 mg	Zenith Labs
Z 2201	Quinidine Sulfate 200 mg	Zenith Labs
Z 2205	Hydrochlorothiazide 50 mg	Zenith Labs
Z 2218	Sulfisoxazole 500 mg	Zenith Labs
Z 2245	Tolbutamide 500 mg	Zenith Labs
Z 2335	Reserpine 0.1 mg, Hydralazine 25 mg, Hydrochlorothiazide 15 mg	Zenith Labs
Z 2338	Hydralazine 10 mg	Zenith Labs
Z 2339	Hydralazine 25 mg	Zenith Labs
Z 2342	Isosorbide Dinitrate 2.5 mg	Zenith Labs
Z 2343	Isosorbide Dinitrate 5 mg	Zenith Labs
Z 2345	Procainamide 250 mg	Zenith Labs
Z 2346	Procainamide 375 mg	Zenith Labs
Z 2347	Procainamide 500 mg	Zenith Labs
Z 2348	Nylidrin 6 mg	Zenith Labs
Z 2349	Nylidrin 12 mg	Zenith Labs
Z 2350	Meclizine 25 mg	Zenith Labs
Z 2359	Quinine Sulfate 200 mg	Zenith Labs
Z 2364	Methocarbamol 500 mg	Zenith Labs
Z 2365	Methocarbamol 750 mg	Zenith Labs
Z 2384	Meclizine 12.5 mg	Zenith Labs
Z 2387	Isoxsuprine 10 mg	Zenith Labs
Z 2388	Isoxsuprine 20 mg	Zenith Labs
Z 2407	Tetracycline 500 mg	Zenith Labs
Z 2416	Tetracycline 250 mg	Zenith Labs
Z 2430	Tetracycline 250 mg	Zenith Labs
Z 2458	Erythromycin 250 mg	Zenith Labs
Z 2484	Triprolidine 2.5 mg, Pseudoephedrine 60 mg	Zenith Labs
Z 2485	Hydrochlorothiazide 100 mg	Zenith Labs
Z 2493	Hydralazine 50 mg	Zenith Labs
Z 2507	Reserpine 0.125 mg, Hydroflumethiazide 50 mg	Zenith Labs
Z 2731	Trimate 400 mg	Zenith Labs
Z 2812	Chlorozoxazone 250 mg, Acetaminphen 300 mg	Zenith Labs
Z 2813	Methocarbamol 400 mg, Aspirin 325 mg	Zenith Labs
Z 2814	Cyclandelate 200 mg	Zenith Labs
Z 2815	Cyclandelate 400 mg	Zenith Labs
Z 2819	Spironolactone 25 mg, Hydrochlorothiazide 25 mg	Zenith Labs
Z 2823	Erythromycin 500 mg	Zenith Labs
Z 2902	Chlorpropamide 250 mg	Zenith Labs

Imprint	Ingredient/Brand Name	Manufacturer
Z 2903	Spironolactone 25 mg	Zenith Labs
Z 2904	Chlorthalidone 100 mg	Zenith Labs
Z 2907	Furosemide 40 mg	Zenith Labs
Z 2908	Furosemide 20 mg	Zenith Labs
Z 2909	Hydroxyzine Pamoate 50 mg	Zenith Labs
Z 2911	Hydroxyzine Pamoate 25 mg	Zenith Labs
Z 2916	Trifluoperazine 1 mg	Zenith Labs
Z 2918	Hydroxyzine 10 mg	Zenith Labs
Z 2919	Hydroxyzine 25 mg	Zenith Labs
Z 2920	Hydroxyzine 50 mg	Zenith Labs
Z 2929	Cyproheptadine 4 mg	Zenith Labs
Z 2931	Methyldopa 250 mg	Zenith Labs
Z 2932	Methyldopa 500 mg	Zenith Labs
Z 2936	Perphenazine 2 mg, Amitriptyline 10 mg	Zenith Labs
Z 2937	Perphenazine 2 mg, Amitriptyline 25 mg	Zenith Labs
Z 2938	Perphenazine 4 mg, Amitriptyline 10 mg	Zenith Labs
Z 2939	Perphenazine 4 mg, Amitriptyline 25 mg	Zenith Labs
Z 2940	Trifluoperazine 2 mg	Zenith Labs
Z 2941	Trifluoperazine 5 mg	Zenith Labs
Z 2942	Trifluoperazine 10 mg	Zenith Labs
Z 2951	Chlorthalidone 50 mg	Zenith Labs
Z 2958	Ergoloid Mesylates 0.5 mg	Zenith Labs
Z 2959	Ergoloid Mesylates 1 mg	Zenith Labs
Z 2960	Chloramphenicol 250 mg	Zenith Labs
Z 2962	Ephedrine, Theophyllne	Zenith Labs
Z 2963	Nitroglycerin 2.5 mg	Zenith Labs
Z 2964	Nitroglycerin 6.5 mg	Zenith Labs
Z 2969	Sulfinpyrazone 200 mg	Zenith Labs
Z 2970	Sulfinpyrazone 100 mg	Zenith Labs
Z 2971	Metronidazole 250 mg	Zenith Labs
Z 2974	Chlorthalidone 25 mg	Zenith Labs
Z 2976	Dipyridamole 50 mg	Zenith Labs
Z 2977	Dipyridamole 75 mg	Zenith Labs
Z 2978	Tolazamide 100 mg	Zenith Labs
Z 2979	Tolazamide 250 mg	Zenith Labs
Z 2980	Tolazamide 500 mg	Zenith Labs
Z 2982	Chlordiazepoxide 5 mg, Clindinium 2.5 mg	Zenith Labs
Z 2984	Doxycycline Hyclate 50 mg	Zenith Labs
Z 2985	Doxycycline Hyclate 100 mg	Zenith Labs
Z 2986	Methyclothiazide 2.5 mg	Zenith Labs
Z 2987	Methyclothiazide 5 mg	Zenith Labs
Z 2992	Dexbrompheniramine 6 mg, Pseudoephedrine 120 mg	Zenith Labs
Z 2994	Dipyridamole 25 mg	Zenith Labs
Z 2999	Chlorthalidone 50 mg	Zenith Labs
Z 3001	Quinine Sulfate 260 mg	Zenith Labs
Z 3007	Metronidazole 500 mg	Zenith Labs
Z 3606	Thioridazine 10 mg	Zenith Labs
Z 3607	Thioridazine 15 mg	Zenith Labs
Z 3608	Thioridazine 25 mg	Zenith Labs
Z 3609	Thioridazine 50 mg	Zenith Labs
Z 3610	Thioridazine 100 mg	Zenith Labs
Z 3614	Propranolol 10 mg	Zenith Labs
Z 3615	Propranolol 20 mg	Zenith Labs
Z 3616	Propranolol 40 mg	Zenith Labs
Z 3617	Propranolol 80 mg	Zenith Labs
Z 3620	Chlorthalidone 25 mg	Zenith Labs

Imprint	Ingredient/Brand Name	Manufacturer
Z 3626	Doxycycline Hyclate 100 mg	Zenith Labs
Z 3632	Hydrochlorothiazide 50 mg, Hydralazine 50 mg	Zenith Labs
Z 3633	Hydrochlorothiazide 25 mg, Hydralazine 25 mg	Zenith Labs
Z 3636	Estrogen 0.3 mg	Zenith Labs
Z 3638	Propranolol 60 mg	Zenith Labs
Z 3643	Nitroglycerin 9 mg	Zenith Labs
Z 3657	Chlorpropamide 100 mg	Zenith Labs
Z 3667 2	Perphenazine 2 mg	Zenith Labs
Z 3668 4	Perphenazine 4 mg	Zenith Labs
Z 3669 8	Perphenazine 8 mg	Zenith Labs
Z 3670	Perphenazine 16 mg	Zenith Labs
Z 3671	Perphenazine 4 mg, Amitriptyline 50 mg	Zenith Labs
Z 3925/2	CONTROLLED - SEE PAGE 190	
Z 3926/5	CONTROLLED - SEE PAGE 205	
Z 3927/10	CONTROLLED - SEE PAGE 209	
Z 3981	CONTROLLED - SEE PAGE 200	
Z 3984/3	CONTROLLED - SEE PAGE 198	
Z 3985/4	CONTROLLED - SEE PAGE 198	
Z 4029	Indomethacin 25 mg	Zenith Labs
Z 4030	Indomethacin 50 mg	Zenith Labs
Z 4038	Phenylbutazone 100 mg	Zenith Labs
Z 4040	Chlorpropamide 100 mg	Zenith Labs
Z 4041	Chlorpropamide 250 mg	Zenith Labs
Z 4051	Disopyramide 100 mg	Zenith Labs
Z 4052	Disopyramide 150 mg	Zenith Labs
Z 4058	Cefadroxil 500 mg	Zenith Labs
Z 4059	Cefadroxil 1000 mg	Zenith Labs
Z 4063	Cephradine 250 mg	Zenith Labs
Z 4064	Cephradine 500 mg	Zenith Labs
Z 4067	Prazosin 1 mg	Zenith Labs
Z 4068	Prazosin 2 mg	Zenith Labs
Z 4069/10	Baclofen 10 mg	Zenith Labs
Z 4073	Cephalexin 250 mg	Zenith Labs
Z 4074	Cephalexin 500 mg	Zenith Labs
Z 4096/10	Baclofen 10 mg	Zenith Labs
Z 4097/20	Baclofen 20 mg	Zenith Labs
Z 4141	Fenoprofen 600 mg	Zenith Labs
Z 4217	Pindolol 5 mg	Zenith Labs
Z 4218	Pindolol 10 mg	Zenith Labs
Z 4229	Triamterene 50 mg, Hydrochlorothiazide 25 mg	Zenith Labs
Z 4280/SR240	Veraoamil SR 240 mg	Zenith Labs
Z 4286/SR180	Verapamil SR 180 mg	Zenith Labs
Z 4760	Cefaclor 250 mg	Zenith Labs
Z 4761	Cefaclor 500 mg	Zenith Labs
Z 4804	CONTROLLED - SEE PAGE 218	
Z 4805	CONTROLLED - SEE PAGE 213	
Z 4806	CONTROLLED - SEE PAGE 221	
Z 4811	CONTROLLED - SEE PAGE 222	
Z 6100	Hydroxyzine 10 mg	Zenith Labs
Z 6200	Hydroxyzine 25 mg	Zenith Labs
Z 6300	Hydroxyzine 50 mg	Zenith Labs
ZANTRYL	CONTROLLED - SEE PAGE 218	
ZAROXOLYN/2 1/2	Zaroxolyn 2.5 mg	Pennwalt Corp
ZAROXOLYN/5	Zaroxolyn 5 mg	Pennwalt Corp
ZAROXOLYN/10	Zaroxolyn 10 mg	Pennwalt Corp
ZEE/A/A	Acetaminophen 325 mg	Zee Medical

Imprint	Ingredient/Brand Name	Manufacturer
ZEE/C/A	Pseudoephedrine 30 mg	Zee Medical
ZEE/D/T	Acetaminophen 325 mg, Phenylpropanolamine	Zee Medical
ZEE/H/F	Aceta 325 mg, Pseudoephedrine 30 mg, Dextromethorphan 10 mg	Zee
ZEE/ P A	Aspirin, Phenacetin, Caffeine, Acetaminophen,	Zee Medical
ZEE/P/C	Aspirin 226.8 mg, Acetaminophen 194.4 mg, Caffeine 32.4 mg	Zee Med
ZEE/S/N	Sodium Chloride 220 mg, Potassium Chloride 15 mg	Zee Medical
ZEE/T/B	Aspirin 325 mg	Zee Medical
ZEE/T/L	Calcium Carbonate 420 mg	Zee Medical
ZEE/X/U	Acetaminophen 500 mg	Zee Medical
ZENITH 2130	Nitrofurantoin Macrocrystals 50 mg	Zenith Labs
ZENITH 2131	Nitrofurantoin Macrocrystals 50 mg	Zenith Labs
ZOVIRAX 200	Zovirax 200 mg	Burroughs Wellcome
ZYLOPRIM 100	Zyloprim 100 mg	Burroughs Wellcome
ZYLOPRIM 300	Zyloprim 300 mg	Burroughs Wellcome

HOW TO USE THE CONTROLLED PRESCRIPTION DRUG SECTION

All of the prescription drugs pictured in this section (pages 184 thru 228) are controlled by the Controlled Substances Act (CSA). To identify a suspected controlled prescription drug, note the imprint on each side of the tablet or capsule. Locate matching imprints in the product marking section (pages 6 thru 181). For tablets which have an imprint on both sides, each side is separated by a slash (/). For instance, if a tablet has "071" on one side and "300" on the other side, the imprint would be represented as "071/300" or "300/071".

If the drug is controlled, the page number on which the tablet or capsule is pictured is included in the imprint listing. Locate a pictured tablet or capsule of approximately the same size, shape and color on that page. When making a comparison, keep in mind that there may be slight color variations between the drug and the photograph due to photography and printing processes. Once the suspected drug has been matched to a picture of the same size, shape and color, the imprint should be compared to those listed for the pictured item. (NOTE: Photos are not available on a limited number of controlled drugs, and this is noted in the imprint listing, if applicable.)

Key to Controlled Prescription Drug Section

❶ C-I C-II C-III C-IV C-V The CSA control status, or schedule of the drug. The relative potential for abuse of the drug is reflected by the schedule; Schedule I drugs having the highest potential, and Schedule V drugs having the lowest. Schedule I drugs have no accepted medical use, and therefore, all controlled prescription drugs fall into Schedules II, III, IV or V. Refer to the section on the *Controlled Substances Act* (pages 2 thru 5) for further information on drug scheduling.

Key to Controlled Prescription Drug Section

❷ **Imprint:** The imprint or product mark(s) appearing on the photographed side of the tablet.

❸ **Reverse side:** The imprint or product mark(s) which appears on the side of the tablet not photographed.

❹ **Brand**: The brand name of the drug, if any. If no brand name is given, the drug is generic.

❺ **Active ingredients:** The active ingredient(s) of the drug and the strength.

❻ **Use:** The page number which contains information on the drug, including an overview, normal use, pharmacology, adverse reactions, overdose, and abuse and dependence. This section is for informational purposes only, and by no means should the information provided be used for medical treatment or emergencies.

❼ **Mfr:** The manufacturer or marketer of the drug.

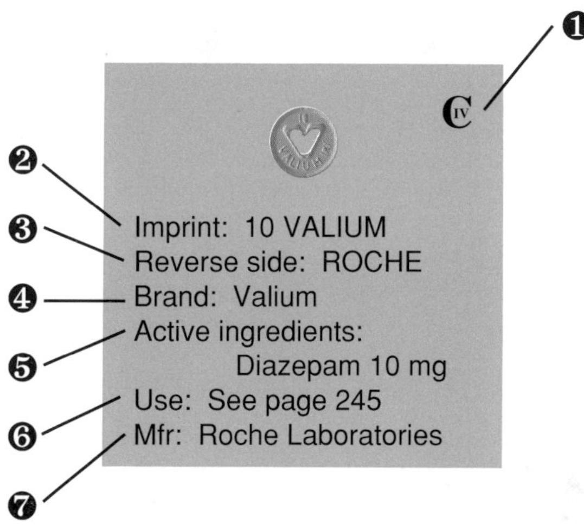

C-IV

Imprint: MP 6
Reverse side: None
Brand: Generic
Active ingredients:
Lorazepam 0.5 mg
Use: See page 262
Mfr: Mutual Pharmaceutical

C-II

Imprint: None
Reverse side: None
Brand: Generic
Active ingredients:
Morphine Sulfate 10 mg
Use: See page 273
Mfr: Eli Lilly and Company

C-II

Imprint: None
Reverse side: None
Brand: Generic
Active ingredients:
Morphine Sulfate 15 mg
Use: See page 273
Mfr: Eli Lilly and Company

C-II

Imprint: None
Reverse side: None
Brand: Generic
Active ingredients:
Morphine Sulfate 30 mg
Use: See page 273
Mfr: Eli Lilly and Company

C-II

Imprint: None
Reverse side: None
Brand: Generic
Active ingredients:
Codeine Phosphate 30 mg
Use: See page 242
Mfr: Eli Lilly and Company

C-IV

Imprint: QPL 156
Reverse side: 0.5
Brand: Loraz
Active ingredients:
Lorazepam 0.5 mg
Use: See page 262
Mfr: Quantum Pharmaceutical

C-IV

Imprint: 59
Reverse side: R
Brand: Generic
Active ingredients:
Lorazepam 0.5 mg
Use: See page 262
Mfr: Rugby Laboratories

C-II

Imprint: None
Reverse side: None
Brand: Generic
Active ingredients:
Codeine Phosphate 60 mg
Use: See page 242
Mfr: Eli Lilly and Company

C-II

Imprint: None
Reverse side: None
Brand: Cocaine HCl Solvet
Active ingredients:
Cocaine HCl 135 mg
Use: See page 241
Mfr: Eli Lilly and Company

C-IV

Imprint: 431
Reverse side: WC
Brand: Generic
Active ingredients:
Lorazepam 0.5 mg
Use: See page 262
Mfr: Warner Chilcott Laboratories

C-IV

Imprint: DAN 5625
Reverse side: 0.5
Brand: Generic
Active ingredients:
Lorazepam 0.5 mg
Use: See page 262
Mfr: Danbury Pharmacal

C-IV

Imprint: 332 0.5
Reverse side: WATSON
Brand: Generic
Active ingredients:
Lorazepam 0.5 mg
Use: See page 262
Mfr: Watson Laboratories

C-IV

Imprint: 57
Reverse side: R
Brand: Generic
Active ingredients:
Lorazepam 0.5 mg
Use: See page 262
Mfr: Purepac Pharmaceutical

C-IV

Imprint: par 206
Reverse side: None
Brand: Generic
Active ingredients:
Lorazepam 0.5 mg
Use: See page 262
Mfr: Par Pharmaceuticals

C-IV

Imprint: 371
Reverse side: b
Brand: Generic
Active ingredients:
Lorazepam 1 mg
Use: See page 262
Mfr: Barr Laboratories

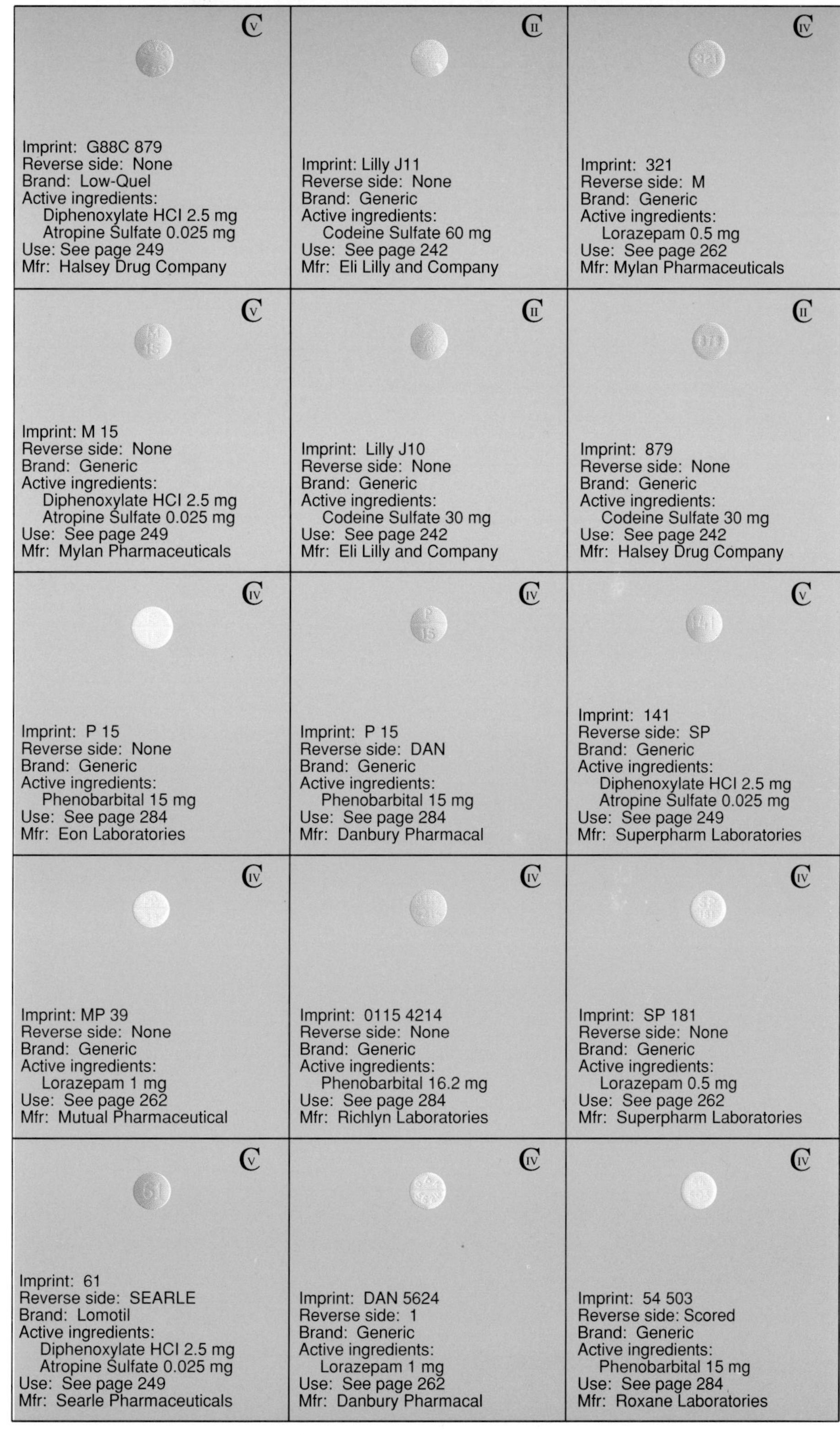

C-V

Imprint: G88C 879
Reverse side: None
Brand: Low-Quel
Active ingredients:
Diphenoxylate HCl 2.5 mg
Atropine Sulfate 0.025 mg
Use: See page 249
Mfr: Halsey Drug Company

C-II

Imprint: Lilly J11
Reverse side: None
Brand: Generic
Active ingredients:
Codeine Sulfate 60 mg
Use: See page 242
Mfr: Eli Lilly and Company

C-IV

Imprint: 321
Reverse side: M
Brand: Generic
Active ingredients:
Lorazepam 0.5 mg
Use: See page 262
Mfr: Mylan Pharmaceuticals

C-V

Imprint: M 15
Reverse side: None
Brand: Generic
Active ingredients:
Diphenoxylate HCl 2.5 mg
Atropine Sulfate 0.025 mg
Use: See page 249
Mfr: Mylan Pharmaceuticals

C-II

Imprint: Lilly J10
Reverse side: None
Brand: Generic
Active ingredients:
Codeine Sulfate 30 mg
Use: See page 242
Mfr: Eli Lilly and Company

C-II

Imprint: 879
Reverse side: None
Brand: Generic
Active ingredients:
Codeine Sulfate 30 mg
Use: See page 242
Mfr: Halsey Drug Company

C-IV

Imprint: P 15
Reverse side: None
Brand: Generic
Active ingredients:
Phenobarbital 15 mg
Use: See page 284
Mfr: Eon Laboratories

C-IV

Imprint: P 15
Reverse side: DAN
Brand: Generic
Active ingredients:
Phenobarbital 15 mg
Use: See page 284
Mfr: Danbury Pharmacal

C-V

Imprint: 141
Reverse side: SP
Brand: Generic
Active ingredients:
Diphenoxylate HCl 2.5 mg
Atropine Sulfate 0.025 mg
Use: See page 249
Mfr: Superpharm Laboratories

C-IV

Imprint: MP 39
Reverse side: None
Brand: Generic
Active ingredients:
Lorazepam 1 mg
Use: See page 262
Mfr: Mutual Pharmaceutical

C-IV

Imprint: 0115 4214
Reverse side: None
Brand: Generic
Active ingredients:
Phenobarbital 16.2 mg
Use: See page 284
Mfr: Richlyn Laboratories

C-IV

Imprint: SP 181
Reverse side: None
Brand: Generic
Active ingredients:
Lorazepam 0.5 mg
Use: See page 262
Mfr: Superpharm Laboratories

C-V

Imprint: 61
Reverse side: SEARLE
Brand: Lomotil
Active ingredients:
Diphenoxylate HCl 2.5 mg
Atropine Sulfate 0.025 mg
Use: See page 249
Mfr: Searle Pharmaceuticals

C-IV

Imprint: DAN 5624
Reverse side: 1
Brand: Generic
Active ingredients:
Lorazepam 1 mg
Use: See page 262
Mfr: Danbury Pharmacal

C-IV

Imprint: 54 503
Reverse side: Scored
Brand: Generic
Active ingredients:
Phenobarbital 15 mg
Use: See page 284
Mfr: Roxane Laboratories

C IV Imprint: 59 Reverse side: R Brand: Generic Active ingredients: Lorazepam 1 mg Use: See page 262 Mfr: Purepac Pharmaceutical	C IV Imprint: 026 Reverse side: R Brand: Generic Active ingredients: Phenobarbital 15 mg Use: See page 284 Mfr: Purepac Pharmaceutical	C IV Imprint: WC 699 Reverse side: None Brand: Generic Active ingredients: Phenobarbital 15 mg Use: See page 284 Mfr: Warner Chilcott Laboratories
C IV Imprint: 91 Reverse side: GG Brand: Generic Active ingredients: Lorazepam 0.5 mg Use: See page 262 Mfr: Geneva Pharmaceuticals	C V Imprint: GG 4 Reverse side: None Brand: Lonox Active ingredients: Diphenoxylate HCl 2.5 mg Atropine Sulfate 0.025 mg Use: See page 249 Mfr: Geneva Pharmaceuticals	C II Imprint: TC Reverse side: a Brand: Desoxyn Active ingredients: Methamphetamine HCl 2.5 mg Use: See page 269 Mfr: Abbott Laboratories
C IV Imprint: HD 565 Reverse side: 0.5 Brand: Generic Active ingredients: Lorazepam 0.5 mg Use: See page 262 Mfr: Halsey Drug Company	C V Imprint: G88C 879 Reverse side: None Brand: Low-Quel Active ingredients: Diphenoxylate HCl 2.5 mg Atropine Sulfate 0.025 mg Use: See page 249 Mfr: Halsey Drug Company	C IV Imprint: 028 Reverse side: R Brand: Generic Active ingredients: Phenobarbital 30 mg Use: See page 284 Mfr: Purepac Pharmaceutical
C IV Imprint: 832 G532C Reverse side: None Brand: Generic Active ingredients: Phenobarbital 30 mg Use: See page 284 Mfr: Pharmaceutical Basics	C IV Imprint: 71 Reverse side: WYETH Brand: Mazanor Active ingredients: Mazindol 1 mg Use: See page 263 Mfr: Wyeth-Ayerst Laboratories	C II Imprint: LEVO-DROMORAN Reverse side: ROCHE Brand: Levo-Dromoran Active ingredients: Levorphanol Tartrate 2 mg Use: See page 261 Mfr: Roche Laboratories
C IV Imprint: 0115 4233 Reverse side: Scored Brand: Generic Active ingredients: Phenobarbital 32.4 mg Use: See page 284 Mfr: Richlyn Laboratories	C IV Imprint: P 30 Reverse side: None Brand: Generic Active ingredients: Phenobarbital 30 mg Use: See page 284 Mfr: Eon Laboratories	C IV Imprint: P 30 Reverse side: DAN Brand: Generic Active ingredients: Phenobarbital 30 mg Use: See page 284 Mfr: Danbury Pharmacal

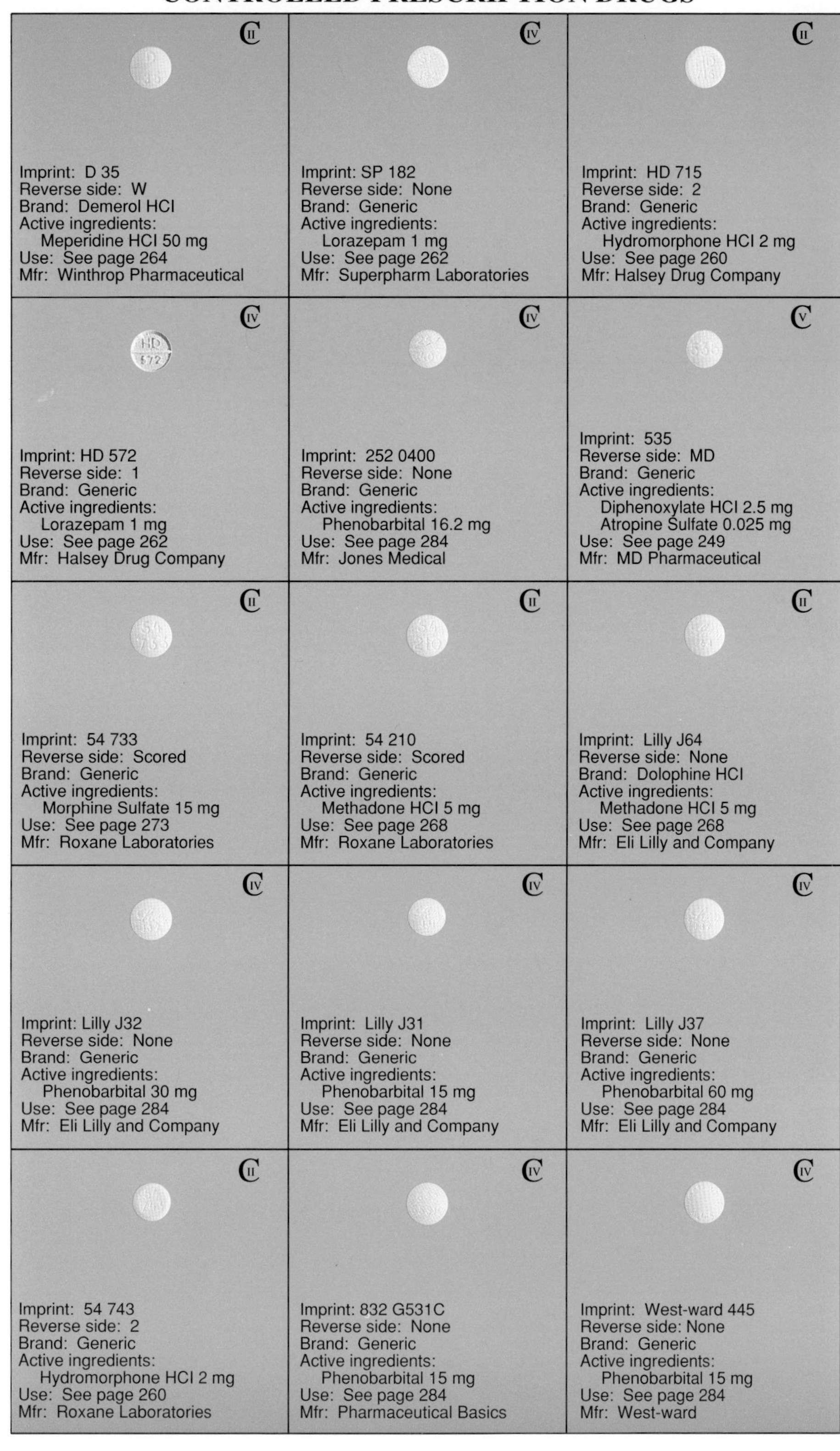

Imprint: D 35
Reverse side: W
Brand: Demerol HCl
Active ingredients:
Meperidine HCl 50 mg
Use: See page 264
Mfr: Winthrop Pharmaceutical

Imprint: SP 182
Reverse side: None
Brand: Generic
Active ingredients:
Lorazepam 1 mg
Use: See page 262
Mfr: Superpharm Laboratories

Imprint: HD 715
Reverse side: 2
Brand: Generic
Active ingredients:
Hydromorphone HCl 2 mg
Use: See page 260
Mfr: Halsey Drug Company

Imprint: HD 572
Reverse side: 1
Brand: Generic
Active ingredients:
Lorazepam 1 mg
Use: See page 262
Mfr: Halsey Drug Company

Imprint: 252 0400
Reverse side: None
Brand: Generic
Active ingredients:
Phenobarbital 16.2 mg
Use: See page 284
Mfr: Jones Medical

Imprint: 535
Reverse side: MD
Brand: Generic
Active ingredients:
Diphenoxylate HCl 2.5 mg
Atropine Sulfate 0.025 mg
Use: See page 249
Mfr: MD Pharmaceutical

Imprint: 54 733
Reverse side: Scored
Brand: Generic
Active ingredients:
Morphine Sulfate 15 mg
Use: See page 273
Mfr: Roxane Laboratories

Imprint: 54 210
Reverse side: Scored
Brand: Generic
Active ingredients:
Methadone HCl 5 mg
Use: See page 268
Mfr: Roxane Laboratories

Imprint: Lilly J64
Reverse side: None
Brand: Dolophine HCl
Active ingredients:
Methadone HCl 5 mg
Use: See page 268
Mfr: Eli Lilly and Company

Imprint: Lilly J32
Reverse side: None
Brand: Generic
Active ingredients:
Phenobarbital 30 mg
Use: See page 284
Mfr: Eli Lilly and Company

Imprint: Lilly J31
Reverse side: None
Brand: Generic
Active ingredients:
Phenobarbital 15 mg
Use: See page 284
Mfr: Eli Lilly and Company

Imprint: Lilly J37
Reverse side: None
Brand: Generic
Active ingredients:
Phenobarbital 60 mg
Use: See page 284
Mfr: Eli Lilly and Company

Imprint: 54 743
Reverse side: 2
Brand: Generic
Active ingredients:
Hydromorphone HCl 2 mg
Use: See page 260
Mfr: Roxane Laboratories

Imprint: 832 G531C
Reverse side: None
Brand: Generic
Active ingredients:
Phenobarbital 15 mg
Use: See page 284
Mfr: Pharmaceutical Basics

Imprint: West-ward 445
Reverse side: None
Brand: Generic
Active ingredients:
Phenobarbital 15 mg
Use: See page 284
Mfr: West-ward

C-IV Imprint: 333 1.0 Reverse side: WATSON Brand: Generic Active ingredients: Lorazepam 1 mg Use: See page 262 Mfr: Watson Laboratories	C-II Imprint: 54 783 Reverse side: Scored Brand: Generic Active ingredients: Codeine Sulfate 30 mg Use: See page 242 Mfr: Roxane Laboratories	C-II Imprint: 54 582 Reverse side: Scored Brand: Roxicodone Active ingredients: Oxycodone HCl 5 mg Use: See page 276 Mfr: Roxane Laboratories
C-II Imprint: 54 613 Reverse side: Scored Brand: Generic Active ingredients: Codeine Sulfate 15 mg Use: See page 242 Mfr: Roxane Laboratories	C-IV Imprint: 57 Reverse side: R Brand: Generic Active ingredients: Lorazepam 1 mg Use: See page 262 Mfr: Rugby Laboratories	C-IV Imprint: M 31 Reverse side: BREON Brand: Mebaral Active ingredients: Mephobarbital 32 mg Use: See page 265 Mfr: Winthrop Pharmaceutical
C-II Imprint: 54 410 Reverse side: Scored Brand: Generic Active ingredients: Levorphanol Tartrate 2 mg Use: See page 261 Mfr: Roxane Laboratories	C-IV Imprint: DAN 5622 Reverse side: 2 Brand: Generic Active ingredients: Lorazepam 2 mg Use: See page 262 Mfr: Danbury Pharmacal	C-IV Imprint: West-ward 450 Reverse side: Scored Brand: Generic Active ingredients: Phenobarbital 30 mg Use: See page 284 Mfr: West-ward
C-II Imprint: 54 609 Reverse side: 4 Brand: Generic Active ingredients: Hydromorphone HCl 4 mg Use: See page 260 Mfr: Roxane Laboratories	C-IV Imprint: par 207 Reverse side: None Brand: Generic Active ingredients: Lorazepam 1 mg Use: See page 262 Mfr: Par Pharmaceuticals	C-II Imprint: HD 717 Reverse side: 4 Brand: Generic Active ingredients: Hydromorphone HCl 4 mg Use: See page 260 Mfr: Halsey Drug Company
C-IV Imprint: 54 572 Reverse side: Scored Brand: Generic Active ingredients: Phenobarbital 30 mg Use: See page 284 Mfr: Roxane Laboratories	C-IV Imprint: WC 700 Reverse side: None Brand: Generic Active ingredients: Phenobarbital 30 mg Use: See page 284 Mfr: Warner Chilcott Laboratories	C-II Imprint: 381 Reverse side: b Brand: Generic Active ingredients: Meperidine HCl 50 mg Use: See page 264 Mfr: Barr Laboratories

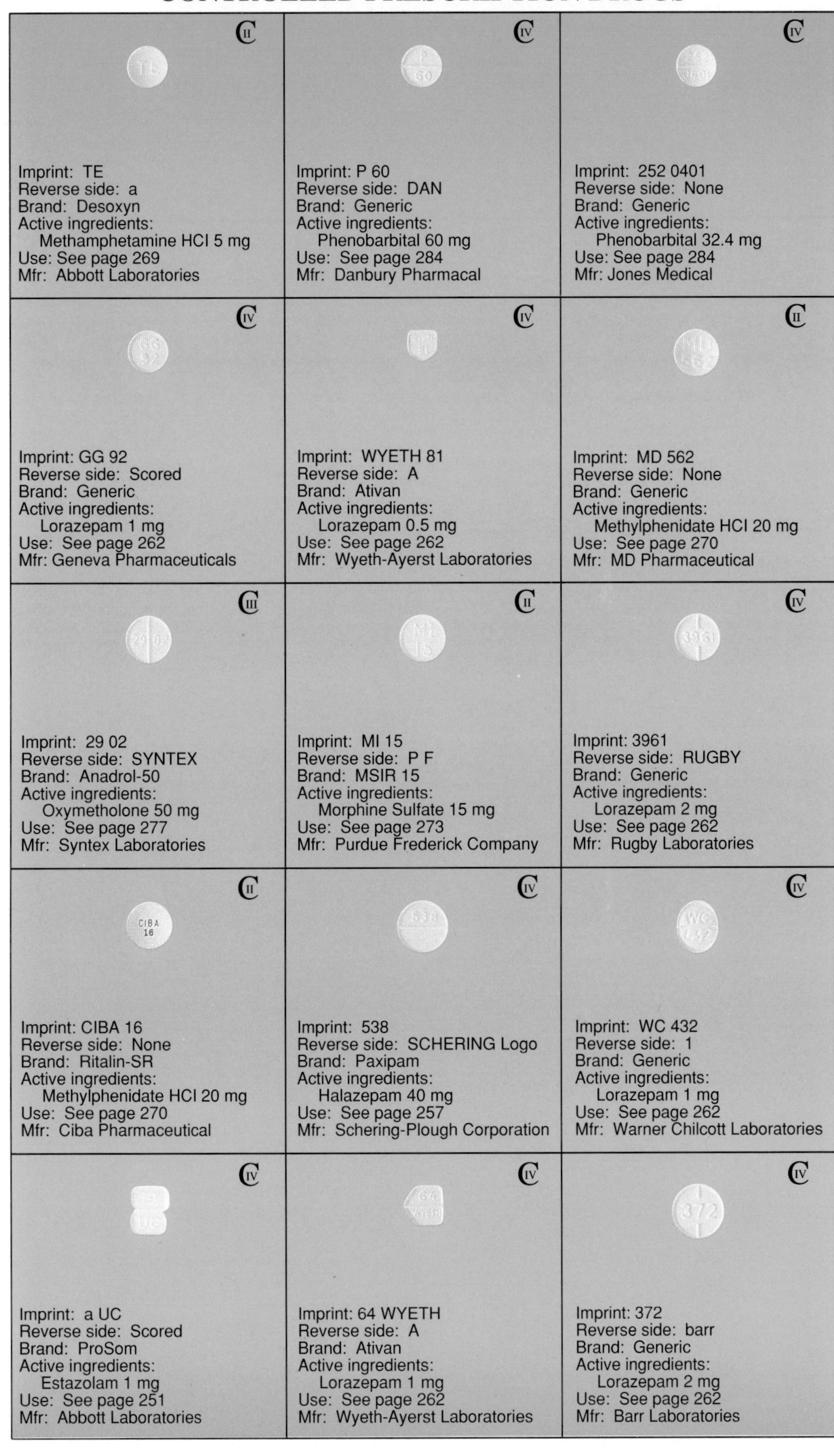

C-II
Imprint: TE
Reverse side: a
Brand: Desoxyn
Active ingredients:
Methamphetamine HCl 5 mg
Use: See page 269
Mfr: Abbott Laboratories

C-IV
Imprint: P 60
Reverse side: DAN
Brand: Generic
Active ingredients:
Phenobarbital 60 mg
Use: See page 284
Mfr: Danbury Pharmacal

C-IV
Imprint: 252 0401
Reverse side: None
Brand: Generic
Active ingredients:
Phenobarbital 32.4 mg
Use: See page 284
Mfr: Jones Medical

C-IV
Imprint: GG 92
Reverse side: Scored
Brand: Generic
Active ingredients:
Lorazepam 1 mg
Use: See page 262
Mfr: Geneva Pharmaceuticals

C-IV
Imprint: WYETH 81
Reverse side: A
Brand: Ativan
Active ingredients:
Lorazepam 0.5 mg
Use: See page 262
Mfr: Wyeth-Ayerst Laboratories

C-II
Imprint: MD 562
Reverse side: None
Brand: Generic
Active ingredients:
Methylphenidate HCl 20 mg
Use: See page 270
Mfr: MD Pharmaceutical

C-III
Imprint: 29 02
Reverse side: SYNTEX
Brand: Anadrol-50
Active ingredients:
Oxymetholone 50 mg
Use: See page 277
Mfr: Syntex Laboratories

C-II
Imprint: MI 15
Reverse side: P F
Brand: MSIR 15
Active ingredients:
Morphine Sulfate 15 mg
Use: See page 273
Mfr: Purdue Frederick Company

C-IV
Imprint: 3961
Reverse side: RUGBY
Brand: Generic
Active ingredients:
Lorazepam 2 mg
Use: See page 262
Mfr: Rugby Laboratories

C-II
Imprint: CIBA 16
Reverse side: None
Brand: Ritalin-SR
Active ingredients:
Methylphenidate HCl 20 mg
Use: See page 270
Mfr: Ciba Pharmaceutical

C-IV
Imprint: 538
Reverse side: SCHERING Logo
Brand: Paxipam
Active ingredients:
Halazepam 40 mg
Use: See page 257
Mfr: Schering-Plough Corporation

C-IV
Imprint: WC 432
Reverse side: 1
Brand: Generic
Active ingredients:
Lorazepam 1 mg
Use: See page 262
Mfr: Warner Chilcott Laboratories

C-IV
Imprint: a UC
Reverse side: Scored
Brand: ProSom
Active ingredients:
Estazolam 1 mg
Use: See page 251
Mfr: Abbott Laboratories

C-IV
Imprint: 64 WYETH
Reverse side: A
Brand: Ativan
Active ingredients:
Lorazepam 1 mg
Use: See page 262
Mfr: Wyeth-Ayerst Laboratories

C-IV
Imprint: 372
Reverse side: barr
Brand: Generic
Active ingredients:
Lorazepam 2 mg
Use: See page 262
Mfr: Barr Laboratories

CIV Imprint: KLONOPIN 2 ROCHE Reverse side: Scored Brand: Klonopin Active ingredients: Clonazepam 2 mg Use: See page 239 Mfr: Roche Laboratories	CIV Imprint: 555 163 Reverse side: barr Brand: Generic Active ingredients: Diazepam 2 mg Use: See page 245 Mfr: Barr Laboratories	CIV Imprint: 832 G533C Reverse side: None Brand: Generic Active ingredients: Phenobarbital 60 mg Use: See page 284 Mfr: Pharmaceutical Basics
CIII Imprint: HYCODAN Reverse side: DuPont Brand: Hycodan Active ingredients: Hydrocodone Bitartrate 5 mg Homatropine MBr 1.5 mg Use: See page 258 Mfr: DuPont Pharmaceuticals	CIV Imprint: MYLAN 457 Reverse side: None Brand: Generic Active ingredients: Lorazepam 1 mg Use: See page 262 Mfr: Mylan Pharmaceuticals	CIV Imprint: Lilly J33 Reverse side: Scored Brand: Generic Active ingredients: Phenobarbital 100 mg Use: See page 284 Mfr: Eli Lilly and Company
CII Imprint: MC Reverse side: a Brand: Desoxyn Gradumet Active ingredients: Methamphetamine HCl 5 mg Use: See page 269 Mfr: Abbott Laboratories	CIV Imprint: WC 607 Reverse side: None Brand: Generic Active ingredients: Phenobarbital 60 mg Use: See page 284 Mfr: Warner Chilcott Laboratories	CIV Imprint: 334 2.0 Reverse side: WATSON Brand: Generic Active ingredients: Lorazepam 2 mg Use: See page 262 Mfr: Watson Laboratories
CIV Imprint: Z 3925 Reverse side: 2 Brand: Generic Active ingredients: Diazepam 2 mg Use: See page 245 Mfr: Zenith Laboratories	CIV Imprint: D 51 Reverse side: LL Brand: Generic Active ingredients: Diazepam 2 mg Use: See page 245 Mfr: Lederle Laboratories	CIV Imprint: M 33 Reverse side: BREON Brand: Mebaral Active ingredients: Mephobarbital 100 mg Use: See page 265 Mfr: Winthrop Pharmaceutical
CIV Imprint: TH Reverse side: a Brand: Cylert Active ingredients: Pemoline 18.75 mg Use: See page 278 Mfr: Abbott Laboratories	CIV Imprint: MYLAN 271 Reverse side: Scored Brand: Generic Active ingredients: Diazepam 2 mg Use: See page 245 Mfr: Mylan Pharmaceuticals	CIV Imprint: WC 698 Reverse side: None Brand: Generic Active ingredients: Phenobarbital 100 mg Use: See page 284 Mfr: Warner Chilcott Laboratories

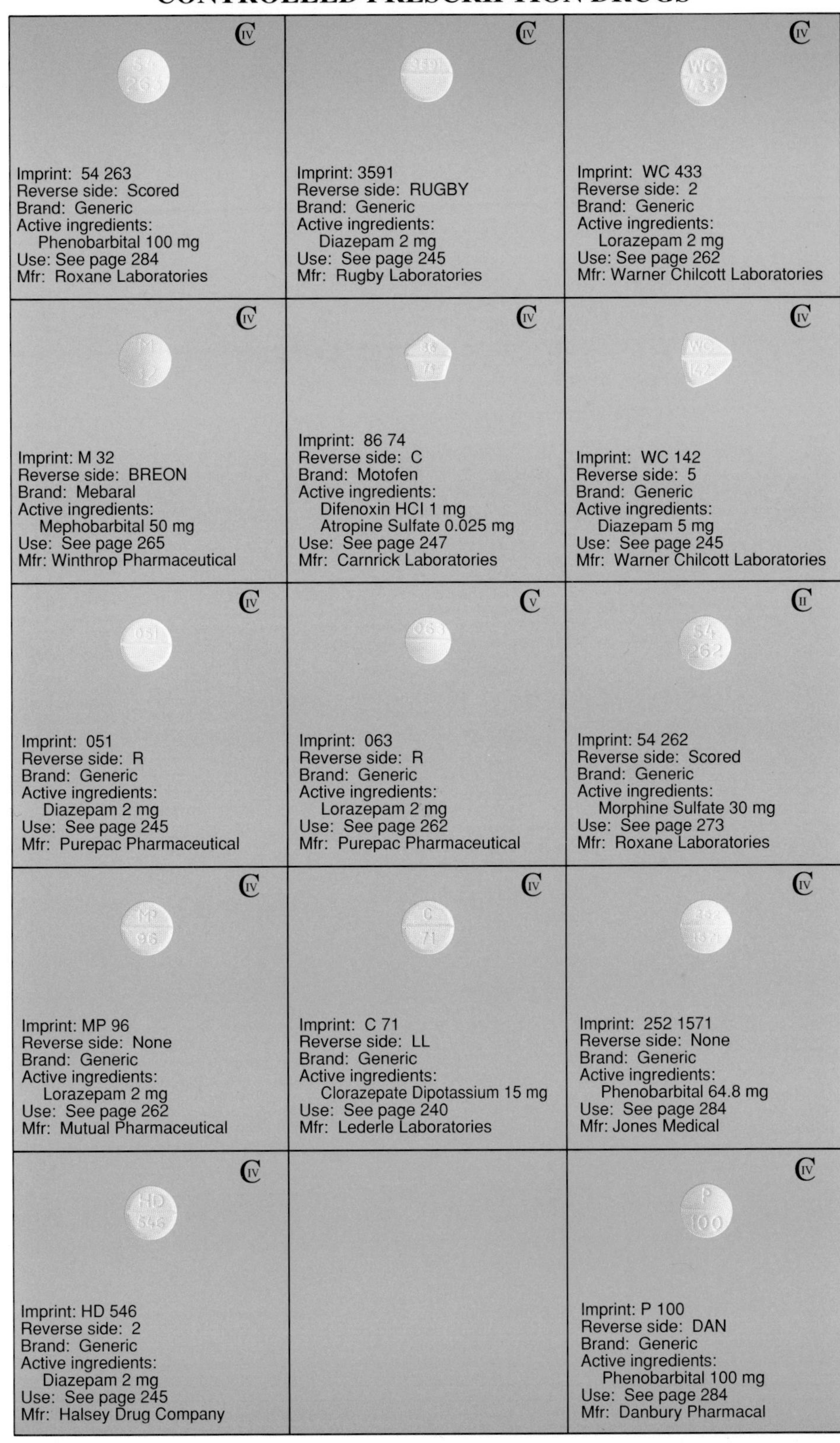
CIV
Imprint: 54 263
Reverse side: Scored
Brand: Generic
Active ingredients:
Phenobarbital 100 mg
Use: See page 284
Mfr: Roxane Laboratories

CIV
Imprint: 3591
Reverse side: RUGBY
Brand: Generic
Active ingredients:
Diazepam 2 mg
Use: See page 245
Mfr: Rugby Laboratories

CIV
Imprint: WC 433
Reverse side: 2
Brand: Generic
Active ingredients:
Lorazepam 2 mg
Use: See page 262
Mfr: Warner Chilcott Laboratories

CIV
Imprint: M 32
Reverse side: BREON
Brand: Mebaral
Active ingredients:
Mephobarbital 50 mg
Use: See page 265
Mfr: Winthrop Pharmaceutical

CIV
Imprint: 86 74
Reverse side: C
Brand: Motofen
Active ingredients:
Difenoxin HCl 1 mg
Atropine Sulfate 0.025 mg
Use: See page 247
Mfr: Carnrick Laboratories

CIV
Imprint: WC 142
Reverse side: 5
Brand: Generic
Active ingredients:
Diazepam 5 mg
Use: See page 245
Mfr: Warner Chilcott Laboratories

CIV
Imprint: 051
Reverse side: R
Brand: Generic
Active ingredients:
Diazepam 2 mg
Use: See page 245
Mfr: Purepac Pharmaceutical

CV
Imprint: 063
Reverse side: R
Brand: Generic
Active ingredients:
Lorazepam 2 mg
Use: See page 262
Mfr: Purepac Pharmaceutical

CII
Imprint: 54 262
Reverse side: Scored
Brand: Generic
Active ingredients:
Morphine Sulfate 30 mg
Use: See page 273
Mfr: Roxane Laboratories

CIV
Imprint: MP 96
Reverse side: None
Brand: Generic
Active ingredients:
Lorazepam 2 mg
Use: See page 262
Mfr: Mutual Pharmaceutical

CIV
Imprint: C 71
Reverse side: LL
Brand: Generic
Active ingredients:
Clorazepate Dipotassium 15 mg
Use: See page 240
Mfr: Lederle Laboratories

CIV
Imprint: 252 1571
Reverse side: None
Brand: Generic
Active ingredients:
Phenobarbital 64.8 mg
Use: See page 284
Mfr: Jones Medical

CIV
Imprint: HD 546
Reverse side: 2
Brand: Generic
Active ingredients:
Diazepam 2 mg
Use: See page 245
Mfr: Halsey Drug Company

CIV
Imprint: P 100
Reverse side: DAN
Brand: Generic
Active ingredients:
Phenobarbital 100 mg
Use: See page 284
Mfr: Danbury Pharmacal

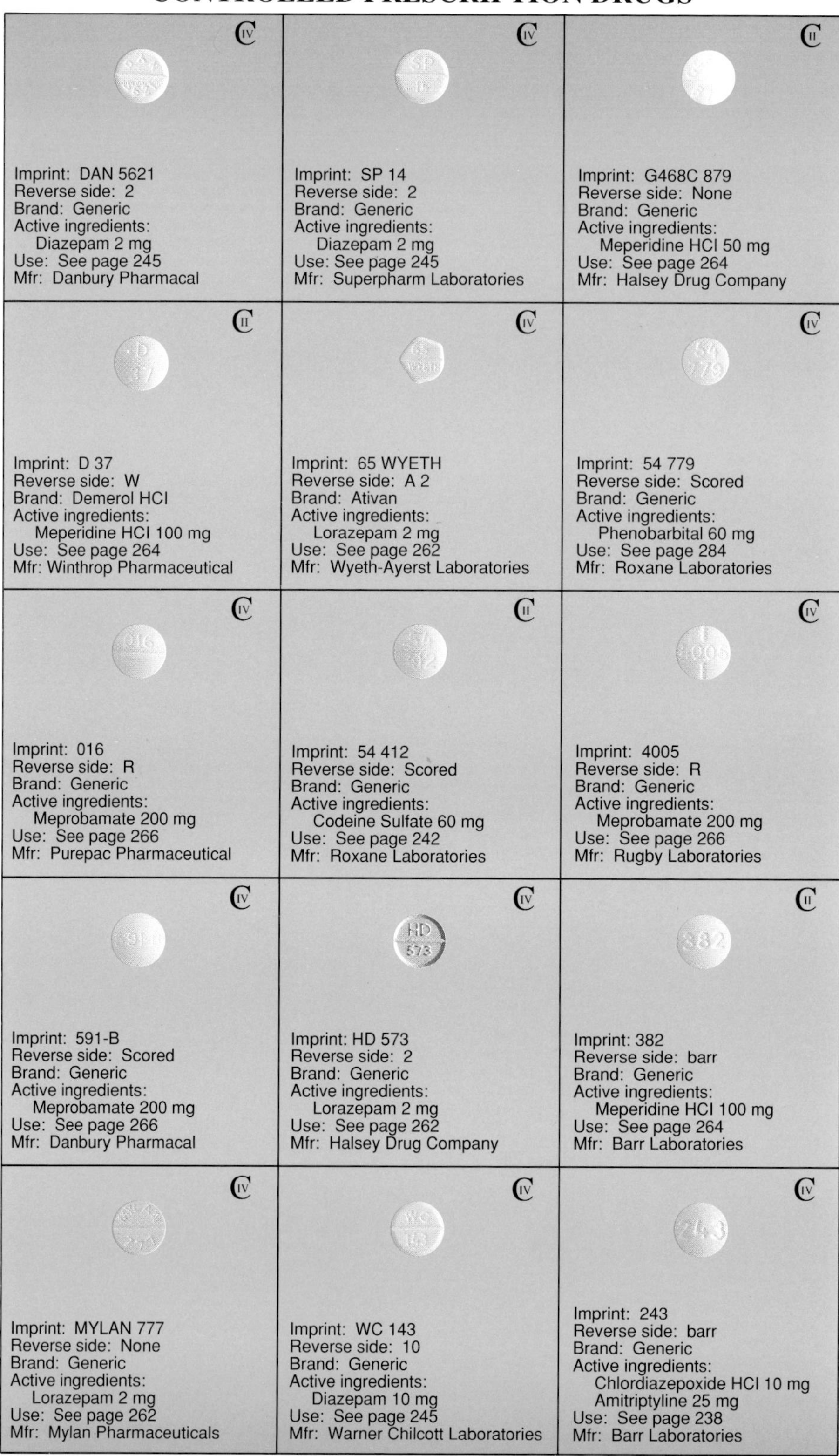

Imprint: DAN 5621
Reverse side: 2
Brand: Generic
Active ingredients:
Diazepam 2 mg
Use: See page 245
Mfr: Danbury Pharmacal

Imprint: SP 14
Reverse side: 2
Brand: Generic
Active ingredients:
Diazepam 2 mg
Use: See page 245
Mfr: Superpharm Laboratories

Imprint: G468C 879
Reverse side: None
Brand: Generic
Active ingredients:
Meperidine HCl 50 mg
Use: See page 264
Mfr: Halsey Drug Company

Imprint: D 37
Reverse side: W
Brand: Demerol HCl
Active ingredients:
Meperidine HCl 100 mg
Use: See page 264
Mfr: Winthrop Pharmaceutical

Imprint: 65 WYETH
Reverse side: A 2
Brand: Ativan
Active ingredients:
Lorazepam 2 mg
Use: See page 262
Mfr: Wyeth-Ayerst Laboratories

Imprint: 54 779
Reverse side: Scored
Brand: Generic
Active ingredients:
Phenobarbital 60 mg
Use: See page 284
Mfr: Roxane Laboratories

Imprint: 016
Reverse side: R
Brand: Generic
Active ingredients:
Meprobamate 200 mg
Use: See page 266
Mfr: Purepac Pharmaceutical

Imprint: 54 412
Reverse side: Scored
Brand: Generic
Active ingredients:
Codeine Sulfate 60 mg
Use: See page 242
Mfr: Roxane Laboratories

Imprint: 4005
Reverse side: R
Brand: Generic
Active ingredients:
Meprobamate 200 mg
Use: See page 266
Mfr: Rugby Laboratories

Imprint: 591-B
Reverse side: Scored
Brand: Generic
Active ingredients:
Meprobamate 200 mg
Use: See page 266
Mfr: Danbury Pharmacal

Imprint: HD 573
Reverse side: 2
Brand: Generic
Active ingredients:
Lorazepam 2 mg
Use: See page 262
Mfr: Halsey Drug Company

Imprint: 382
Reverse side: barr
Brand: Generic
Active ingredients:
Meperidine HCl 100 mg
Use: See page 264
Mfr: Barr Laboratories

Imprint: MYLAN 777
Reverse side: None
Brand: Generic
Active ingredients:
Lorazepam 2 mg
Use: See page 262
Mfr: Mylan Pharmaceuticals

Imprint: WC 143
Reverse side: 10
Brand: Generic
Active ingredients:
Diazepam 10 mg
Use: See page 245
Mfr: Warner Chilcott Laboratories

Imprint: 243
Reverse side: barr
Brand: Generic
Active ingredients:
Chlordiazepoxide HCl 10 mg
Amitriptyline 25 mg
Use: See page 238
Mfr: Barr Laboratories

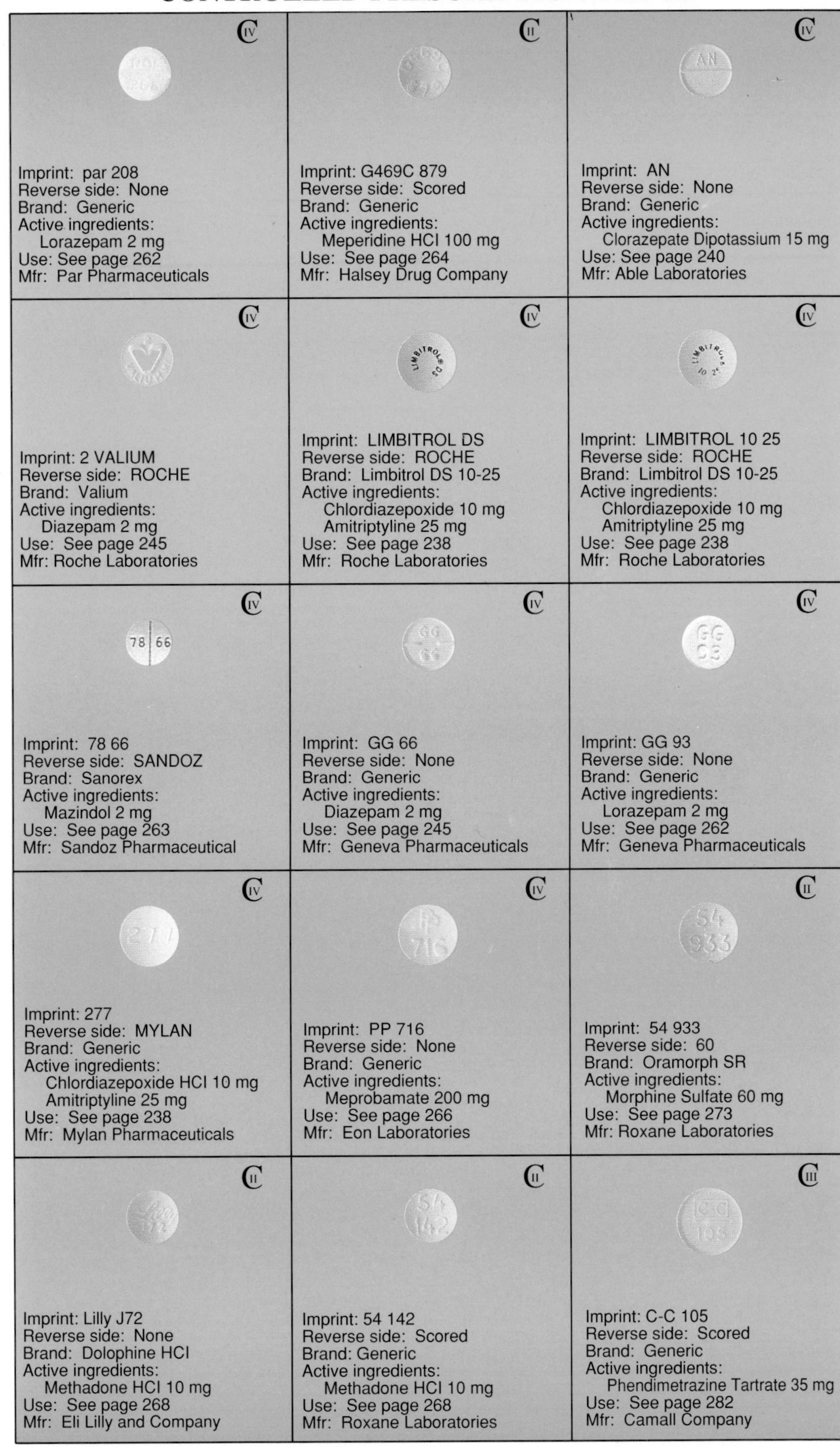

Imprint: par 208
Reverse side: None
Brand: Generic
Active ingredients:
Lorazepam 2 mg
Use: See page 262
Mfr: Par Pharmaceuticals

Imprint: G469C 879
Reverse side: Scored
Brand: Generic
Active ingredients:
Meperidine HCl 100 mg
Use: See page 264
Mfr: Halsey Drug Company

Imprint: AN
Reverse side: None
Brand: Generic
Active ingredients:
Clorazepate Dipotassium 15 mg
Use: See page 240
Mfr: Able Laboratories

Imprint: 2 VALIUM
Reverse side: ROCHE
Brand: Valium
Active ingredients:
Diazepam 2 mg
Use: See page 245
Mfr: Roche Laboratories

Imprint: LIMBITROL DS
Reverse side: ROCHE
Brand: Limbitrol DS 10-25
Active ingredients:
Chlordiazepoxide 10 mg
Amitriptyline 25 mg
Use: See page 238
Mfr: Roche Laboratories

Imprint: LIMBITROL 10 25
Reverse side: ROCHE
Brand: Limbitrol DS 10-25
Active ingredients:
Chlordiazepoxide 10 mg
Amitriptyline 25 mg
Use: See page 238
Mfr: Roche Laboratories

Imprint: 78 66
Reverse side: SANDOZ
Brand: Sanorex
Active ingredients:
Mazindol 2 mg
Use: See page 263
Mfr: Sandoz Pharmaceutical

Imprint: GG 66
Reverse side: None
Brand: Generic
Active ingredients:
Diazepam 2 mg
Use: See page 245
Mfr: Geneva Pharmaceuticals

Imprint: GG 93
Reverse side: None
Brand: Generic
Active ingredients:
Lorazepam 2 mg
Use: See page 262
Mfr: Geneva Pharmaceuticals

Imprint: 277
Reverse side: MYLAN
Brand: Generic
Active ingredients:
Chlordiazepoxide HCl 10 mg
Amitriptyline 25 mg
Use: See page 238
Mfr: Mylan Pharmaceuticals

Imprint: PP 716
Reverse side: None
Brand: Generic
Active ingredients:
Meprobamate 200 mg
Use: See page 266
Mfr: Eon Laboratories

Imprint: 54 933
Reverse side: 60
Brand: Oramorph SR
Active ingredients:
Morphine Sulfate 60 mg
Use: See page 273
Mfr: Roxane Laboratories

Imprint: Lilly J72
Reverse side: None
Brand: Dolophine HCl
Active ingredients:
Methadone HCl 10 mg
Use: See page 268
Mfr: Eli Lilly and Company

Imprint: 54 142
Reverse side: Scored
Brand: Generic
Active ingredients:
Methadone HCl 10 mg
Use: See page 268
Mfr: Roxane Laboratories

Imprint: C-C 105
Reverse side: Scored
Brand: Generic
Active ingredients:
Phendimetrazine Tartrate 35 mg
Use: See page 282
Mfr: Camall Company

CONTROLLED PRESCRIPTION DRUGS

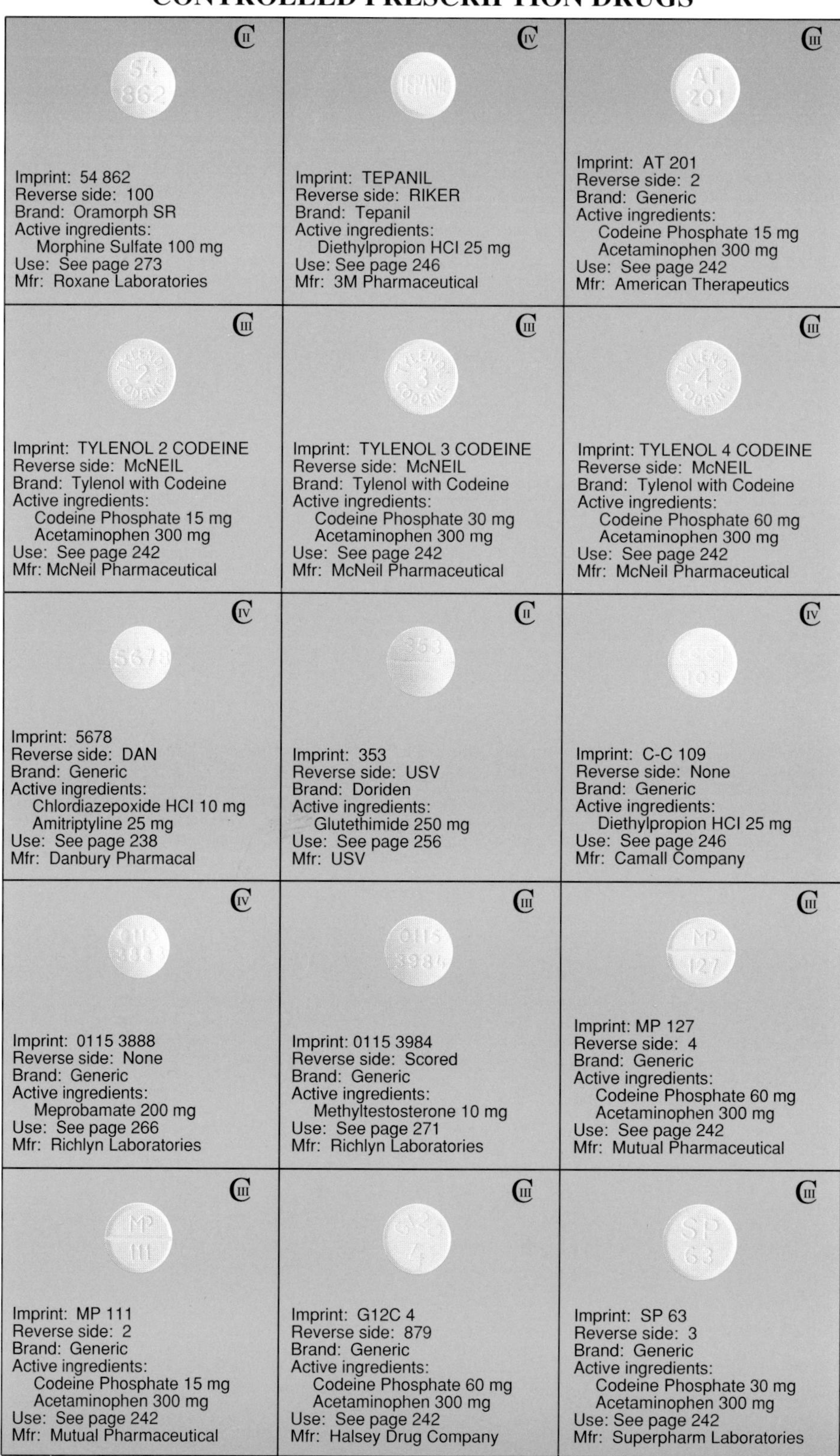

Imprint: 54 862
Reverse side: 100
Brand: Oramorph SR
Active ingredients:
Morphine Sulfate 100 mg
Use: See page 273
Mfr: Roxane Laboratories

Imprint: TEPANIL
Reverse side: RIKER
Brand: Tepanil
Active ingredients:
Diethylpropion HCl 25 mg
Use: See page 246
Mfr: 3M Pharmaceutical

Imprint: AT 201
Reverse side: 2
Brand: Generic
Active ingredients:
Codeine Phosphate 15 mg
Acetaminophen 300 mg
Use: See page 242
Mfr: American Therapeutics

Imprint: TYLENOL 2 CODEINE
Reverse side: McNEIL
Brand: Tylenol with Codeine
Active ingredients:
Codeine Phosphate 15 mg
Acetaminophen 300 mg
Use: See page 242
Mfr: McNeil Pharmaceutical

Imprint: TYLENOL 3 CODEINE
Reverse side: McNEIL
Brand: Tylenol with Codeine
Active ingredients:
Codeine Phosphate 30 mg
Acetaminophen 300 mg
Use: See page 242
Mfr: McNeil Pharmaceutical

Imprint: TYLENOL 4 CODEINE
Reverse side: McNEIL
Brand: Tylenol with Codeine
Active ingredients:
Codeine Phosphate 60 mg
Acetaminophen 300 mg
Use: See page 242
Mfr: McNeil Pharmaceutical

Imprint: 5678
Reverse side: DAN
Brand: Generic
Active ingredients:
Chlordiazepoxide HCl 10 mg
Amitriptyline 25 mg
Use: See page 238
Mfr: Danbury Pharmacal

Imprint: 353
Reverse side: USV
Brand: Doriden
Active ingredients:
Glutethimide 250 mg
Use: See page 256
Mfr: USV

Imprint: C-C 109
Reverse side: None
Brand: Generic
Active ingredients:
Diethylpropion HCl 25 mg
Use: See page 246
Mfr: Camall Company

Imprint: 0115 3888
Reverse side: None
Brand: Generic
Active ingredients:
Meprobamate 200 mg
Use: See page 266
Mfr: Richlyn Laboratories

Imprint: 0115 3984
Reverse side: Scored
Brand: Generic
Active ingredients:
Methyltestosterone 10 mg
Use: See page 271
Mfr: Richlyn Laboratories

Imprint: MP 127
Reverse side: 4
Brand: Generic
Active ingredients:
Codeine Phosphate 60 mg
Acetaminophen 300 mg
Use: See page 242
Mfr: Mutual Pharmaceutical

Imprint: MP 111
Reverse side: 2
Brand: Generic
Active ingredients:
Codeine Phosphate 15 mg
Acetaminophen 300 mg
Use: See page 242
Mfr: Mutual Pharmaceutical

Imprint: G12C 4
Reverse side: 879
Brand: Generic
Active ingredients:
Codeine Phosphate 60 mg
Acetaminophen 300 mg
Use: See page 242
Mfr: Halsey Drug Company

Imprint: SP 63
Reverse side: 3
Brand: Generic
Active ingredients:
Codeine Phosphate 30 mg
Acetaminophen 300 mg
Use: See page 242
Mfr: Superpharm Laboratories

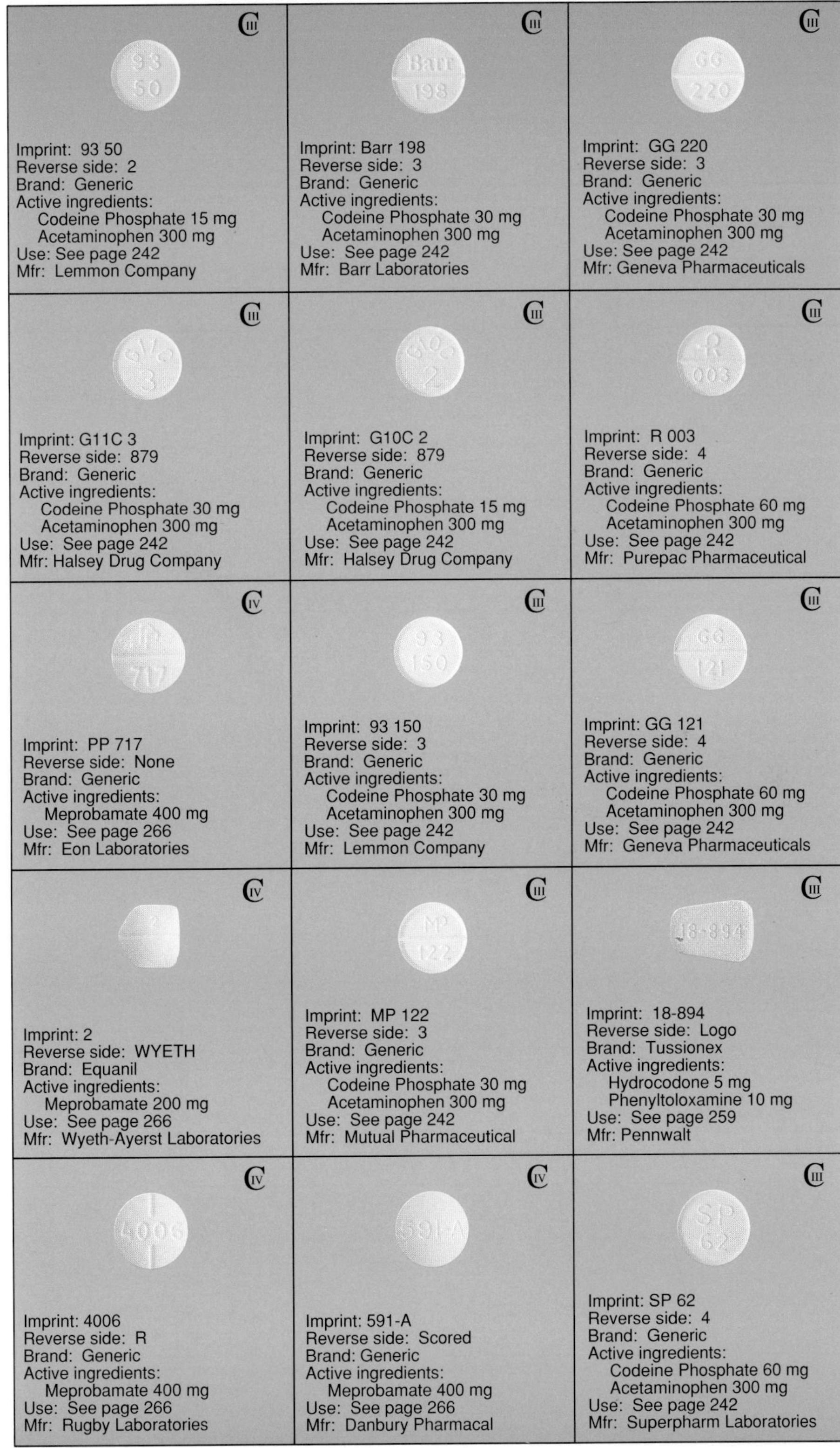

CIII
Imprint: 93 50
Reverse side: 2
Brand: Generic
Active ingredients:
Codeine Phosphate 15 mg
Acetaminophen 300 mg
Use: See page 242
Mfr: Lemmon Company

CIII
Imprint: Barr 198
Reverse side: 3
Brand: Generic
Active ingredients:
Codeine Phosphate 30 mg
Acetaminophen 300 mg
Use: See page 242
Mfr: Barr Laboratories

CIII
Imprint: GG 220
Reverse side: 3
Brand: Generic
Active ingredients:
Codeine Phosphate 30 mg
Acetaminophen 300 mg
Use: See page 242
Mfr: Geneva Pharmaceuticals

CIII
Imprint: G11C 3
Reverse side: 879
Brand: Generic
Active ingredients:
Codeine Phosphate 30 mg
Acetaminophen 300 mg
Use: See page 242
Mfr: Halsey Drug Company

CIII
Imprint: G10C 2
Reverse side: 879
Brand: Generic
Active ingredients:
Codeine Phosphate 15 mg
Acetaminophen 300 mg
Use: See page 242
Mfr: Halsey Drug Company

CIII
Imprint: R 003
Reverse side: 4
Brand: Generic
Active ingredients:
Codeine Phosphate 60 mg
Acetaminophen 300 mg
Use: See page 242
Mfr: Purepac Pharmaceutical

CIV
Imprint: PP 717
Reverse side: None
Brand: Generic
Active ingredients:
Meprobamate 400 mg
Use: See page 266
Mfr: Eon Laboratories

CIII
Imprint: 93 150
Reverse side: 3
Brand: Generic
Active ingredients:
Codeine Phosphate 30 mg
Acetaminophen 300 mg
Use: See page 242
Mfr: Lemmon Company

CIII
Imprint: GG 121
Reverse side: 4
Brand: Generic
Active ingredients:
Codeine Phosphate 60 mg
Acetaminophen 300 mg
Use: See page 242
Mfr: Geneva Pharmaceuticals

CIV
Imprint: 2
Reverse side: WYETH
Brand: Equanil
Active ingredients:
Meprobamate 200 mg
Use: See page 266
Mfr: Wyeth-Ayerst Laboratories

CIII
Imprint: MP 122
Reverse side: 3
Brand: Generic
Active ingredients:
Codeine Phosphate 30 mg
Acetaminophen 300 mg
Use: See page 242
Mfr: Mutual Pharmaceutical

CIII
Imprint: 18-894
Reverse side: Logo
Brand: Tussionex
Active ingredients:
Hydrocodone 5 mg
Phenyltoloxamine 10 mg
Use: See page 259
Mfr: Pennwalt

CIV
Imprint: 4006
Reverse side: R
Brand: Generic
Active ingredients:
Meprobamate 400 mg
Use: See page 266
Mfr: Rugby Laboratories

CIV
Imprint: 591-A
Reverse side: Scored
Brand: Generic
Active ingredients:
Meprobamate 400 mg
Use: See page 266
Mfr: Danbury Pharmacal

CIII
Imprint: SP 62
Reverse side: 4
Brand: Generic
Active ingredients:
Codeine Phosphate 60 mg
Acetaminophen 300 mg
Use: See page 242
Mfr: Superpharm Laboratories

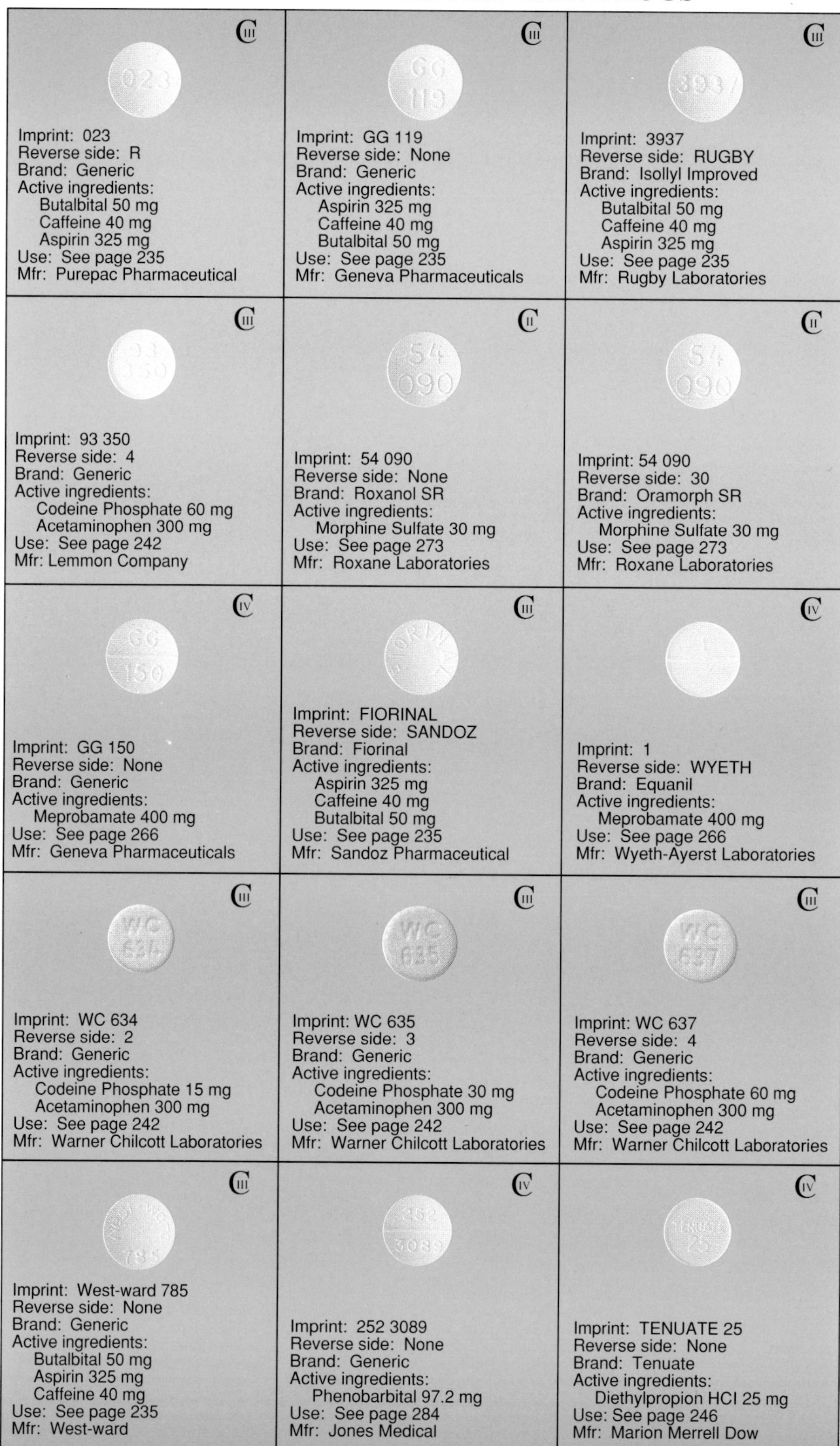

C III
Imprint: 023
Reverse side: R
Brand: Generic
Active ingredients:
Butalbital 50 mg
Caffeine 40 mg
Aspirin 325 mg
Use: See page 235
Mfr: Purepac Pharmaceutical

C III
Imprint: GG 119
Reverse side: None
Brand: Generic
Active ingredients:
Aspirin 325 mg
Caffeine 40 mg
Butalbital 50 mg
Use: See page 235
Mfr: Geneva Pharmaceuticals

C III
Imprint: 3937
Reverse side: RUGBY
Brand: Isollyl Improved
Active ingredients:
Butalbital 50 mg
Caffeine 40 mg
Aspirin 325 mg
Use: See page 235
Mfr: Rugby Laboratories

C III
Imprint: 93 350
Reverse side: 4
Brand: Generic
Active ingredients:
Codeine Phosphate 60 mg
Acetaminophen 300 mg
Use: See page 242
Mfr: Lemmon Company

C II
Imprint: 54 090
Reverse side: None
Brand: Roxanol SR
Active ingredients:
Morphine Sulfate 30 mg
Use: See page 273
Mfr: Roxane Laboratories

C II
Imprint: 54 090
Reverse side: 30
Brand: Oramorph SR
Active ingredients:
Morphine Sulfate 30 mg
Use: See page 273
Mfr: Roxane Laboratories

C IV
Imprint: GG 150
Reverse side: None
Brand: Generic
Active ingredients:
Meprobamate 400 mg
Use: See page 266
Mfr: Geneva Pharmaceuticals

C III
Imprint: FIORINAL
Reverse side: SANDOZ
Brand: Fiorinal
Active ingredients:
Aspirin 325 mg
Caffeine 40 mg
Butalbital 50 mg
Use: See page 235
Mfr: Sandoz Pharmaceutical

C IV
Imprint: 1
Reverse side: WYETH
Brand: Equanil
Active ingredients:
Meprobamate 400 mg
Use: See page 266
Mfr: Wyeth-Ayerst Laboratories

C III
Imprint: WC 634
Reverse side: 2
Brand: Generic
Active ingredients:
Codeine Phosphate 15 mg
Acetaminophen 300 mg
Use: See page 242
Mfr: Warner Chilcott Laboratories

C III
Imprint: WC 635
Reverse side: 3
Brand: Generic
Active ingredients:
Codeine Phosphate 30 mg
Acetaminophen 300 mg
Use: See page 242
Mfr: Warner Chilcott Laboratories

C III
Imprint: WC 637
Reverse side: 4
Brand: Generic
Active ingredients:
Codeine Phosphate 60 mg
Acetaminophen 300 mg
Use: See page 242
Mfr: Warner Chilcott Laboratories

C III
Imprint: West-ward 785
Reverse side: None
Brand: Generic
Active ingredients:
Butalbital 50 mg
Aspirin 325 mg
Caffeine 40 mg
Use: See page 235
Mfr: West-ward

C IV
Imprint: 252 3089
Reverse side: None
Brand: Generic
Active ingredients:
Phenobarbital 97.2 mg
Use: See page 284
Mfr: Jones Medical

C IV
Imprint: TENUATE 25
Reverse side: None
Brand: Tenuate
Active ingredients:
Diethylpropion HCl 25 mg
Use: See page 246
Mfr: Marion Merrell Dow

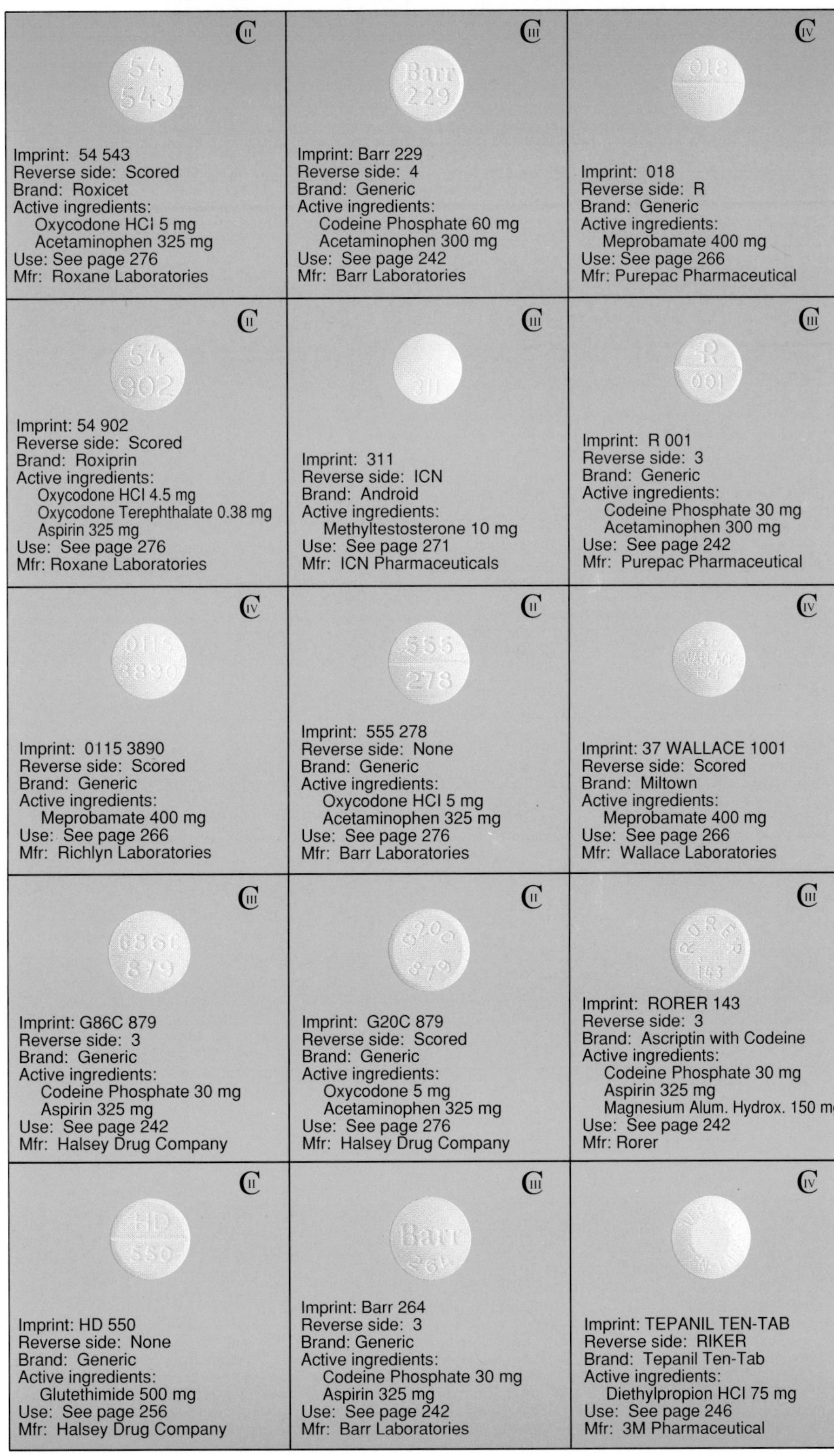

CII
Imprint: 54 543
Reverse side: Scored
Brand: Roxicet
Active ingredients:
Oxycodone HCl 5 mg
Acetaminophen 325 mg
Use: See page 276
Mfr: Roxane Laboratories

CIII
Imprint: Barr 229
Reverse side: 4
Brand: Generic
Active ingredients:
Codeine Phosphate 60 mg
Acetaminophen 300 mg
Use: See page 242
Mfr: Barr Laboratories

CIV
Imprint: 018
Reverse side: R
Brand: Generic
Active ingredients:
Meprobamate 400 mg
Use: See page 266
Mfr: Purepac Pharmaceutical

CII
Imprint: 54 902
Reverse side: Scored
Brand: Roxiprin
Active ingredients:
Oxycodone HCl 4.5 mg
Oxycodone Terephthalate 0.38 mg
Aspirin 325 mg
Use: See page 276
Mfr: Roxane Laboratories

CIII
Imprint: 311
Reverse side: ICN
Brand: Android
Active ingredients:
Methyltestosterone 10 mg
Use: See page 271
Mfr: ICN Pharmaceuticals

CIII
Imprint: R 001
Reverse side: 3
Brand: Generic
Active ingredients:
Codeine Phosphate 30 mg
Acetaminophen 300 mg
Use: See page 242
Mfr: Purepac Pharmaceutical

CIV
Imprint: 0115 3890
Reverse side: Scored
Brand: Generic
Active ingredients:
Meprobamate 400 mg
Use: See page 266
Mfr: Richlyn Laboratories

CII
Imprint: 555 278
Reverse side: None
Brand: Generic
Active ingredients:
Oxycodone HCl 5 mg
Acetaminophen 325 mg
Use: See page 276
Mfr: Barr Laboratories

CIV
Imprint: 37 WALLACE 1001
Reverse side: Scored
Brand: Miltown
Active ingredients:
Meprobamate 400 mg
Use: See page 266
Mfr: Wallace Laboratories

CIII
Imprint: G86C 879
Reverse side: 3
Brand: Generic
Active ingredients:
Codeine Phosphate 30 mg
Aspirin 325 mg
Use: See page 242
Mfr: Halsey Drug Company

CII
Imprint: G20C 879
Reverse side: Scored
Brand: Generic
Active ingredients:
Oxycodone 5 mg
Acetaminophen 325 mg
Use: See page 276
Mfr: Halsey Drug Company

CIII
Imprint: RORER 143
Reverse side: 3
Brand: Ascriptin with Codeine
Active ingredients:
Codeine Phosphate 30 mg
Aspirin 325 mg
Magnesium Alum. Hydrox. 150 mg
Use: See page 242
Mfr: Rorer

CII
Imprint: HD 550
Reverse side: None
Brand: Generic
Active ingredients:
Glutethimide 500 mg
Use: See page 256
Mfr: Halsey Drug Company

CIII
Imprint: Barr 264
Reverse side: 3
Brand: Generic
Active ingredients:
Codeine Phosphate 30 mg
Aspirin 325 mg
Use: See page 242
Mfr: Barr Laboratories

CIV
Imprint: TEPANIL TEN-TAB
Reverse side: RIKER
Brand: Tepanil Ten-Tab
Active ingredients:
Diethylpropion HCl 75 mg
Use: See page 246
Mfr: 3M Pharmaceutical

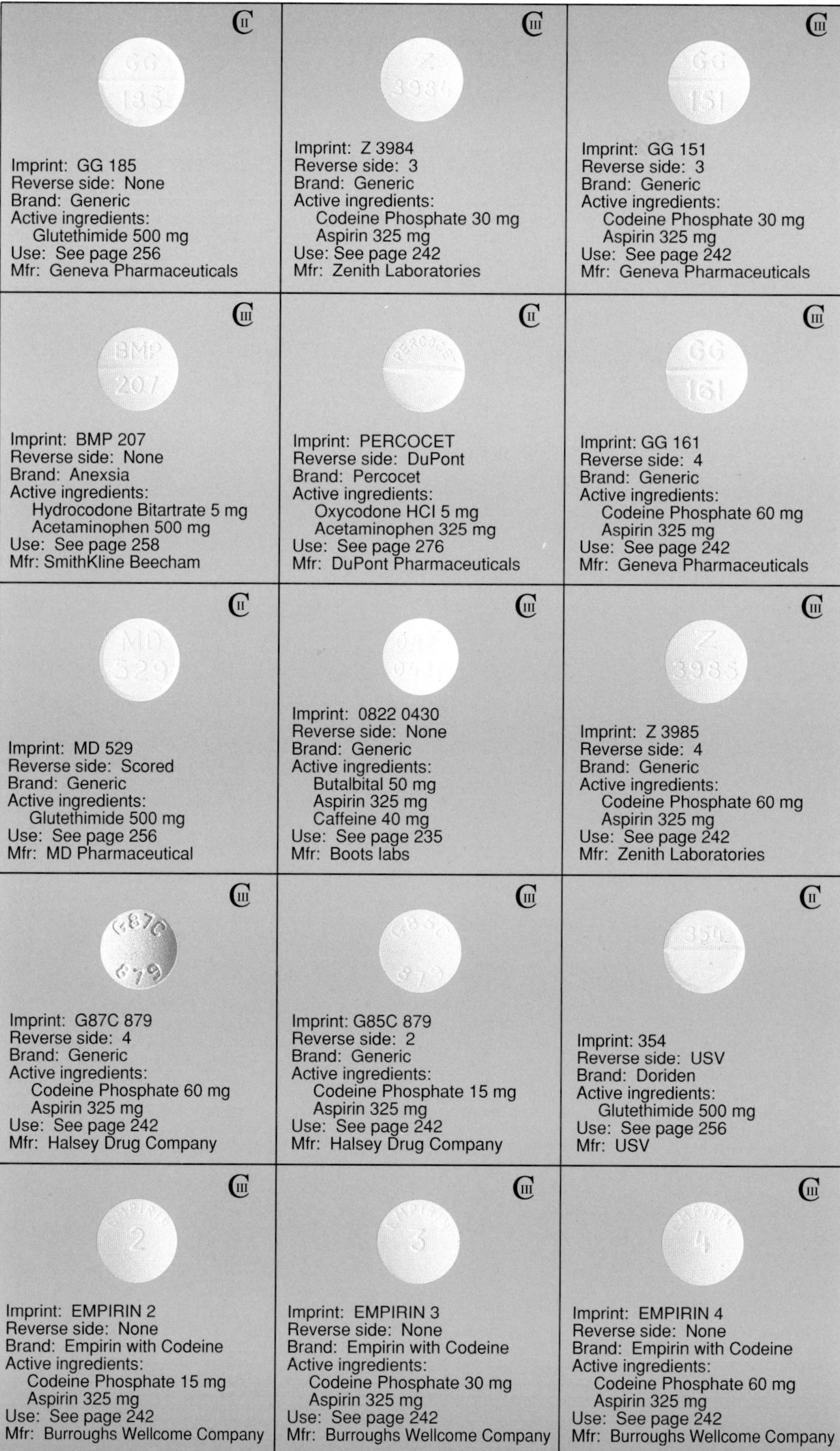

C-II
Imprint: GG 185
Reverse side: None
Brand: Generic
Active ingredients:
Glutethimide 500 mg
Use: See page 256
Mfr: Geneva Pharmaceuticals

C-III
Imprint: Z 3984
Reverse side: 3
Brand: Generic
Active ingredients:
Codeine Phosphate 30 mg
Aspirin 325 mg
Use: See page 242
Mfr: Zenith Laboratories

C-III
Imprint: GG 151
Reverse side: 3
Brand: Generic
Active ingredients:
Codeine Phosphate 30 mg
Aspirin 325 mg
Use: See page 242
Mfr: Geneva Pharmaceuticals

C-III
Imprint: BMP 207
Reverse side: None
Brand: Anexsia
Active ingredients:
Hydrocodone Bitartrate 5 mg
Acetaminophen 500 mg
Use: See page 258
Mfr: SmithKline Beecham

C-II
Imprint: PERCOCET
Reverse side: DuPont
Brand: Percocet
Active ingredients:
Oxycodone HCl 5 mg
Acetaminophen 325 mg
Use: See page 276
Mfr: DuPont Pharmaceuticals

C-III
Imprint: GG 161
Reverse side: 4
Brand: Generic
Active ingredients:
Codeine Phosphate 60 mg
Aspirin 325 mg
Use: See page 242
Mfr: Geneva Pharmaceuticals

C-II
Imprint: MD 529
Reverse side: Scored
Brand: Generic
Active ingredients:
Glutethimide 500 mg
Use: See page 256
Mfr: MD Pharmaceutical

C-III
Imprint: 0822 0430
Reverse side: None
Brand: Generic
Active ingredients:
Butalbital 50 mg
Aspirin 325 mg
Caffeine 40 mg
Use: See page 235
Mfr: Boots labs

C-III
Imprint: Z 3985
Reverse side: 4
Brand: Generic
Active ingredients:
Codeine Phosphate 60 mg
Aspirin 325 mg
Use: See page 242
Mfr: Zenith Laboratories

C-III
Imprint: G87C 879
Reverse side: 4
Brand: Generic
Active ingredients:
Codeine Phosphate 60 mg
Aspirin 325 mg
Use: See page 242
Mfr: Halsey Drug Company

C-III
Imprint: G85C 879
Reverse side: 2
Brand: Generic
Active ingredients:
Codeine Phosphate 15 mg
Aspirin 325 mg
Use: See page 242
Mfr: Halsey Drug Company

C-II
Imprint: 354
Reverse side: USV
Brand: Doriden
Active ingredients:
Glutethimide 500 mg
Use: See page 256
Mfr: USV

C-III
Imprint: EMPIRIN 2
Reverse side: None
Brand: Empirin with Codeine
Active ingredients:
Codeine Phosphate 15 mg
Aspirin 325 mg
Use: See page 242
Mfr: Burroughs Wellcome Company

C-III
Imprint: EMPIRIN 3
Reverse side: None
Brand: Empirin with Codeine
Active ingredients:
Codeine Phosphate 30 mg
Aspirin 325 mg
Use: See page 242
Mfr: Burroughs Wellcome Company

C-III
Imprint: EMPIRIN 4
Reverse side: None
Brand: Empirin with Codeine
Active ingredients:
Codeine Phosphate 60 mg
Aspirin 325 mg
Use: See page 242
Mfr: Burroughs Wellcome Company

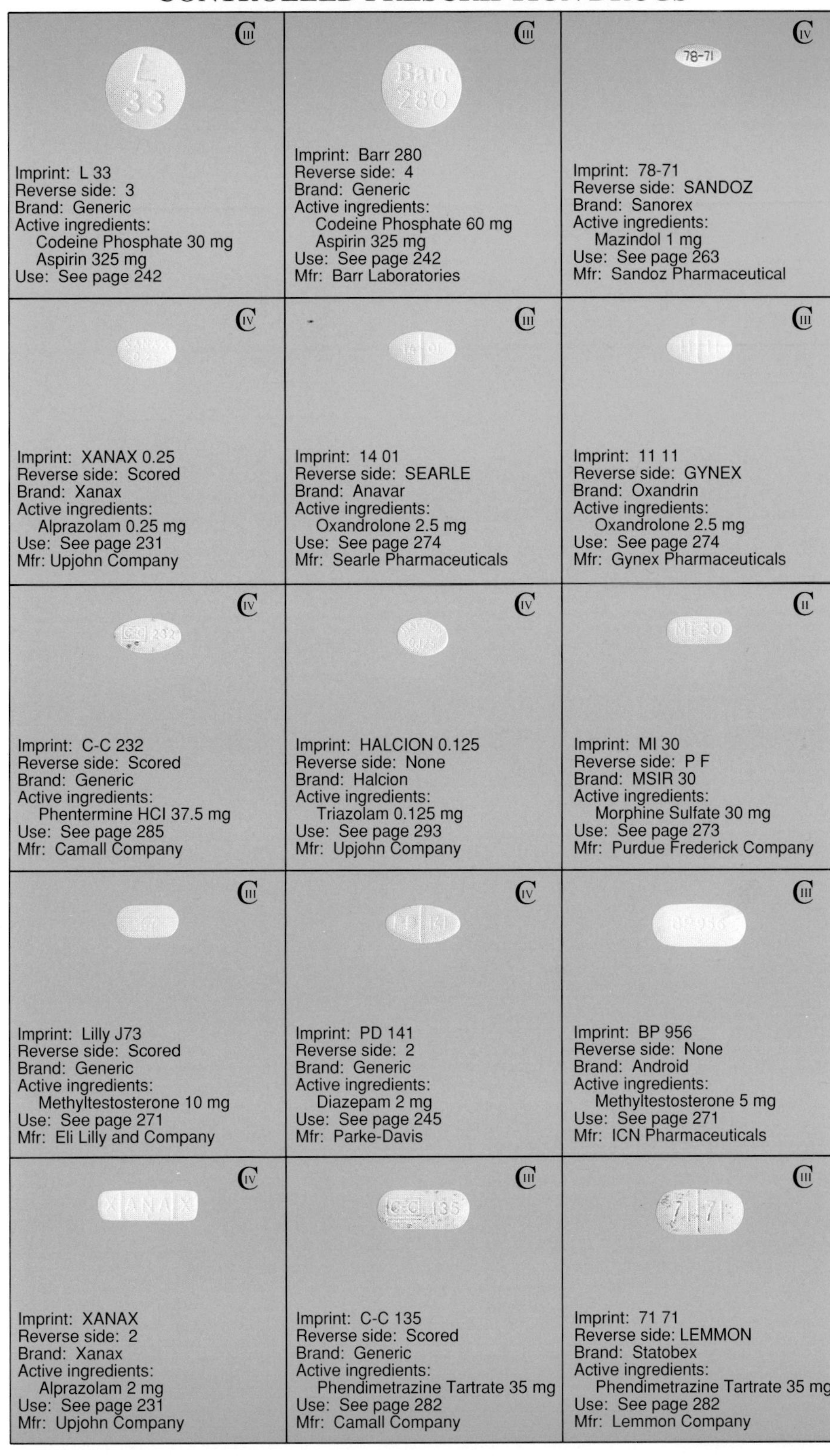

Imprint: L 33
Reverse side: 3
Brand: Generic
Active ingredients:
Codeine Phosphate 30 mg
Aspirin 325 mg
Use: See page 242

Imprint: Barr 280
Reverse side: 4
Brand: Generic
Active ingredients:
Codeine Phosphate 60 mg
Aspirin 325 mg
Use: See page 242
Mfr: Barr Laboratories

Imprint: 78-71
Reverse side: SANDOZ
Brand: Sanorex
Active ingredients:
Mazindol 1 mg
Use: See page 263
Mfr: Sandoz Pharmaceutical

Imprint: XANAX 0.25
Reverse side: Scored
Brand: Xanax
Active ingredients:
Alprazolam 0.25 mg
Use: See page 231
Mfr: Upjohn Company

Imprint: 14 01
Reverse side: SEARLE
Brand: Anavar
Active ingredients:
Oxandrolone 2.5 mg
Use: See page 274
Mfr: Searle Pharmaceuticals

Imprint: 11 11
Reverse side: GYNEX
Brand: Oxandrin
Active ingredients:
Oxandrolone 2.5 mg
Use: See page 274
Mfr: Gynex Pharmaceuticals

Imprint: C-C 232
Reverse side: Scored
Brand: Generic
Active ingredients:
Phentermine HCl 37.5 mg
Use: See page 285
Mfr: Camall Company

Imprint: HALCION 0.125
Reverse side: None
Brand: Halcion
Active ingredients:
Triazolam 0.125 mg
Use: See page 293
Mfr: Upjohn Company

Imprint: MI 30
Reverse side: P F
Brand: MSIR 30
Active ingredients:
Morphine Sulfate 30 mg
Use: See page 273
Mfr: Purdue Frederick Company

Imprint: Lilly J73
Reverse side: Scored
Brand: Generic
Active ingredients:
Methyltestosterone 10 mg
Use: See page 271
Mfr: Eli Lilly and Company

Imprint: PD 141
Reverse side: 2
Brand: Generic
Active ingredients:
Diazepam 2 mg
Use: See page 245
Mfr: Parke-Davis

Imprint: BP 956
Reverse side: None
Brand: Android
Active ingredients:
Methyltestosterone 5 mg
Use: See page 271
Mfr: ICN Pharmaceuticals

Imprint: XANAX
Reverse side: 2
Brand: Xanax
Active ingredients:
Alprazolam 2 mg
Use: See page 231
Mfr: Upjohn Company

Imprint: C-C 135
Reverse side: Scored
Brand: Generic
Active ingredients:
Phendimetrazine Tartrate 35 mg
Use: See page 282
Mfr: Camall Company

Imprint: 71 71
Reverse side: LEMMON
Brand: Statobex
Active ingredients:
Phendimetrazine Tartrate 35 mg
Use: See page 282
Mfr: Lemmon Company

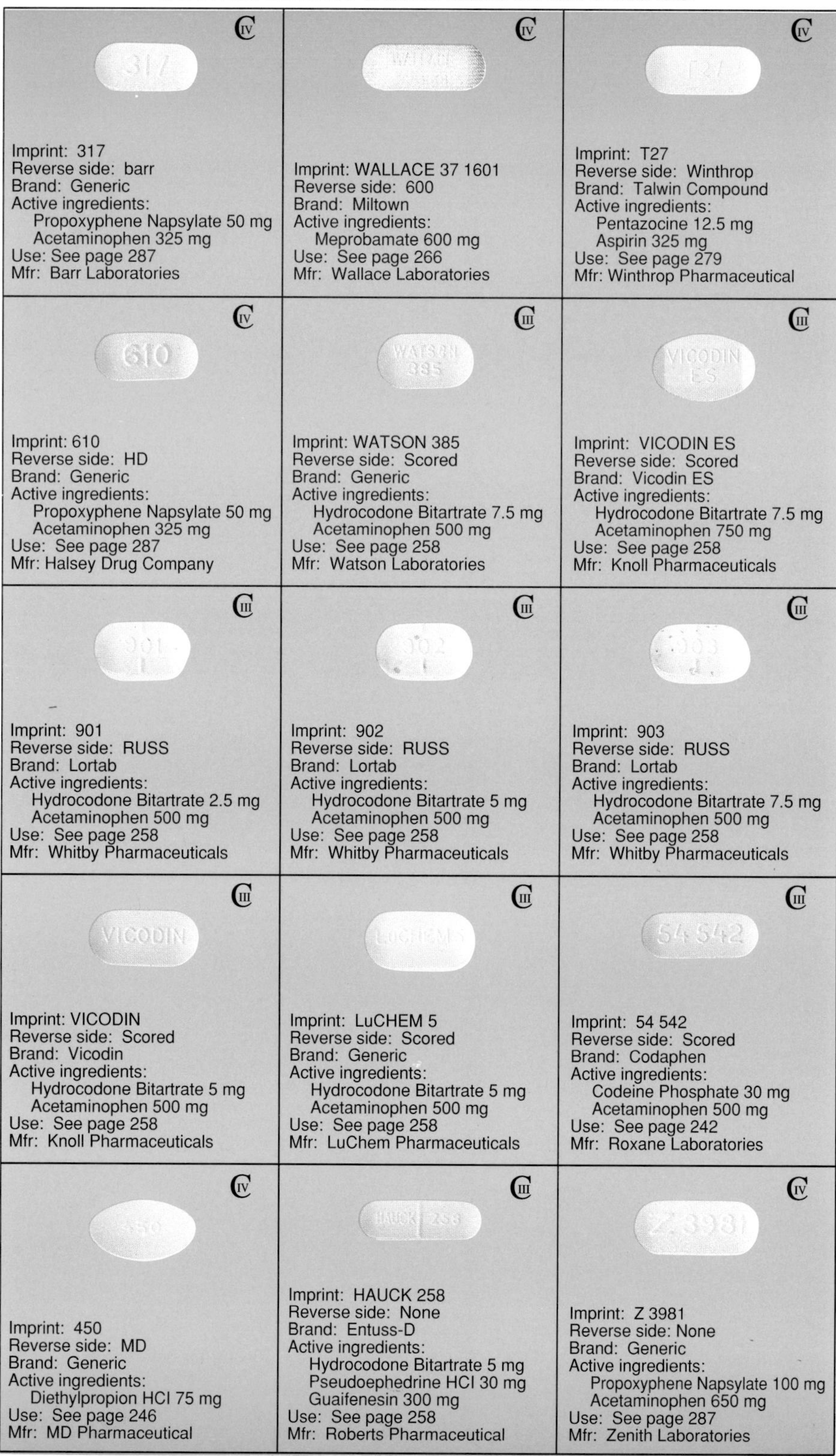
CIV
317
Imprint: 317
Reverse side: barr
Brand: Generic
Active ingredients:
Propoxyphene Napsylate 50 mg
Acetaminophen 325 mg
Use: See page 287
Mfr: Barr Laboratories
CIV
Imprint: WALLACE 37 1601
Reverse side: 600
Brand: Miltown
Active ingredients:
Meprobamate 600 mg
Use: See page 266
Mfr: Wallace Laboratories
CIV
T27
Imprint: T27
Reverse side: Winthrop
Brand: Talwin Compound
Active ingredients:
Pentazocine 12.5 mg
Aspirin 325 mg
Use: See page 279
Mfr: Winthrop Pharmaceutical
CIV
610
Imprint: 610
Reverse side: HD
Brand: Generic
Active ingredients:
Propoxyphene Napsylate 50 mg
Acetaminophen 325 mg
Use: See page 287
Mfr: Halsey Drug Company
CIII
WATSON 385
Imprint: WATSON 385
Reverse side: Scored
Brand: Generic
Active ingredients:
Hydrocodone Bitartrate 7.5 mg
Acetaminophen 500 mg
Use: See page 258
Mfr: Watson Laboratories
CIII
VICODIN ES
Imprint: VICODIN ES
Reverse side: Scored
Brand: Vicodin ES
Active ingredients:
Hydrocodone Bitartrate 7.5 mg
Acetaminophen 750 mg
Use: See page 258
Mfr: Knoll Pharmaceuticals
CIII
Imprint: 901
Reverse side: RUSS
Brand: Lortab
Active ingredients:
Hydrocodone Bitartrate 2.5 mg
Acetaminophen 500 mg
Use: See page 258
Mfr: Whitby Pharmaceuticals
CIII
Imprint: 902
Reverse side: RUSS
Brand: Lortab
Active ingredients:
Hydrocodone Bitartrate 5 mg
Acetaminophen 500 mg
Use: See page 258
Mfr: Whitby Pharmaceuticals
CIII
Imprint: 903
Reverse side: RUSS
Brand: Lortab
Active ingredients:
Hydrocodone Bitartrate 7.5 mg
Acetaminophen 500 mg
Use: See page 258
Mfr: Whitby Pharmaceuticals
CIII
VICODIN
Imprint: VICODIN
Reverse side: Scored
Brand: Vicodin
Active ingredients:
Hydrocodone Bitartrate 5 mg
Acetaminophen 500 mg
Use: See page 258
Mfr: Knoll Pharmaceuticals
CIII
Imprint: LuCHEM 5
Reverse side: Scored
Brand: Generic
Active ingredients:
Hydrocodone Bitartrate 5 mg
Acetaminophen 500 mg
Use: See page 258
Mfr: LuChem Pharmaceuticals
CIII
54 542
Imprint: 54 542
Reverse side: Scored
Brand: Codaphen
Active ingredients:
Codeine Phosphate 30 mg
Acetaminophen 500 mg
Use: See page 242
Mfr: Roxane Laboratories
CIV
Imprint: 450
Reverse side: MD
Brand: Generic
Active ingredients:
Diethylpropion HCl 75 mg
Use: See page 246
Mfr: MD Pharmaceutical
CIII
Imprint: HAUCK 258
Reverse side: None
Brand: Entuss-D
Active ingredients:
Hydrocodone Bitartrate 5 mg
Pseudoephedrine HCl 30 mg
Guaifenesin 300 mg
Use: See page 258
Mfr: Roberts Pharmaceutical
CIV
Z 3981
Imprint: Z 3981
Reverse side: None
Brand: Generic
Active ingredients:
Propoxyphene Napsylate 100 mg
Acetaminophen 650 mg
Use: See page 287
Mfr: Zenith Laboratories

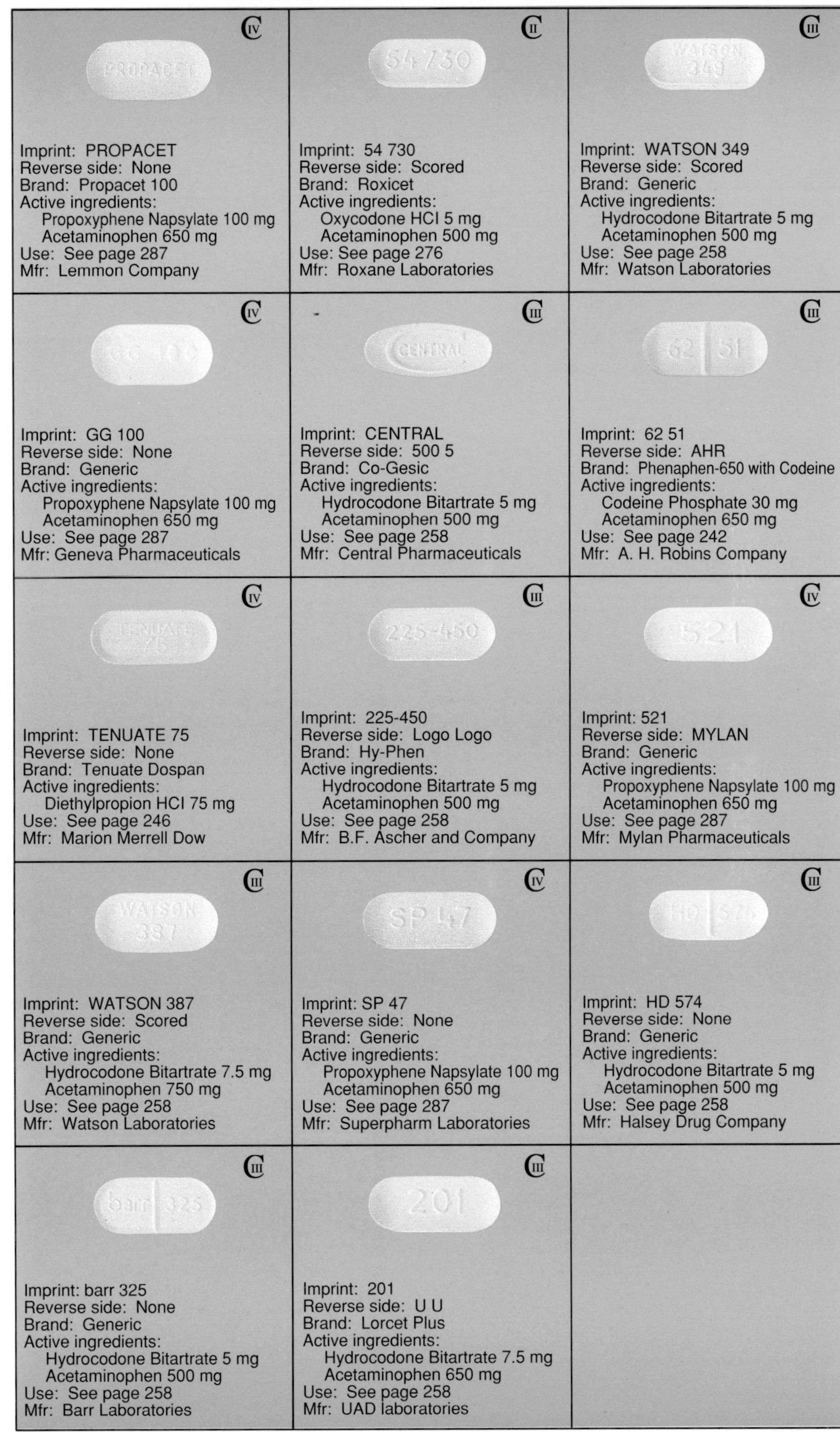

CIV

Imprint: PROPACET
Reverse side: None
Brand: Propacet 100
Active ingredients:
Propoxyphene Napsylate 100 mg
Acetaminophen 650 mg
Use: See page 287
Mfr: Lemmon Company

CII

Imprint: 54 730
Reverse side: Scored
Brand: Roxicet
Active ingredients:
Oxycodone HCl 5 mg
Acetaminophen 500 mg
Use: See page 276
Mfr: Roxane Laboratories

CIII

Imprint: WATSON 349
Reverse side: Scored
Brand: Generic
Active ingredients:
Hydrocodone Bitartrate 5 mg
Acetaminophen 500 mg
Use: See page 258
Mfr: Watson Laboratories

CIV

Imprint: GG 100
Reverse side: None
Brand: Generic
Active ingredients:
Propoxyphene Napsylate 100 mg
Acetaminophen 650 mg
Use: See page 287
Mfr: Geneva Pharmaceuticals

CIII

Imprint: CENTRAL
Reverse side: 500 5
Brand: Co-Gesic
Active ingredients:
Hydrocodone Bitartrate 5 mg
Acetaminophen 500 mg
Use: See page 258
Mfr: Central Pharmaceuticals

CIII

Imprint: 62 51
Reverse side: AHR
Brand: Phenaphen-650 with Codeine
Active ingredients:
Codeine Phosphate 30 mg
Acetaminophen 650 mg
Use: See page 242
Mfr: A. H. Robins Company

CIV

Imprint: TENUATE 75
Reverse side: None
Brand: Tenuate Dospan
Active ingredients:
Diethylpropion HCl 75 mg
Use: See page 246
Mfr: Marion Merrell Dow

CIII

Imprint: 225-450
Reverse side: Logo Logo
Brand: Hy-Phen
Active ingredients:
Hydrocodone Bitartrate 5 mg
Acetaminophen 500 mg
Use: See page 258
Mfr: B.F. Ascher and Company

CIV

Imprint: 521
Reverse side: MYLAN
Brand: Generic
Active ingredients:
Propoxyphene Napsylate 100 mg
Acetaminophen 650 mg
Use: See page 287
Mfr: Mylan Pharmaceuticals

CIII

Imprint: WATSON 387
Reverse side: Scored
Brand: Generic
Active ingredients:
Hydrocodone Bitartrate 7.5 mg
Acetaminophen 750 mg
Use: See page 258
Mfr: Watson Laboratories

CIV

Imprint: SP 47
Reverse side: None
Brand: Generic
Active ingredients:
Propoxyphene Napsylate 100 mg
Acetaminophen 650 mg
Use: See page 287
Mfr: Superpharm Laboratories

CIII

Imprint: HD 574
Reverse side: None
Brand: Generic
Active ingredients:
Hydrocodone Bitartrate 5 mg
Acetaminophen 500 mg
Use: See page 258
Mfr: Halsey Drug Company

CIII

Imprint: barr 325
Reverse side: None
Brand: Generic
Active ingredients:
Hydrocodone Bitartrate 5 mg
Acetaminophen 500 mg
Use: See page 258
Mfr: Barr Laboratories

CIII

Imprint: 201
Reverse side: U U
Brand: Lorcet Plus
Active ingredients:
Hydrocodone Bitartrate 7.5 mg
Acetaminophen 650 mg
Use: See page 258
Mfr: UAD laboratories

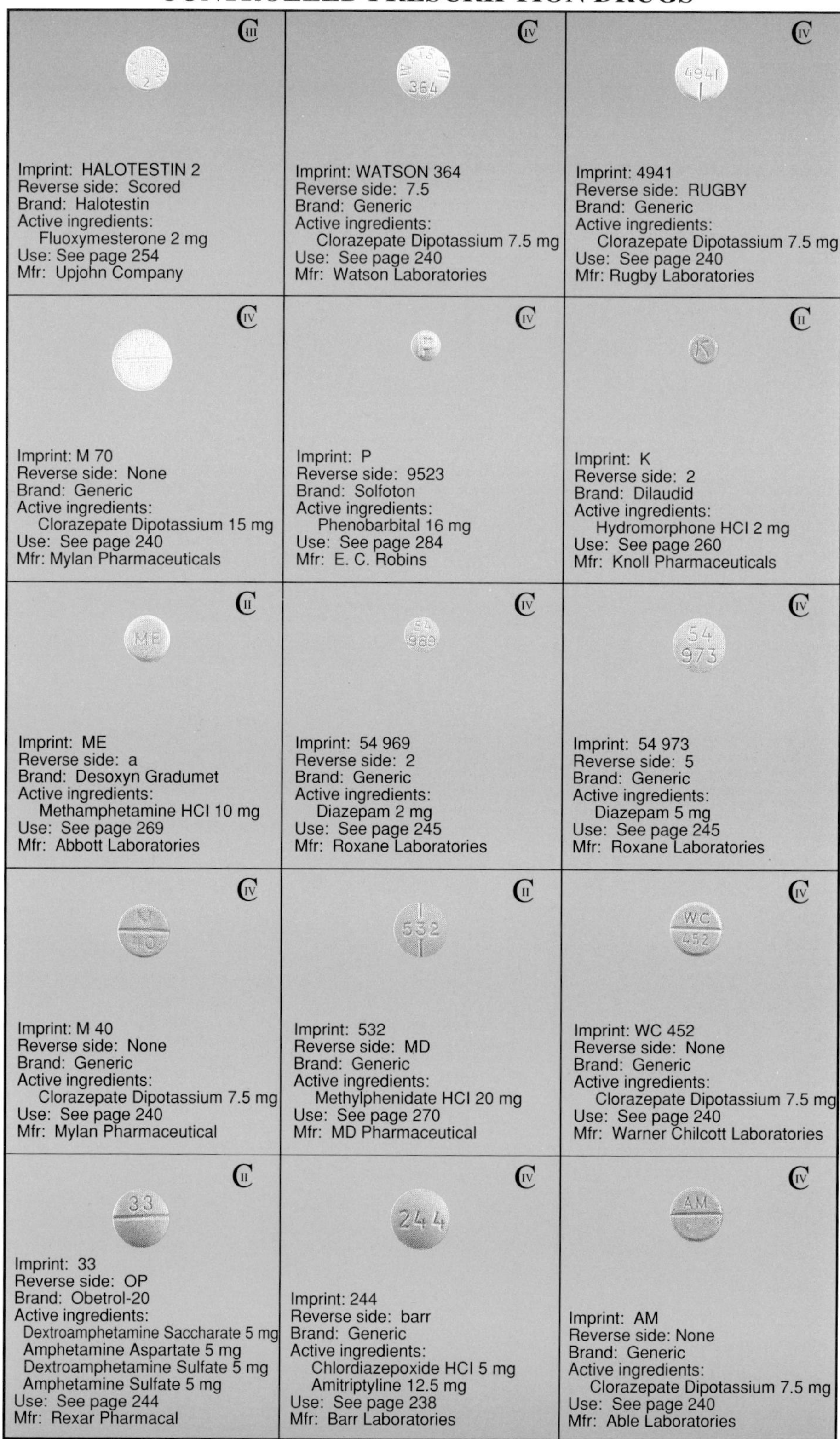

CIII
Imprint: HALOTESTIN 2
Reverse side: Scored
Brand: Halotestin
Active ingredients:
Fluoxymesterone 2 mg
Use: See page 254
Mfr: Upjohn Company

CIV
Imprint: WATSON 364
Reverse side: 7.5
Brand: Generic
Active ingredients:
Clorazepate Dipotassium 7.5 mg
Use: See page 240
Mfr: Watson Laboratories

CIV
Imprint: 4941
Reverse side: RUGBY
Brand: Generic
Active ingredients:
Clorazepate Dipotassium 7.5 mg
Use: See page 240
Mfr: Rugby Laboratories

CIV
Imprint: M 70
Reverse side: None
Brand: Generic
Active ingredients:
Clorazepate Dipotassium 15 mg
Use: See page 240
Mfr: Mylan Pharmaceuticals

CIV
Imprint: P
Reverse side: 9523
Brand: Solfoton
Active ingredients:
Phenobarbital 16 mg
Use: See page 284
Mfr: E. C. Robins

CII
Imprint: K
Reverse side: 2
Brand: Dilaudid
Active ingredients:
Hydromorphone HCl 2 mg
Use: See page 260
Mfr: Knoll Pharmaceuticals

CII
Imprint: ME
Reverse side: a
Brand: Desoxyn Gradumet
Active ingredients:
Methamphetamine HCl 10 mg
Use: See page 269
Mfr: Abbott Laboratories

CIV
Imprint: 54 969
Reverse side: 2
Brand: Generic
Active ingredients:
Diazepam 2 mg
Use: See page 245
Mfr: Roxane Laboratories

CIV
Imprint: 54 973
Reverse side: 5
Brand: Generic
Active ingredients:
Diazepam 5 mg
Use: See page 245
Mfr: Roxane Laboratories

CIV
Imprint: M 40
Reverse side: None
Brand: Generic
Active ingredients:
Clorazepate Dipotassium 7.5 mg
Use: See page 240
Mfr: Mylan Pharmaceutical

CII
Imprint: 532
Reverse side: MD
Brand: Generic
Active ingredients:
Methylphenidate HCl 20 mg
Use: See page 270
Mfr: MD Pharmaceutical

CIV
Imprint: WC 452
Reverse side: None
Brand: Generic
Active ingredients:
Clorazepate Dipotassium 7.5 mg
Use: See page 240
Mfr: Warner Chilcott Laboratories

CII
Imprint: 33
Reverse side: OP
Brand: Obetrol-20
Active ingredients:
Dextroamphetamine Saccharate 5 mg
Amphetamine Aspartate 5 mg
Dextroamphetamine Sulfate 5 mg
Amphetamine Sulfate 5 mg
Use: See page 244
Mfr: Rexar Pharmacal

CIV
Imprint: 244
Reverse side: barr
Brand: Generic
Active ingredients:
Chlordiazepoxide HCl 5 mg
Amitriptyline 12.5 mg
Use: See page 238
Mfr: Barr Laboratories

CIV
Imprint: AM
Reverse side: None
Brand: Generic
Active ingredients:
Clorazepate Dipotassium 7.5 mg
Use: See page 240
Mfr: Able Laboratories

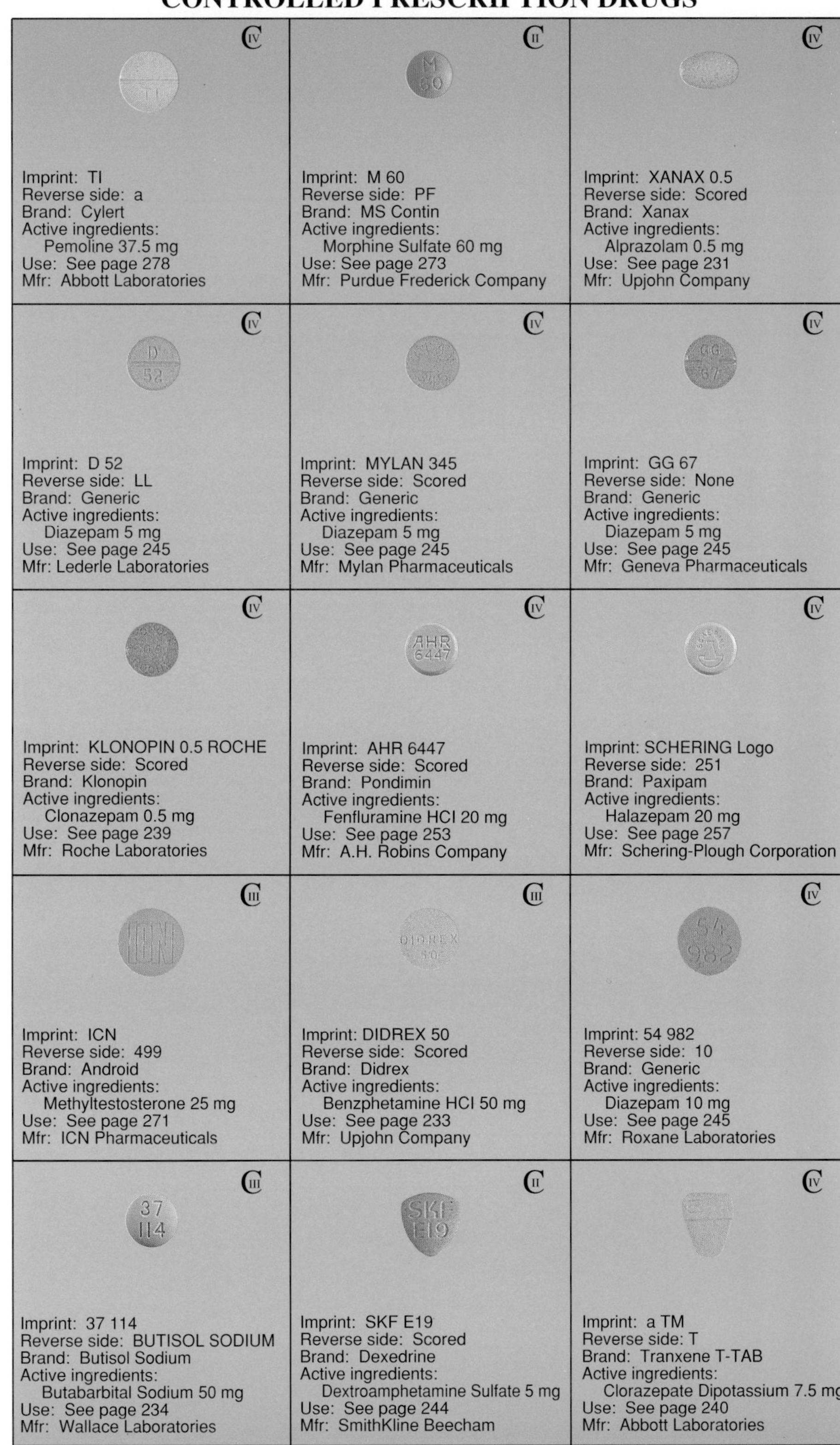

C IV Imprint: TI Reverse side: a Brand: Cylert Active ingredients: Pemoline 37.5 mg Use: See page 278 Mfr: Abbott Laboratories	C II Imprint: M 60 Reverse side: PF Brand: MS Contin Active ingredients: Morphine Sulfate 60 mg Use: See page 273 Mfr: Purdue Frederick Company	C IV Imprint: XANAX 0.5 Reverse side: Scored Brand: Xanax Active ingredients: Alprazolam 0.5 mg Use: See page 231 Mfr: Upjohn Company
C IV Imprint: D 52 Reverse side: LL Brand: Generic Active ingredients: Diazepam 5 mg Use: See page 245 Mfr: Lederle Laboratories	C IV Imprint: MYLAN 345 Reverse side: Scored Brand: Generic Active ingredients: Diazepam 5 mg Use: See page 245 Mfr: Mylan Pharmaceuticals	C IV Imprint: GG 67 Reverse side: None Brand: Generic Active ingredients: Diazepam 5 mg Use: See page 245 Mfr: Geneva Pharmaceuticals
C IV Imprint: KLONOPIN 0.5 ROCHE Reverse side: Scored Brand: Klonopin Active ingredients: Clonazepam 0.5 mg Use: See page 239 Mfr: Roche Laboratories	C IV Imprint: AHR 6447 Reverse side: Scored Brand: Pondimin Active ingredients: Fenfluramine HCl 20 mg Use: See page 253 Mfr: A.H. Robins Company	C IV Imprint: SCHERING Logo Reverse side: 251 Brand: Paxipam Active ingredients: Halazepam 20 mg Use: See page 257 Mfr: Schering-Plough Corporation
C III Imprint: ICN Reverse side: 499 Brand: Android Active ingredients: Methyltestosterone 25 mg Use: See page 271 Mfr: ICN Pharmaceuticals	C III Imprint: DIDREX 50 Reverse side: Scored Brand: Didrex Active ingredients: Benzphetamine HCl 50 mg Use: See page 233 Mfr: Upjohn Company	C IV Imprint: 54 982 Reverse side: 10 Brand: Generic Active ingredients: Diazepam 10 mg Use: See page 245 Mfr: Roxane Laboratories
C III Imprint: 37 114 Reverse side: BUTISOL SODIUM Brand: Butisol Sodium Active ingredients: Butabarbital Sodium 50 mg Use: See page 234 Mfr: Wallace Laboratories	C II Imprint: SKF E19 Reverse side: Scored Brand: Dexedrine Active ingredients: Dextroamphetamine Sulfate 5 mg Use: See page 244 Mfr: SmithKline Beecham	C IV Imprint: a TM Reverse side: T Brand: Tranxene T-TAB Active ingredients: Clorazepate Dipotassium 7.5 mg Use: See page 240 Mfr: Abbott Laboratories

CONTROLLED PRESCRIPTION DRUGS

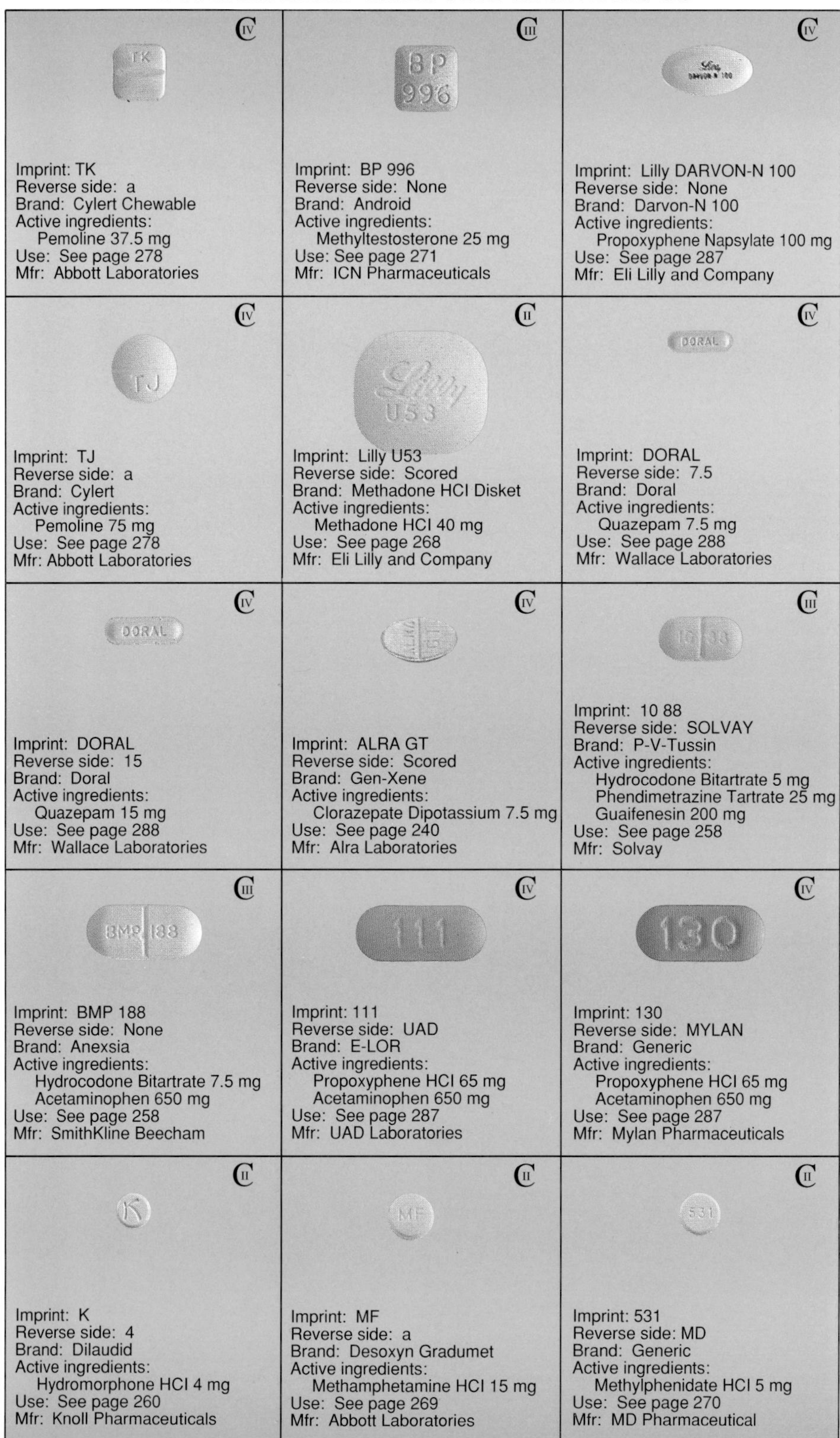

C-IV
Imprint: TK
Reverse side: a
Brand: Cylert Chewable
Active ingredients:
Pemoline 37.5 mg
Use: See page 278
Mfr: Abbott Laboratories

C-III
Imprint: BP 996
Reverse side: None
Brand: Android
Active ingredients:
Methyltestosterone 25 mg
Use: See page 271
Mfr: ICN Pharmaceuticals

C-IV
Imprint: Lilly DARVON-N 100
Reverse side: None
Brand: Darvon-N 100
Active ingredients:
Propoxyphene Napsylate 100 mg
Use: See page 287
Mfr: Eli Lilly and Company

C-IV
Imprint: TJ
Reverse side: a
Brand: Cylert
Active ingredients:
Pemoline 75 mg
Use: See page 278
Mfr: Abbott Laboratories

C-II
Imprint: Lilly U53
Reverse side: Scored
Brand: Methadone HCl Disket
Active ingredients:
Methadone HCl 40 mg
Use: See page 268
Mfr: Eli Lilly and Company

C-IV
Imprint: DORAL
Reverse side: 7.5
Brand: Doral
Active ingredients:
Quazepam 7.5 mg
Use: See page 288
Mfr: Wallace Laboratories

C-IV
Imprint: DORAL
Reverse side: 15
Brand: Doral
Active ingredients:
Quazepam 15 mg
Use: See page 288
Mfr: Wallace Laboratories

C-IV
Imprint: ALRA GT
Reverse side: Scored
Brand: Gen-Xene
Active ingredients:
Clorazepate Dipotassium 7.5 mg
Use: See page 240
Mfr: Alra Laboratories

C-III
Imprint: 10 88
Reverse side: SOLVAY
Brand: P-V-Tussin
Active ingredients:
Hydrocodone Bitartrate 5 mg
Phendimetrazine Tartrate 25 mg
Guaifenesin 200 mg
Use: See page 258
Mfr: Solvay

C-III
Imprint: BMP 188
Reverse side: None
Brand: Anexsia
Active ingredients:
Hydrocodone Bitartrate 7.5 mg
Acetaminophen 650 mg
Use: See page 258
Mfr: SmithKline Beecham

C-IV
Imprint: 111
Reverse side: UAD
Brand: E-LOR
Active ingredients:
Propoxyphene HCl 65 mg
Acetaminophen 650 mg
Use: See page 287
Mfr: UAD Laboratories

C-IV
Imprint: 130
Reverse side: MYLAN
Brand: Generic
Active ingredients:
Propoxyphene HCl 65 mg
Acetaminophen 650 mg
Use: See page 287
Mfr: Mylan Pharmaceuticals

C-II
Imprint: K
Reverse side: 4
Brand: Dilaudid
Active ingredients:
Hydromorphone HCl 4 mg
Use: See page 260
Mfr: Knoll Pharmaceuticals

C-II
Imprint: MF
Reverse side: a
Brand: Desoxyn Gradumet
Active ingredients:
Methamphetamine HCl 15 mg
Use: See page 269
Mfr: Abbott Laboratories

C-II
Imprint: 531
Reverse side: MD
Brand: Generic
Active ingredients:
Methylphenidate HCl 5 mg
Use: See page 270
Mfr: MD Pharmaceutical

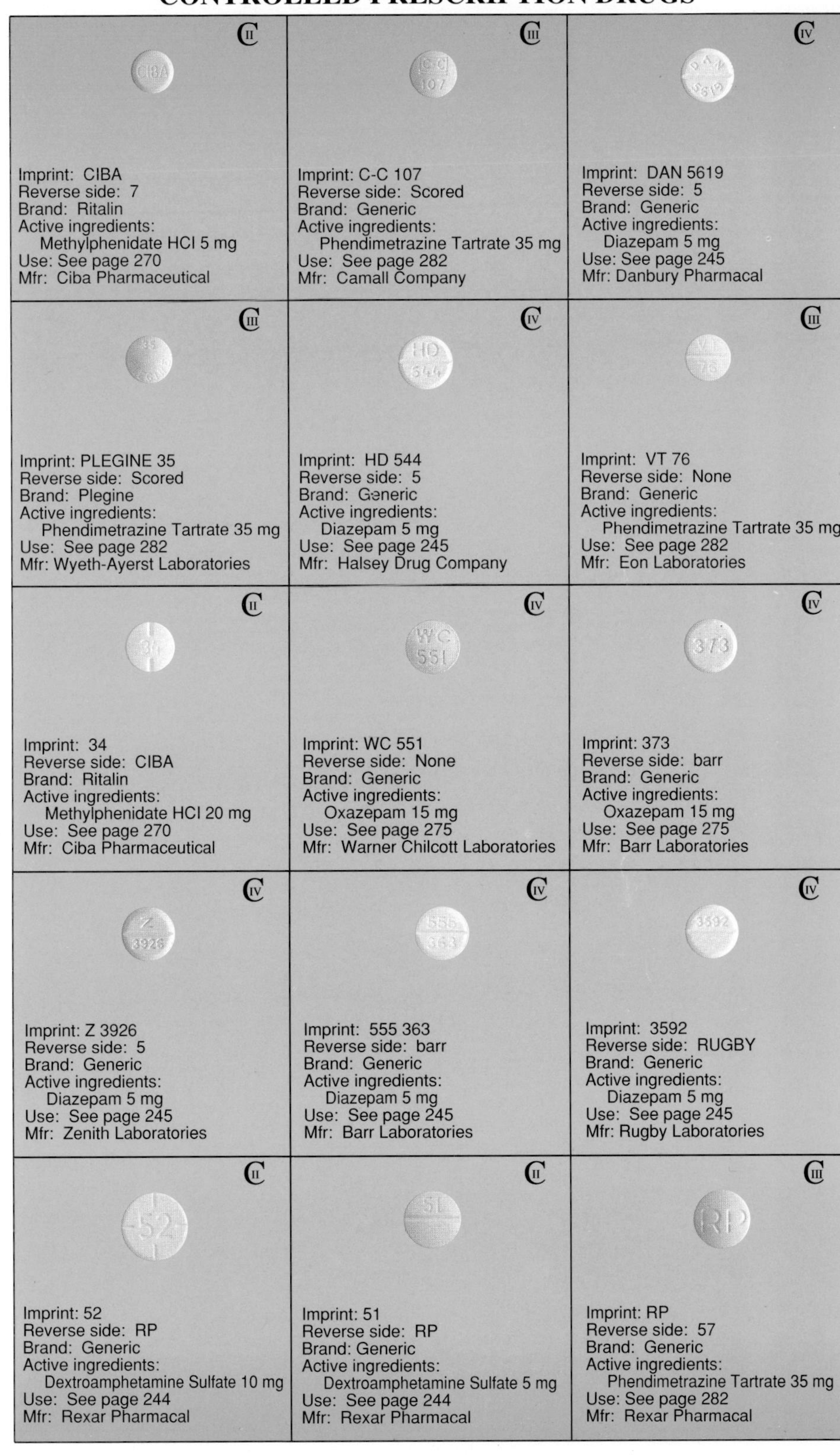

CII

Imprint: CIBA
Reverse side: 7
Brand: Ritalin
Active ingredients:
Methylphenidate HCl 5 mg
Use: See page 270
Mfr: Ciba Pharmaceutical

CIII

Imprint: C-C 107
Reverse side: Scored
Brand: Generic
Active ingredients:
Phendimetrazine Tartrate 35 mg
Use: See page 282
Mfr: Camall Company

CIV

Imprint: DAN 5619
Reverse side: 5
Brand: Generic
Active ingredients:
Diazepam 5 mg
Use: See page 245
Mfr: Danbury Pharmacal

CIII

Imprint: PLEGINE 35
Reverse side: Scored
Brand: Plegine
Active ingredients:
Phendimetrazine Tartrate 35 mg
Use: See page 282
Mfr: Wyeth-Ayerst Laboratories

CIV

Imprint: HD 544
Reverse side: 5
Brand: Generic
Active ingredients:
Diazepam 5 mg
Use: See page 245
Mfr: Halsey Drug Company

CIII

Imprint: VT 76
Reverse side: None
Brand: Generic
Active ingredients:
Phendimetrazine Tartrate 35 mg
Use: See page 282
Mfr: Eon Laboratories

CII

Imprint: 34
Reverse side: CIBA
Brand: Ritalin
Active ingredients:
Methylphenidate HCl 20 mg
Use: See page 270
Mfr: Ciba Pharmaceutical

CIV

Imprint: WC 551
Reverse side: None
Brand: Generic
Active ingredients:
Oxazepam 15 mg
Use: See page 275
Mfr: Warner Chilcott Laboratories

CIV

Imprint: 373
Reverse side: barr
Brand: Generic
Active ingredients:
Oxazepam 15 mg
Use: See page 275
Mfr: Barr Laboratories

CIV

Imprint: Z 3926
Reverse side: 5
Brand: Generic
Active ingredients:
Diazepam 5 mg
Use: See page 245
Mfr: Zenith Laboratories

CIV

Imprint: 555 363
Reverse side: barr
Brand: Generic
Active ingredients:
Diazepam 5 mg
Use: See page 245
Mfr: Barr Laboratories

CIV

Imprint: 3592
Reverse side: RUGBY
Brand: Generic
Active ingredients:
Diazepam 5 mg
Use: See page 245
Mfr: Rugby Laboratories

CII

Imprint: 52
Reverse side: RP
Brand: Generic
Active ingredients:
Dextroamphetamine Sulfate 10 mg
Use: See page 244
Mfr: Rexar Pharmacal

CII

Imprint: 51
Reverse side: RP
Brand: Generic
Active ingredients:
Dextroamphetamine Sulfate 5 mg
Use: See page 244
Mfr: Rexar Pharmacal

CIII

Imprint: RP
Reverse side: 57
Brand: Generic
Active ingredients:
Phendimetrazine Tartrate 35 mg
Use: See page 282
Mfr: Rexar Pharmacal

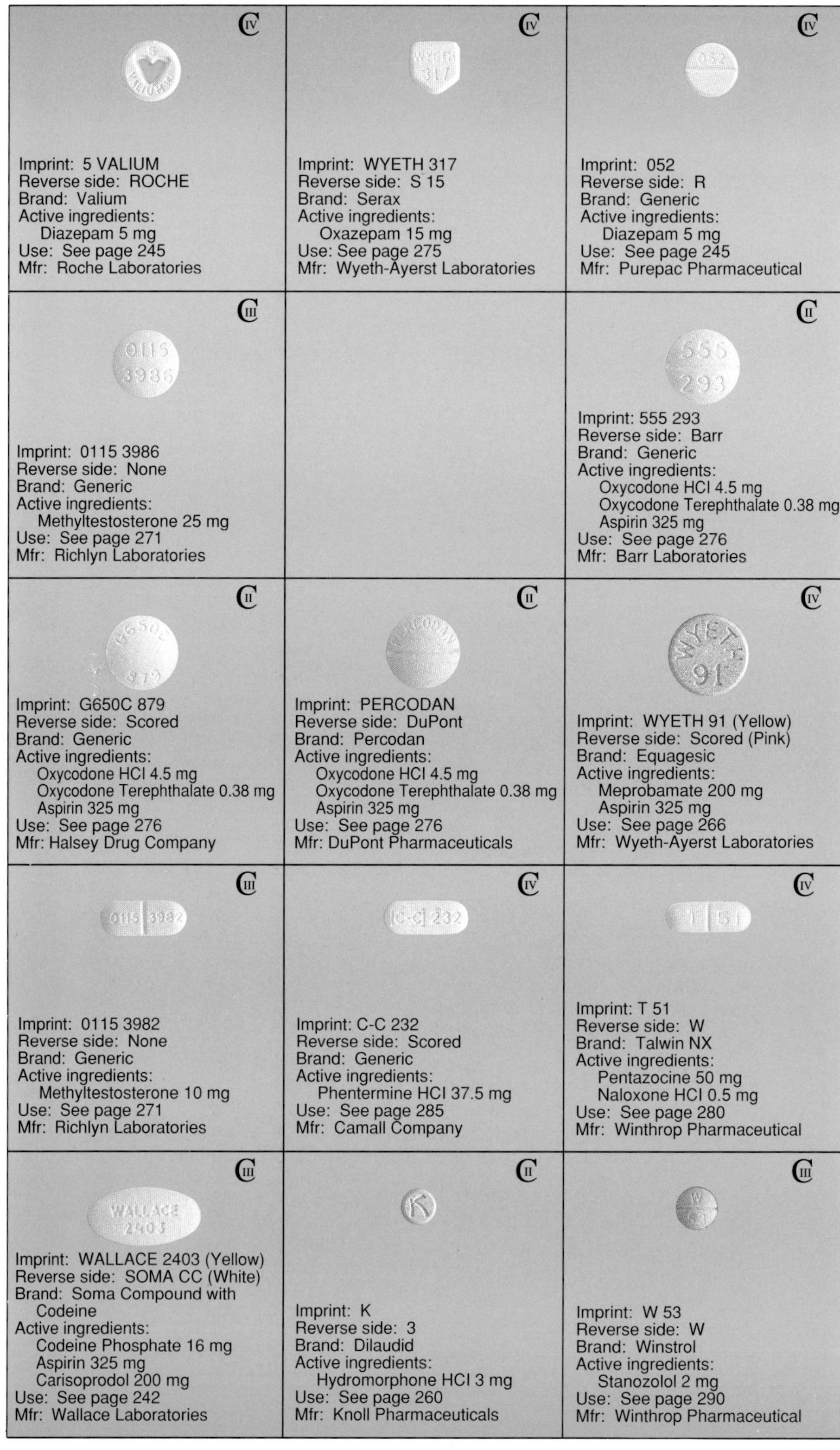

CIV
Imprint: 5 VALIUM
Reverse side: ROCHE
Brand: Valium
Active ingredients:
Diazepam 5 mg
Use: See page 245
Mfr: Roche Laboratories

CIV
Imprint: WYETH 317
Reverse side: S 15
Brand: Serax
Active ingredients:
Oxazepam 15 mg
Use: See page 275
Mfr: Wyeth-Ayerst Laboratories

CIV
Imprint: 052
Reverse side: R
Brand: Generic
Active ingredients:
Diazepam 5 mg
Use: See page 245
Mfr: Purepac Pharmaceutical

CIII
Imprint: 0115 3986
Reverse side: None
Brand: Generic
Active ingredients:
Methyltestosterone 25 mg
Use: See page 271
Mfr: Richlyn Laboratories

CII
Imprint: 555 293
Reverse side: Barr
Brand: Generic
Active ingredients:
Oxycodone HCl 4.5 mg
Oxycodone Terephthalate 0.38 mg
Aspirin 325 mg
Use: See page 276
Mfr: Barr Laboratories

CII
Imprint: G650C 879
Reverse side: Scored
Brand: Generic
Active ingredients:
Oxycodone HCl 4.5 mg
Oxycodone Terephthalate 0.38 mg
Aspirin 325 mg
Use: See page 276
Mfr: Halsey Drug Company

CII
Imprint: PERCODAN
Reverse side: DuPont
Brand: Percodan
Active ingredients:
Oxycodone HCl 4.5 mg
Oxycodone Terephthalate 0.38 mg
Aspirin 325 mg
Use: See page 276
Mfr: DuPont Pharmaceuticals

CIV
Imprint: WYETH 91 (Yellow)
Reverse side: Scored (Pink)
Brand: Equagesic
Active ingredients:
Meprobamate 200 mg
Aspirin 325 mg
Use: See page 266
Mfr: Wyeth-Ayerst Laboratories

CIII
Imprint: 0115 3982
Reverse side: None
Brand: Generic
Active ingredients:
Methyltestosterone 10 mg
Use: See page 271
Mfr: Richlyn Laboratories

CIV
Imprint: C-C 232
Reverse side: Scored
Brand: Generic
Active ingredients:
Phentermine HCl 37.5 mg
Use: See page 285
Mfr: Camall Company

CIV
Imprint: T 51
Reverse side: W
Brand: Talwin NX
Active ingredients:
Pentazocine 50 mg
Naloxone HCl 0.5 mg
Use: See page 280
Mfr: Winthrop Pharmaceutical

CIII
Imprint: WALLACE 2403 (Yellow)
Reverse side: SOMA CC (White)
Brand: Soma Compound with Codeine
Active ingredients:
Codeine Phosphate 16 mg
Aspirin 325 mg
Carisoprodol 200 mg
Use: See page 242
Mfr: Wallace Laboratories

CII
Imprint: K
Reverse side: 3
Brand: Dilaudid
Active ingredients:
Hydromorphone HCl 3 mg
Use: See page 260
Mfr: Knoll Pharmaceuticals

CIII
Imprint: W 53
Reverse side: W
Brand: Winstrol
Active ingredients:
Stanozolol 2 mg
Use: See page 290
Mfr: Winthrop Pharmaceutical

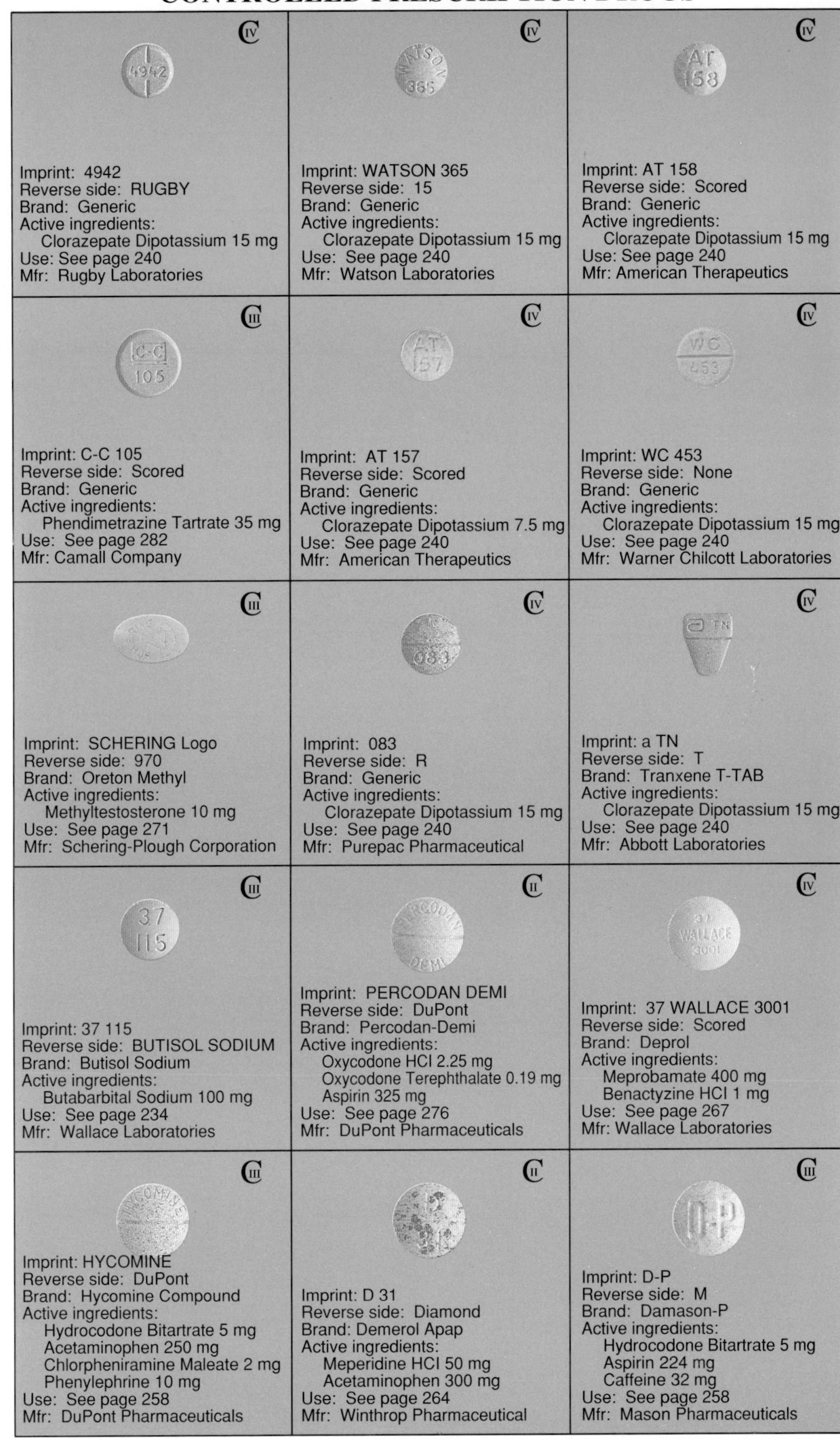

C-IV
Imprint: 4942
Reverse side: RUGBY
Brand: Generic
Active ingredients:
Clorazepate Dipotassium 15 mg
Use: See page 240
Mfr: Rugby Laboratories

C-IV
Imprint: WATSON 365
Reverse side: 15
Brand: Generic
Active ingredients:
Clorazepate Dipotassium 15 mg
Use: See page 240
Mfr: Watson Laboratories

C-IV
Imprint: AT 158
Reverse side: Scored
Brand: Generic
Active ingredients:
Clorazepate Dipotassium 15 mg
Use: See page 240
Mfr: American Therapeutics

C-III
Imprint: C-C 105
Reverse side: Scored
Brand: Generic
Active ingredients:
Phendimetrazine Tartrate 35 mg
Use: See page 282
Mfr: Camall Company

C-IV
Imprint: AT 157
Reverse side: Scored
Brand: Generic
Active ingredients:
Clorazepate Dipotassium 7.5 mg
Use: See page 240
Mfr: American Therapeutics

C-IV
Imprint: WC 453
Reverse side: None
Brand: Generic
Active ingredients:
Clorazepate Dipotassium 15 mg
Use: See page 240
Mfr: Warner Chilcott Laboratories

C-III
Imprint: SCHERING Logo
Reverse side: 970
Brand: Oreton Methyl
Active ingredients:
Methyltestosterone 10 mg
Use: See page 271
Mfr: Schering-Plough Corporation

C-IV
Imprint: 083
Reverse side: R
Brand: Generic
Active ingredients:
Clorazepate Dipotassium 15 mg
Use: See page 240
Mfr: Purepac Pharmaceutical

C-IV
Imprint: a TN
Reverse side: T
Brand: Tranxene T-TAB
Active ingredients:
Clorazepate Dipotassium 15 mg
Use: See page 240
Mfr: Abbott Laboratories

C-III
Imprint: 37 115
Reverse side: BUTISOL SODIUM
Brand: Butisol Sodium
Active ingredients:
Butabarbital Sodium 100 mg
Use: See page 234
Mfr: Wallace Laboratories

C-II
Imprint: PERCODAN DEMI
Reverse side: DuPont
Brand: Percodan-Demi
Active ingredients:
Oxycodone HCl 2.25 mg
Oxycodone Terephthalate 0.19 mg
Aspirin 325 mg
Use: See page 276
Mfr: DuPont Pharmaceuticals

C-IV
Imprint: 37 WALLACE 3001
Reverse side: Scored
Brand: Deprol
Active ingredients:
Meprobamate 400 mg
Benactyzine HCl 1 mg
Use: See page 267
Mfr: Wallace Laboratories

C-III
Imprint: HYCOMINE
Reverse side: DuPont
Brand: Hycomine Compound
Active ingredients:
Hydrocodone Bitartrate 5 mg
Acetaminophen 250 mg
Chlorpheniramine Maleate 2 mg
Phenylephrine 10 mg
Use: See page 258
Mfr: DuPont Pharmaceuticals

C-II
Imprint: D 31
Reverse side: Diamond
Brand: Demerol Apap
Active ingredients:
Meperidine HCl 50 mg
Acetaminophen 300 mg
Use: See page 264
Mfr: Winthrop Pharmaceutical

C-III
Imprint: D-P
Reverse side: M
Brand: Damason-P
Active ingredients:
Hydrocodone Bitartrate 5 mg
Aspirin 224 mg
Caffeine 32 mg
Use: See page 258
Mfr: Mason Pharmaceuticals

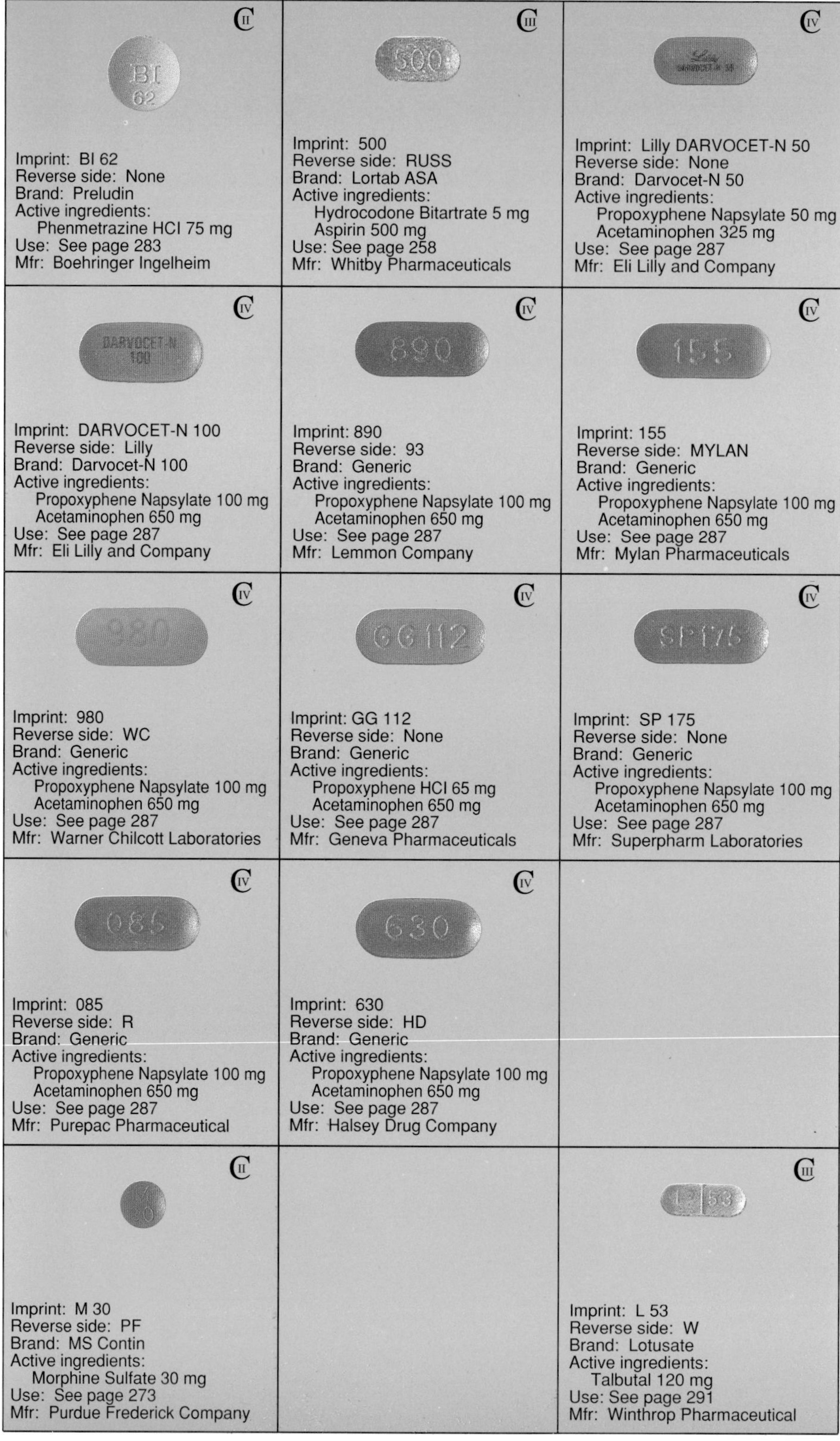

C-II
Imprint: BI 62
Reverse side: None
Brand: Preludin
Active ingredients:
Phenmetrazine HCl 75 mg
Use: See page 283
Mfr: Boehringer Ingelheim

C-III
Imprint: 500
Reverse side: RUSS
Brand: Lortab ASA
Active ingredients:
Hydrocodone Bitartrate 5 mg
Aspirin 500 mg
Use: See page 258
Mfr: Whitby Pharmaceuticals

C-IV
Imprint: Lilly DARVOCET-N 50
Reverse side: None
Brand: Darvocet-N 50
Active ingredients:
Propoxyphene Napsylate 50 mg
Acetaminophen 325 mg
Use: See page 287
Mfr: Eli Lilly and Company

C-IV
Imprint: DARVOCET-N 100
Reverse side: Lilly
Brand: Darvocet-N 100
Active ingredients:
Propoxyphene Napsylate 100 mg
Acetaminophen 650 mg
Use: See page 287
Mfr: Eli Lilly and Company

C-IV
Imprint: 890
Reverse side: 93
Brand: Generic
Active ingredients:
Propoxyphene Napsylate 100 mg
Acetaminophen 650 mg
Use: See page 287
Mfr: Lemmon Company

C-IV
Imprint: 155
Reverse side: MYLAN
Brand: Generic
Active ingredients:
Propoxyphene Napsylate 100 mg
Acetaminophen 650 mg
Use: See page 287
Mfr: Mylan Pharmaceuticals

C-IV
Imprint: 980
Reverse side: WC
Brand: Generic
Active ingredients:
Propoxyphene Napsylate 100 mg
Acetaminophen 650 mg
Use: See page 287
Mfr: Warner Chilcott Laboratories

C-IV
Imprint: GG 112
Reverse side: None
Brand: Generic
Active ingredients:
Propoxyphene HCl 65 mg
Acetaminophen 650 mg
Use: See page 287
Mfr: Geneva Pharmaceuticals

C-IV
Imprint: SP 175
Reverse side: None
Brand: Generic
Active ingredients:
Propoxyphene Napsylate 100 mg
Acetaminophen 650 mg
Use: See page 287
Mfr: Superpharm Laboratories

C-IV
Imprint: 085
Reverse side: R
Brand: Generic
Active ingredients:
Propoxyphene Napsylate 100 mg
Acetaminophen 650 mg
Use: See page 287
Mfr: Purepac Pharmaceutical

C-IV
Imprint: 630
Reverse side: HD
Brand: Generic
Active ingredients:
Propoxyphene Napsylate 100 mg
Acetaminophen 650 mg
Use: See page 287
Mfr: Halsey Drug Company

C-II
Imprint: M 30
Reverse side: PF
Brand: MS Contin
Active ingredients:
Morphine Sulfate 30 mg
Use: See page 273
Mfr: Purdue Frederick Company

C-III
Imprint: L 53
Reverse side: W
Brand: Lotusate
Active ingredients:
Talbutal 120 mg
Use: See page 291
Mfr: Winthrop Pharmaceutical

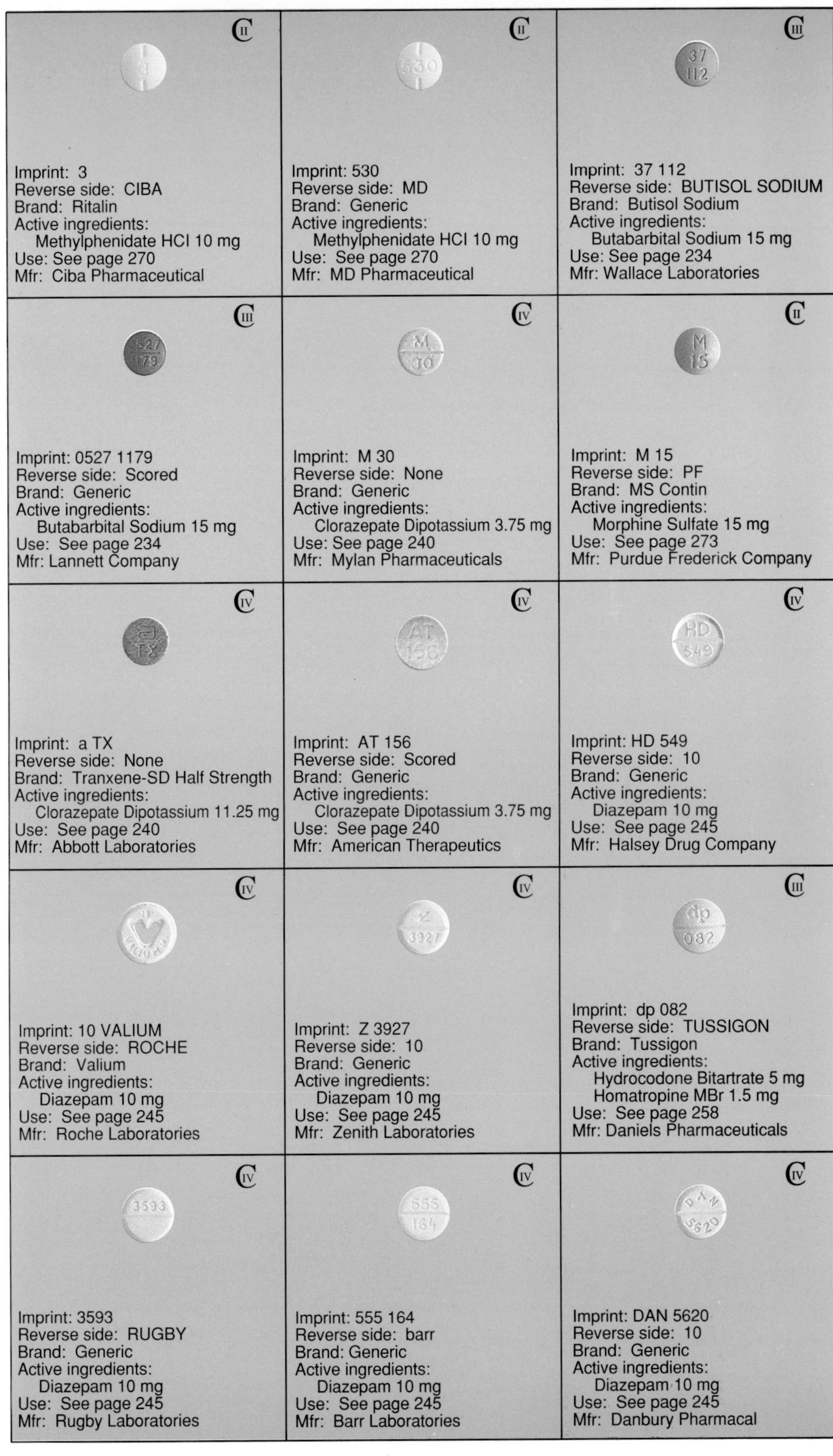

C-II Imprint: 3 Reverse side: CIBA Brand: Ritalin Active ingredients: Methylphenidate HCl 10 mg Use: See page 270 Mfr: Ciba Pharmaceutical	C-II Imprint: 530 Reverse side: MD Brand: Generic Active ingredients: Methylphenidate HCl 10 mg Use: See page 270 Mfr: MD Pharmaceutical	C-III Imprint: 37 112 Reverse side: BUTISOL SODIUM Brand: Butisol Sodium Active ingredients: Butabarbital Sodium 15 mg Use: See page 234 Mfr: Wallace Laboratories
C-III Imprint: 0527 1179 Reverse side: Scored Brand: Generic Active ingredients: Butabarbital Sodium 15 mg Use: See page 234 Mfr: Lannett Company	C-IV Imprint: M 30 Reverse side: None Brand: Generic Active ingredients: Clorazepate Dipotassium 3.75 mg Use: See page 240 Mfr: Mylan Pharmaceuticals	C-II Imprint: M 15 Reverse side: PF Brand: MS Contin Active ingredients: Morphine Sulfate 15 mg Use: See page 273 Mfr: Purdue Frederick Company
C-IV Imprint: a TX Reverse side: None Brand: Tranxene-SD Half Strength Active ingredients: Clorazepate Dipotassium 11.25 mg Use: See page 240 Mfr: Abbott Laboratories	C-IV Imprint: AT 156 Reverse side: Scored Brand: Generic Active ingredients: Clorazepate Dipotassium 3.75 mg Use: See page 240 Mfr: American Therapeutics	C-IV Imprint: HD 549 Reverse side: 10 Brand: Generic Active ingredients: Diazepam 10 mg Use: See page 245 Mfr: Halsey Drug Company
C-IV Imprint: 10 VALIUM Reverse side: ROCHE Brand: Valium Active ingredients: Diazepam 10 mg Use: See page 245 Mfr: Roche Laboratories	C-IV Imprint: Z 3927 Reverse side: 10 Brand: Generic Active ingredients: Diazepam 10 mg Use: See page 245 Mfr: Zenith Laboratories	C-III Imprint: dp 082 Reverse side: TUSSIGON Brand: Tussigon Active ingredients: Hydrocodone Bitartrate 5 mg Homatropine MBr 1.5 mg Use: See page 258 Mfr: Daniels Pharmaceuticals
C-IV Imprint: 3593 Reverse side: RUGBY Brand: Generic Active ingredients: Diazepam 10 mg Use: See page 245 Mfr: Rugby Laboratories	C-IV Imprint: 555 164 Reverse side: barr Brand: Generic Active ingredients: Diazepam 10 mg Use: See page 245 Mfr: Barr Laboratories	C-IV Imprint: DAN 5620 Reverse side: 10 Brand: Generic Active ingredients: Diazepam 10 mg Use: See page 245 Mfr: Danbury Pharmacal

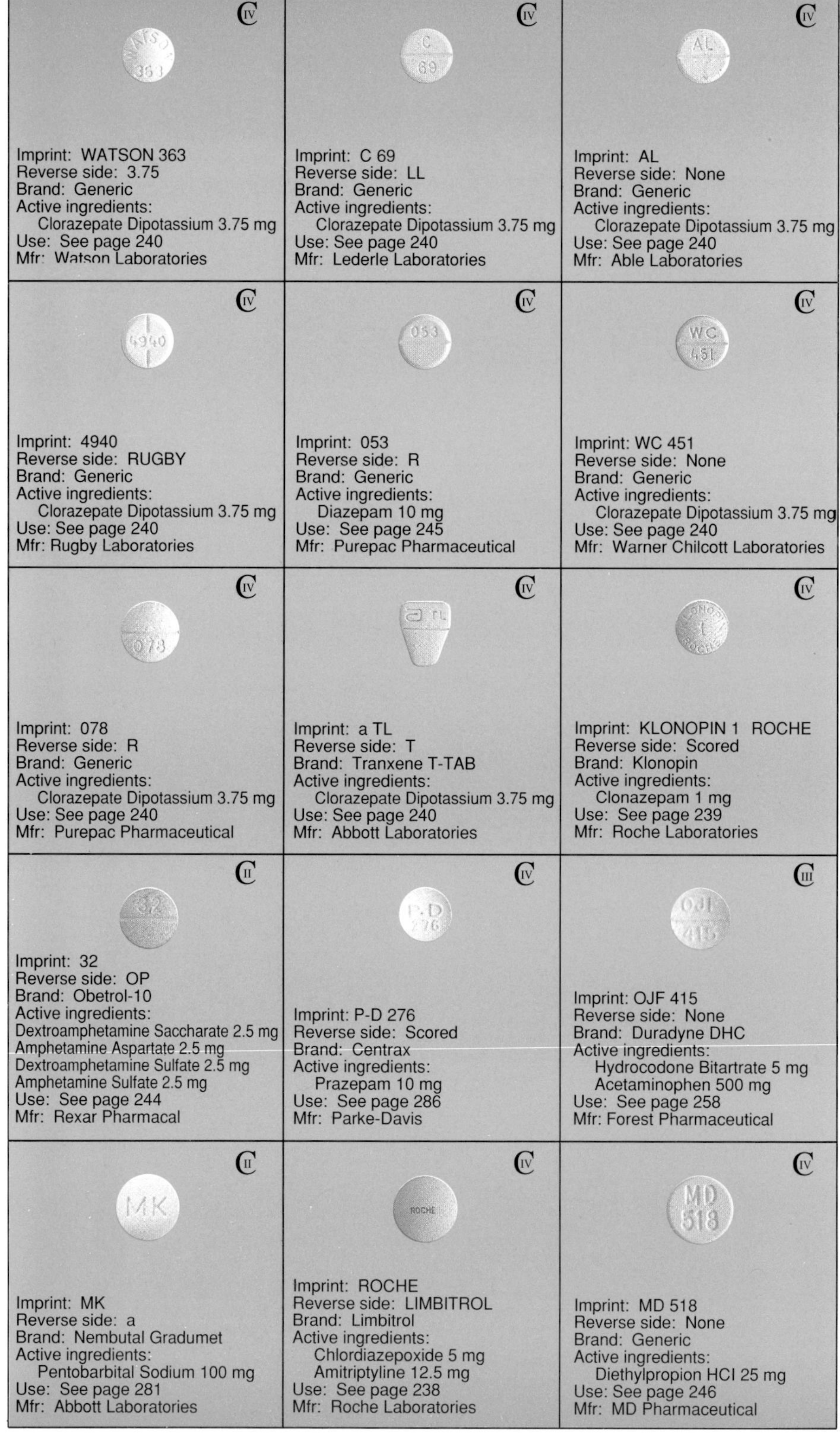

C-IV Imprint: WATSON 363 Reverse side: 3.75 Brand: Generic Active ingredients: Clorazepate Dipotassium 3.75 mg Use: See page 240 Mfr: Watson Laboratories	C-IV Imprint: C 69 Reverse side: LL Brand: Generic Active ingredients: Clorazepate Dipotassium 3.75 mg Use: See page 240 Mfr: Lederle Laboratories	C-IV Imprint: AL Reverse side: None Brand: Generic Active ingredients: Clorazepate Dipotassium 3.75 mg Use: See page 240 Mfr: Able Laboratories
C-IV Imprint: 4940 Reverse side: RUGBY Brand: Generic Active ingredients: Clorazepate Dipotassium 3.75 mg Use: See page 240 Mfr: Rugby Laboratories	C-IV Imprint: 053 Reverse side: R Brand: Generic Active ingredients: Diazepam 10 mg Use: See page 245 Mfr: Purepac Pharmaceutical	C-IV Imprint: WC 451 Reverse side: None Brand: Generic Active ingredients: Clorazepate Dipotassium 3.75 mg Use: See page 240 Mfr: Warner Chilcott Laboratories
C-IV Imprint: 078 Reverse side: R Brand: Generic Active ingredients: Clorazepate Dipotassium 3.75 mg Use: See page 240 Mfr: Purepac Pharmaceutical	C-IV Imprint: a TL Reverse side: T Brand: Tranxene T-TAB Active ingredients: Clorazepate Dipotassium 3.75 mg Use: See page 240 Mfr: Abbott Laboratories	C-IV Imprint: KLONOPIN 1 ROCHE Reverse side: Scored Brand: Klonopin Active ingredients: Clonazepam 1 mg Use: See page 239 Mfr: Roche Laboratories
C-II Imprint: 32 Reverse side: OP Brand: Obetrol-10 Active ingredients: Dextroamphetamine Saccharate 2.5 mg Amphetamine Aspartate 2.5 mg Dextroamphetamine Sulfate 2.5 mg Amphetamine Sulfate 2.5 mg Use: See page 244 Mfr: Rexar Pharmacal	C-IV Imprint: P-D 276 Reverse side: Scored Brand: Centrax Active ingredients: Prazepam 10 mg Use: See page 286 Mfr: Parke-Davis	C-III Imprint: OJF 415 Reverse side: None Brand: Duradyne DHC Active ingredients: Hydrocodone Bitartrate 5 mg Acetaminophen 500 mg Use: See page 258 Mfr: Forest Pharmaceutical
C-II Imprint: MK Reverse side: a Brand: Nembutal Gradumet Active ingredients: Pentobarbital Sodium 100 mg Use: See page 281 Mfr: Abbott Laboratories	C-IV Imprint: ROCHE Reverse side: LIMBITROL Brand: Limbitrol Active ingredients: Chlordiazepoxide 5 mg Amitriptyline 12.5 mg Use: See page 238 Mfr: Roche Laboratories	C-IV Imprint: MD 518 Reverse side: None Brand: Generic Active ingredients: Diethylpropion HCl 25 mg Use: See page 246 Mfr: MD Pharmaceutical

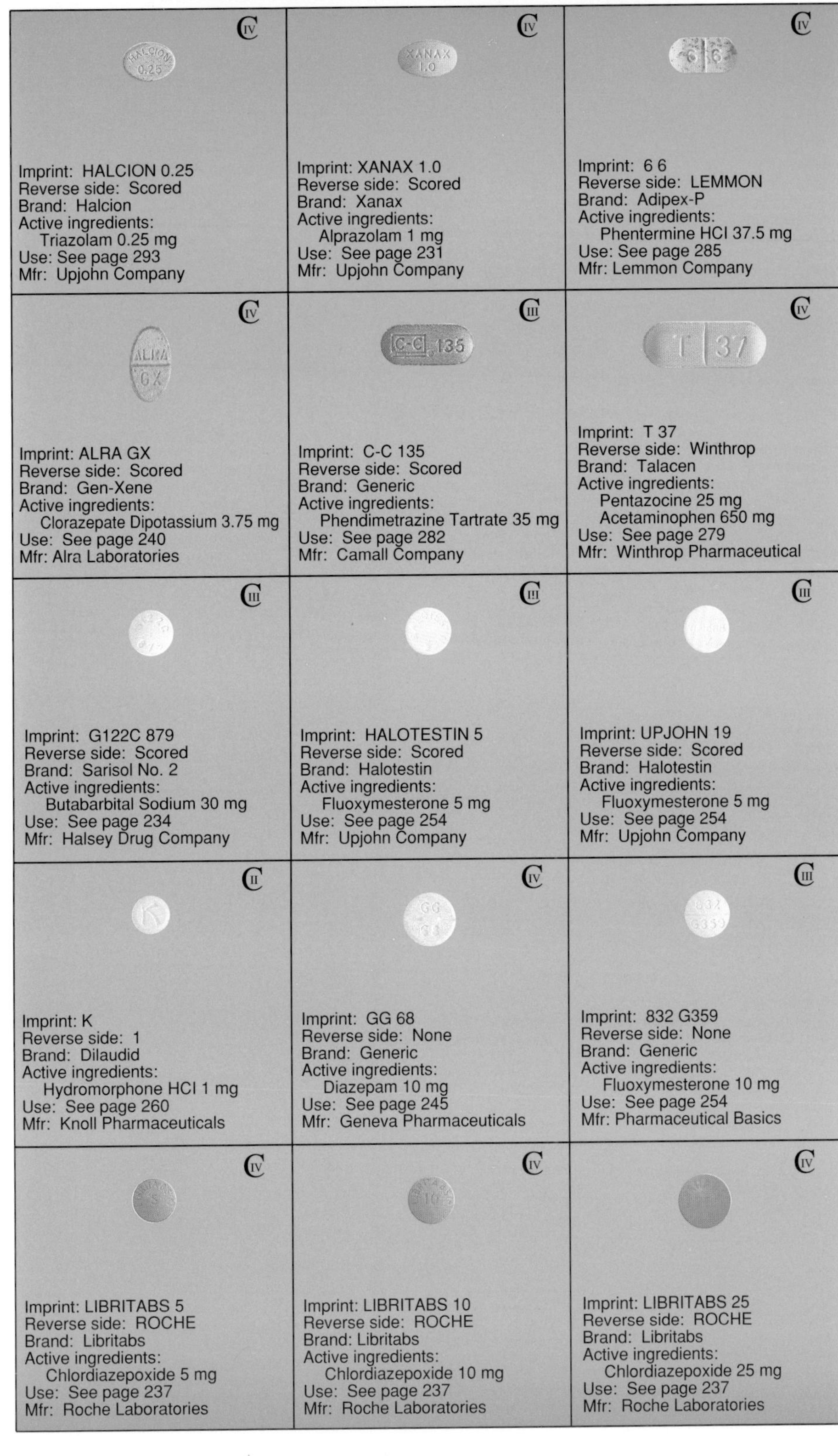

CIV Imprint: HALCION 0.25 Reverse side: Scored Brand: Halcion Active ingredients: Triazolam 0.25 mg Use: See page 293 Mfr: Upjohn Company	CIV Imprint: XANAX 1.0 Reverse side: Scored Brand: Xanax Active ingredients: Alprazolam 1 mg Use: See page 231 Mfr: Upjohn Company	CIV Imprint: 6 6 Reverse side: LEMMON Brand: Adipex-P Active ingredients: Phentermine HCl 37.5 mg Use: See page 285 Mfr: Lemmon Company
CIV Imprint: ALRA GX Reverse side: Scored Brand: Gen-Xene Active ingredients: Clorazepate Dipotassium 3.75 mg Use: See page 240 Mfr: Alra Laboratories	CIII Imprint: C-C 135 Reverse side: Scored Brand: Generic Active ingredients: Phendimetrazine Tartrate 35 mg Use: See page 282 Mfr: Camall Company	CIV Imprint: T 37 Reverse side: Winthrop Brand: Talacen Active ingredients: Pentazocine 25 mg Acetaminophen 650 mg Use: See page 279 Mfr: Winthrop Pharmaceutical
CIII Imprint: G122C 879 Reverse side: Scored Brand: Sarisol No. 2 Active ingredients: Butabarbital Sodium 30 mg Use: See page 234 Mfr: Halsey Drug Company	CIII Imprint: HALOTESTIN 5 Reverse side: Scored Brand: Halotestin Active ingredients: Fluoxymesterone 5 mg Use: See page 254 Mfr: Upjohn Company	CIII Imprint: UPJOHN 19 Reverse side: Scored Brand: Halotestin Active ingredients: Fluoxymesterone 5 mg Use: See page 254 Mfr: Upjohn Company
CII Imprint: K Reverse side: 1 Brand: Dilaudid Active ingredients: Hydromorphone HCl 1 mg Use: See page 260 Mfr: Knoll Pharmaceuticals	CIV Imprint: GG 68 Reverse side: None Brand: Generic Active ingredients: Diazepam 10 mg Use: See page 245 Mfr: Geneva Pharmaceuticals	CIII Imprint: 832 G359 Reverse side: None Brand: Generic Active ingredients: Fluoxymesterone 10 mg Use: See page 254 Mfr: Pharmaceutical Basics
CIV Imprint: LIBRITABS 5 Reverse side: ROCHE Brand: Libritabs Active ingredients: Chlordiazepoxide 5 mg Use: See page 237 Mfr: Roche Laboratories	CIV Imprint: LIBRITABS 10 Reverse side: ROCHE Brand: Libritabs Active ingredients: Chlordiazepoxide 10 mg Use: See page 237 Mfr: Roche Laboratories	CIV Imprint: LIBRITABS 25 Reverse side: ROCHE Brand: Libritabs Active ingredients: Chlordiazepoxide 25 mg Use: See page 237 Mfr: Roche Laboratories

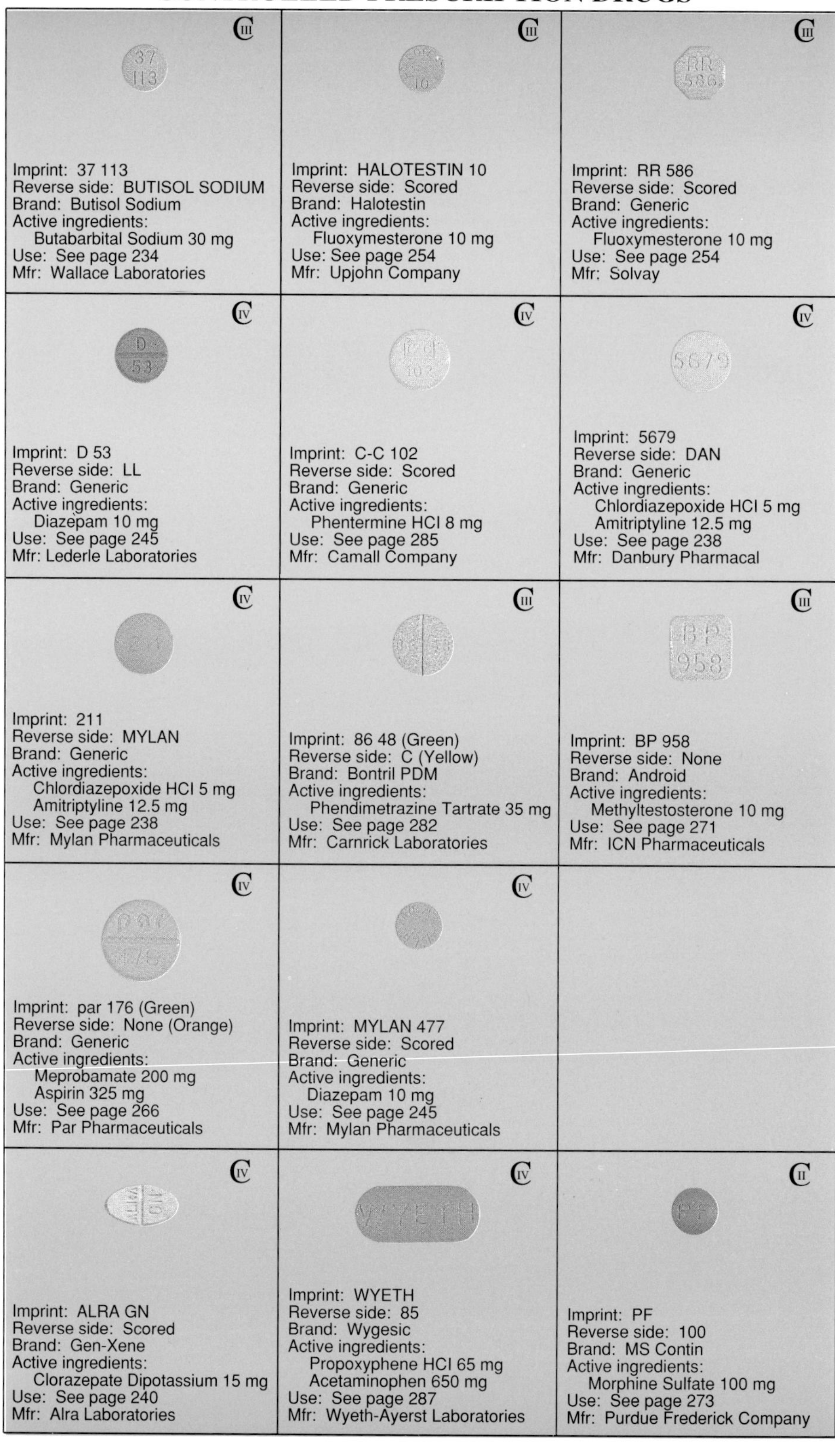

C III

Imprint: 37 113
Reverse side: BUTISOL SODIUM
Brand: Butisol Sodium
Active ingredients:
Butabarbital Sodium 30 mg
Use: See page 234
Mfr: Wallace Laboratories

C III

Imprint: HALOTESTIN 10
Reverse side: Scored
Brand: Halotestin
Active ingredients:
Fluoxymesterone 10 mg
Use: See page 254
Mfr: Upjohn Company

C III

Imprint: RR 586
Reverse side: Scored
Brand: Generic
Active ingredients:
Fluoxymesterone 10 mg
Use: See page 254
Mfr: Solvay

C IV

Imprint: D 53
Reverse side: LL
Brand: Generic
Active ingredients:
Diazepam 10 mg
Use: See page 245
Mfr: Lederle Laboratories

C IV

Imprint: C-C 102
Reverse side: Scored
Brand: Generic
Active ingredients:
Phentermine HCl 8 mg
Use: See page 285
Mfr: Camall Company

C IV

Imprint: 5679
Reverse side: DAN
Brand: Generic
Active ingredients:
Chlordiazepoxide HCl 5 mg
Amitriptyline 12.5 mg
Use: See page 238
Mfr: Danbury Pharmacal

C IV

Imprint: 211
Reverse side: MYLAN
Brand: Generic
Active ingredients:
Chlordiazepoxide HCl 5 mg
Amitriptyline 12.5 mg
Use: See page 238
Mfr: Mylan Pharmaceuticals

C III

Imprint: 86 48 (Green)
Reverse side: C (Yellow)
Brand: Bontril PDM
Active ingredients:
Phendimetrazine Tartrate 35 mg
Use: See page 282
Mfr: Carnrick Laboratories

C III

Imprint: BP 958
Reverse side: None
Brand: Android
Active ingredients:
Methyltestosterone 10 mg
Use: See page 271
Mfr: ICN Pharmaceuticals

C IV

Imprint: par 176 (Green)
Reverse side: None (Orange)
Brand: Generic
Active ingredients:
Meprobamate 200 mg
Aspirin 325 mg
Use: See page 266
Mfr: Par Pharmaceuticals

C IV

Imprint: MYLAN 477
Reverse side: Scored
Brand: Generic
Active ingredients:
Diazepam 10 mg
Use: See page 245
Mfr: Mylan Pharmaceuticals

C IV

Imprint: ALRA GN
Reverse side: Scored
Brand: Gen-Xene
Active ingredients:
Clorazepate Dipotassium 15 mg
Use: See page 240
Mfr: Alra Laboratories

C IV

Imprint: WYETH
Reverse side: 85
Brand: Wygesic
Active ingredients:
Propoxyphene HCl 65 mg
Acetaminophen 650 mg
Use: See page 287
Mfr: Wyeth-Ayerst Laboratories

C II

Imprint: PF
Reverse side: 100
Brand: MS Contin
Active ingredients:
Morphine Sulfate 100 mg
Use: See page 273
Mfr: Purdue Frederick Company

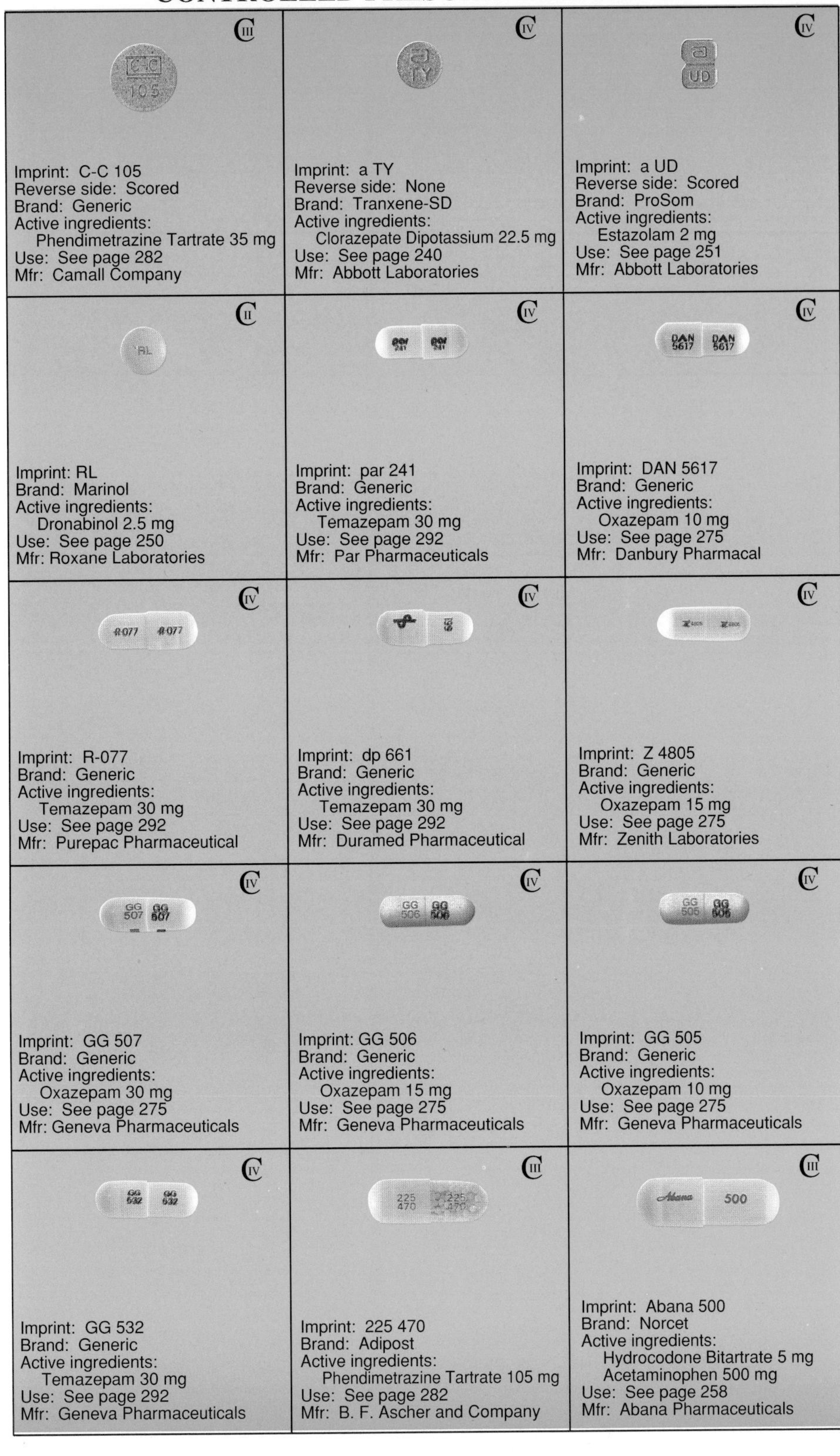

C-III

Imprint: C-C 105
Reverse side: Scored
Brand: Generic
Active ingredients:
Phendimetrazine Tartrate 35 mg
Use: See page 282
Mfr: Camall Company

C-IV

Imprint: a TY
Reverse side: None
Brand: Tranxene-SD
Active ingredients:
Clorazepate Dipotassium 22.5 mg
Use: See page 240
Mfr: Abbott Laboratories

C-IV

Imprint: a UD
Reverse side: Scored
Brand: ProSom
Active ingredients:
Estazolam 2 mg
Use: See page 251
Mfr: Abbott Laboratories

C-II

Imprint: RL
Brand: Marinol
Active ingredients:
Dronabinol 2.5 mg
Use: See page 250
Mfr: Roxane Laboratories

C-IV

Imprint: par 241
Brand: Generic
Active ingredients:
Temazepam 30 mg
Use: See page 292
Mfr: Par Pharmaceuticals

C-IV

Imprint: DAN 5617
Brand: Generic
Active ingredients:
Oxazepam 10 mg
Use: See page 275
Mfr: Danbury Pharmacal

C-IV

Imprint: R-077
Brand: Generic
Active ingredients:
Temazepam 30 mg
Use: See page 292
Mfr: Purepac Pharmaceutical

C-IV

Imprint: dp 661
Brand: Generic
Active ingredients:
Temazepam 30 mg
Use: See page 292
Mfr: Duramed Pharmaceutical

C-IV

Imprint: Z 4805
Brand: Generic
Active ingredients:
Oxazepam 15 mg
Use: See page 275
Mfr: Zenith Laboratories

C-IV

Imprint: GG 507
Brand: Generic
Active ingredients:
Oxazepam 30 mg
Use: See page 275
Mfr: Geneva Pharmaceuticals

C-IV

Imprint: GG 506
Brand: Generic
Active ingredients:
Oxazepam 15 mg
Use: See page 275
Mfr: Geneva Pharmaceuticals

C-IV

Imprint: GG 505
Brand: Generic
Active ingredients:
Oxazepam 10 mg
Use: See page 275
Mfr: Geneva Pharmaceuticals

C-IV

Imprint: GG 532
Brand: Generic
Active ingredients:
Temazepam 30 mg
Use: See page 292
Mfr: Geneva Pharmaceuticals

C-III

Imprint: 225 470
Brand: Adipost
Active ingredients:
Phendimetrazine Tartrate 105 mg
Use: See page 282
Mfr: B. F. Ascher and Company

C-III

Imprint: Abana 500
Brand: Norcet
Active ingredients:
Hydrocodone Bitartrate 5 mg
Acetaminophen 500 mg
Use: See page 258
Mfr: Abana Pharmaceuticals

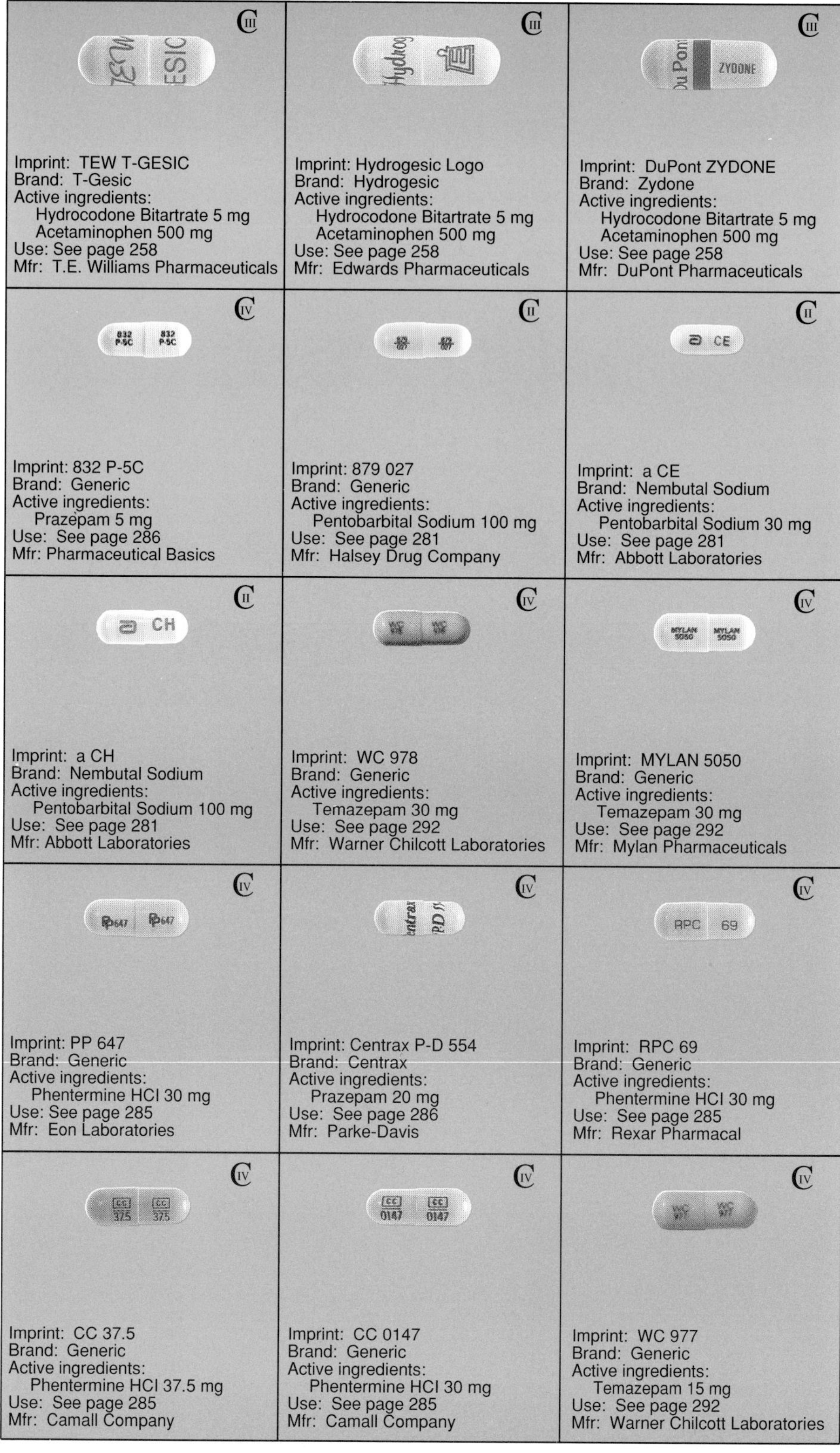

C III
Imprint: TEW T-GESIC
Brand: T-Gesic
Active ingredients:
Hydrocodone Bitartrate 5 mg
Acetaminophen 500 mg
Use: See page 258
Mfr: T.E. Williams Pharmaceuticals

C III
Imprint: Hydrogesic Logo
Brand: Hydrogesic
Active ingredients:
Hydrocodone Bitartrate 5 mg
Acetaminophen 500 mg
Use: See page 258
Mfr: Edwards Pharmaceuticals

C III
Imprint: DuPont ZYDONE
Brand: Zydone
Active ingredients:
Hydrocodone Bitartrate 5 mg
Acetaminophen 500 mg
Use: See page 258
Mfr: DuPont Pharmaceuticals

C IV
Imprint: 832 P-5C
Brand: Generic
Active ingredients:
Prazepam 5 mg
Use: See page 286
Mfr: Pharmaceutical Basics

C II
Imprint: 879 027
Brand: Generic
Active ingredients:
Pentobarbital Sodium 100 mg
Use: See page 281
Mfr: Halsey Drug Company

C II
Imprint: a CE
Brand: Nembutal Sodium
Active ingredients:
Pentobarbital Sodium 30 mg
Use: See page 281
Mfr: Abbott Laboratories

C II
Imprint: a CH
Brand: Nembutal Sodium
Active ingredients:
Pentobarbital Sodium 100 mg
Use: See page 281
Mfr: Abbott Laboratories

C IV
Imprint: WC 978
Brand: Generic
Active ingredients:
Temazepam 30 mg
Use: See page 292
Mfr: Warner Chilcott Laboratories

C IV
Imprint: MYLAN 5050
Brand: Generic
Active ingredients:
Temazepam 30 mg
Use: See page 292
Mfr: Mylan Pharmaceuticals

C IV
Imprint: PP 647
Brand: Generic
Active ingredients:
Phentermine HCl 30 mg
Use: See page 285
Mfr: Eon Laboratories

C IV
Imprint: Centrax P-D 554
Brand: Centrax
Active ingredients:
Prazepam 20 mg
Use: See page 286
Mfr: Parke-Davis

C IV
Imprint: RPC 69
Brand: Generic
Active ingredients:
Phentermine HCl 30 mg
Use: See page 285
Mfr: Rexar Pharmacal

C IV
Imprint: CC 37.5
Brand: Generic
Active ingredients:
Phentermine HCl 37.5 mg
Use: See page 285
Mfr: Camall Company

C IV
Imprint: CC 0147
Brand: Generic
Active ingredients:
Phentermine HCl 30 mg
Use: See page 285
Mfr: Camall Company

C IV
Imprint: WC 977
Brand: Generic
Active ingredients:
Temazepam 15 mg
Use: See page 292
Mfr: Warner Chilcott Laboratories

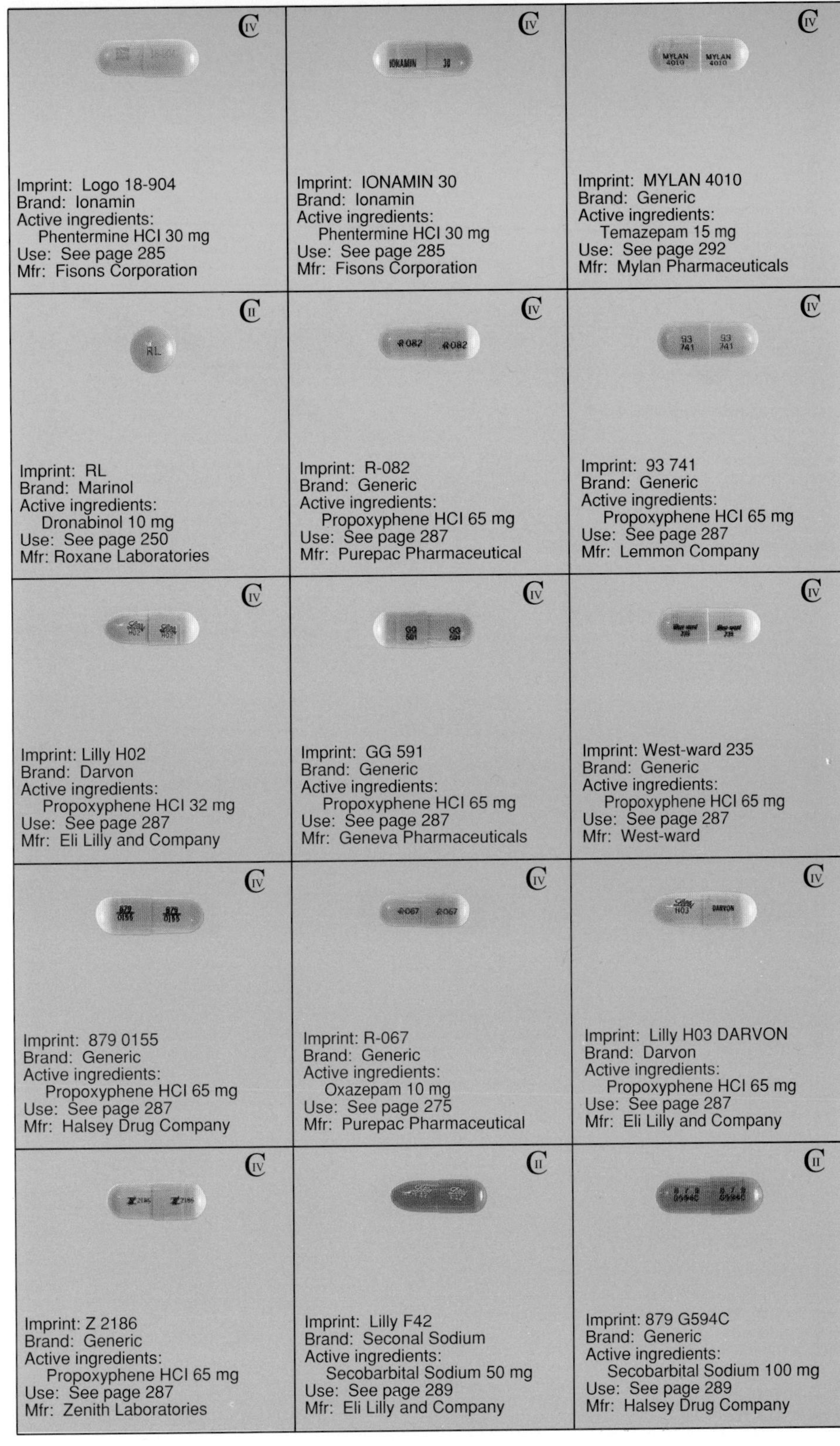

C-IV Imprint: Logo 18-904 Brand: Ionamin Active ingredients: Phentermine HCl 30 mg Use: See page 285 Mfr: Fisons Corporation	C-IV Imprint: IONAMIN 30 Brand: Ionamin Active ingredients: Phentermine HCl 30 mg Use: See page 285 Mfr: Fisons Corporation	C-IV Imprint: MYLAN 4010 Brand: Generic Active ingredients: Temazepam 15 mg Use: See page 292 Mfr: Mylan Pharmaceuticals
C-II Imprint: RL Brand: Marinol Active ingredients: Dronabinol 10 mg Use: See page 250 Mfr: Roxane Laboratories	C-IV Imprint: R-082 Brand: Generic Active ingredients: Propoxyphene HCl 65 mg Use: See page 287 Mfr: Purepac Pharmaceutical	C-IV Imprint: 93 741 Brand: Generic Active ingredients: Propoxyphene HCl 65 mg Use: See page 287 Mfr: Lemmon Company
C-IV Imprint: Lilly H02 Brand: Darvon Active ingredients: Propoxyphene HCl 32 mg Use: See page 287 Mfr: Eli Lilly and Company	C-IV Imprint: GG 591 Brand: Generic Active ingredients: Propoxyphene HCl 65 mg Use: See page 287 Mfr: Geneva Pharmaceuticals	C-IV Imprint: West-ward 235 Brand: Generic Active ingredients: Propoxyphene HCl 65 mg Use: See page 287 Mfr: West-ward
C-IV Imprint: 879 0155 Brand: Generic Active ingredients: Propoxyphene HCl 65 mg Use: See page 287 Mfr: Halsey Drug Company	C-IV Imprint: R-067 Brand: Generic Active ingredients: Oxazepam 10 mg Use: See page 275 Mfr: Purepac Pharmaceutical	C-IV Imprint: Lilly H03 DARVON Brand: Darvon Active ingredients: Propoxyphene HCl 65 mg Use: See page 287 Mfr: Eli Lilly and Company
C-IV Imprint: Z 2186 Brand: Generic Active ingredients: Propoxyphene HCl 65 mg Use: See page 287 Mfr: Zenith Laboratories	C-II Imprint: Lilly F42 Brand: Seconal Sodium Active ingredients: Secobarbital Sodium 50 mg Use: See page 289 Mfr: Eli Lilly and Company	C-II Imprint: 879 G594C Brand: Generic Active ingredients: Secobarbital Sodium 100 mg Use: See page 289 Mfr: Halsey Drug Company

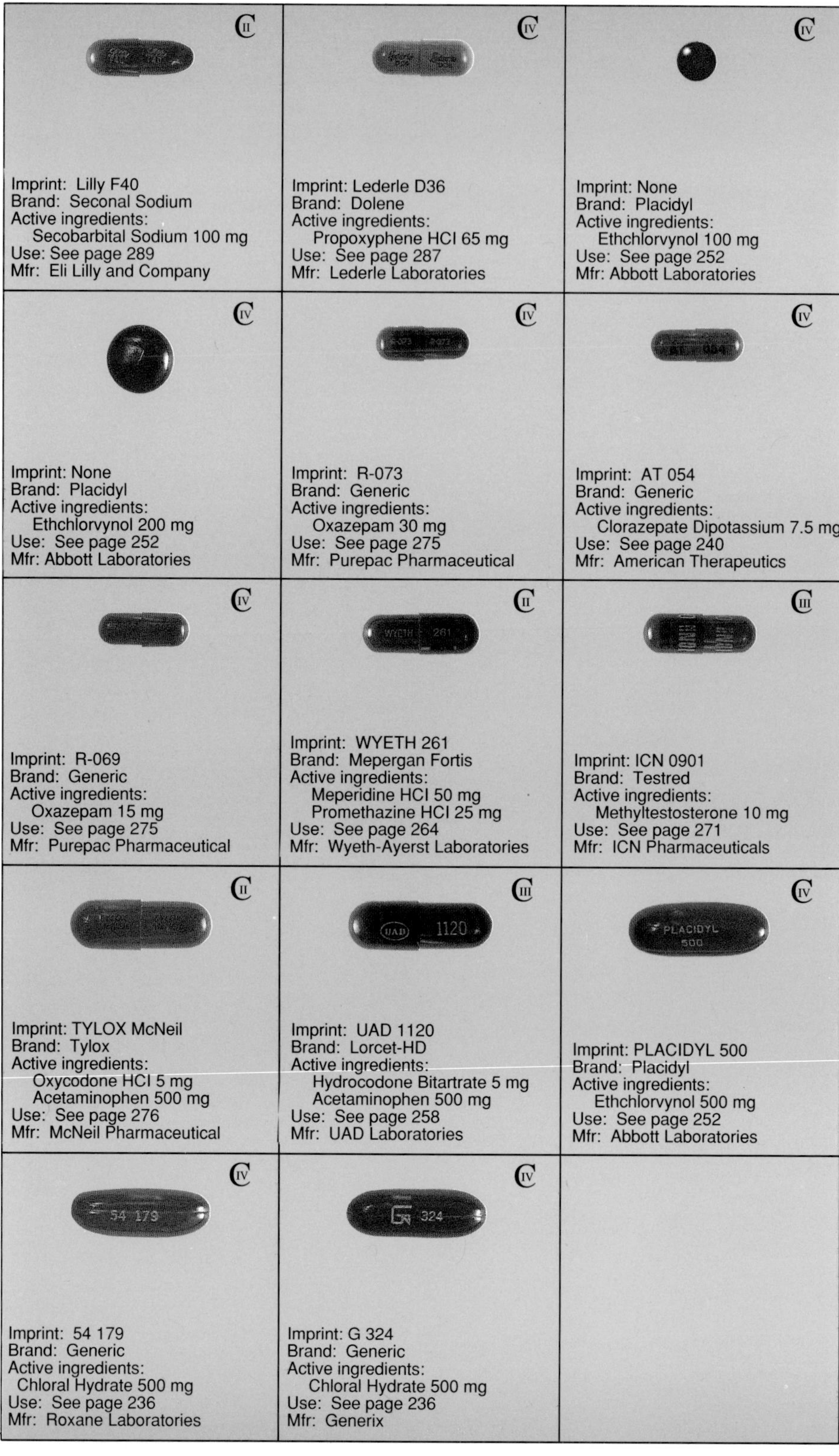

C-II
Imprint: Lilly F40
Brand: Seconal Sodium
Active ingredients:
Secobarbital Sodium 100 mg
Use: See page 289
Mfr: Eli Lilly and Company

C-IV
Imprint: Lederle D36
Brand: Dolene
Active ingredients:
Propoxyphene HCl 65 mg
Use: See page 287
Mfr: Lederle Laboratories

C-IV
Imprint: None
Brand: Placidyl
Active ingredients:
Ethchlorvynol 100 mg
Use: See page 252
Mfr: Abbott Laboratories

C-IV
Imprint: None
Brand: Placidyl
Active ingredients:
Ethchlorvynol 200 mg
Use: See page 252
Mfr: Abbott Laboratories

C-IV
Imprint: R-073
Brand: Generic
Active ingredients:
Oxazepam 30 mg
Use: See page 275
Mfr: Purepac Pharmaceutical

C-IV
Imprint: AT 054
Brand: Generic
Active ingredients:
Clorazepate Dipotassium 7.5 mg
Use: See page 240
Mfr: American Therapeutics

C-IV
Imprint: R-069
Brand: Generic
Active ingredients:
Oxazepam 15 mg
Use: See page 275
Mfr: Purepac Pharmaceutical

C-II
Imprint: WYETH 261
Brand: Mepergan Fortis
Active ingredients:
Meperidine HCl 50 mg
Promethazine HCl 25 mg
Use: See page 264
Mfr: Wyeth-Ayerst Laboratories

C-III
Imprint: ICN 0901
Brand: Testred
Active ingredients:
Methyltestosterone 10 mg
Use: See page 271
Mfr: ICN Pharmaceuticals

C-II
Imprint: TYLOX McNeil
Brand: Tylox
Active ingredients:
Oxycodone HCl 5 mg
Acetaminophen 500 mg
Use: See page 276
Mfr: McNeil Pharmaceutical

C-III
Imprint: UAD 1120
Brand: Lorcet-HD
Active ingredients:
Hydrocodone Bitartrate 5 mg
Acetaminophen 500 mg
Use: See page 258
Mfr: UAD Laboratories

C-IV
Imprint: PLACIDYL 500
Brand: Placidyl
Active ingredients:
Ethchlorvynol 500 mg
Use: See page 252
Mfr: Abbott Laboratories

C-IV
Imprint: 54 179
Brand: Generic
Active ingredients:
Chloral Hydrate 500 mg
Use: See page 236
Mfr: Roxane Laboratories

C-IV
Imprint: G 324
Brand: Generic
Active ingredients:
Chloral Hydrate 500 mg
Use: See page 236
Mfr: Generix

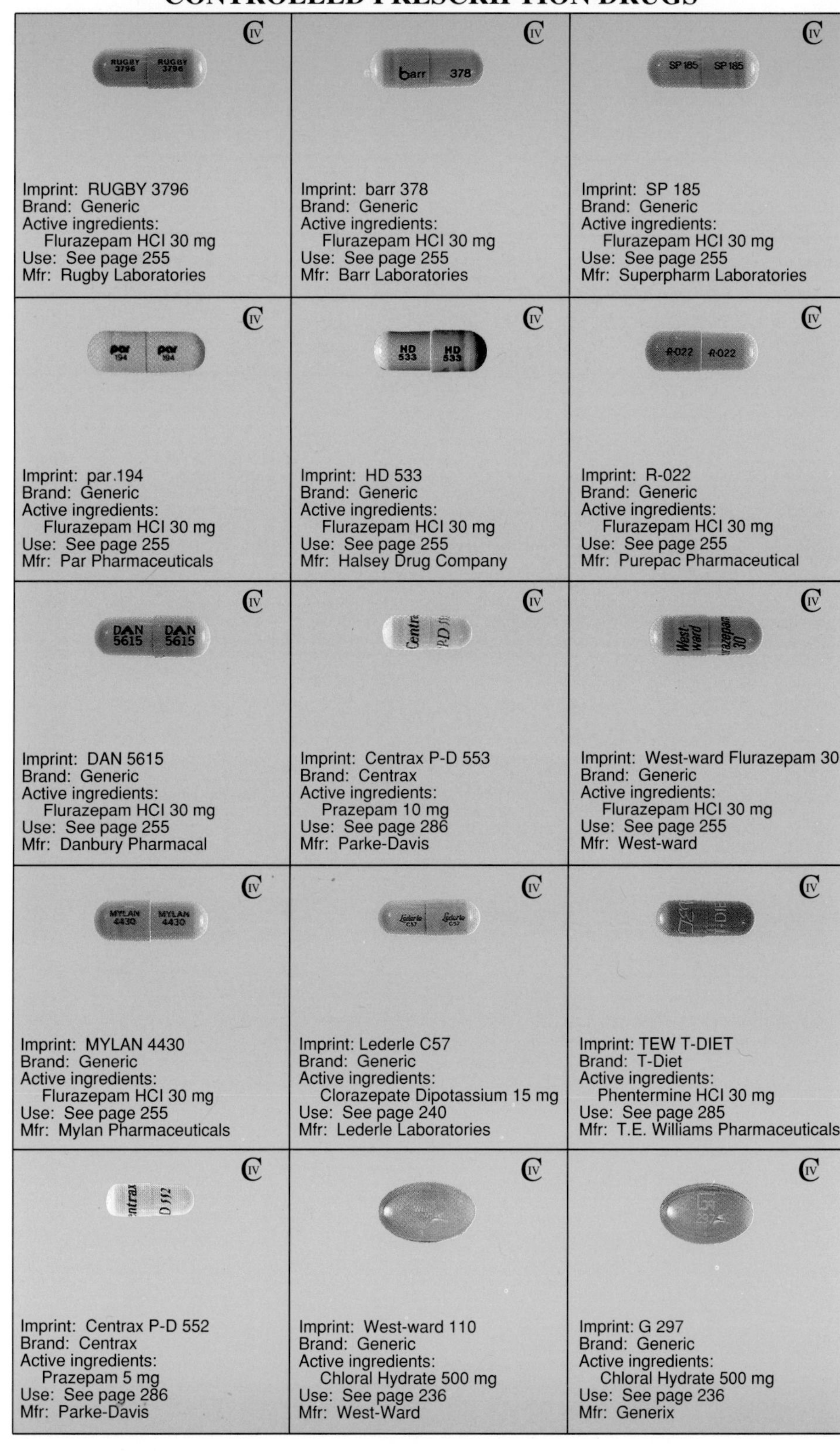

Imprint: RUGBY 3796
Brand: Generic
Active ingredients:
Flurazepam HCl 30 mg
Use: See page 255
Mfr: Rugby Laboratories

Imprint: barr 378
Brand: Generic
Active ingredients:
Flurazepam HCl 30 mg
Use: See page 255
Mfr: Barr Laboratories

Imprint: SP 185
Brand: Generic
Active ingredients:
Flurazepam HCl 30 mg
Use: See page 255
Mfr: Superpharm Laboratories

Imprint: par.194
Brand: Generic
Active ingredients:
Flurazepam HCl 30 mg
Use: See page 255
Mfr: Par Pharmaceuticals

Imprint: HD 533
Brand: Generic
Active ingredients:
Flurazepam HCl 30 mg
Use: See page 255
Mfr: Halsey Drug Company

Imprint: R-022
Brand: Generic
Active ingredients:
Flurazepam HCl 30 mg
Use: See page 255
Mfr: Purepac Pharmaceutical

Imprint: DAN 5615
Brand: Generic
Active ingredients:
Flurazepam HCl 30 mg
Use: See page 255
Mfr: Danbury Pharmacal

Imprint: Centrax P-D 553
Brand: Centrax
Active ingredients:
Prazepam 10 mg
Use: See page 286
Mfr: Parke-Davis

Imprint: West-ward Flurazepam 30
Brand: Generic
Active ingredients:
Flurazepam HCl 30 mg
Use: See page 255
Mfr: West-ward

Imprint: MYLAN 4430
Brand: Generic
Active ingredients:
Flurazepam HCl 30 mg
Use: See page 255
Mfr: Mylan Pharmaceuticals

Imprint: Lederle C57
Brand: Generic
Active ingredients:
Clorazepate Dipotassium 15 mg
Use: See page 240
Mfr: Lederle Laboratories

Imprint: TEW T-DIET
Brand: T-Diet
Active ingredients:
Phentermine HCl 30 mg
Use: See page 285
Mfr: T.E. Williams Pharmaceuticals

Imprint: Centrax P-D 552
Brand: Centrax
Active ingredients:
Prazepam 5 mg
Use: See page 286
Mfr: Parke-Davis

Imprint: West-ward 110
Brand: Generic
Active ingredients:
Chloral Hydrate 500 mg
Use: See page 236
Mfr: West-Ward

Imprint: G 297
Brand: Generic
Active ingredients:
Chloral Hydrate 500 mg
Use: See page 236
Mfr: Generix

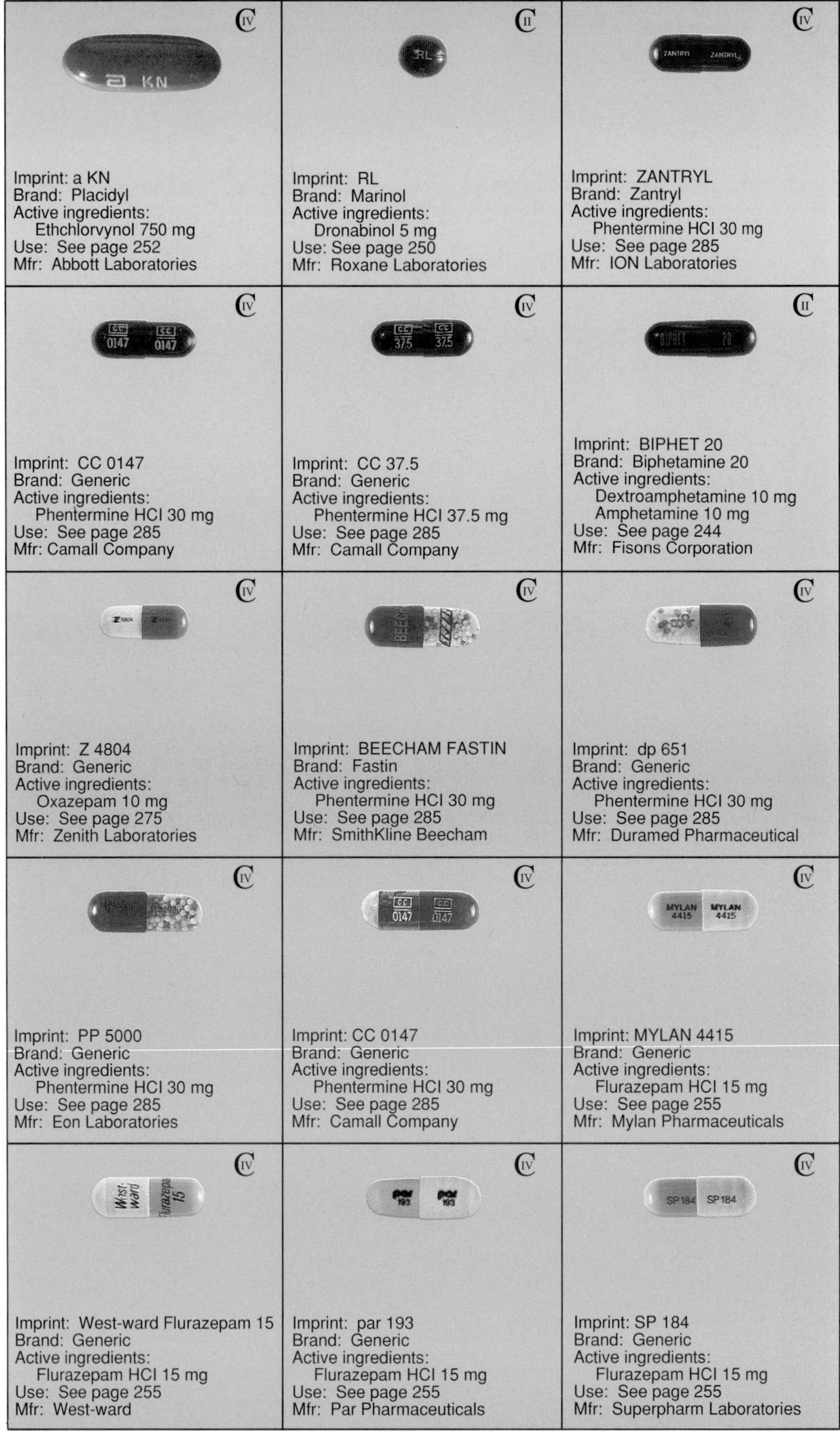

CIV
Imprint: a KN
Brand: Placidyl
Active ingredients:
Ethchlorvynol 750 mg
Use: See page 252
Mfr: Abbott Laboratories

CII
Imprint: RL
Brand: Marinol
Active ingredients:
Dronabinol 5 mg
Use: See page 250
Mfr: Roxane Laboratories

CIV
Imprint: ZANTRYL
Brand: Zantryl
Active ingredients:
Phentermine HCl 30 mg
Use: See page 285
Mfr: ION Laboratories

CIV
Imprint: CC 0147
Brand: Generic
Active ingredients:
Phentermine HCl 30 mg
Use: See page 285
Mfr: Camall Company

CIV
Imprint: CC 37.5
Brand: Generic
Active ingredients:
Phentermine HCl 37.5 mg
Use: See page 285
Mfr: Camall Company

CII
Imprint: BIPHET 20
Brand: Biphetamine 20
Active ingredients:
Dextroamphetamine 10 mg
Amphetamine 10 mg
Use: See page 244
Mfr: Fisons Corporation

CIV
Imprint: Z 4804
Brand: Generic
Active ingredients:
Oxazepam 10 mg
Use: See page 275
Mfr: Zenith Laboratories

CIV
Imprint: BEECHAM FASTIN
Brand: Fastin
Active ingredients:
Phentermine HCl 30 mg
Use: See page 285
Mfr: SmithKline Beecham

CIV
Imprint: dp 651
Brand: Generic
Active ingredients:
Phentermine HCl 30 mg
Use: See page 285
Mfr: Duramed Pharmaceutical

CIV
Imprint: PP 5000
Brand: Generic
Active ingredients:
Phentermine HCl 30 mg
Use: See page 285
Mfr: Eon Laboratories

CIV
Imprint: CC 0147
Brand: Generic
Active ingredients:
Phentermine HCl 30 mg
Use: See page 285
Mfr: Camall Company

CIV
Imprint: MYLAN 4415
Brand: Generic
Active ingredients:
Flurazepam HCl 15 mg
Use: See page 255
Mfr: Mylan Pharmaceuticals

CIV
Imprint: West-ward Flurazepam 15
Brand: Generic
Active ingredients:
Flurazepam HCl 15 mg
Use: See page 255
Mfr: West-ward

CIV
Imprint: par 193
Brand: Generic
Active ingredients:
Flurazepam HCl 15 mg
Use: See page 255
Mfr: Par Pharmaceuticals

CIV
Imprint: SP 184
Brand: Generic
Active ingredients:
Flurazepam HCl 15 mg
Use: See page 255
Mfr: Superpharm Laboratories

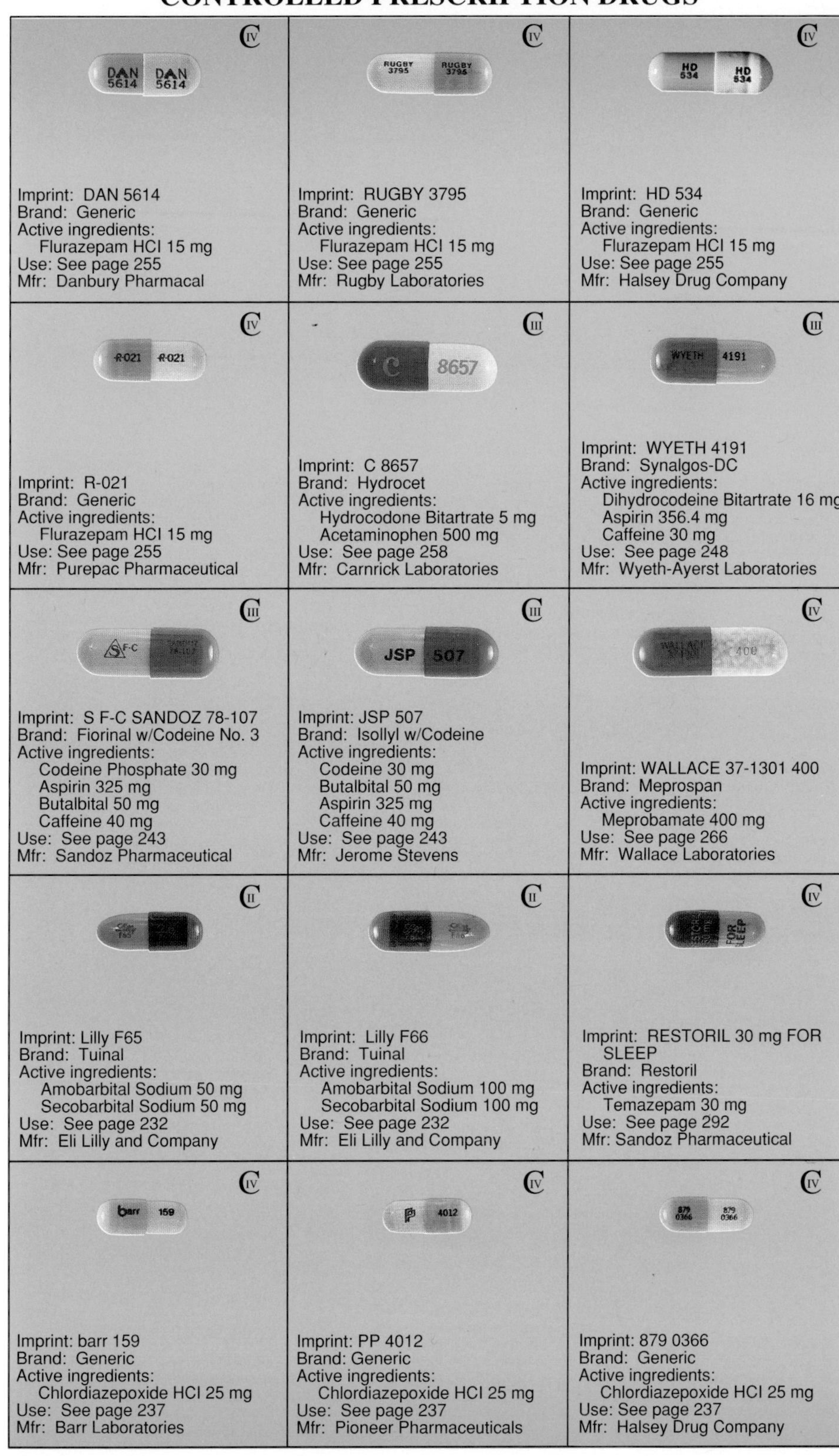

CIV Imprint: DAN 5614 Brand: Generic Active ingredients: Flurazepam HCl 15 mg Use: See page 255 Mfr: Danbury Pharmacal	CIV Imprint: RUGBY 3795 Brand: Generic Active ingredients: Flurazepam HCl 15 mg Use: See page 255 Mfr: Rugby Laboratories	CIV Imprint: HD 534 Brand: Generic Active ingredients: Flurazepam HCl 15 mg Use: See page 255 Mfr: Halsey Drug Company
CIV Imprint: R-021 Brand: Generic Active ingredients: Flurazepam HCl 15 mg Use: See page 255 Mfr: Purepac Pharmaceutical	CIII Imprint: C 8657 Brand: Hydrocet Active ingredients: Hydrocodone Bitartrate 5 mg Acetaminophen 500 mg Use: See page 258 Mfr: Carnrick Laboratories	CIII Imprint: WYETH 4191 Brand: Synalgos-DC Active ingredients: Dihydrocodeine Bitartrate 16 mg Aspirin 356.4 mg Caffeine 30 mg Use: See page 248 Mfr: Wyeth-Ayerst Laboratories
CIII Imprint: S F-C SANDOZ 78-107 Brand: Fiorinal w/Codeine No. 3 Active ingredients: Codeine Phosphate 30 mg Aspirin 325 mg Butalbital 50 mg Caffeine 40 mg Use: See page 243 Mfr: Sandoz Pharmaceutical	CIII Imprint: JSP 507 Brand: Isollyl w/Codeine Active ingredients: Codeine 30 mg Butalbital 50 mg Aspirin 325 mg Caffeine 40 mg Use: See page 243 Mfr: Jerome Stevens	CIV Imprint: WALLACE 37-1301 400 Brand: Meprospan Active ingredients: Meprobamate 400 mg Use: See page 266 Mfr: Wallace Laboratories
CII Imprint: Lilly F65 Brand: Tuinal Active ingredients: Amobarbital Sodium 50 mg Secobarbital Sodium 50 mg Use: See page 232 Mfr: Eli Lilly and Company	CII Imprint: Lilly F66 Brand: Tuinal Active ingredients: Amobarbital Sodium 100 mg Secobarbital Sodium 100 mg Use: See page 232 Mfr: Eli Lilly and Company	CIV Imprint: RESTORIL 30 mg FOR SLEEP Brand: Restoril Active ingredients: Temazepam 30 mg Use: See page 292 Mfr: Sandoz Pharmaceutical
CIV Imprint: barr 159 Brand: Generic Active ingredients: Chlordiazepoxide HCl 25 mg Use: See page 237 Mfr: Barr Laboratories	CIV Imprint: PP 4012 Brand: Generic Active ingredients: Chlordiazepoxide HCl 25 mg Use: See page 237 Mfr: Pioneer Pharmaceuticals	CIV Imprint: 879 0366 Brand: Generic Active ingredients: Chlordiazepoxide HCl 25 mg Use: See page 237 Mfr: Halsey Drug Company

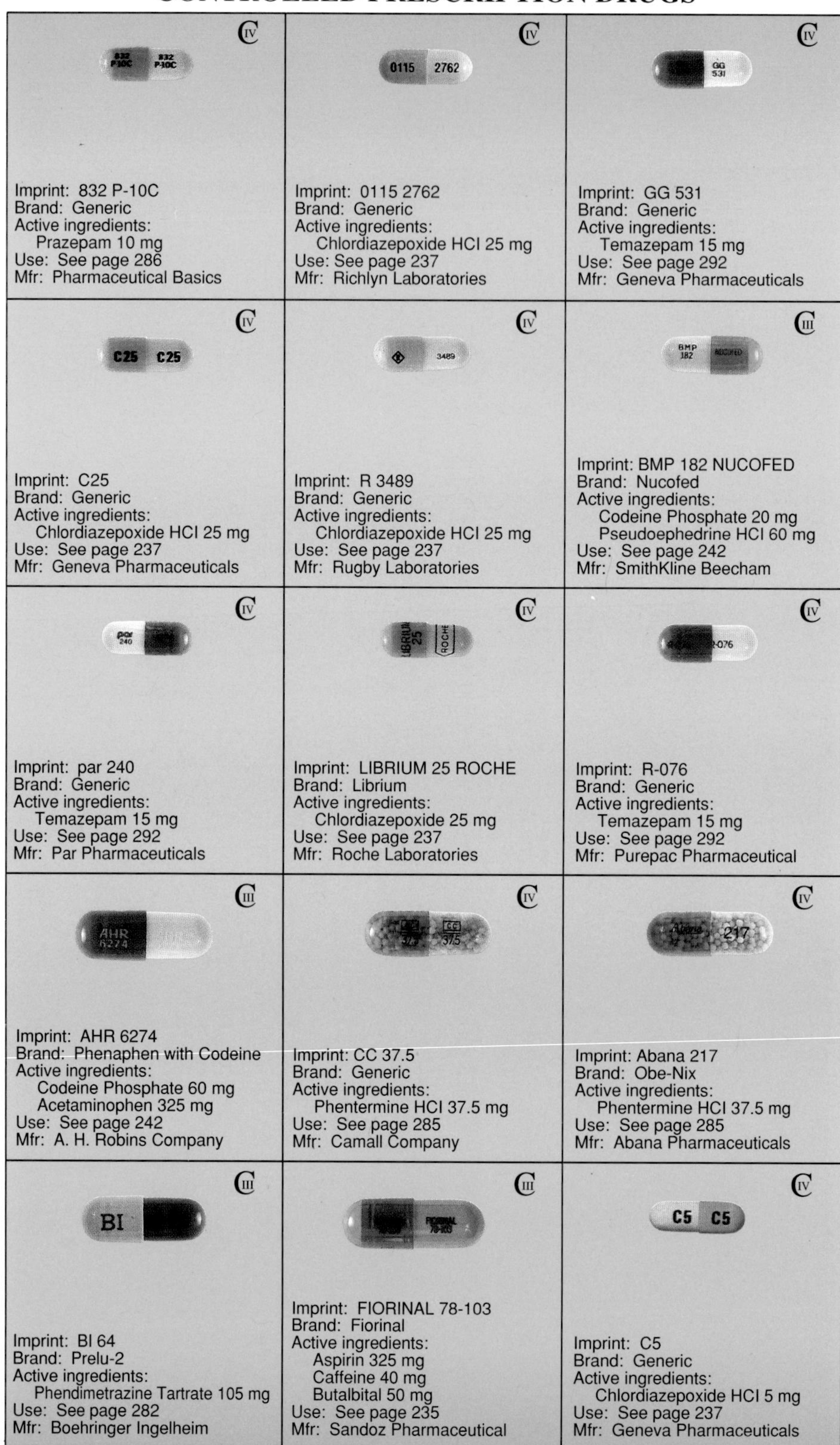

CIV
Imprint: 832 P-10C
Brand: Generic
Active ingredients:
Prazepam 10 mg
Use: See page 286
Mfr: Pharmaceutical Basics

CIV
Imprint: 0115 2762
Brand: Generic
Active ingredients:
Chlordiazepoxide HCl 25 mg
Use: See page 237
Mfr: Richlyn Laboratories

CIV
Imprint: GG 531
Brand: Generic
Active ingredients:
Temazepam 15 mg
Use: See page 292
Mfr: Geneva Pharmaceuticals

CIV
Imprint: C25
Brand: Generic
Active ingredients:
Chlordiazepoxide HCl 25 mg
Use: See page 237
Mfr: Geneva Pharmaceuticals

CIV
Imprint: R 3489
Brand: Generic
Active ingredients:
Chlordiazepoxide HCl 25 mg
Use: See page 237
Mfr: Rugby Laboratories

CIII
Imprint: BMP 182 NUCOFED
Brand: Nucofed
Active ingredients:
Codeine Phosphate 20 mg
Pseudoephedrine HCl 60 mg
Use: See page 242
Mfr: SmithKline Beecham

CIV
Imprint: par 240
Brand: Generic
Active ingredients:
Temazepam 15 mg
Use: See page 292
Mfr: Par Pharmaceuticals

CIV
Imprint: LIBRIUM 25 ROCHE
Brand: Librium
Active ingredients:
Chlordiazepoxide 25 mg
Use: See page 237
Mfr: Roche Laboratories

CIV
Imprint: R-076
Brand: Generic
Active ingredients:
Temazepam 15 mg
Use: See page 292
Mfr: Purepac Pharmaceutical

CIII
Imprint: AHR 6274
Brand: Phenaphen with Codeine
Active ingredients:
Codeine Phosphate 60 mg
Acetaminophen 325 mg
Use: See page 242
Mfr: A. H. Robins Company

CIV
Imprint: CC 37.5
Brand: Generic
Active ingredients:
Phentermine HCl 37.5 mg
Use: See page 285
Mfr: Camall Company

CIV
Imprint: Abana 217
Brand: Obe-Nix
Active ingredients:
Phentermine HCl 37.5 mg
Use: See page 285
Mfr: Abana Pharmaceuticals

CIII
Imprint: BI 64
Brand: Prelu-2
Active ingredients:
Phendimetrazine Tartrate 105 mg
Use: See page 282
Mfr: Boehringer Ingelheim

CIII
Imprint: FIORINAL 78-103
Brand: Fiorinal
Active ingredients:
Aspirin 325 mg
Caffeine 40 mg
Butalbital 50 mg
Use: See page 235
Mfr: Sandoz Pharmaceutical

CIV
Imprint: C5
Brand: Generic
Active ingredients:
Chlordiazepoxide HCl 5 mg
Use: See page 237
Mfr: Geneva Pharmaceuticals

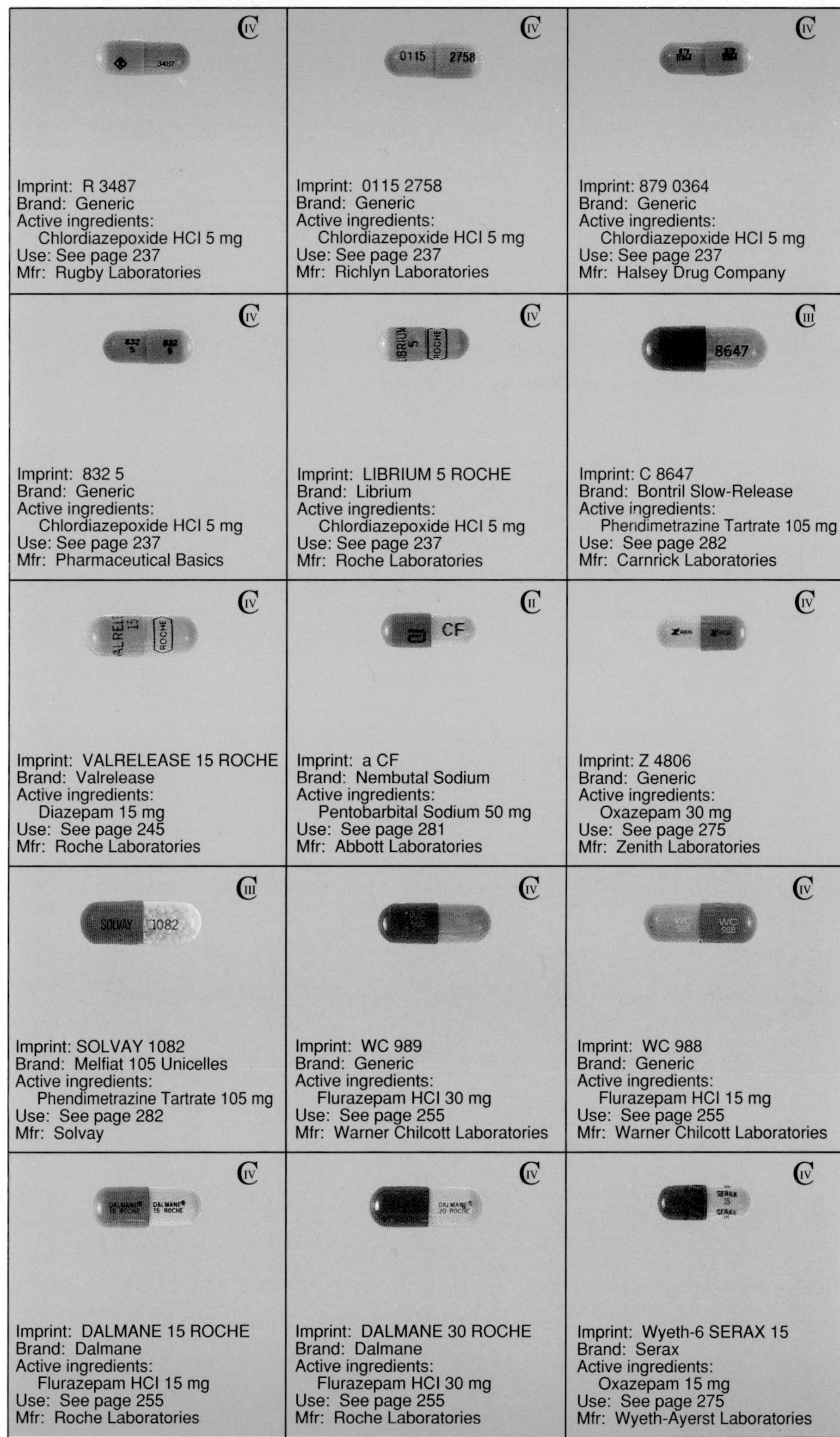

C IV
Imprint: R 3487
Brand: Generic
Active ingredients:
Chlordiazepoxide HCl 5 mg
Use: See page 237
Mfr: Rugby Laboratories

C IV
Imprint: 0115 2758
Brand: Generic
Active ingredients:
Chlordiazepoxide HCl 5 mg
Use: See page 237
Mfr: Richlyn Laboratories

C IV
Imprint: 879 0364
Brand: Generic
Active ingredients:
Chlordiazepoxide HCl 5 mg
Use: See page 237
Mfr: Halsey Drug Company

C IV
Imprint: 832 5
Brand: Generic
Active ingredients:
Chlordiazepoxide HCl 5 mg
Use: See page 237
Mfr: Pharmaceutical Basics

C IV
Imprint: LIBRIUM 5 ROCHE
Brand: Librium
Active ingredients:
Chlordiazepoxide HCl 5 mg
Use: See page 237
Mfr: Roche Laboratories

C III
Imprint: C 8647
Brand: Bontril Slow-Release
Active ingredients:
Phendimetrazine Tartrate 105 mg
Use: See page 282
Mfr: Carnrick Laboratories

C IV
Imprint: VALRELEASE 15 ROCHE
Brand: Valrelease
Active ingredients:
Diazepam 15 mg
Use: See page 245
Mfr: Roche Laboratories

C II
Imprint: a CF
Brand: Nembutal Sodium
Active ingredients:
Pentobarbital Sodium 50 mg
Use: See page 281
Mfr: Abbott Laboratories

C IV
Imprint: Z 4806
Brand: Generic
Active ingredients:
Oxazepam 30 mg
Use: See page 275
Mfr: Zenith Laboratories

C III
Imprint: SOLVAY 1082
Brand: Melfiat 105 Unicelles
Active ingredients:
Phendimetrazine Tartrate 105 mg
Use: See page 282
Mfr: Solvay

C IV
Imprint: WC 989
Brand: Generic
Active ingredients:
Flurazepam HCl 30 mg
Use: See page 255
Mfr: Warner Chilcott Laboratories

C IV
Imprint: WC 988
Brand: Generic
Active ingredients:
Flurazepam HCl 15 mg
Use: See page 255
Mfr: Warner Chilcott Laboratories

C IV
Imprint: DALMANE 15 ROCHE
Brand: Dalmane
Active ingredients:
Flurazepam HCl 15 mg
Use: See page 255
Mfr: Roche Laboratories

C IV
Imprint: DALMANE 30 ROCHE
Brand: Dalmane
Active ingredients:
Flurazepam HCl 30 mg
Use: See page 255
Mfr: Roche Laboratories

C IV
Imprint: Wyeth-6 SERAX 15
Brand: Serax
Active ingredients:
Oxazepam 15 mg
Use: See page 275
Mfr: Wyeth-Ayerst Laboratories

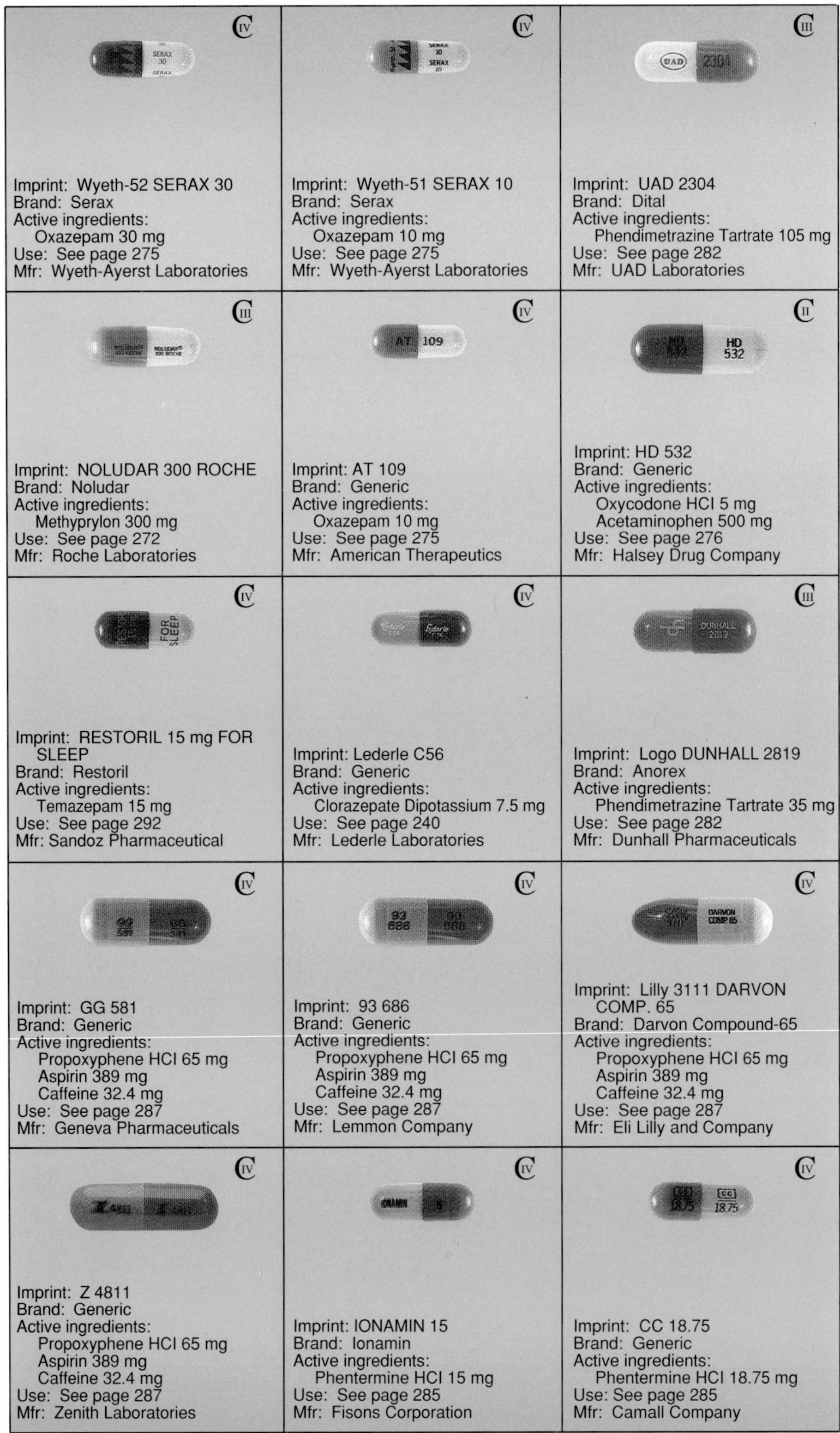

C IV Imprint: Wyeth-52 SERAX 30 Brand: Serax Active ingredients: Oxazepam 30 mg Use: See page 275 Mfr: Wyeth-Ayerst Laboratories	C IV Imprint: Wyeth-51 SERAX 10 Brand: Serax Active ingredients: Oxazepam 10 mg Use: See page 275 Mfr: Wyeth-Ayerst Laboratories	C III Imprint: UAD 2304 Brand: Dital Active ingredients: Phendimetrazine Tartrate 105 mg Use: See page 282 Mfr: UAD Laboratories
C III Imprint: NOLUDAR 300 ROCHE Brand: Noludar Active ingredients: Methyprylon 300 mg Use: See page 272 Mfr: Roche Laboratories	C IV Imprint: AT 109 Brand: Generic Active ingredients: Oxazepam 10 mg Use: See page 275 Mfr: American Therapeutics	C II Imprint: HD 532 Brand: Generic Active ingredients: Oxycodone HCl 5 mg Acetaminophen 500 mg Use: See page 276 Mfr: Halsey Drug Company
C IV Imprint: RESTORIL 15 mg FOR SLEEP Brand: Restoril Active ingredients: Temazepam 15 mg Use: See page 292 Mfr: Sandoz Pharmaceutical	C IV Imprint: Lederle C56 Brand: Generic Active ingredients: Clorazepate Dipotassium 7.5 mg Use: See page 240 Mfr: Lederle Laboratories	C III Imprint: Logo DUNHALL 2819 Brand: Anorex Active ingredients: Phendimetrazine Tartrate 35 mg Use: See page 282 Mfr: Dunhall Pharmaceuticals
C IV Imprint: GG 581 Brand: Generic Active ingredients: Propoxyphene HCl 65 mg Aspirin 389 mg Caffeine 32.4 mg Use: See page 287 Mfr: Geneva Pharmaceuticals	C IV Imprint: 93 686 Brand: Generic Active ingredients: Propoxyphene HCl 65 mg Aspirin 389 mg Caffeine 32.4 mg Use: See page 287 Mfr: Lemmon Company	C IV Imprint: Lilly 3111 DARVON COMP. 65 Brand: Darvon Compound-65 Active ingredients: Propoxyphene HCl 65 mg Aspirin 389 mg Caffeine 32.4 mg Use: See page 287 Mfr: Eli Lilly and Company
C IV Imprint: Z 4811 Brand: Generic Active ingredients: Propoxyphene HCl 65 mg Aspirin 389 mg Caffeine 32.4 mg Use: See page 287 Mfr: Zenith Laboratories	C IV Imprint: IONAMIN 15 Brand: Ionamin Active ingredients: Phentermine HCl 15 mg Use: See page 285 Mfr: Fisons Corporation	C IV Imprint: CC 18.75 Brand: Generic Active ingredients: Phentermine HCl 18.75 mg Use: See page 285 Mfr: Camall Company

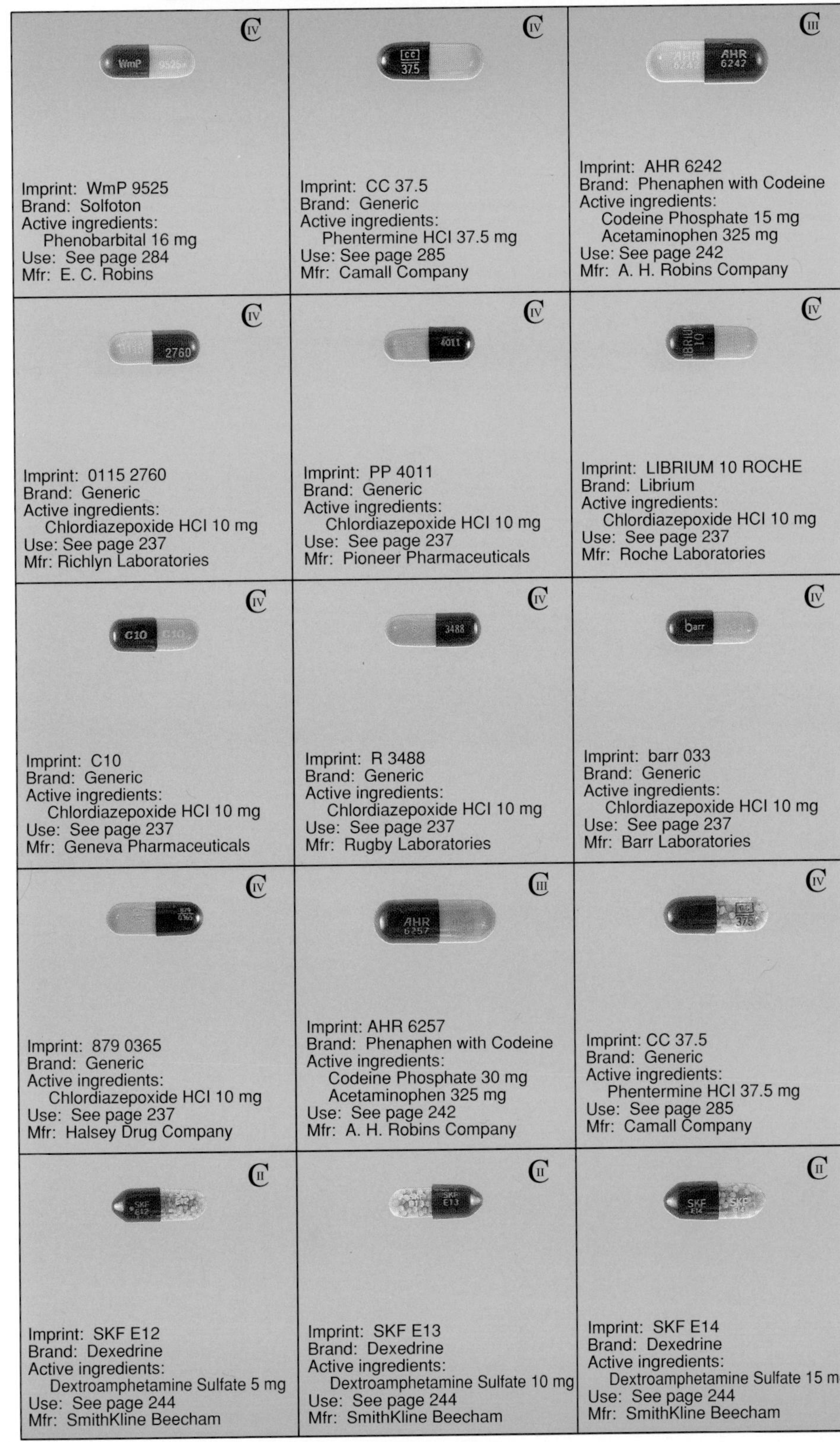

Imprint: WmP 9525
Brand: Solfoton
Active ingredients:
Phenobarbital 16 mg
Use: See page 284
Mfr: E. C. Robins

Imprint: CC 37.5
Brand: Generic
Active ingredients:
Phentermine HCl 37.5 mg
Use: See page 285
Mfr: Camall Company

Imprint: AHR 6242
Brand: Phenaphen with Codeine
Active ingredients:
Codeine Phosphate 15 mg
Acetaminophen 325 mg
Use: See page 242
Mfr: A. H. Robins Company

Imprint: 0115 2760
Brand: Generic
Active ingredients:
Chlordiazepoxide HCl 10 mg
Use: See page 237
Mfr: Richlyn Laboratories

Imprint: PP 4011
Brand: Generic
Active ingredients:
Chlordiazepoxide HCl 10 mg
Use: See page 237
Mfr: Pioneer Pharmaceuticals

Imprint: LIBRIUM 10 ROCHE
Brand: Librium
Active ingredients:
Chlordiazepoxide HCl 10 mg
Use: See page 237
Mfr: Roche Laboratories

Imprint: C10
Brand: Generic
Active ingredients:
Chlordiazepoxide HCl 10 mg
Use: See page 237
Mfr: Geneva Pharmaceuticals

Imprint: R 3488
Brand: Generic
Active ingredients:
Chlordiazepoxide HCl 10 mg
Use: See page 237
Mfr: Rugby Laboratories

Imprint: barr 033
Brand: Generic
Active ingredients:
Chlordiazepoxide HCl 10 mg
Use: See page 237
Mfr: Barr Laboratories

Imprint: 879 0365
Brand: Generic
Active ingredients:
Chlordiazepoxide HCl 10 mg
Use: See page 237
Mfr: Halsey Drug Company

Imprint: AHR 6257
Brand: Phenaphen with Codeine
Active ingredients:
Codeine Phosphate 30 mg
Acetaminophen 325 mg
Use: See page 242
Mfr: A. H. Robins Company

Imprint: CC 37.5
Brand: Generic
Active ingredients:
Phentermine HCl 37.5 mg
Use: See page 285
Mfr: Camall Company

Imprint: SKF E12
Brand: Dexedrine
Active ingredients:
Dextroamphetamine Sulfate 5 mg
Use: See page 244
Mfr: SmithKline Beecham

Imprint: SKF E13
Brand: Dexedrine
Active ingredients:
Dextroamphetamine Sulfate 10 mg
Use: See page 244
Mfr: SmithKline Beecham

Imprint: SKF E14
Brand: Dexedrine
Active ingredients:
Dextroamphetamine Sulfate 15 mg
Use: See page 244
Mfr: SmithKline Beecham

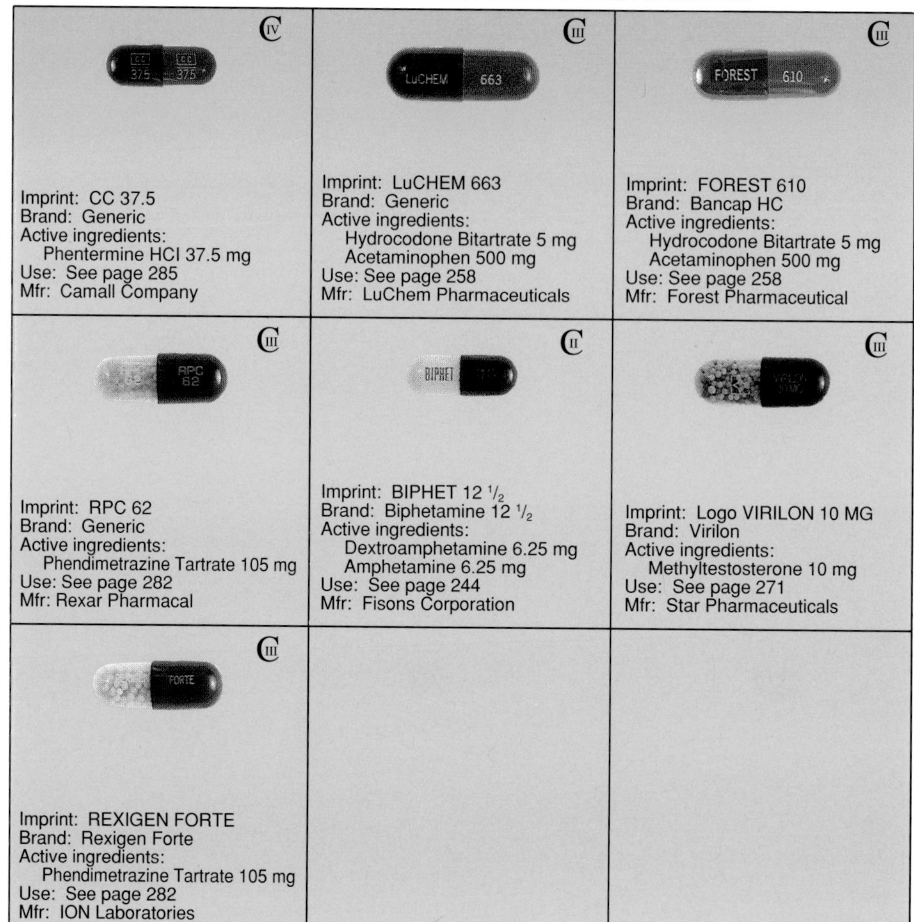

CIV

Imprint: CC 37.5
Brand: Generic
Active ingredients:
Phentermine HCl 37.5 mg
Use: See page 285
Mfr: Camall Company

CIII

Imprint: LuCHEM 663
Brand: Generic
Active ingredients:
Hydrocodone Bitartrate 5 mg
Acetaminophen 500 mg
Use: See page 258
Mfr: LuChem Pharmaceuticals

CIII

Imprint: FOREST 610
Brand: Bancap HC
Active ingredients:
Hydrocodone Bitartrate 5 mg
Acetaminophen 500 mg
Use: See page 258
Mfr: Forest Pharmaceutical

CIII

Imprint: RPC 62
Brand: Generic
Active ingredients:
Phendimetrazine Tartrate 105 mg
Use: See page 282
Mfr: Rexar Pharmacal

CII

Imprint: BIPHET 12 $^1/_2$
Brand: Biphetamine 12 $^1/_2$
Active ingredients:
Dextroamphetamine 6.25 mg
Amphetamine 6.25 mg
Use: See page 244
Mfr: Fisons Corporation

CIII

Imprint: Logo VIRILON 10 MG
Brand: Virilon
Active ingredients:
Methyltestosterone 10 mg
Use: See page 271
Mfr: Star Pharmaceuticals

CIII

Imprint: REXIGEN FORTE
Brand: Rexigen Forte
Active ingredients:
Phendimetrazine Tartrate 105 mg
Use: See page 282
Mfr: ION Laboratories

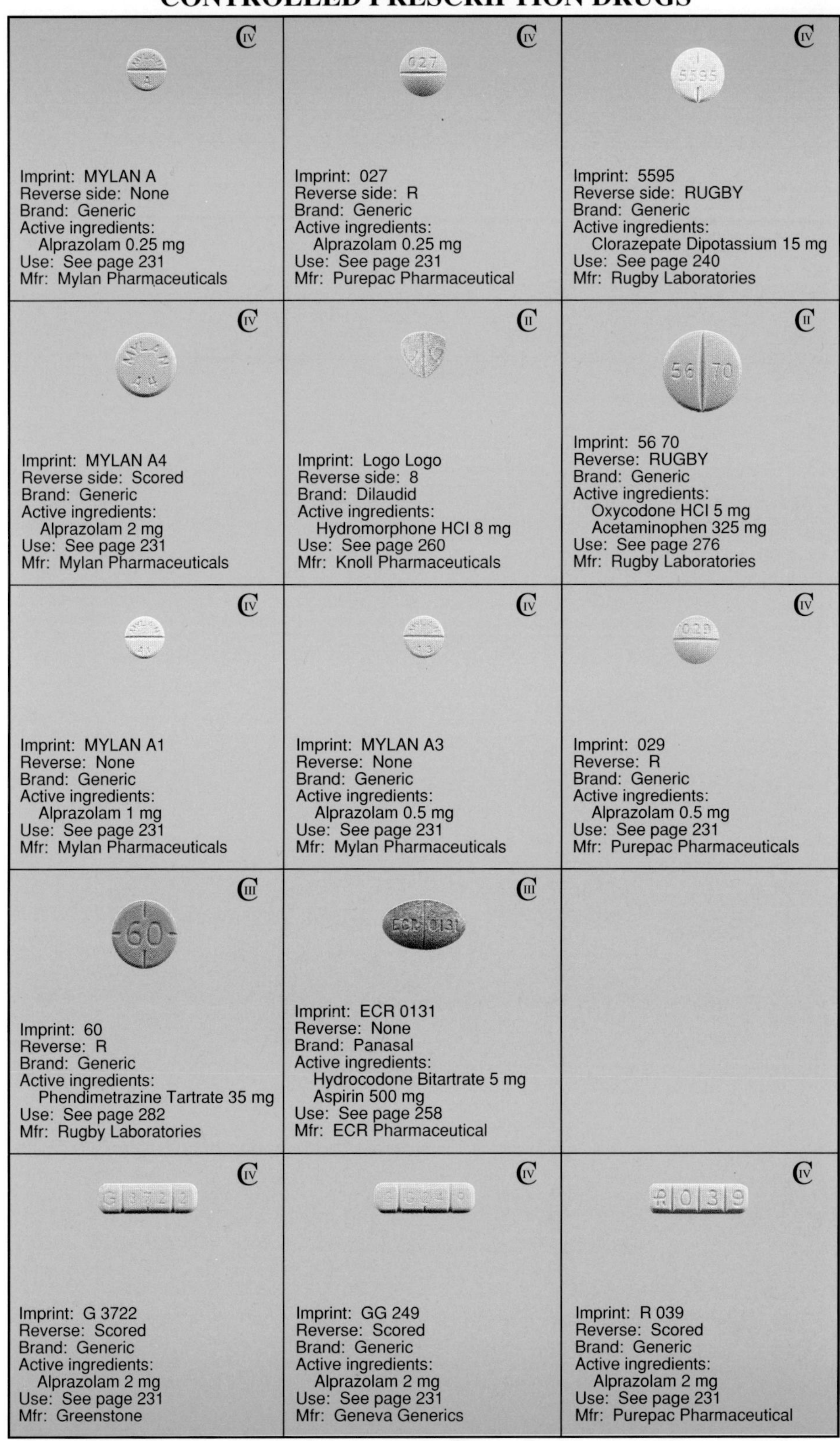

CIV

Imprint: MYLAN A
Reverse side: None
Brand: Generic
Active ingredients:
Alprazolam 0.25 mg
Use: See page 231
Mfr: Mylan Pharmaceuticals

CIV

Imprint: 027
Reverse side: R
Brand: Generic
Active ingredients:
Alprazolam 0.25 mg
Use: See page 231
Mfr: Purepac Pharmaceutical

CIV

Imprint: 5595
Reverse side: RUGBY
Brand: Generic
Active ingredients:
Clorazepate Dipotassium 15 mg
Use: See page 240
Mfr: Rugby Laboratories

CIV

Imprint: MYLAN A4
Reverse side: Scored
Brand: Generic
Active ingredients:
Alprazolam 2 mg
Use: See page 231
Mfr: Mylan Pharmaceuticals

CII

Imprint: Logo Logo
Reverse side: 8
Brand: Dilaudid
Active ingredients:
Hydromorphone HCl 8 mg
Use: See page 260
Mfr: Knoll Pharmaceuticals

CII

Imprint: 56 70
Reverse: RUGBY
Brand: Generic
Active ingredients:
Oxycodone HCl 5 mg
Acetaminophen 325 mg
Use: See page 276
Mfr: Rugby Laboratories

CIV

Imprint: MYLAN A1
Reverse: None
Brand: Generic
Active ingredients:
Alprazolam 1 mg
Use: See page 231
Mfr: Mylan Pharmaceuticals

CIV

Imprint: MYLAN A3
Reverse: None
Brand: Generic
Active ingredients:
Alprazolam 0.5 mg
Use: See page 231
Mfr: Mylan Pharmaceuticals

CIV

Imprint: 029
Reverse: R
Brand: Generic
Active ingredients:
Alprazolam 0.5 mg
Use: See page 231
Mfr: Purepac Pharmaceuticals

CIII

Imprint: 60
Reverse: R
Brand: Generic
Active ingredients:
Phendimetrazine Tartrate 35 mg
Use: See page 282
Mfr: Rugby Laboratories

CIII

Imprint: ECR 0131
Reverse: None
Brand: Panasal
Active ingredients:
Hydrocodone Bitartrate 5 mg
Aspirin 500 mg
Use: See page 258
Mfr: ECR Pharmaceutical

CIV

Imprint: G 3722
Reverse: Scored
Brand: Generic
Active ingredients:
Alprazolam 2 mg
Use: See page 231
Mfr: Greenstone

CIV

Imprint: GG 249
Reverse: Scored
Brand: Generic
Active ingredients:
Alprazolam 2 mg
Use: See page 231
Mfr: Geneva Generics

CIV

Imprint: R 039
Reverse: Scored
Brand: Generic
Active ingredients:
Alprazolam 2 mg
Use: See page 231
Mfr: Purepac Pharmaceutical

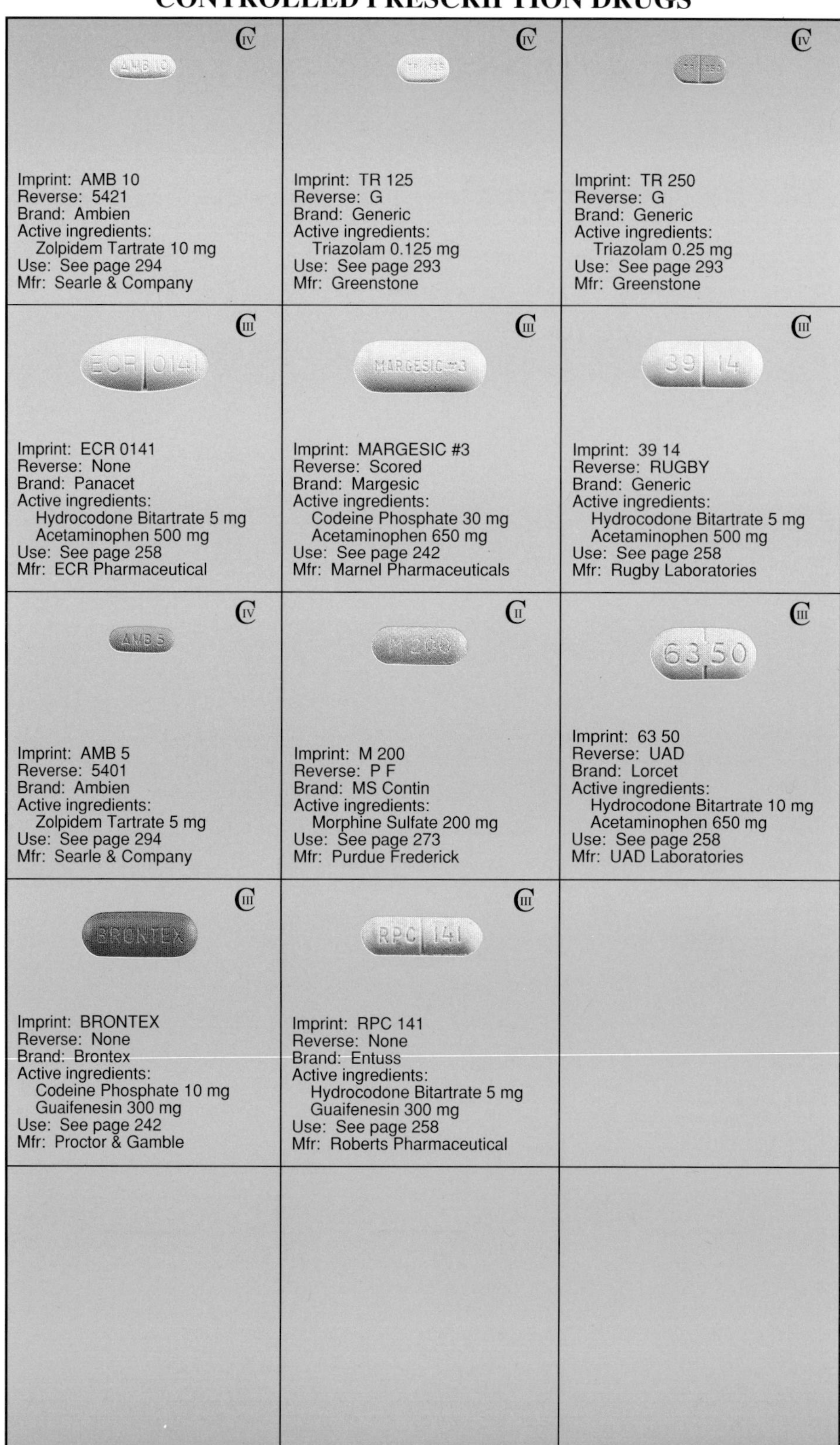

C IV

Imprint: AMB 10
Reverse: 5421
Brand: Ambien
Active ingredients:
Zolpidem Tartrate 10 mg
Use: See page 294
Mfr: Searle & Company

C IV

Imprint: TR 125
Reverse: G
Brand: Generic
Active ingredients:
Triazolam 0.125 mg
Use: See page 293
Mfr: Greenstone

C IV

Imprint: TR 250
Reverse: G
Brand: Generic
Active ingredients:
Triazolam 0.25 mg
Use: See page 293
Mfr: Greenstone

C III

Imprint: ECR 0141
Reverse: None
Brand: Panacet
Active ingredients:
Hydrocodone Bitartrate 5 mg
Acetaminophen 500 mg
Use: See page 258
Mfr: ECR Pharmaceutical

C III

Imprint: MARGESIC #3
Reverse: Scored
Brand: Margesic
Active ingredients:
Codeine Phosphate 30 mg
Acetaminophen 650 mg
Use: See page 242
Mfr: Marnel Pharmaceuticals

C III

Imprint: 39 14
Reverse: RUGBY
Brand: Generic
Active ingredients:
Hydrocodone Bitartrate 5 mg
Acetaminophen 500 mg
Use: See page 258
Mfr: Rugby Laboratories

C IV

Imprint: AMB 5
Reverse: 5401
Brand: Ambien
Active ingredients:
Zolpidem Tartrate 5 mg
Use: See page 294
Mfr: Searle & Company

C II

Imprint: M 200
Reverse: P F
Brand: MS Contin
Active ingredients:
Morphine Sulfate 200 mg
Use: See page 273
Mfr: Purdue Frederick

C III

Imprint: 63 50
Reverse: UAD
Brand: Lorcet
Active ingredients:
Hydrocodone Bitartrate 10 mg
Acetaminophen 650 mg
Use: See page 258
Mfr: UAD Laboratories

C III

Imprint: BRONTEX
Reverse: None
Brand: Brontex
Active ingredients:
Codeine Phosphate 10 mg
Guaifenesin 300 mg
Use: See page 242
Mfr: Proctor & Gamble

C III

Imprint: RPC 141
Reverse: None
Brand: Entuss
Active ingredients:
Hydrocodone Bitartrate 5 mg
Guaifenesin 300 mg
Use: See page 258
Mfr: Roberts Pharmaceutical

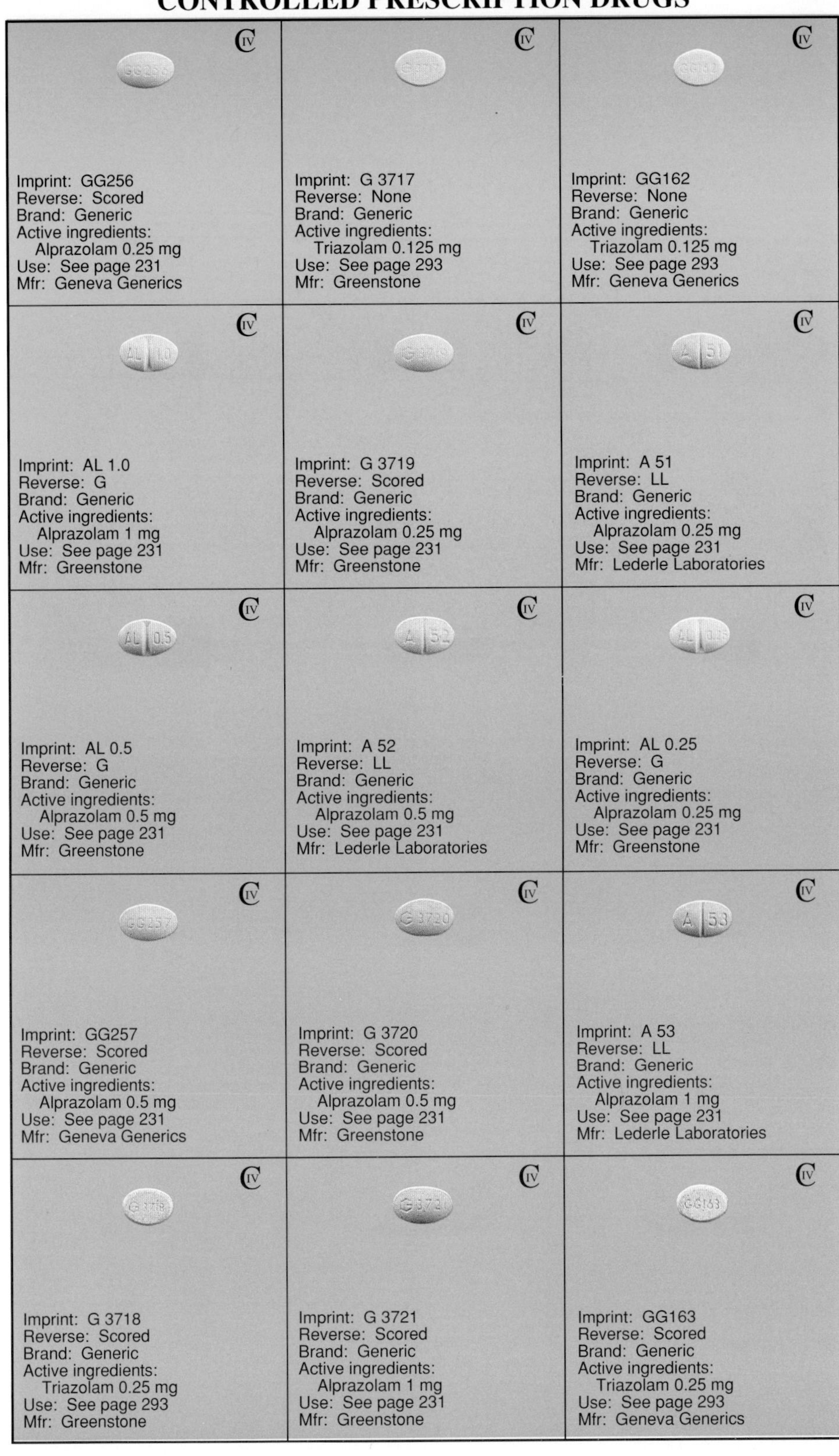

Imprint: GG256
Reverse: Scored
Brand: Generic
Active ingredients:
Alprazolam 0.25 mg
Use: See page 231
Mfr: Geneva Generics

Imprint: G 3717
Reverse: None
Brand: Generic
Active ingredients:
Triazolam 0.125 mg
Use: See page 293
Mfr: Greenstone

Imprint: GG162
Reverse: None
Brand: Generic
Active ingredients:
Triazolam 0.125 mg
Use: See page 293
Mfr: Geneva Generics

Imprint: AL 1.0
Reverse: G
Brand: Generic
Active ingredients:
Alprazolam 1 mg
Use: See page 231
Mfr: Greenstone

Imprint: G 3719
Reverse: Scored
Brand: Generic
Active ingredients:
Alprazolam 0.25 mg
Use: See page 231
Mfr: Greenstone

Imprint: A 51
Reverse: LL
Brand: Generic
Active ingredients:
Alprazolam 0.25 mg
Use: See page 231
Mfr: Lederle Laboratories

Imprint: AL 0.5
Reverse: G
Brand: Generic
Active ingredients:
Alprazolam 0.5 mg
Use: See page 231
Mfr: Greenstone

Imprint: A 52
Reverse: LL
Brand: Generic
Active ingredients:
Alprazolam 0.5 mg
Use: See page 231
Mfr: Lederle Laboratories

Imprint: AL 0.25
Reverse: G
Brand: Generic
Active ingredients:
Alprazolam 0.25 mg
Use: See page 231
Mfr: Greenstone

Imprint: GG257
Reverse: Scored
Brand: Generic
Active ingredients:
Alprazolam 0.5 mg
Use: See page 231
Mfr: Geneva Generics

Imprint: G 3720
Reverse: Scored
Brand: Generic
Active ingredients:
Alprazolam 0.5 mg
Use: See page 231
Mfr: Greenstone

Imprint: A 53
Reverse: LL
Brand: Generic
Active ingredients:
Alprazolam 1 mg
Use: See page 231
Mfr: Lederle Laboratories

Imprint: G 3718
Reverse: Scored
Brand: Generic
Active ingredients:
Triazolam 0.25 mg
Use: See page 293
Mfr: Greenstone

Imprint: G 3721
Reverse: Scored
Brand: Generic
Active ingredients:
Alprazolam 1 mg
Use: See page 231
Mfr: Greenstone

Imprint: GG163
Reverse: Scored
Brand: Generic
Active ingredients:
Triazolam 0.25 mg
Use: See page 293
Mfr: Geneva Generics

CONTROLLED PRESCRIPTION DRUGS

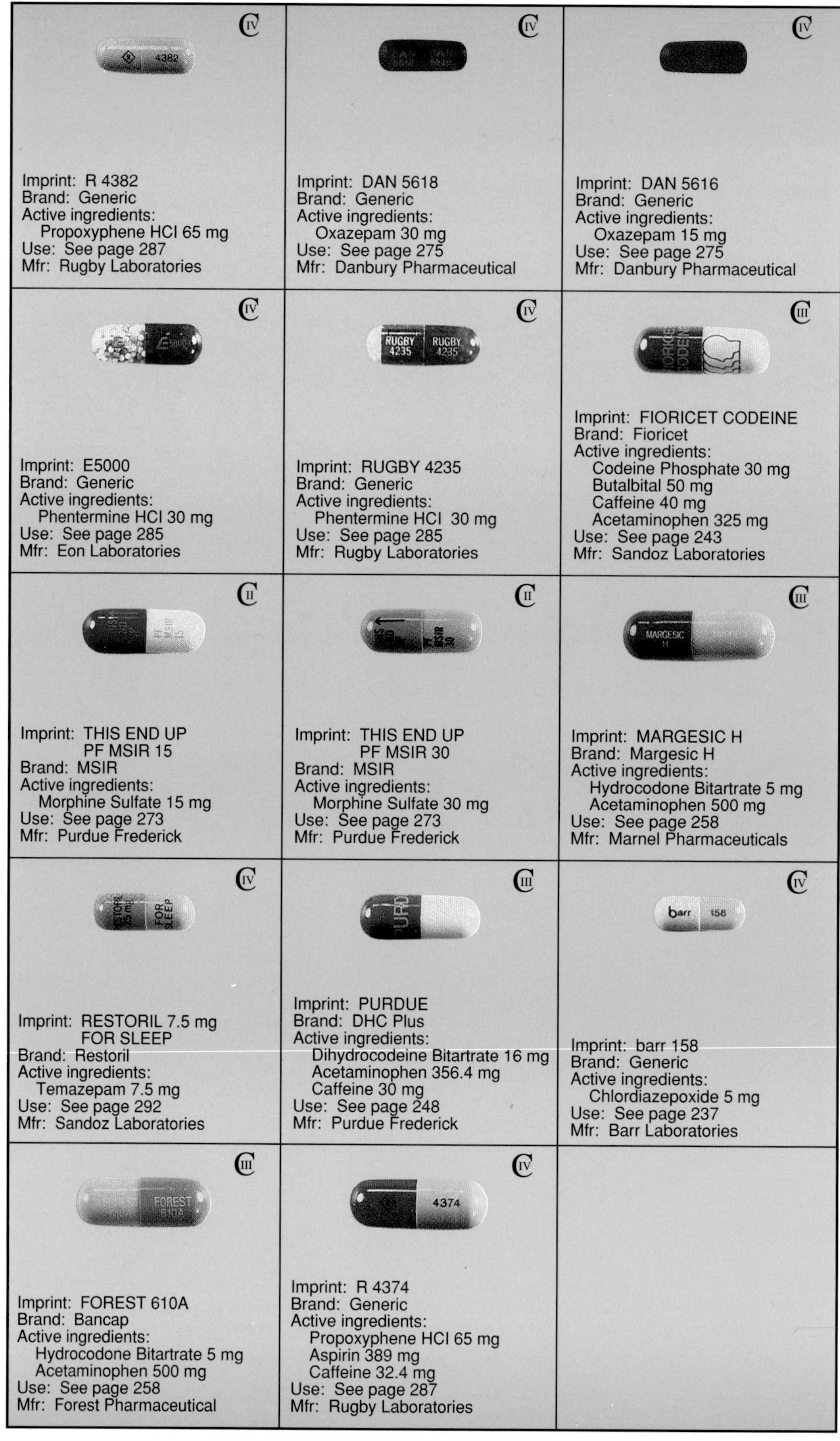

CIV
Imprint: R 4382
Brand: Generic
Active ingredients:
Propoxyphene HCl 65 mg
Use: See page 287
Mfr: Rugby Laboratories

CIV
Imprint: DAN 5618
Brand: Generic
Active ingredients:
Oxazepam 30 mg
Use: See page 275
Mfr: Danbury Pharmaceutical

CIV
Imprint: DAN 5616
Brand: Generic
Active ingredients:
Oxazepam 15 mg
Use: See page 275
Mfr: Danbury Pharmaceutical

CIV
Imprint: E5000
Brand: Generic
Active ingredients:
Phentermine HCl 30 mg
Use: See page 285
Mfr: Eon Laboratories

CIV
Imprint: RUGBY 4235
Brand: Generic
Active ingredients:
Phentermine HCl 30 mg
Use: See page 285
Mfr: Rugby Laboratories

CIII
Imprint: FIORICET CODEINE
Brand: Fioricet
Active ingredients:
Codeine Phosphate 30 mg
Butalbital 50 mg
Caffeine 40 mg
Acetaminophen 325 mg
Use: See page 243
Mfr: Sandoz Laboratories

CII
Imprint: THIS END UP
PF MSIR 15
Brand: MSIR
Active ingredients:
Morphine Sulfate 15 mg
Use: See page 273
Mfr: Purdue Frederick

CII
Imprint: THIS END UP
PF MSIR 30
Brand: MSIR
Active ingredients:
Morphine Sulfate 30 mg
Use: See page 273
Mfr: Purdue Frederick

CIII
Imprint: MARGESIC H
Brand: Margesic H
Active ingredients:
Hydrocodone Bitartrate 5 mg
Acetaminophen 500 mg
Use: See page 258
Mfr: Marnel Pharmaceuticals

CIV
Imprint: RESTORIL 7.5 mg
FOR SLEEP
Brand: Restoril
Active ingredients:
Temazepam 7.5 mg
Use: See page 292
Mfr: Sandoz Laboratories

CIII
Imprint: PURDUE
Brand: DHC Plus
Active ingredients:
Dihydrocodeine Bitartrate 16 mg
Acetaminophen 356.4 mg
Caffeine 30 mg
Use: See page 248
Mfr: Purdue Frederick

CIV
Imprint: barr 158
Brand: Generic
Active ingredients:
Chlordiazepoxide 5 mg
Use: See page 237
Mfr: Barr Laboratories

CIII
Imprint: FOREST 610A
Brand: Bancap
Active ingredients:
Hydrocodone Bitartrate 5 mg
Acetaminophen 500 mg
Use: See page 258
Mfr: Forest Pharmaceutical

CIV
Imprint: R 4374
Brand: Generic
Active ingredients:
Propoxyphene HCl 65 mg
Aspirin 389 mg
Caffeine 32.4 mg
Use: See page 287
Mfr: Rugby Laboratories

CONTROLLED PRESCRIPTION DRUGS USE, EFFECTS AND ABUSE

Information in this section was compiled by Mr. Casey Clark, R.Ph. Mr. Clark graduated from the University of Colorado School of Pharmacy in 1978 and is currently the Clinical Coordinator of Pharmacy Services at Aurora Presbyterian Hospital in Aurora, Colorado. Mr. Clark is the founder and director of the nonprofit organization, A Chronicle On Drug Abuse, headquartered in Aurora, Colorado. This organization has been recognized for its innovative approach to drug education. He and his program have reached hundreds of thousands of students in virtually every school in Colorado and Wyoming. In recognition of his work and accomplishments, Mr. Clark has received dozens of awards, among them the University of Colorado Distinguished Service Award (1988), the USA Today Drugbuster Award (Colorado Nominee 1989), the National Pharmacist of the Year Award from the Pharmacists Against Drug Abuse Foundation (1990), the National U.S. Pharmacists/Searle Community Service Award (1991) and the National Drug Abuse Education Award given by NARD and Parke-Davis (1993). His assistance in completing this book is greatly appreciated.

The Drug Monographs (pages 231 thru 294) are divided into seven sections to assist you with specific desired information. The OVERVIEW is a consolidated summary of the entire drug monograph. Due to space limitations, we were not able to include all information about each drug, but we have tried to provide you with the most pertinent knowledge. It is not our intention that this manual be used as a reference for medical treatment. These monographs are only designed to provide the reader with some of the normal uses, drug actions and visual and physical effects which might be observed. A glossary and a list of references have been provided for your convenience.

Casey F. Clark, R.Ph

GLOSSARY

Anabolic - process of constructive metabolism (eg. muscle growth)
Anaphylaxis - extreme allergic reaction (can lead to death)
Androgenic - producing masculine characteristics
Anesthetic - causes a loss of feeling or sensation to pain
Angioedema - swelling of blood vessels (eg. neck, throat, tongue)
Anorexigenic - producing a diminished appetite
Anxiolytic - agents which work to relieve anxiety
Ataxia - loss of muscular coordination
Cardiovascular - pertaining to the heart and blood vessels
Cerebellum - chief role, unconscious control of muscle movements
Cerebral cortex - site of thought processing and intellect
Cerebral infarct - ruptured blood vessel in the brain (stroke)
Cerebrum - largest part of brain, includes the cerebral cortex, hypothalamus, thalamus and more
CNS - central nervous system (spinal cord & all brain structures)
Dermatitis - vast array of skin inflammations
Epiphyseal growth plates - end of the long bones where further growth occurs
Hemolytic - breaking down of red blood cells (releases hemoglobin)
Hypersomnia - excessive sleep
Hyper/hypotension - high or low blood pressure
Hyper/hypothermia - high or low body temperature
Hypogonadism - decreased activity of the gonads with retardation of growth and sexual development
Hypothalamus - involved with vast array of reflexes including, emotion, motivation, hunger and thirst, body temperature
Libido - sexual desire
Limbic - involved with motivational behavior and emotion
Medulla - controls respiration, swallowing, cardiovascular and functions
Miosis - contraction of the pupils of the eyes
Mydriasis - dilatation of the pupils of the eyes
Myoclonic seizure - seizure of an entire muscle or muscle group
Narcissism - love of one's self
Narcolepsy - uncontrollable desire to sleep
Palpitation - rapid heartbeat felt by the individual
Psychomotor seizure - seizure of cerebral motor or psychic activity
Pulmonary edema - fluid overload in the lungs
Reticular activating system - network of brain tissue connecting parts of the cortex, thalamus, hypothalamus, etc.
Somnolence - sleepiness; unnatural drowsiness
Subcortical levels of the CNS - contribute to muscle movements
Tachycardia - excessive heart rate (pulse greater than 100)

REFERENCES

A Chronicle On Drug Abuse - DRUG FACT SHEETS 1990
American Hospital Formulary Service 1994
(DRUG) Facts and Comparison 1994
Goodman & Gilman's The Pharmacological Basis of Therapeutics 1990
Handbook of Clinical Drug Data 7th Edition 1989
Martindale - The Extra Pharmacopoeia 29th Edition 1989
Micromedex/Poisindex 1994

ALPRAZOLAM (Xanax)
Drug Class: Benzodiazepine

HOW SUPPLIED

Tablets: 0.25mg, 0.5mg, 1mg, 2mg

OVERVIEW

Alprazolam is used for anxiety, depression, panic disorders and premenstrual syndrome. Drowsiness, confusion, slurred speech and ataxia are common side effects, but paradoxically, anger and hostility has been witnessed. Alprazolam is ten times more potent than diazepam and shows a greater risk of withdrawal than other benzodiazepines. Withdrawal leads to confusion, agitation, vomiting, sweating and possibly, seizures, rebound anxiety or psychotic symptoms.

INDICATIONS (NORMAL USE)

Alprazolam is indicated for the short-term relief of symptoms of anxiety, insomnia and panic disorders. Unlike diazepam or other benzodiazepines, it also possesses antidepressant activity and may be used for depression. Occasionally, alprazolam has been used for premenstrual syndrome.

PHARMACOLOGY

Alprazolam is about ten times more potent than diazepam and has a much shorter half-life. Its effects appear to be mediated through the inhibitory neurotransmitter gamma-aminobutyric acid (GABA) which, like all benzodiazepines, enhances the drug's affinity for certain sites within the limbic, thalamic and hypothalamic areas of the brain. It is this inhibition or blocking of the arousal components of these areas which produces the sedative and hypnotic activity. The anxiolytic, antidepressive and paradoxical CNS stimulatory effects are postulated to result from the release of previously suppressed responses (disinhibition) in much the same manner in which alcohol can effect an individual.

ADVERSE REACTION AND OVERDOSE

The most common adverse effects which can be visually observed are: drowsiness, ataxia, fatigue, confusion, weakness and dizziness. Amnesia, blurred vision, slurred speech or stuttering can occur. Paradoxical CNS stimulation can present as restlessness, hyperactivity, mania or possibly, extreme anger and hostility. Acute overdose will generally result in somnolence or coma with respiratory depression. Cardiac or respiratory arrest may result if concurrent ingestion of alcohol or other CNS depressants has occurred.

DRUG ABUSE AND DEPENDENCE

Ingestion of high doses of alprazolam following the taking of methadone has been reported. The combination produces a "high" without pronounced sedation. Nonopiate-drug abusers are also experimenting with alprazolam. The usual urine toxicology screens for benzodiazepines often give false-negative results for alprazolam because of extremely low concentrations of the metabolites excreted, thus making abuse difficult to detect. Physical dependence can occur and due to alprazolams short half-life, withdrawal symptoms may peak within 24-72 hours, much sooner than seen with diazepam (5-8 days). Confusion, agitation, hallucination and life-threatening grand mal seizures are all possible after abrupt withdrawal. Less serious withdrawal symptoms include tremors, abdominal cramps, vomiting and sweating. As with all benzodiazepines, individuals using the drug for anxiety may experience a significant rebound in anxiety after the medication is discontinued which can be easily mistaken for drug withdrawal.

∎

AMOBARBITAL/SECOBARBITAL (Tuinal)
Drug Class: Barbiturate

HOW SUPPLIED
Capsules: 50mg/50mg and 100mg/100mg

OVERVIEW
Amobarbital/secobarbital (Tuinal) is a barbiturate hypnotic primarily indicated for the short-term treatment of insomnia. Drowsiness may be preceded with a period of euphoria, excitement and confusion before its desired sedative actions take effect. Its effects have often been mistakenly attributed to alcohol consumption. The most common side effects include excess sedation, respiratory depression, confusion, ataxia and skin rashes. Overdoses can lead to further respiratory and cardiovascular depression, a fall in blood pressure, shock, coma and ensuing death. Tuinal is addictive and withdrawal symptoms are very similar to those seen with alcohol abstinence and may be life threatening.

INDICATIONS (NORMAL USE)
Tuinal is indicated for the short-term treatment of insomnia.

PHARMACOLOGY
Amobarbital and secobarbital are substituted pyrimidine derivatives. Like all barbiturates, the basic structure of each is barbituric acid. Tuinal, a combination product, acts throughout the CNS and reversibly depresses the activity of all excitable tissues. It is particularly active at the midbrain reticular formation which is specifically concerned with the arousal mechanism. All barbiturates are capable of producing a progressive degree of CNS depression - from mild sedation to hypnosis to deep coma to death. Tuinal has no analgesic effects and may actually increase the reaction to painful stimuli such as an injury.

ADVERSE REACTION AND OVERDOSE
The most common adverse effects are excess sedation, confusion, ataxia, respiratory depression and allergic skin reactions which may be serious. Neuralgic or arthralgic pain, nausea and vomiting are less common. Pupils are usually slightly constricted but may be dilated with severe overdoses. The more alarming effects of reduced blood pressure, body temperature, profound respiratory and cardiovascular depression can lead to coma and death. Paradoxical reactions include a period of euphoria, excitement and possibly, irritability prior to the time the desired sedative actions take effect.

DRUG ABUSE AND DEPENDENCE
Physical dependence to barbiturates like Tuinal is more apt to occur than with other sedative hypnotics such as benzodiazepines. Withdrawal symptoms are similar to those of alcohol abstinence and will usually begin in the first 12-24 hours. Tuinal has a relatively long half-life of 14-42 hours and therefore, symptoms may not peak for several days. Classic symptoms include: weakness, apprehension, anxiety, nausea, vomiting, tremors, abdominal pains, insomnia and tachycardia. Hallucinations, delirium tremors and life-threatening convulsions are possible.

▮

BENZPHETAMINE (Didrex)
Drug Class: Cerebral Stimulant/Amphetamine

HOW SUPPLIED
Tablets: 25mg and 50mg

OVERVIEW
Benzphetamine is an amphetamine congener which is indicated in the short-term therapy (a few weeks) of exogenous obesity. It is abused for it's stimulant activities. The drug's anorexigenic effect appears to be related to CNS stimulation and not to increased metabolic effects or due to appetite suppression. Common side effects include: flushing, hyperexcitability, palpitations, nervousness, insomnia, tremors, mydriasis, increased blood pressure and heart rate and nausea and vomiting. Overdoses can result in death due to convulsions and coma which is frequently associated with a cerebral hemorrhage (stroke). Psychological addiction can occur, but withdrawal symptoms are not medically significant except that severe depression or suicidal ideation may appear.

INDICATIONS (NORMAL USE)
Benzphetamine is indicated as an adjunct to dietary measures in the short-term therapy of exogenous obesity.

PHARMACOLOGY
Benzphetamine, like amphetamine, is a sympathomimetic amine which has greater CNS stimulant activity than epinephrine and ephedrine. It appears to work by enhancing the release of norepinephrine which causes numerous effects including CNS and respiratory stimulation and increased blood pressure. The main site of action is the cerebral cortex and possibly the reticular-activating system which together account for increased motor activity, mental alertness and mild euphoria. Psychic stimulation and excitability over fatigue are also related to the drug's action on the CNS.

ADVERSE REACTION AND OVERDOSE
The most common adverse effects include excitability, nervousness, increased blood pressure and heart rate, as well as those listed in the Overview. Additional adverse effects are increased respiration and libido. Increased mental alertness can be hazardous because the individual is in a hyperexcitatory state and may use poor judgement or overreact. NOTE: As found with all stimulants, including the amphetamines and amphetamine congeners, drug-induced anorexia can lead to unhealthy weight reduction. Overdoses may be manifested initially by increased heart rate, blood pressure and respiration with subsequent cardiac arrhythmias, stroke, coma and death. Hallucinations, delirium, paranoia and combativeness may also be warning signs of an overdose.

DRUG ABUSE AND DEPENDENCE
Physical addiction to benzphetamine due to pharmacological action does not occur, but psychological addiction does. It is not as potent as amphetamine or some of the related drugs, but is still subjected to abuse. Benzphetamine's stimulatory effects may persist for about four hours. Although true physical withdrawal symptoms do not occur, sleep disturbances, including insomnia and hypersomnia, and irritability, severe depression and suicidal ideation can necessitate careful supervision.

▮

BUTABARBITAL (Butisol)
Drug Class: Barbiturate

HOW SUPPLIED

Tablets: 15mg, 30mg, 50mg and 100mg
Oral Elixir: 30mg/5ml and 33.3mg/5ml
*Available in nonproprietary name

OVERVIEW

Butabarbital is a barbiturate hypnotic primarily indicated for the relieving of anxiety and providing sedation preoperatively. Drowsiness may be preceded with a period of euphoria, excitement and confusion before its desired sedative actions take effect. Its effects have often been mistakenly attributed to alcohol consumption. The most common side effects include excess sedation, respiratory depression, confusion, ataxia and skin rashes. Overdoses can lead to further respiratory and cardiovascular depression, a fall in blood pressure, shock, coma and ensuing death. Butabarbital is addictive and withdrawal symptoms are very similar to those seen with alcohol abstinence and may be life threatening.

INDICATIONS (NORMAL USE)

Butabarbital is indicated preoperatively to control anxiety and provide sedation. It has also been used as an hypnotic in the short-term treatment of insomnia.

PHARMACOLOGY

Butabarbital is a substituted pyrimidine derivative. Like all barbiturates, the basic structure is barbituric acid. Butabarbital acts throughout the CNS and reversibly depresses the activity of all excitable tissues. It is particularly active at the midbrain reticular formation which is specifically concerned with the arousal mechanism. All barbiturates are capable of producing a progressive degree of CNS depression - from mild sedation to hypnosis to deep coma to death. Butabarbital has no analgesic effects and may actually increase the reaction to painful stimuli such as an injury.

ADVERSE REACTION AND OVERDOSE

The most common adverse effects are excess sedation, confusion, ataxia, respiratory depression and allergic skin reactions which may be serious. Neuralgic or arthralgic pain, nausea and vomiting are less common. Pupils are usually slightly constricted but may be dilated with severe overdoses. The more alarming effects of reduced blood pressure, body temperature, profound respiratory and cardiovascular depression can lead to coma and death. Paradoxical reactions include a period of euphoria, excitement and possibly, irritability prior to the time the desired sedative actions take effect. Butabarbital, like pentobarbital, has the yellow dye, tartrazine, which can induce allergic reaction such as bronchial asthma in the susceptible individual.

DRUG ABUSE AND DEPENDENCE

Physical dependence to barbiturates like butabarbital is more apt to occur than with other sedative hypnotics such as benzodiazepines. Withdrawal symptoms are similar to those of alcohol abstinence and will usually begin in the first 12-24 hours. Butabarbital has a relatively long half-life of 34-42 hours and therefore, symptoms may not peak for several days. Classic symptoms include: weakness, apprehension, anxiety, nausea, vomiting, tremors, abdominal pains, insomnia and tachycardia. Hallucinations, delirium tremors and life-threatening convulsions are possible.

BUTALBITAL/ASPIRIN/CAFFEINE (Fiorinal)
Drug Class: Barbiturate

HOW SUPPLIED

Tablets: 50mg with 325mg aspirin and 40mg caffeine
*Available in nonproprietary name

OVERVIEW

Butalbital is a barbiturate sedative contained in Fiorinal along with aspirin and caffeine and is used for tension headaches. Drowsiness may be preceded with a period of euphoria, excitement and confusion before its desired sedative actions take effect. The most common side effects include excess sedation, respiratory depression, confusion, ataxia and skin rashes. Overdoses can lead to further respiratory and cardiovascular depression, a fall in blood pressure, shock, coma and ensuing death. Butalbital is less addictive than other barbiturates, but withdrawal symptoms are very similar to those seen with alcohol abstinence.

INDICATIONS (NORMAL USE)

Butalbital/aspirin/caffeine (Fiorinal) is indicated for the relief of symptoms associated with tension or muscle contraction headaches. It has also been tried for migraine headaches.

PHARMACOLOGY

Butalbital is a substituted pyrimidine derivative. Like all barbiturates, the basic structure is barbituric acid. Butalbital acts throughout the CNS and reversibly depresses the activity of all excitable tissues. It is particularly active at the midbrain reticular formation which is specifically concerned with the arousal mechanism. All barbiturates are capable of producing a progressive degree of CNS depression - from mild sedation to hypnosis to deep coma to death. Butalbital has no analgesic effects but is used for its anxiolytic and muscle relaxant effects in combination with aspirin for tension headaches.

ADVERSE REACTION AND OVERDOSE

The most common adverse effects are excess sedation, confusion, ataxia, respiratory depression, nausea, vomiting and allergic skin reactions which may be serious. Pupils are usually slightly constricted but may be dilated with severe overdoses. The more alarming effects of reduced blood pressure, body temperature, profound respiratory and cardiovascular depression can lead to coma and death. Paradoxical reactions include a period of euphoria, excitement and possibly, irritability. Aspirin overdose can lead to bleeding abnormalities, hyperthermia and convulsions, while caffeine can cause insomnia, tremors and tachycardia.

DRUG ABUSE AND DEPENDENCE

Physical dependence to Fiorinal does occur at times. Withdrawal symptoms are similar to those of alcohol abstinence and will usually begin in the first 12-24 hours and symptoms may not peak for several days. Classic symptoms include: weakness, apprehension, anxiety, nausea, vomiting, tremors, abdominal pains, insomnia and tachycardia. Hallucinations, delirium tremors and life-threatening convulsions are possible.

CHLORAL HYDRATE (Noctec)
Drug Class: Sedative/Hypnotic

HOW SUPPLED
Capsules: 200mg and 500mg
Oral Solution: 250mg/5ml and 500mg/5ml
Suppositories: 325mg, 500mg and 650mg
*Available in nonproprietary name

OVERVIEW
Chloral hydrate is a sedative hypnotic which has CNS depressant effects similar to barbiturates. It is primarily indicated for the short-term treatment of insomnia and as a mild sedative. It's depressant actions are greatly enhanced in combination with alcohol (known as a Mickey Finn). The most common side effects include excess sedation, nausea, vomiting, diarrhea, and confusion. Overdoses can lead to excessive respiratory and cardiovascular depression, a fall in blood pressure, shock, coma and ensuing death. Chloral hydrate is addictive with prolonged use and withdrawal symptoms are very similar to those seen with alcohol or barbiturate abstinence and may be life threatening.

INDICATIONS (NORMAL USE)
Chloral hydrate is indicated as an hypnotic in the short-term treatment of insomnia. It is also used preoperatively to allay anxiety and produce sedation. It is often used in elderly patients and children because it appears to possess fewer paradoxical excitatory effects when compared to sedatives such as barbiturates. Occasionally it is used to reduce anxiety when withdrawing from other drugs such as opiates or barbiturates.

PHARMACOLOGY
Chloral hydrate is trichloroacetaldehyde which is metabolized to trichloroethanol, thought to be the active constituent. It's action is similar to that of alcohol (ethanol, which is non-chlorinated). It's exact mechanism of action is unknown, but is most likely concerned with the arousal center as is alcohol's effects. It is capable of producing a progressive degree of CNS depression - from mild sedation to hypnosis to deep coma to death. Unlike the barbiturates and some of the other hypnotics such as glutethimide, chloral hydrate does not seem to effect REM sleep and there is no rebound effects when the drug is withdrawn.

ADVERSE REACTION AND OVERDOSE
The most common adverse effects are excess sedation, confusion, nausea, vomiting and diarrhea. Sometimes, ataxia, respiratory depression and serious allergic skin reactions may occur. The liquid is known to be a topical irritant to mucosal tissue, as well as cutaneous tissue. The more alarming effects of reduced blood pressure, body temperature, profound respiratory and cardiovascular depression can lead to coma and death. Very rarely there may be paradoxical reactions such as excitement and nightmares.

DRUG ABUSE AND DEPENDENCE
Physical dependence to chloral hydrate is very similar to that of chronic alcoholism but may develop within a matter of only two to three weeks of use. Withdrawal symptoms are also similar and usually begin in the first 12-24 hours. Chloral hydrate has a moderate half-life of 8-11 hours and therefore may not peak for several days. Classic symptoms include: weakness, apprehension, anxiety, nausea, vomiting, tremors, abdominal pains, insomnia and tachycardia. Hallucinations, delirium tremors and life-threatening convulsions are possible.

CHLORDIAZEPOXIDE (Librium)
Drug Class: Benzodiazepine

HOW SUPPLIED

Capsules: 5mg, 10mg, and 25mg
Tablets: 5mg, 10mg, and 25mg
Injection: 100mg ampule
* Available by nonproprietary name

OVERVIEW

Chlordiazepoxide is used for anxiety disorders, preoperatively to relieve anxiety and tension and for the management of agitation associated with acute alcohol withdrawal. Drowsiness, confusion, slurred speech and ataxia are common side effects, but paradoxically, anger and hostility has been witnessed. Withdrawal may lead to confusion, agitation, vomiting, sweating and possibly, seizures. These symptoms and rebound anxiety are possible, but they are much less frequent and milder than occurs with alprazolam and lorazepam.

INDICATIONS (NORMAL USE)

Chlordiazepoxide is indicated for the management of anxiety disorders or the short-term relief of symptoms of anxiety. It is also used preoperatively to relieve anxiety and tension and has been utilized widely for the management of acute alcohol withdrawal to reduce, prevent or reduce the frequency and severity of the delirium tremors (DT's)

PHARMACOLOGY

Chlordiazepoxide has one of the longer half-lives of the benzodiazepine class. Its effects appear to be mediated through the inhibitory neurotransmitter gamma-aminobutyric acid (GABA) which, like all benzodiazepines, enhances the drug's affinity for certain sites within the limbic, thalamic and hypothalamic areas of the brain. It is this inhibition or blocking of the arousal components of these areas which produces the sedative and hypnotic activity. The anxiolytic and paradoxical CNS stimulatory effects are postulated to result from the release of previously suppressed responses (disinhibition) in much the same manner in which alcohol can effect an individual.

ADVERSE REACTION AND OVERDOSE

The most common adverse effects which can be visually observed are drowsiness, ataxia, fatigue, confusion, weakness and dizziness. Amnesia, blurred vision and slurred speech can occur. Paradoxical CNS stimulation can present as restlessness, hyperactivity, mania or possibly, extreme anger and hostility. Acute overdose will generally result in somnolence or coma with respiratory depression. Cardiac or respiratory arrest may result if concurrent ingestion of alcohol or other CNS depressants has occurred, but this is unlikely with chlordiazepoxide.

DRUG ABUSE AND DEPENDENCE

Physical dependence can occur and due to chlordiazepoxide's long half-life, withdrawal symptoms may not peak for 5-8 days. Confusion, agitation, hallucinations and seizures are all possible after abrupt withdrawal. Less serious withdrawal symptoms include tremors, abdominal cramps, vomiting and sweating. As with all benzodiazepines, individuals using the drug for anxiety may experience a significant rebound in anxiety after the medication is discontinued which can be easily mistaken for drug withdrawal. The capsule's powder is soluble in water and, along with the injectable form may be abused by the intravenous route also.

▮

CHLORDIAZEPOXIDE PLUS AMITRIPTYLINE (Limbitrol)

Drug Class: Benzodiazepine/Tricyclic Antidepressant

HOW SUPPLIED

Tablets: Limbitrol (5 mg/12.5 mg)
Limbitrol DS (10 mg/25 mg)

OVERVIEW

Limbitrol is used for moderate to severe depression associated with moderate to severe anxiety. While drowsiness, confusion, slurred speech and ataxia are the most common side effects of the chlordiazepoxide component, the amitriptyline can cause a wide range of adverse effects including blurred vision, dry mouth, insomnia, agitation, tremors, rigidity and numerous other reactions. Decreased blood pressure and cardiac arrhythmias, along with other cardiovascular complications such as palpitations, tachycardia or fibrillations can lead to sudden death. Because of the tricyclic component of Limbitrol, abusing this drug can be extremely dangerous, especially in cases of overdose.

INDICATIONS (NORMAL USE)

Limbitrol is indicated for the management of moderate to severe depression associated with moderate to severe anxiety. It has been used for insomnia, feelings of guilt or worthlessness, agitation, psychic and somatic anxiety, suicidal ideation and anorexia.

PHARMACOLOGY

The chlordiazepoxide component has been thoroughly discussed in the preceding section explaining it's action. (Please refer to the monograph on chlordiazepoxide.) Amitriptyline, like all the tricyclic antidepressants, appear to work by blocking the reuptake of various neurotransmitter back into the brain cell at the neuronal membrane. Thus, the transmitters, norepinephrine and serotonin are potentiated. It is this action which most likely accounts for the antidepressant activity.

ADVERSE REACTION AND OVERDOSE

The most common adverse effects which can be visually observed are drowsiness, ataxia, fatigue, confusion, weakness, dizziness, blurred vision (due to mydriasis) and slurred speech. Paradoxical CNS stimulation can present as restlessness, hyperactivity, mania or possibly, extreme anger and hostility. Acute overdose will generally result in somnolence or coma with respiratory depression. Cardiac arrest resulting from a variety of cardiovascular effects such as arrhythmias, palpitations, tachycardia, bradycardia, and ventricular fibrillation can all lead to sudden death.

DRUG ABUSE AND DEPENDENCE

Physical dependence is not likely to occur since the chlordiazepoxide dosage is relatively small. The adverse effects of the amitriptyline component are most likely to manifest an undesirable outcome before a dependency problem arises. However, Limbitrol has been abused on a limited basis for the delusional and hallucinogenic effects which it can possess.

CLONAZEPAM (Klonopin)
Drug Class: Benzodiazepine

HOW SUPPLIED
Tablets: 0.5mg, 1mg and 2mg

OVERVIEW
Clonazepam is primarily used as an anticonvulsant in the prophylactic management of various types of seizure disorders. Drowsiness, confusion, slurred speech and ataxia are common side effects, but paradoxically, behavioral disturbances including aggression, irritability, anger and hostility have occurred, especially in children. Withdrawal leads to confusion, agitation, vomiting, sweating and possibly, seizures, rebound anxiety or psychotic symptoms. Compared to other benzodiazepines, clonazepam is found to have a much more limited abuse potential.

INDICATIONS (NORMAL USE)
Clonazepam is indicated for the prophylactic management of a variety of seizure disorders including petit mal epilepsy, myoclonic seizures and psychomotor seizures. It has also been useful for partial (focal) seizures and some cases of infantile spasms.

PHARMACOLOGY
Clonazepam's action appears to be mediated through the inhibitory neurotransmitter gamma-aminobutyric acid (GABA) which, like all benzodiazepines, enhances the drug's affinity for certain sites within the limbic, thalamic and hypothalamic areas of the brain. Clonazepam primarily acts at the limbic and subcortical levels of the CNS and it is inhibition or blocking of the arousal components of these areas which produces the anti-seizure and sedative effects. Any anxiolytic and paradoxical CNS stimulatory effects which the drug possesses is postulated to result from the release of previously suppressed responses (disinhibition) in much the same manner in which alcohol can effect an individual.

ADVERSE REACTION AND OVERDOSE
The most common adverse effects which can be visually observed are: drowsiness, ataxia, fatigue, confusion, weakness and dizziness. Amnesia, blurred vision and slurred speech can occur. Paradoxical CNS stimulation can present as restlessness, hyperactivity, mania or possibly, extreme anger and hostility. Acute overdose will generally result in somnolence or coma with respiratory depression. Concomitant ingestion of alcohol or other CNS depressants may aggravate symptoms.

DRUG ABUSE AND DEPENDENCE
Physical dependence can occur and due to clonazepam's long half-life (19-39 hours), withdrawal symptoms may not peak for 4-7 days. Confusion, agitation, hallucinations and seizures are all possible after abrupt withdrawal. Less serious withdrawal symptoms include tremors, abdominal cramps, vomiting and sweating. Though clonazepam is not prescribed for anxiety, as with all benzodiazepines, individuals may experience a significant rebound in anxiety after the medication is discontinued which can be easily mistaken for drug withdrawal. ** Note: Clonazepam and all benzodiazepines which have longer half-lives are less likely than benzodiazepines with shorter half-lives to cause serious withdrawal symptoms though it is possible.

▮

CLORAZEPATE DIPOTASSIUM (Tranxene)
Drug Class: Benzodiazepine

HOW SUPPLIED

Capsules: 3.75mg, 7.5mg, and 15mg
Tablets: 3.75mg, 7.5mg, 11.25mg, 15mg and 22.5mg
*Available by nonproprietary name

OVERVIEW

Clorazepate is used in the management of acute alcohol withdrawal, partial seizures, and for anxiety disorders. Drowsiness, confusion, slurred speech and ataxia are common side effects, but paradoxically, anger and hostility has been witnessed. Withdrawal leads to confusion, agitation, vomiting, sweating and possibly, seizures, rebound anxiety or psychotic symptoms. The powder in the capsules is soluble in water and might be abused by the intravenous route as well.

INDICATIONS (NORMAL USE)

Clorazepate is indicated for the management of acute alcohol withdrawal, as an adjunct in the treatment of partial seizures, and for anxiety disorders or the short-term relief of symptoms of anxiety.

PHARMACOLOGY

Clorazepate's action appears to be mediated through the inhibitory neurotransmitter gamma-aminobutyric acid (GABA) which, like all benzodiazepines, enhances the drug's affinity for certain sites within the limbic, thalamic and hypothalamic areas of the brain. It is this inhibition or blocking of the arousal components of these areas which produces the anti-seizure, sedative and hypnotic activity. The anxiolytic and paradoxical CNS stimulatory effects are postulated to result from the release of previously suppressed responses (disinhibition) in much the same manner in which alcohol can effect an individual.

ADVERSE REACTION AND OVERDOSE

The most common adverse effects which can be visually observed are: drowsiness, ataxia, fatigue, confusion, weakness and dizziness. Amnesia, blurred vision and slurred speech can occur. Paradoxical CNS stimulation can present as restlessness, hyperactivity, mania or possibly, extreme anger and hostility. Acute overdose will generally result in somnolence or coma with respiratory depression. Concomitant ingestion of alcohol or other CNS depressants may aggravate symptoms.

DRUG ABUSE AND DEPENDENCE

Physical dependence can occur and due to clorazepate's long half-life, withdrawal symptoms may not peak for 4-7 days. Confusion, agitation, hallucinations and seizures are all possible after abrupt withdrawal. Less serious withdrawal symptoms include tremors, abdominal cramps, vomiting and sweating. As with all benzodiazepines, individuals using the drug for anxiety may experience a significant rebound in anxiety after the medication is discontinued which can be easily mistaken for drug withdrawal.
** Note: Clorazepate and all benzodiazepines which have longer half-lives, i.e., diazepam, chlordiazepoxide, flurazepam, halazepam, prazepam and quazepam are less likely than benzodiazepines with shorter half-lives to cause serious withdrawal symptoms, though it is possible.

COCAINE

Drug Class: Local Anesthetic

HOW SUPPLIED

Topical Solution: 4% and 10% 4ml bottles
Crystals and powder
135mg Soluble Tablet
*Available by nonproprietary name

OVERVIEW

Cocaine is a naturally occurring alkaloid found in the leaves of Erythroxylum coca. Medically it is used as a local anesthetic agent and for the drug's intense vasoconstriction on the mucous membranes of the nose and mouth to deaden the pain and reduce bleeding. Cocaine is abused for its stimulant effects on the CNS which produces a mood elevation and euphoria that can cause an overwhelming desire to continue use of the drug. The most common side effects include increased heart rate, blood pressure and body temperature along with weight loss, nausea and vomiting - the eyes are frequently dilated. Psychotic states and hallucinations (so-called "cocaine bugs") are relatively common occurrences. Death may occur from a single dose or overdosing can lead to convulsions, coma and death. Cocaine is extremely psychologically addicting and is known to be somewhat physically addicting with some withdrawal symptoms being evident, particularly fatigue, irritability and depression ("cocaine blues").

INDICATIONS (NORMAL USE)

Cocaine is used as a local anesthetic and to inhibit bleeding by constricting blood vessels on the mucous membranes of the nose and throat, and also on minor lacerations requiring stitches.

PHARMACOLOGY

Cocaine blocks the initiation or conduction of nerve impulses following local application and it is this action which makes it useful as an anesthetic. Cocaine is also a powerful vasoconstrictor which decreases bleeding, but also accounts for increased body temperature since it prevents the routine heat loss by blood vessels. Its CNS stimulating and addicting effects are due to its interference with the normal reuptake of norepinephrine and dopamine at nerve terminals in the brain. (See Dependence below)

ADVERSE REACTION AND OVERDOSE

Cocaine is a CNS stimulant comparable to amphetamines and produces hyper-stimulation lasting about 30 minutes. Nervousness, tremors and convulsions are possible. Basically, all body systems are put in overdrive and overdoses can lead to death as a result of cardiac or respiratory arrest, cerebral infarcts or convulsions. A single 20mg dose of cocaine has caused death due to the drug's compromising the normal electrical conduction of the heart. Habitual "snorting" of cocaine can cause tissue damage to the mucous membranes of the nose resulting in a loss of smell, symptoms like those of a chronic cold and possibly, perforation of the nasal septum. Hallucinations and psychotic behavior are common findings.

DRUG ABUSE AND DEPENDENCE

Cocaine's addicting qualities appear to focus around the so-called "pleasure centers" of the brain where basic instinctive drives such as hunger, thirst and sexual desires are reinforced. These "drives", mediated by dopamine, are replaced with the drive to obtain more cocaine which blocks dopamine's normal reuptake and continues the CNS stimulation at the expense of natural occurring dopamine which is severely depleted. Higher doses or more frequent use of cocaine are required to satisfy the user's desired effects and to stave off severe depression, the "cocaine blues". Fatigue, lassitude and irritability are also withdrawal symptoms seen with abrupt cessation yet, gradual withdrawal from cocaine is not necessary or recommended.

CODEINE (Tylenol or Empirin with Codeine)
Drug Class: Opiate Agonist

HOW SUPPLIED
Tablets: 30mg, and 60mg
Soluble Tablets: 15mg, 30mg, and 60mg
Injection: 15mg/ml, 30mg/ml and 60mg/ml syringes
Combination Tablets: 15mg, 30mg, and 60mg with acetaminophen 300mg
15mg, 30mg, and 60mg with aspirin 325mg
Combination Capsules: 30mg and 60mg with acetaminophen 325mg
* Available by nonproprietary name and other combinations

OVERVIEW
Codeine is an opioid analgesic used for relieving mild to moderate pain. Like morphine, it is one of the principal alkaloids of opium. Drowsiness, confusion, nausea, vomiting and miosis are the most common side effects. Although less potent than morphine, on an equianalgesic dose codeine also decreases heart rate and blood pressure, along with respiratory depression which can be life threatening. It too possesses euphoric effects which make it addictive and withdrawal symptoms can be severe.

INDICATIONS (NORMAL USE)
Codeine is indicated for the symptomatic relief of mild to moderate pain of numerous types. It has also been used as a cough suppressant, and occasionally as an agent for diarrhea. It is usually used in combination with other analgesics such as acetaminophen and aspirin or in a vast variety of cold and cough preparations.

PHARMACOLOGY
Codeine's action appears to be mediated through the stimulation of several types of opioid receptors throughout the CNS. The opioids possess some of the same properties which the naturally occurring peptides in the body, enkephalins, endorphins and dynorphins, can elicit to reduce pain and produce endogenous euphoria. Codeine acts on the four main opioid receptors, (mu, kappa, delta and sigma) which each activate various responses ranging from analgesia, sedation, miosis and respiratory depression to euphoria, hallucination and dependence, but none of these actions are to the same degree as morphine. Codeine is considered a CNS depressant.

ADVERSE REACTION AND OVERDOSE
The most common adverse effects are nausea, vomiting, drowsiness, confusion, miosis and facial flushing. Paradoxical effects include: ataxia and restlessness. Due to opiates' histamine-releasing effects, rash, itching and significant dermatitis has occurred. With overdoses, more serious adverse effects such as decreases in heart rate, blood pressure, body temperature and respirations can lead to circulatory and respiratory failure with ensuing coma and death. Aspirin and acetaminophen overdoses in combination products can cause death due to an assortment of complications including bleeding abnormalities and liver toxicity.

DRUG ABUSE AND DEPENDENCE
Physical dependence does occur but is not as common a finding with codeine as morphine or related opiate agonists since codeine produces less euphoria. Withdrawal symptoms usually begin within a few hours due to a short half-life (2-4 hours) and peak within 36-72 hours. Classic symptoms include yawning, mydriasis, muscle tremors, sweating, runny nose and watery eyes, diarrhea, nausea, vomiting, abdominal cramping and other abstinence symptoms are similar to morphine.

CODEINE/BUTALBITAL (Fioricet and Fiorinal with Codeine)
Drug Class: Opiate Agonist/Barbiturate

HOW SUPPLIED

Capsules: 30 mg codeine and 50 mg butalbital with 40 mg caffeine and 325 mg acetaminophen or 325 mg aspirin
*Available by nonproprietary name and other combinations

OVERVIEW

Codeine is an opioid analgesic used for relieving mild to moderate pain. Like morphine, it is one of the principal alkaloids of opium. Drowsiness, confusion, nausea, vomiting and miosis are the most common side effects. Although less potent than morphine, on an equianalgesic dose codeine also decreases heart rate and blood pressure, along with respiratory depression which can be life threatening. It too possesses euphoric effects which make it addictive and withdrawal symptoms can be severe. Butalbital is a barbiturate with sedative and hypnotic action. This combination is frequently used for migraine or vascular headaches.

INDICATIONS (NORMAL USE)

Codeine/Butalbital is indicated for the symptomatic relief of mild to moderate pain especially that of migraine or vascular headaches.

PHARMACOLOGY

Codeine's action appears to be mediated through the stimulation of several types of opioid receptors throughout the CNS. Codeine acts on the four main opioid receptors, (mu, kappa, delta and sigma) which each activate various responses ranging from analgesia, sedation, miosis and respiratory depression to euphoria, hallucination and dependence, but none of these actions are to the same degree as morphine. Codeine is considered a CNS depressant. Butalbital's action is not completely known but is thought to depend on a particular site of sensitivity in the polysynaptic midbrain reticular formation which is concerned with the arousal mechanism.

ADVERSE REACTION AND OVERDOSE

The most common adverse effects are nausea, vomiting, drowsiness, confusion, miosis and facial flushing. Paradoxical effects include: ataxia and restlessness. Due to opiates' histamine-releasing effects, rash, itching and significant dermatitis has occurred. With overdoses, more serious adverse effects such as decreases in heart rate, blood pressure, body temperature and respirations can lead to circulatory and respiratory failure with ensuing coma and death. Butalbital causes many of the same adverse effects as codeine and can especially depress respiration further. Again, the aspirin and acetaminophen overdoses in combination products can cause death due to an assortment of complications including bleeding abnormalities and liver toxicity.

DRUG ABUSE AND DEPENDENCE

Because of the combination products' assortment of adverse effects, physical dependence is not as common, but certainly can occur. Both codeine and butalbital can result in dependence which is somewhat more complicated since codeine has a short half-life (2-4 hours) and butalbital has a much longer half-life of 34-42 hours. Withdrawal symptoms are usually not as severe since high doses do not often occur (The toxic effects of aspirin and acetaminophen would arise most likely before pronounced addiction.) Classic symptoms include yawning, mydriasis, muscle tremors, sweating, runny nose and watery eyes, diarrhea, nausea, vomiting and abdominal cramping.

DEXTROAMPHETAMINE (Dexedrine)
Drug Class: Cerebral Stimulant/Amphetamine

HOW SUPPLIED

Tablets: 5mg* and 10mg*
Capsules: 5mg, 10mg, 15mg
Combination Capsules: 6.25mg with 6.25mg amphetamine
10mg with 10mg amphetamine
(Biphetamine 12.5 and 20)
Other combination - Obetrol 10 & 20
*Available by nonproprietary name

OVERVIEW

Dextroamphetamine is an isomer of amphetamine which is indicated in the short-term therapy (a few weeks) of exogenous obesity, narcolepsy and attention deficit disorders. It is abused for it's stimulant activities. Common side effects include: flushing, hyperexcitability, palpitations, nervousness, insomnia, tremors, mydriasis, increased blood pressure and heart rate and nausea and vomiting. Overdoses can result in death due to convulsions and coma which is frequently associated with a cerebral hemorrhage (stroke). Psychological addiction can occur, but withdrawal symptoms are not medically significant except that severe depression or suicidal ideation may appear.

INDICATIONS (NORMAL USE)

Dextroamphetamine alone and in combination products listed above is indicated for narcolepsy, attention deficit disorders (ADD or hyperactivity) in children and as an adjunct to dietary measures in the short-term therapy of exogenous obesity.

PHARMACOLOGY

Dextroamphetamine is a sympathomimetic amine which has greater CNS stimulant activity than epinephrine and ephedrine. It appears to work by enhancing the release of norepinephrine which causes numerous effects including CNS and respiratory stimulation and increased blood pressure. The main site of action is the cerebral cortex and possibly the reticular-activating system which together account for increased motor activity, mental alertness and euphoria. Psychic stimulation and excitability over fatigue are also related to the drug's action on the CNS.

ADVERSE REACTION AND OVERDOSE

The most common adverse effects include excitability, nervousness, increased blood pressure and heart rate, as well as those listed in the Overview. Additional adverse effects are increased respiration and libido. Increased mental alertness can be hazardous because the individual is in a hyperexcitatory state and may use poor judgement or overreact. Continued use results in a loss of libido and mental alertness. Overdoses may be manifested initially by increased heart rate, blood pressure and respiration with subsequent cardiac arrhythmias, stroke, coma and death. Hallucinations, delirium, paranoia and combativeness may also be warning signs of an overdose.

DRUG ABUSE AND DEPENDENCE

Physical addiction to dextroamphetamine due to pharmacological action does not occur, but psychological addiction does. It has a very high abuse potential. Dextroamphetamine's stimulatory effects may persist for about 4-24 hours depending on amount and extended release form. Although true physical withdrawal symptoms do not occur, sleep disturbances, including insomnia and hypersomnia, and irritability, severe depression and suicidal ideation can necessitate careful supervision.

▮

DIAZEPAM (Valium)
Drug Class: Benzodiazepine

HOW SUPPLIED

Tablets: 2mg, 5mg, 10mg
Capsules: 15mg, (Valrelease)
Oral Solution: 5mg/ml
5mg/5ml
Oral suspension: 5mg/5ml
Injection: 5mg/ml in 2ml ampules or 10mg vials
Disposable syringe: 2ml Tel E-Ject
*Available by nonproprietary name

OVERVIEW

Diazepam is used for anxiety, as a muscle relaxant, for insomnia and seizures. It is a CNS depressant. Drowsiness, confusion, slurred speech or ataxia are generally seen, but paradoxically, agitation with hallucinations and rage can occur. Withdrawal leads to tremors, convulsions, muscle cramps, vomiting and sweating. 4%-6% of adults have abused the benzodiazepines.

INDICATIONS (NORMAL USE)

Diazepam is indicated for the short-term relief of symptoms of anxiety, insomnia and panic disorders. It is also used as an anticonvulsant and as a skeletal muscle relaxant in numerous types of muscle spasticity. Occasionally, diazepam has been used in acute alcohol withdrawal to provide symptomatic relief from acute agitation and the DT's (delirium tremors).

PHARMACOLOGY

The effects of diazepam appear to be mediated through the inhibitory neurotransmitter gamma-aminobutyric acid (GABA) which enhances diazepam's affinity for certain sites within the limbic, thalamic and hypothalamic areas of the brain. It is this inhibition or blocking of the arousal components of these areas which produces the sedative, hypnotic, skeletal muscle relaxant and anticonvulsant effects of diazepam. The anxiolytic and paradoxical CNS stimulatory effects are postulated to result from release of previously suppressed responses (disinhibition) in much the same manner in which alcohol can effect an individual.

ADVERSE REACTION AND OVERDOSE

The most common adverse effects which can be visually observed are an extension of the pharmacological actions of diazepam and include drowsiness, ataxia, fatigue, confusion, weakness, dizziness, vertigo and syncope. Amnesia, blurred vision and slurred speech can also occur. Paradoxical CNS stimulation can be manifested by talkativeness, restlessness, hyperactivity, mania or even acute rage. Acute overdose will generally result in extreme somnolence or coma with respiratory depression. Concurrent ingestion of alcohol or other CNS depressants can further exacerbate this action leading to cardiac or respiratory arrest.

DRUG ABUSE AND DEPENDENCE

Approximately 4%-6% of adults have abused a sedative drug for nonmedical use. Diazepam, having the highest lipophilicity of all the benzodiazepines, is one of the fastest acting and therefore, has a greater appeal on the illicit market. Physical dependence can occur. Due to the long half-life of the drug, withdrawal symptoms may not peak until 5-8 days after diazepam has been discontinued. Withdrawal symptoms are similar to those seen with alcohol and barbiturates: convulsions, tremors, abdominal and muscle cramps, vomiting and sweating. Individuals who have taken diazepam for the treatment of anxiety often experience a rebound increase in anxiety after the drug is discontinued, which can be easily mistaken for drug withdrawal.

▮

DIETHYLPROPION (Tenuate)
Drug Class: Cerebral Stimulant/Amphetamine

HOW SUPPLIED

Tablets: 25mg and 75mg
*Available by nonproprietary name

OVERVIEW

Diethylpropion is an amphetamine congener which is indicated in the short-term therapy (a few weeks) of exogenous obesity. It is abused for it's stimulant activities, but is much less active than dextroamphetamine. The drug's anorexigenic effect appears to be related to CNS stimulation and not to increased metabolic effects or due to appetite suppression. Common side effects include: flushing, hyperexcitability, palpitations, nervousness, insomnia, tremors, mydriasis, increased blood pressure and heart rate and nausea and vomiting. Overdoses can result in death due to convulsions and coma which is frequently associated with a cerebral hemorrhage (stroke). Psychological addiction can occur, but withdrawal symptoms are not medically significant except that severe depression or suicidal ideation may appear.

INDICATIONS (NORMAL USE)

Diethylpropion is indicated as an adjunct to dietary measures in the short-term therapy of exogenous obesity.

PHARMACOLOGY

Diethylpropion, like amphetamine, is a sympathomimetic amine which has greater CNS stimulant activity than epinephrine and ephedrine. It appears to work by enhancing the release of norepinephrine which causes numerous effects including CNS and respiratory stimulation and increased blood pressure; however, this pressure effect is much less potent than dextroamphetamine. The main site of action is the cerebral cortex and possibly the reticular-activating system which together account for increased motor activity, mental alertness and mild euphoria. Psychic stimulation and excitability over fatigue are also related to the drug's action on the CNS.

ADVERSE REACTION AND OVERDOSE

The most common adverse effects include excitability, nervousness, increased blood pressure and heart rate, as well as those listed in the Overview. Additional adverse effects are increased respiration and libido. Increased mental alertness can be hazardous because the individual is in a hyperexcitatory state and may use poor judgement or overreact. Overdoses may be manifested initially by increased heart rate, blood pressure and respiration with subsequent cardiac arrhythmias, stroke, coma and death. Hallucination, delirium, paranoia and combativeness may also be warning signs of an overdose.

DRUG ABUSE AND DEPENDENCE

Physical addiction to diethylpropion due to pharmacological action does not occur, but psychological addiction does. It is not as potent as amphetamine or some of the related drugs and its limited availability decreases its area of abuse. Diethylpropion's stimulatory effects may persist for about 4-24 hours depending on dose and extended release form. Although true physical withdrawal symptoms do not occur, sleep disturbances, including insomnia and hypersomnia, and irritability, severe depression and suicidal ideation can necessitate careful supervision.

DIFENOXIN (Motofen)
Drug Class: Opiate Agonist

HOW SUPPLIED
Combination Tablets: 1mg with atropine sulfate 0.025mg

OVERVIEW
Difenoxin is the principle metabolite of diphenoxylate which is a synthetic opioid agonist structurally related to meperidine, but has little to no analgesic effect. It is indicated as adjunctive therapy in the treatment of diarrhea. Usually, 10-20 tablets are required to produce euphoria. Difenoxin's most common side effects include dizziness, drowsiness, nausea, vomiting and abdominal discomfort. (See Adverse Reactions And Overdose for atropine's effects.) Overdoses are difficult to manage since the toxic effects of each ingredient peaks at different times and have opposite actions on the heart and respiratory system.

INDICATIONS (NORMAL USE)
Difenoxin/Atropine (Motofen) is indicated for the adjunctive treatment of diarrhea.

PHARMACOLOGY
While difenoxin possesses some activity with the stimulation of opioid receptors throughout the CNS, its principle action is on the smooth muscles of the intestinal tract. It inhibits gastrointestinal (GI) motility and excess GI propulsion. As an opiate agonist, it also possesses some of the same properties of the naturally occurring peptides in the body, enkephalins, endorphins and dynorphins which can produce euphoria. Difenoxin effects the four opioid receptors much differently than morphine and has little to no analgesic effect and less euphoria. However, like morphine, it can cause constipation. As with all opioids, difenoxin is a CNS depressant.

ADVERSE REACTION AND OVERDOSE
The most common adverse effects are nausea, vomiting, abdominal discomfort, dizziness, drowsiness and confusion. Paradoxical effects include: agitation, insomnia and increased heart rate. Atropine, which is an anticholinergic drug that has been purported to produce some hallucinatory effects, was added to the commercial preparation of difenoxin to discourage deliberate overdose because of its numerous unpleasant side effects which include: blurred vision, dry mouth, thirst, hyperthermia, increased heart rate, urinary retention and flushing. Severe overdoses can lead to respiratory depression, seizures, coma and death.

DRUG ABUSE AND DEPENDENCE
Difenoxin has a half-life between 3-14 hours. Withdrawal symptoms are rare since few individuals abuse this combination product due to its many adverse effects. When it does occur, the abstinence syndrome is less intense and subsides within 4-6 days. The classic symptoms for opiate withdrawal will become apparent after the effects of atropine are no longer present, usually within 24 hours, and include: yawning, muscle tremors, sweating, runny nose and watery eyes, nausea, vomiting and abdominal cramping. In contrast to an overdose, increases in heart rate, blood pressure, body temperature and respirations may occur. Insomnia and gooseflesh may also occur.

DIHYDROCODEINE (Synalgos-DC)
Drug Class: Opiate Agonist

HOW SUPPLIED

Combination Capsules: 16mg with aspirin 356.4mg and caffeine 30mg
*Available by nonproprietary name and many other combinations

OVERVIEW

Dihydrocodeine is a semisynthetic opioid analgesic used for relieving moderate to moderately severe pain. It is an analogue of codeine, but is approximately twice as potent. Drowsiness, confusion, nausea, vomiting and miosis are the most common side effects. Although less potent than morphine, on an equianalgesic dose dihydrocodeine also decreases heart rate and blood pressure, along with respiratory depression which can be life threatening. Euphoric effects, addiction potential and withdrawal symptoms can occur, but are less pronounced than with morphine.

INDICATIONS (NORMAL USE)

Dihydrocodeine is indicated for the symptomatic relief of moderate to moderately severe pain of numerous types including dislocations, sprains, neuralgias and various other injuries and headaches. It has a limited use in the U.S. where it is found in combination with aspirin and caffeine.

PHARMACOLOGY

Dihydrocodeine's action appears to be mediated through the stimulation of several types of opioid receptors throughout the CNS. The opioids possess some of the same properties which the naturally occurring peptides in the body, enkephalins, endorphins and dynorphins, can elicit to reduce pain and produce endogenous euphoria. Dihydrocodeine acts on the four main opioid receptors, (mu, kappa, delta and sigma) which each activate various responses ranging from analgesia, sedation, miosis, and respiratory depression, to euphoria, hallucination and dependence, but none of these actions are to the same degree as morphine. Dihydrocodeine is considered a CNS depressant.

ADVERSE REACTION AND OVERDOSE

The most common adverse effects are nausea, vomiting, drowsiness, confusion, miosis and facial flushing. Paradoxical effects include ataxia and restlessness. Due to opiates' histamine-releasing effects, rash, itching and significant dermatitis has occurred. With overdoses, more serious adverse effects such as decreases in heart rate, blood pressure, body temperature and respirations can lead to circulatory and respiratory failure with ensuing coma and death. Aspirin overdoses in combination products can cause death due to an assortment of complications including bleeding abnormalities.

DRUG ABUSE AND DEPENDENCE

Physical dependence does occur but is not as common a finding with dihydrocodeine as morphine or related opiate agonists since it produces less euphoria. Withdrawal symptoms may begin within a few hours due to a relatively short half-life (2-4 hours) and peak within 2-4 days. Classic symptoms include yawning, mydriasis, muscle tremors, sweating, runny nose and watery eyes, diarrhea, nausea, vomiting, abdominal cramping and other abstinence symptoms are similar to codeine or morphine.

DIPHENOXYLATE (Lomotil)
Drug Class: Opiate Agonist

HOW SUPPLIED

Combination Tablets: 2.5mg with atropine sulfate 0.025mg
Combination Oral Solution: 2.5mg and 0.025mg atropine sulfate/5ml
*Available by nonproprietary name.

OVERVIEW

Diphenoxylate is a synthetic opioid agonist structurally related to meperidine, but has little to no analgesic effect. It is indicated as adjunctive therapy in the treatment of diarrhea. Very high doses, 40-60mg (15-25 tablets) are required to produce euphoria. Diphenoxylate's most common side effects include dizziness, drowsiness, nausea, vomiting and abdominal discomfort. (See Adverse Reaction And Overdose for atropine's effects.) Overdoses are difficult to manage since the toxic effects of each ingredient peaks at different times and have opposite actions on the heart and respiratory system.

INDICATIONS (NORMAL USE)

Diphenoxylate is indicated for the adjunctive treatment of diarrhea.

PHARMACOLOGY

While diphenoxylate possesses some activity with the stimulation of opioid receptors throughout the CNS, its principle action is on the smooth muscles of the intestinal tract. It inhibits gastrointestinal (GI) motility and excess GI propulsion. As an opiate agonist, it also possesses some of the same properties of the naturally occurring peptides in the body, enkephalins, endorphins and dynorphins which can produce euphoria. Diphenoxylate effects the four opioid receptors much differently than morphine and has little to no analgesic effect and less euphoria. However, like morphine, it can cause constipation. As with all opioids, diphenoxylate is a CNS depressant.

ADVERSE REACTION AND OVERDOSE

The most common adverse effects are nausea, vomiting, abdominal discomfort, dizziness, drowsiness and confusion. Paradoxical effects include agitation, insomnia and increased heart rate. Atropine, which is an anticholinergic drug that has been purported to produce some hallucinatory effects, was added to the commercial preparation of diphenoxylate to discourage deliberate overdose because of its numerous unpleasant side effects which include blurred vision, dry mouth, thirst, hyperthermia, increased heart rate, urinary retention and flushing. Severe overdoses can lead to respiratory depression, seizures, coma and death.

DRUG ABUSE AND DEPENDENCE

Diphenoxylate has a short half-life (2-3 hours) with its active metabolite's half-life being 3-14 hours. Withdrawal symptoms are rare since few individuals abuse this combination product due to its many adverse effects. When it does occur, the abstinence syndrome is less intense and subsides within 4-6 days. The classic symptoms for opiate withdrawal will become apparent after the effects of atropine are no longer present, usually within 24 hours, and include yawning, muscle tremors, sweating, runny nose and watery eyes, nausea, vomiting and abdominal cramping. In contrast to an overdose, increases in heart rate, blood pressure, body temperature and respirations may occur. Insomnia and goose-flesh may also occur.

DRONABINOL (Marinol)
Drug Class: Antiemetic

HOW SUPPLIED

Capsules: 2.5mg, 5mg, and 10mg

OVERVIEW

Dronabinol, delta-9-tetrahydrocannabinol (THC), is naturally occurring and is extracted from Cannabis sativa L. (marijuana). Medically it is indicated as an antiemetic with cancer chemotherapy patients and with AIDS related anorexia. The drug's antiemetic effects appear to be related to binding of receptors in the forebrain and indirect inhibition of the vomiting center in the medulla. The most common side effects include reddened conjunctiva (the classic red eyes of marijuana users), euphoria, confusion, ataxia, depersonalization, dizziness, tachycardia and low blood pressure are possible. Paranoia and abnormal thinking are relatively common. Though there is some evidence of physical addiction, the drug's psychological dependence due to its psychoactive effects is the primary reason for abuse. However, Marinol's expense, limited availability and easy access to cultivated marijuana limits its misuse. There are some mild withdrawal symptoms. Overdoses are not known to be life-threatening.

INDICATIONS (NORMAL USE)

Dronabinol is indicated for nausea and vomiting associated with cancer chemotherapy in patients who have failed to respond to conventional antiemetic treatments. It has also been used as an appetite stimulant in anorexia associated with weight loss in patients with AIDS.

PHARMACOLOGY

Dronabinol is an orally active cannabinoid which has complex effects on the CNS resulting in reversible effects on appetite, mood, cognition, memory and perception. Its antiemetic effects appear to be the result of the drug's inhibition of the vomiting center in the medulla. Like THC from marijuana use, dronabinol is extremely fat-soluble and thus will concentrate in fatty areas of the body including the brain and sexual glands. It has a long half-life and may result in detection of THC in the urine or blood being evident for weeks to several months after discontinuation.

ADVERSE REACTION AND OVERDOSE

Dronabinol's psychoactive effects account for many of its CNS adverse reactions including: euphoria, hallucinations, paranoia, amnesia, somnolence and abnormal thinking. All of these phenomena appear to be dose-related, increasing in frequency with higher doses. Visual difficulties, red eyes, nausea and vomiting, dry mouth, urinary retention, ataxia, tachycardia and inconsistent blood pressures (low or high) are also seen. Severe overdose may lead to exacerbation of previously mentioned effects along with panic reactions or possibly seizures in individuals with existing seizure disorders. Overdoses are not considered life-threatening.

DRUG ABUSE AND DEPENDENCE

Dronabinol, as the active ingredient of marijuana, is highly psychoactive and therefore can be addictive to susceptible individuals. However, addiction to dronabinol capsules is not found to be very common and has only been seen after prolonged use of high doses. Withdrawal from high doses has caused irritability, insomnia, sweating, "hot flashes", loose stools and anorexia in some instances. Most of these symptoms resolved after 48 hours, but disruption of normal sleep continued for several weeks.

■

ESTAZOLAM (Pro-Som)
Drug Class: Benzodiazepine

HOW SUPPLIED
Tablets: 1mg and 2mg

OVERVIEW
Estazolam is used as an hypnotic in the short-term management of insomnia. It is similar to temazepam, but more potent on a mg per mg basis. Drowsiness, confusion, slurred speech and ataxia are possible side effects. Paradoxical agitation, anger and hostility have been observed. Abrupt withdrawal is often characterized by rebound insomnia and anxiety. Dependency and withdrawal can occur.

INDICATIONS (NORMAL USE)
Estazolam is indicated as an hypnotic in the short-term management of insomnia.

PHARMACOLOGY
Estazolam's action appears to be mediated through the inhibitory neurotransmitter gamma-aminobutyric acid (GABA) which, like all benzodiazepines, enhances the drug's affinity for certain sites within the limbic, thalamic and hypothalamic areas of the brain. It is this inhibition or blocking of the arousal components of these areas which produces the sedative and hypnotic activity. The paradoxical CNS stimulatory effects are postulated to result from the release of previously suppressed responses (disinhibition) in much the same manner in which alcohol can effect an individual.

ADVERSE REACTION AND OVERDOSE
The most common adverse effects which can be visually observed are extreme drowsiness, ataxia, fatigue, confusion, weakness and dizziness. Amnesia, blurred vision and slurred speech can occur. Paradoxical CNS stimulation, agitation, restlessness and hyperactivity are less common than seen with triazolam or some of the other shorter acting benzodiazepines like alprazolam and lorazepam. Acute overdose will generally result in somnolence or coma with respiratory depression. Concomitant ingestion of alcohol or other CNS depressants may aggravate symptoms.

DRUG ABUSE AND DEPENDENCE
Physical dependence can occur and withdrawal symptoms may not peak for 24-72 hours since estazolam has an intermediate half-life. Rebound insomnia and anxiety, agitation, confusion, rigidity of limbs, hallucinations and seizures are all possible after abrupt withdrawal. Less serious withdrawal symptoms include tremors, abdominal cramps, vomiting and sweating.

ETHCHLORVYNOL (Placidyl)
Drug Class: Sedative/Hypnotic

HOW SUPPLIED
Capsules: 200mg, 500mg, and 750mg
*Available in nonproprietary name

OVERVIEW
Ethchlorvynol is an hypnotic which has CNS depressant effects similar to barbiturates and chloral hydrate. It is primarily indicated for the short-term (1 week) treatment of insomnia. Its effects have often been mistakenly attributed to alcohol consumption. The most common side effects include excess sedation, blurred vision, nausea, vomiting, confusion, respiratory depression and ataxia. Overdoses can lead to further respiratory and cardiovascular depression, a fall in blood pressure, shock, coma and ensuing death. Ethchlorvynol is addictive with prolonged use and withdrawal symptoms are very similar to those seen with barbiturate abstinence and may be life threatening.

INDICATIONS (NORMAL USE)
Ethchlorvynol is indicated as an hypnotic in the short-term treatment of insomnia. Occasionally it has been used routinely for it's sedative effects.

PHARMACOLOGY
Ethchlorvynol is not structurally related to any of the sedatives/hypnotics. It is a chlorinated tertiary acetylenic carbinol that acts on the CNS as a depressant to excitable tissues. It's exact mechanism of action is unknown, but is most likely concerned with the arousal center. It is capable of producing a progressive degree of CNS depression - from mild sedation to hypnosis to deep coma to death.

ADVERSE REACTION AND OVERDOSE
The most common adverse effects are excess sedation, confusion, nausea, vomiting, blurred vision, ataxia, respiratory depression and allergic skin reactions which may be serious. The more alarming effects of reduced blood pressure, body temperature, profound respiratory and cardiovascular depression can lead to coma and death, as can pulmonary edema which has occurred when the contents of the capsules are dissolved and injected by IV drug abusers. Paradoxical reactions include a period of excitement, hysteria and profound muscle weakness. Ethchlorvynol 750mg capsule has the yellow dye, tartrazine, which can induce allergic reactions such as bronchial asthma in the susceptible individual.

DRUG ABUSE AND DEPENDENCE
Physical dependence to ethchlorvynol is very similar to that of barbiturates. Withdrawal symptoms are also similar and usually begin in the first 12-24 hours. Ethchlorvynol has a relatively long half-life of 10-20 hours (sometimes up to 105 hours) and therefore, symptoms may not peak for several days. Classic symptoms include: weakness, apprehension, anxiety, nausea, vomiting, tremors, abdominal pains, insomnia and tachycardia. Hallucinations, delirium tremors and life-threatening convulsions are possible.

FENFLURAMINE (Pondimin)
Drug Class: Cerebral Stimulant/Amphetamine

HOW SUPPLIED

Tablets: 20mg

OVERVIEW

Fenfluramine is an amphetamine congener which is indicated in the short-term therapy (a few weeks) of exogenous obesity. It is abused for it's stimulant activities, but is much less active than dextroamphetamine. The drug's anorexigenic effect appears to be related to CNS stimulation and not to increased metabolic effects or due to appetite suppression. Common side effects include: flushing, hyperexcitability, palpitations, nervousness, insomnia, tremors, mydriasis, increased blood pressure and heart rate and nausea and vomiting. Overdoses can result in death due to convulsions and coma which is frequently associated with a cerebral hemorrhage (stroke). Psychological addiction can occur, but withdrawal symptoms are not medically significant except that severe depression or suicidal ideation may appear.

INDICATIONS (NORMAL USE)

Fenfluramine is indicated as an adjunct to dietary measures in the short-term therapy of exogenous obesity.

PHARMACOLOGY

Fenfluramine, like amphetamine, is a sympathomimetic amine which has greater CNS stimulant activity than epinephrine and ephedrine. It appears to work by enhancing the release of norepinephrine which causes numerous effects including CNS and respiratory stimulation and increased blood pressure; however, this pressure effect is 10-20 times less potent than dextroamphetamine. The main site of action is the cerebral cortex and possibly the reticular-activating system which together account for increased motor activity, mental alertness and mild euphoria. Psychic stimulation and excitability over fatigue are also related to the drug's action on the CNS.

ADVERSE REACTION AND OVERDOSE

The most common adverse effects include excitability, nervousness, increased blood pressure and heart rate, as well as those listed in the Overview. Additional adverse effects are increased respiration and libido. Increased mental alertness can be hazardous because the individual is in a hyperexcitatory state and may use poor judgement or overreact. Overdoses may be manifested initially by increased heart rate, blood pressure and respiration with subsequent cardiac arrhythmias, stroke, coma and death. Hallucinations, delirium, paranoia and combativeness, may also be warning signs of an overdose.

DRUG ABUSE AND DEPENDENCE

Physical addiction to fenfluramine due to pharmacological action does not occur, but psychological addiction does. It is not as potent as amphetamine or some of the related drugs and its limited availability decreases its area of abuse. Fenfluramine's stimulatory effects may persist for about four hours. Although true physical withdrawal symptoms do not occur, sleep disturbances, including insomnia and hypersomnia, and irritability, severe depression and suicidal ideation can necessitate careful supervision. ▮

FLUOXYMESTERONE (Halotestin)
Drug Class: Androgen

HOW SUPPLIED

Tablets: 2mg, 5mg and 10mg
Combination Tablet: 1mg with 0.02mg ethinyl estradiol
*Available by nonproprietary name

OVERVIEW

Fluoxymesterone is a synthetic androgenic, anabolic steroid, hormone. It is primarily indicated for the management of hypogonadism to replace testosterone deficiency in males and to stimulate puberty in carefully selected males with delayed puberty. It is also used to treat inoperable breast cancer in women. Athletes, bodybuilders, weight lifters and physical laborers have used it to add muscle mass. It's most common side effects include increased hair growth and general masculinization, but it also leads to testicular atrophy, breast enlargement and premature baldness in men. It is known to increase aggression and antisocial behavior ("roid rage"). Liver damage or cancer and increased cardiovascular disease are possible. Though not physically addicting, there is some mood elevation. There is no known withdrawal.

INDICATIONS (NORMAL USE)

Fluoxymesterone is indicated for the management of hypogonadism to replace testosterone deficiency in males and stimulate puberty when clinically necessary. It is used for inoperable breast cancer in women and sometimes for painful, postpartum breast engorgement and certain types of aggravating symptoms of menopause.

PHARMACOLOGY

Fluoxymesterone is a synthetic androgenic hormone. The endogenous androgens are essential hormones that are responsible for normal growth and development of the male sex organs and for maintenance of secondary sex characteristics. Like testosterone, it causes retention of nitrogen, potassium, phosphorous and sodium which are subsequently used for protein anabolism; thus promoting an increase in muscle mass and edema (water weight gain). The androgens stimulate the closure of the epiphyseal growth plates and can cause premature termination of the growth process if used inappropriately in prepubertal children.

ADVERSE REACTION AND OVERDOSE

Hormones work by a biofeedback mechanism. If an individual is taking excessive doses of anabolic steroids, the body stops producing testosterone which after time, leads to male eunuchs with characteristics of testicular atrophy (a wasting or diminution of testicle size), aspermia which can cause male infertility, enlarged prostrate and the above mentioned. Serious hemolytic effects and cancer of the liver are possible with excess use. Inappropriate aggressive behavior has also been witnessed. Women will have irregular menstrual cycles, masculinization with excess hair growth, clitoral enlargement, acne and deepening of their voice, many of these changes are permanent.

DRUG ABUSE AND DEPENDENCE

Fluoxymesterone is not physically addicting, but some individuals experience a mood elevation. Initial excitation, including increased libido (which is later followed by impotence), may be appealing to the abuser and thus may contribute to continued use. Enhanced physical appearance may lead to narcissism (love of ones self)and this may account for a degree of psychological addiction. To attain the enhanced performance or physique the abuser desires, dosages of 10 to 1,000-fold that of therapeutic dosages are used. There is no known physical withdrawal.

FLURAZEPAM (Dalmane)
Drug Class: Benzodiazepine

HOW SUPPLIED
Capsules: 15mg and 30mg
*Available by nonproprietary name

OVERVIEW
Flurazepam is used as an hypnotic in the short-term management of insomnia. It was the first benzodiazepine to be approved in the U.S. as an hypnotic. Drowsiness, confusion, slurred speech and ataxia are possible side effects. Paradoxical agitation, anger and hostility have been observed. Abrupt withdrawal is often characterized by rebound insomnia and anxiety. Dependency and withdrawal can occur.

INDICATIONS (NORMAL USE)
Flurazepam is indicated as an hypnotic in the short-term management of insomnia.

PHARMACOLOGY
Flurazepam's action appears to be mediated through the inhibitory neurotransmitter gamma-aminobutyric acid (GABA) which, like all benzodiazepines, enhances the drug's affinity for certain sites within the limbic, thalamic and hypothalamic areas of the brain. It is this inhibition or blocking of the arousal components of these areas which produces the sedative and hypnotic activity. The paradoxical CNS stimulatory effects are postulated to result from the release of previously suppressed responses (disinhibition) in much the same manner in which alcohol can effect an individual.

ADVERSE REACTION AND OVERDOSE
The most common adverse effects which can be visually observed are extreme drowsiness, ataxia, fatigue, confusion, weakness and dizziness. Amnesia, blurred vision and slurred speech can occur. Paradoxical CNS stimulation, agitation, restlessness and hyperactivity are less common than seen with triazolam. Acute overdose will generally result in somnolence or coma with respiratory depression. Concomitant ingestion of alcohol or other CNS depressants may aggravate symptoms.

DRUG ABUSE AND DEPENDENCE
Physical dependence can occur and due to flurazepam's long half-life, withdrawal symptoms may not peak for 5-7 days. Rebound insomnia and anxiety, agitation, confusion, rigidity of limbs, hallucinations and seizures are all possible after abrupt withdrawal. Less serious withdrawal symptoms include tremors, abdominal cramps, vomiting and sweating. The capsule's powder is soluble in water and could be abused intravenously. ** An important reminder: The oral overdose of flurazepam, as well as any benzodiazepines, when taken alone is rarely lethal, but can be particularly dangerous if taken with alcohol, barbiturates, opioids or any additional CNS depressant.

▮

GLUTETHIMIDE (Doriden)
Drug Class: Sedative/Hypnotic

HOW SUPPLIED

Tablets: 250mg and 500mg
*Available in nonproprietary name

OVERVIEW

Glutethimide is an hypnotic which has CNS depressant effects similar to barbiturates and methyprylon. It is primarily indicated for the short-term (one week) treatment of insomnia, but it's high abuse potential and the fact that it offers no hypnotic or sedative advantages over other similar medications has limited it's use in recent years. On the street it is known as "loads". Its effects are particularly enhanced by alcohol consumption. The most common side effects include excess sedation, blurred vision, mydriasis, nausea, vomiting, confusion, skin rashes, respiratory depression and ataxia. Overdoses can lead to further respiratory and cardiovascular depression, a fall in blood pressure, shock, coma and ensuing death. Glutethimide is addictive with prolonged use and withdrawal symptoms are very similar to those seen with barbiturate abstinence and may be life threatening.

INDICATIONS (NORMAL USE)

Glutethimide is indicated as an hypnotic in the short-term treatment of insomnia. It was formerly used as a routine sedative and preoperatively in the first stages of labor to induce sleep.

PHARMACOLOGY

Glutethimide is structurally related to methyprylon, both being a piperidinedione derivative. It's exact mechanism of action is unknown, but is most likely concerned with the arousal center, and thus has very similar CNS depressant effects to those of barbiturates. It is capable of producing a progressive degree of CNS depression - from mild sedation to hypnosis to deep coma to death. In addition, glutethimide has anticholinergic actions which are responsible for the mydriasis, dry mouth and urinary retention effects. Like barbiturates, the usual hypnotic doses of glutethimide significantly suppress rapid eye movement (REM) or dreaming stage of sleep.

ADVERSE REACTION AND OVERDOSE

The most common adverse effects are excess sedation, confusion, nausea, mydriasis, blurred vision, ataxia, respiratory depression and allergic skin reactions which may be serious. The more alarming effects of reduced blood pressure, body temperature, profound respiratory and cardiovascular depression can lead to coma and death. Paradoxical reactions include excitement, headache and vertigo.

DRUG ABUSE AND DEPENDENCE

Physical dependence to glutethimide is very similar to that of barbiturates. Withdrawal symptoms are also similar and usually begin in the first 12-24 hours. Glutethimide has a moderate half-life of 10-12 hours. Symptoms may not peak for several days and may be accompanied by REM rebound resulting in markedly increased dreaming or nightmares. Classic withdrawal symptoms include: weakness, apprehension, anxiety, nausea, vomiting, tremors, abdominal pains, insomnia and tachycardia. Hallucinations, delirium tremors and life-threatening convulsions are possible.

HALAZEPAM (Paxipam)
Drug Class: Benzodiazepine

HOW SUPPLIED

Tablets: 20mg and 40mg

OVERVIEW

Halazepam is used in the management of anxiety or for the short-term relief of symptoms of anxiety. Drowsiness, confusion, slurred speech and ataxia are possible side effects. The use of halazepam is very limited and therefore, some side effects including paradoxical excitation may not have been documented. However, since halazepam shares similar chemical and therapeutic properties, one would expect actions to closely mimic those seen with diazepam.

INDICATIONS (NORMAL USE)

Halazepam is indicated for the management of anxiety disorders and the short-term relief of symptoms of anxiety.

PHARMACOLOGY

Halazepam's action appears to be mediated through the inhibitory neurotransmitter gamma-aminobutyric acid (GABA) which, like all benzodiazepines, enhances the drug's affinity for certain sites within the limbic, thalamic and hypothalamic areas of the brain. It is this inhibition or blocking of the arousal components of these areas which produces the sedative and hypnotic activity. The anxiolytic and paradoxical CNS stimulatory effects are postulated to result from the release of previously suppressed responses (disinhibition) in much the same manner in which alcohol can effect an individual.

ADVERSE REACTION AND OVERDOSE

The most common adverse effects which can be visually observed are drowsiness, ataxia, fatigue, confusion, weakness and dizziness. Amnesia, blurred vision and slurred speech can occur. Paradoxical CNS stimulation is not as common as seen with other benzodiazepines but can present as restlessness, hyperactivity, mania or possibly extreme anger and hostility. Acute overdose will generally result in somnolence or coma with respiratory depression. Concomitant ingestion of alcohol or other CNS depressants may aggravate symptoms.

DRUG ABUSE AND DEPENDENCE

Physical dependence can occur and like diazepam, halazepam has a relatively long half-life. Withdrawal symptoms may not peak for 4-8 days. Confusion, agitation, rigidity of limbs, hallucinations and seizures are all possible after abrupt withdrawal. Less serious withdrawal symptoms include tremors, abdominal cramps, vomiting and sweating. As with all benzodiazepines, individuals using the drug for anxiety may experience a significant rebound in anxiety after the medication is discontinued which can be easily mistaken for drug withdrawal.

HYDROCODONE (Vicodin, Lortab)
Drug Class: Opiate Agonist

HOW SUPPLIED

Combination Tablets: 2.5mg, 5mg, 7.5mg, and 10mg with acetaminophen or aspirin (500mg-750mg)
Combination Capsules: 5mg with acetaminophen 500mg
Combination Solution: 2.5mg & 120mg acetaminophen/5ml
*Available by nonproprietary name and many other combinations

OVERVIEW

Hydrocodone is an opioid analgesic used for relieving moderate to moderately severe pain. It is an analogue of codeine, but is approximately six times more potent. Drowsiness, confusion, nausea, vomiting and miosis are the most common side effects. Although less potent than morphine, on an equianalgesic dose hydrocodone also decreases heart rate and blood pressure, along with respiratory depression which can be life threatening. It too possesses euphoric effects which make it addictive and withdrawal symptoms can be severe.

INDICATIONS (NORMAL USE)

Hydrocodone is indicated for the symptomatic relief of moderate to moderately severe pain of numerous types. It has also been used as a cough suppressant or in combination with other antitussives or expectorants for the symptomatic relief of nonproductive coughs. It is usually used in combination with other analgesics such as acetaminophen and aspirin or in a vast variety of cold and cough preparations.

PHARMACOLOGY

Hydrocodone's action appears to be mediated through the stimulation of several types of opioid receptors throughout the CNS. The opioids possess some of the same properties which the naturally occurring peptides in the body, enkephalins, endorphins and dynorphins, can elicit to reduce pain and produce endogenous euphoria. Hydrocodone acts on the four main opioid receptors, (mu, kappa, delta and sigma) which each activate various responses ranging from analgesia, sedation, miosis and respiratory depression to euphoria, hallucination and dependence, but none of these actions are to the same degree as morphine. Hydrocodone is considered a CNS depressant.

ADVERSE REACTION AND OVERDOSE

The most common adverse effects are nausea, vomiting, drowsiness, confusion, miosis and facial flushing. Paradoxical effects include ataxia and restlessness. Due to opiates' histamine-releasing effects, rash, itching and significant dermatitis has occurred. With overdoses, more serious adverse effects such as decreases in heart rate, blood pressure, body temperature and respirations can lead to circulatory and respiratory failure with ensuing coma and death. Aspirin and acetaminophen overdoses in combination products can cause death due to an assortment of complications including bleeding abnormalities and liver toxicity.

DRUG ABUSE AND DEPENDENCE

Physical dependence does occur but is not as common a finding with hydrocodone as morphine or related opiate agonists since it produces less euphoria. Withdrawal symptoms usually begin within a few hours due to a short half-life (3-4 hours) and peak within 36-72 hours. Classic symptoms include yawning, mydriasis, muscle tremors, sweating, runny nose and watery eyes, diarrhea, nausea, vomiting, abdominal cramping and other abstinence symptoms are similar to codeine or morphine.

HYDROCODONE RESIN/PHENYLTOLOXAMINE (Tussionex Tablet)
Drug Class: Opiate Agonist

HOW SUPPLIED

Tablet: 5mg hydrocodone resin & 10mg phenyltoloxamine (Marketed in Canada)
Combination Suspension: 10mg & 8mg chlorpheniramine/5ml

OVERVIEW

Both forms of (Tussionex) are combinations of an opioid analgesic and antihistamine in a long acting formulation (resin complex). They are indicated for relieving irritant coughs and moderate to moderately severe pain. The hydrocodone component is an analogue of codeine, but is approximately six times more potent. Drowsiness, confusion, nausea, vomiting and miosis are the most common side effects. Although less potent than morphine, on an equianalgesic dose hydrocodone also decreases heart rate and blood pressure, along with respiratory depression which can be life threatening. It too possesses euphoric effects which make it addictive and withdrawal symptoms can be severe. The tablets are not marketed in the U.S., but are available in Canada. Both the tablets and the old formulation of Tussionex Suspension are likely to be circulating in the U.S. despite no longer being produced in this country.

INDICATIONS (NORMAL USE)

Tussionex is indicated for the symptomatic relief of irritant coughs and has also been used for moderate to moderately severe pain of numerous types.

PHARMACOLOGY

Hydrocodone's action appears to be mediated through the stimulation of several types of opioid receptors throughout the CNS. The opioids possess some of the same properties which the naturally occurring peptides in the body, enkephalins, endorphins and dynorphins, can elicit to reduce pain and produce endogenous euphoria. Hydrocodone acts on the four main opioid receptors, (mu, kappa, delta and sigma) which each activate various responses ranging form analgesia, sedation, miosis and respiratory depression to euphoria, hallucination and dependence, but none of these actions are to the same degree as morphine. Hydrocodone is considered a CNS depressant.

ADVERSE REACTION AND OVERDOSE

The most common adverse effects are nausea, vomiting, drowsiness, confusion, miosis and facial flushing. Paradoxical effects include ataxia and restlessness. Due to opiates' histamine-releasing effects, rash, itching and significant dermatitis has occurred. With overdoses, more serious adverse effects such as decreases in heart rate, blood pressure, body temperature and respirations can lead to circulatory and respiratory failure with ensuing coma and death. Deaths from pulmonary edema have been reported with the old suspension formulation and the tablets which contains hydrocodone and phenyltoloxamine, also an antihistamine. These products are likely to be available in some areas.

DRUG ABUSE AND DEPENDENCE

Physical dependence does occur. Tussionex's long duration of action contributes to its abuse since its psychotropic effects last up to eight hours. Withdrawal symptoms are usually delayed for 12-24 hours due to the long-acting formulation; however, the abstinence course will generally follow that seen with the other hydrocodone preparations and will peak within 36-72 hours. Classic symptoms include yawning, mydriasis, muscle tremors, sweating, runny nose and watery eyes, diarrhea, nausea, vomiting, abdominal cramping and other abstinence symptoms are similar to codeine or morphine.

HYDROMORPHONE (Dilaudid)
Drug Class: Opiate Agonist

HOW SUPPLIED

Tablets: 1mg, 2mg, 3mg, 4mg, and 8mg
Oral Solution: 5mg/5ml
Suppositories: 3mg
Injection: 1mg/ml, 2mg/ml and 4mg/ml syringes
2mg/ml and 10mg/ml ampules and vials
30mg/30ml infusion syringe
Combination Solution: 1mg & 100mg guaifenesin/5ml
*Available by nonproprietary name

OVERVIEW

Hydromorphone is a semisynthetic opioid analgesic used for relieving moderate to severe pain and as a cough suppressant. It is structurally very similar to morphine with the only difference being the substitution of an oxygen for hydroxyl group and hydrogenation of one of the double bonds. These differences make the drug 6-8 times more potent than morphine. Drowsiness, confusion, nausea, vomiting and miosis are the most common side effects. Decreased heart rate and blood pressure, along with respiratory depression can be life threatening. It's euphoric effects make hydromorphone highly addictive and withdrawal symptoms can be severe.

INDICATIONS (NORMAL USE)

Hydromorphone is indicated for the symptomatic relief of moderate to severe pain associated with cancer, heart attacks, surgeries and trauma. The high potency hydromorphone, (i.e. 10mg/ml), has been particularly useful for patients who have developed opiate tolerance, and therefore require higher doses to relieve pain. It is also used as a cough suppressant.

PHARMACOLOGY

Hydromorphone's action is nearly identical to morphine's which appears to be mediated through the stimulation of several of the four types of opioid receptors found in the CNS. The opioids possess some of the same properties which the naturally occurring peptides in the body, enkephalins, endorphins and dynorphins, can elicit to reduce pain and produce endogenous euphoria. The opioid receptors each activate various responses ranging from analgesia, sedation, miosis and respiratory depression to euphoria, hallucination and dependence. Hydromorphone is a CNS depressant.

ADVERSE REACTION AND OVERDOSE

The most common adverse effects are nausea, vomiting, drowsiness, confusion, miosis and facial flushing. Paradoxical effects include restlessness, muscle rigidity and mood changes. Due to opiates' histamine-releasing effects, rash, itching and significant dermatitis has occurred. With overdoses more serious adverse effects, such as decreases in heart rate, blood pressure, body temperature and respirations can lead to circulatory and respiratory failure with ensuing coma and death.

DRUG ABUSE AND DEPENDENCE

Physical dependence is a common finding with hydromorphone. Withdrawal symptoms usually begin within a few hours due to a short half-life (1.5-2 hours) and peak within 36-72 hours. Classic symptoms include yawning, mydriasis, muscle tremors, sweating, runny nose and watery eyes, diarrhea, nausea, vomiting and abdominal cramping. In contrast to an overdose, increases in heart rate, blood pressure, body temperature and respirations will occur. Insomnia and goose-flesh are also common findings.

▮

LEVORPHANOL (Levo-Dromoran)
Drug Class: Opiate Agonist

HOW SUPPLIED

Tablet: 2mg
Injection: 2mg/ml ampule and vial

OVERVIEW

Levorphanol is a synthetic opioid analgesic similar in action to morphine and hydromorphone. It is used for relieving moderate to severe pain. Drowsiness, confusion, nausea and vomiting are the most common side effects. Like the opioids mentioned above, it causes similar decreases in heart rate, blood pressure and respiration, which can be life-threatening. Levorphanol can cause dependence and withdrawal symptoms do occur.

INDICATIONS (NORMAL USE)

Levorphanol is indicated for the symptomatic relief of moderate to severe pain often associated with surgeries, labor and trauma. It has been used for intractable pain in the terminally ill and also for preoperative sedation.

PHARMACOLOGY

Levorphanol's action appears to be mediated through the stimulation of several types of opioid receptors throughout the CNS. The opioids possess some of the same properties which the naturally occurring peptides in the body, enkephalins, endorphins and dynorphins, can elicit to reduce pain and produce endogenous euphoria. Levorphanol effects the four opioid receptors in such a way as to possibly cause more sedation and smooth muscle stimulation than morphine, but less constipation, nausea and vomiting. As with all opioids, levorphanol is a CNS depressant.

ADVERSE REACTION AND OVERDOSE

The most common adverse effects are nausea, vomiting, drowsiness and confusion. Paradoxical effects include agitation, muscle rigidity, tremors and seizures. Due to both its histamine-releasing effects and sulfite containing preservative, rash, itching and anaphylaxis and asthmatic episodes can be precipitated. Overdoses can lead to respiratory depression with accompanying decreases in heart rate, blood pressure and body temperature. Ensuing coma and death can occur.

DRUG ABUSE AND DEPENDENCE

Levorphanol has a half-life similar to morphine (2-3 hours), but has a somewhat longer duration of action. Onset of withdrawal symptoms would be delayed slightly, perhaps 4-8 hours. The abstinence syndrome is less intense and subsides within 4-5 days. Classic symptoms include yawning, muscle tremors, sweating, runny nose and watery eyes, nausea, vomiting and abdominal cramping. In contrast to an overdose, increases in heart rate, blood pressure, body temperature and respirations may occur. Insomnia and goose-flesh are also common findings.

∎

LORAZEPAM (Ativan)
Drug Class: Benzodiazepine

HOW SUPPLIED

Tablets: 0.5mg, 1mg, and 2mg
Oral Solution: 2mg/ml (Lorazepam Intensol)
Injection: 2mg/ml and 4mg/ml syringe; 2mg/ml 30ml vial
*Available by nonproprietary name

OVERVIEW

Lorazepam is used for anxiety, anxiety-depressive disorder and acute alcohol withdrawal. Drowsiness, confusion, slurred speech and ataxia are common side effects, but paradoxically, anger and hostility has been witnessed. Withdrawal leads to confusion, agitation, vomiting, sweating and possibly, seizures, rebound anxiety or psychotic symptoms.

INDICATIONS (NORMAL USE)

Lorazepam is indicated for the short-term relief of symptoms of anxiety or anxiety associated with depressive disorders. It is used preoperatively to produce sedation, relieve anxiety and provide anterograde amnesia for patients preferring diminished recall after surgery. It has been used for the management of agitation associated with acute alcohol withdrawal.

PHARMACOLOGY

Lorazepam's action appears to be mediated through the inhibitory neurotransmitter gamma-aminobutyric acid (GABA) which, like all benzodiazepines, enhances the drug's affinity for certain sites within the limbic, thalamic and hypothalamic areas of the brain. It is this inhibition or blocking of the arousal components of these areas which produces the sedative and hypnotic activity. The anxiolytic and paradoxical CNS stimulatory effects are postulated to result from the release of previously suppressed responses (disinhibition) in much the same manner in which alcohol can effect an individual.

ADVERSE REACTION AND OVERDOSE

The most common adverse effects which can be visually observed are drowsiness, ataxia, fatigue, confusion weakness and dizziness. Amnesia, blurred vision and slurred speech can occur. Paradoxical CNS stimulation is not as common as seen with other benzodiazepines but can present as restlessness, hyperactivity, mania or possibly, extreme anger and hostility. Acute overdose will generally result in somnolence or coma with respiratory depression. Concomitant ingestion of alcohol or other CNS depressants may aggravate symptoms.

DRUG ABUSE AND DEPENDENCE

Physical dependence can occur and due to lorazepam's short half-life, withdrawal symptoms may peak within 24-72 hours, much sooner than seen with diazepam (5-8 days). Confusion, agitation, rigidity of limbs, hallucinations and seizures are all possible after abrupt withdrawal. Less serious withdrawal symptoms include tremors, abdominal cramps, vomiting and sweating. As with all benzodiazepines, individuals using the drug for anxiety may experience a significant rebound in anxiety after the medication is discontinued which can be easily mistaken for drug withdrawal.
** Note: Lorazepam, along with alprazolam and triazolam seem to exhibit more serious withdrawal symptoms than other benzodiazepines.

MAZINDOL (Sanorex)
Drug Class: Cerebral Stimulant

HOW SUPPLIED

Tablets: 1mg Mazanor or Sanorex
2mg Sanorex

OVERVIEW

Mazindol is a stimulant structurally unrelated to amphetamines but possessing similar, but much milder properties. It is indicated as an adjunct to dietary measures in the short-term therapy of exogenous obesity. It is abused for it's stimulant activities. Common side effects include palpitations, nervousness, insomnia, tremors, increased blood pressure and heart rate and nausea and vomiting. Although overdoses can result in death due to convulsions and coma, it is unlikely except in extreme cases. Psychological addiction can occur, but withdrawal symptoms are not medically significant except that severe depression or suicidal ideation may appear.

INDICATIONS (NORMAL USE)

Mazindol is indicated as an adjunct to dietary measures in the short-term therapy of exogenous obesity.

PHARMACOLOGY

Mazindol is an imidazoisoindol derivative anorexigenic agent which has some stimulant properties similar to amphetamines. The exact mechanism of action, as well as it's sites of actions in the CNS have not been determined, but the drug is thought to act in the limbic region of the brain and prevent the reuptake of norepinephrine. This action causes CNS, cardiac and respiratory stimulation and increased blood pressure. Mazindol may also cause some psychic stimulation and excitability over fatigue which one would assume is related to the drug's action on the CNS.

ADVERSE REACTION AND OVERDOSE

The most common adverse effects include excitability, nervousness, increased blood pressure, respiration and heart rate, as well as those listed in the Overview. Overdoses may be manifested initially by increased heart rate, blood pressure and respiration with subsequent cardiac arrhythmias, stroke, coma and death although all of these effects are less than observed with amphetamines. As found with all of the stimulants, drug-induced anorexia can result in unhealthy weight reduction. Hallucinations, delirium, paranoia and combativeness may also be warning signs of an overdose.

DRUG ABUSE AND DEPENDENCE

The abuse potential of mazindol in humans has not been determined; however, the possibility of physical or psychological addiction should be considered. Mazindol's stimulatory effects may persist for about 8-15 hours depending on dose. Although true physical withdrawal symptoms do not occur, sleep disturbances (insomnia and hypersomnia), irritability and mental depression have occurred.

▮

MEPERIDINE (Demerol)
Drug Class: Opiate Agonist

HOW SUPPLIED

Tablets: 50mg and 100mg
Oral Solution: 50mg/5ml
Injection: 25mg/50mg/75mg and 100mg/ml syringes, ampules & vials
10mg/ml 30ml infusion syringe
Combination Capsules: 50 mg with promethazine 25mg (Mepergan Fortis)
Injection: 25mg with promethazine 25mg (Mepergan)
*Available by nonproprietary name and some other combinations

OVERVIEW

Meperidine, like methadone, is a synthetic opioid analgesic. It is used for relieving moderate to severe pain. Drowsiness, confusion, nausea and vomiting are the most common side effects. Pupil effects can vary from miosis to mydriasis to no change. The sedative and euphoric effects of meperidine may be greater than morphine when equianalgesic doses are compared. It causes similar decreases in heart rate, blood pressure and respiration which can be life-threatening. It can cause seizures and is more likely to cause anaphylaxis than other opioids. Though not as severe as morphine, dependence and withdrawal symptoms do occur.

INDICATIONS (NORMAL USE)

Meperidine is indicated for the symptomatic relief of moderate to severe pain often associated with surgeries, labor and trauma. It has been used for preoperative sedation, to allay anxiety, and in patients with acute pulmonary edema in contrast to methadone which can cause pulmonary edema. It has been used to relieve pain associated with heart attacks, but since it can paradoxically stimulate the heart at times it is not often utilized.

PHARMACOLOGY

Meperidine's action appears to be mediated through the stimulation of several types of opioid receptors throughout the CNS. The opioids possess some of the same properties which the naturally occurring peptides in the body, enkephalins, endorphins and dynorphins, can elicit to reduce pain and produce endogenous euphoria. Meperidine effects the four opioid receptors in such a way as to possibly cause more sedation and euphoria than morphine, but less constipation and cough suppressant activity compared to the naturally occurring opioids. As with all opioids, meperidine is a CNS depressant.

ADVERSE REACTION AND OVERDOSE

The most common adverse effects are nausea, vomiting, drowsiness and confusion. Paradoxical effects include agitation, muscle rigidity, tremors and seizures. Due to both its histamine-releasing effects and sulfite containing preservative, rash, itching and anaphylaxis and asthmatic episodes can be precipitated. Overdoses can lead to respiratory depression with accompanying decreases in heart rate, blood pressure and body temperature. Ensuing coma and death can occur.

DRUG ABUSE AND DEPENDENCE

Meperidine has a short half-life (12 minutes-3 hours) and thus, it has a shorter duration of action and a more rapid onset of withdrawal symptoms (3-4 hours). The abstinence syndrome is less intense and subsides within 4-5 days. Classic symptoms include yawning, muscle tremors, sweating, runny nose and watery eyes, nausea, vomiting, and abdominal cramping. In contrast to an overdose, increases in heart rate, blood pressure, body temperature and respirations may occur. Insomnia and goose-flesh are also common findings.

▮

MEPHOBARBITAL (Mebaral)
Drug Class: Barbiturate

HOW SUPPLIED
Tablets: 32mg, 50mg and 100mg

OVERVIEW
Mephobarbital is a barbiturate hypnotic primarily indicated in the prophylactic management of epilepsy and occasionally for sedation. Drowsiness may be preceded with a period of euphoria, excitement and confusion. Its effects have often been mistakenly attributed to alcohol consumption. The most common side effects include excess sedation, respiratory depression, confusion, ataxia and skin rashes. Overdoses can lead to further respiratory and cardiovascular depression, a fall in blood pressure, shock, coma and ensuing death. Mephobarbital is less addictive than other barbiturates, but can have withdrawal symptoms similar to those seen with alcohol abstinence.

INDICATIONS (NORMAL USE)
Mephobarbital is indicated in the prophylactic management of epilepsy. It has also been used to provide sedation.

PHARMACOLOGY
Mephobarbital is a substituted pyrimidine derivative. Like all barbiturates, the basic structure is barbituric acid. Nearly 75% of the drug is converted to phenobarbital in the body in the first 24 hours and thus accounts for its activity as an anticonvulsant agent. Mephobarbital acts throughout the CNS and reversibly depresses the activity of all excitable tissues. It is particularly active at the midbrain reticular formation which is specifically concerned with the arousal mechanism. All barbiturates are capable of producing a progressive degree of CNS depression - from mild sedation to hypnosis to deep coma to death. Mephobarbital has no analgesic effects and may actually increase the reaction to painful stimuli such as an injury.

ADVERSE REACTION AND OVERDOSE
The most common adverse effects are excess sedation, confusion, ataxia, respiratory depression and allergic skin reactions which may be serious. Neuralgic or arthralgic pain, nausea and vomiting are less common. Pupils are usually slightly constricted but may be dilated with severe overdoses. The more alarming effects of reduced blood pressure, body temperature, profound respiratory and cardiovascular depression can lead to coma and death. Paradoxical reactions include a period of euphoria, excitement and possibly, irritability prior to the time the desired sedative actions take effect.

DRUG ABUSE AND DEPENDENCE
Physical dependence to barbiturates like mephobarbital is less likely to occur than with other barbiturates. Withdrawal symptoms are similar to those of alcohol abstinence and will usually begin in the first couple of days. Mephobarbital has a very long half-life of 48-120 hours and therefore, symptoms may not peak for several days. Classic symptoms include weakness, apprehension, anxiety, nausea, vomiting, tremors, abdominal pains, insomnia and tachycardia. Hallucinations, delirium tremors and life-threatening convulsions are possible.

▮

MEPROBAMATE (Equanil/Miltown)
Drug Class: Anxiolytic

HOW SUPPLIED

Tablets: 200mg, 400mg, and 600mg
Combination Tablets: 200mg with 325mg aspirin (Equagesic)
Capsules: 200mg and 400mg with 0.45mg conjugated estrogen (PMB/Melprem)
*Available in nonproprietary name

OVERVIEW

Meprobamate is a carbamate derivative which has CNS depressant effects similar to barbiturates, but not as pronounced. It is primarily indicated for the management of anxiety disorders and has been used to promote sleep in the anxious, tense patient. The most common side effects include excess sedation, nausea, dizziness, slurred speech, ataxia and euphoria. Overdoses can lead to excessive respiratory and cardiovascular depression, a fall in blood pressure, shock, coma and ensuing death. Meprobamate is addictive with prolonged use and withdrawal symptoms are very similar to those seen with barbiturate abstinence and may be life threatening.

INDICATIONS (NORMAL USE)

Meprobamate is indicated in the management of anxiety disorders. It has been used preoperatively to relieve anxiety and promote sedation. It has also been used as a muscle relaxant, alone or in combination with an analgesic.

PHARMACOLOGY

Meprobamate is a carbamate derivative which apparently acts at multiple sites in the CNS including the hypothalamus, thalamus and limbic system which is involved with emotions. The drug's skeletal muscle relaxant effects are probably due to it's sedative effects. It may induce convulsions in patient's with a history of epilepsy, and in high doses is capable of producing a progressive degree of CNS depression - from mild sedation to hypnosis to deep coma to death.

ADVERSE REACTION AND OVERDOSE

The most common adverse effects are excess sedation, dizziness, nausea, vomiting, ataxia, euphoria, slurred speech and impaired vision. Respiratory depression, bronchospasm, anaphylaxis and allergic skin reactions have occurred and may be serious. The more alarming effects of reduced blood pressure, body temperature, profound respiratory and cardiovascular depression can lead to coma and death. Paradoxical reactions include a period of palpitations and tachycardia (racing heart). An aspirin overdose which may occur in combination products can lead to bleeding abnormalities, hyperthermia and convulsions.

DRUG ABUSE AND DEPENDENCE

Physical dependence to meprobamate is very similar to that of barbiturates but requires higher doses and more prolonged use. Withdrawal symptoms are also similar and usually begin in the first 12-24 hours. Meprobamate has a moderate half-life of 10-11 hours, but symptoms usually peak within 12-48 hours. Classic symptoms include weakness, apprehension, anxiety, nausea, muscle twitches, vomiting, tremors, abdominal pains, insomnia and psychotic behavior resembling delirium tremors. Life-threatening convulsions are possible, but is rarely seen.

▮

MEPROBAMATE/BENACTYZINE (Deprol)

Drug Class: Anxiolytic/Antidepressant

HOW SUPPLIED

Tablets: 400mg meprobamate with 1mg benactyzine

OVERVIEW

Meprobamate is a carbamate derivative which has CNS depressant effects similar to barbiturates, but not as pronounced. Benactyzine is a mild antidepressant which has anticholinergic effects which cause, most notably, blurred vision and dry mouth. Deprol is primarily indicated in the management of less severe depressions that are accompanied by anxiety, insomnia or agitation. The most common side effects include excess sedation, nausea, dizziness, slurred speech, ataxia and euphoria. Overdoses can lead to excessive respiratory and cardiovascular depression, a fall in blood pressure, shock, coma and ensuing death. Meprobamate is addictive with prolonged use and withdrawal symptoms are very similar to those seen with barbiturate abstinence and may be life threatening. Benactyzine is not known to be addictive when used alone.

INDICATIONS (NORMAL USE)

Meprobamate/benactyzine (Deprol) is indicated in the management of depression, both acute and chronic. It is most useful in less severe depressions which are associated with anxiety, insomnia and agitation.

PHARMACOLOGY

Meprobamate is a carbamate derivative which apparently acts at multiple sites in the CNS including the hypothalamus, thalamus and limbic system which is involved with emotions. The drug's skeletal muscle relaxant effects are probably due to it's sedative effects. Benactyzine's mechanism of action is unknown, but probably blocks the reuptake of neurotransmitters such as norepinephrine and serotonin which are essential for emotional stability. The meprobamate component of Deprol may induce convulsions in patient's with a history of epilepsy and in high doses, is capable of producing a progressive degree of CNS depression - from mild sedation to hypnosis to deep coma to death.

ADVERSE REACTION AND OVERDOSE

The most common adverse effects are excess sedation, dizziness, nausea, vomiting, ataxia, euphoria, slurred speech, dry mouth and impaired vision. Respiratory depression, bronchospasm, anaphylaxis and allergic skin reactions have occurred and may be serious. The more alarming effects of reduced blood pressure, body temperature, profound respiratory and cardiovascular depression can lead to coma and death. Paradoxical reactions include a period of palpitations and tachycardia (racing heart). Benactyzine can also result in thought-blocking, a feeling of depersonalization and aggravation of anxiety in high doses.

DRUG ABUSE AND DEPENDENCE

Physical dependence to Deprol is primarily due to the meprobamate and is thus, very similar to that of barbiturates but requires higher doses and more prolonged use. Withdrawal symptoms are also similar and usually begin in the first 12-24 hours. Meprobamate has a moderate half-life of 10-11 hours, but symptoms usually peak within 12-48 hours. Classic symptoms include weakness, apprehension, anxiety, nausea, muscle twitches, vomiting, tremors, abdominal pains, insomnia and psychotic behavior resembling delirium tremors. Life-threatening convulsions are possible, but is rarely seen. ∎

METHADONE (Dolophine)
Drug Class: Opiate Agonist

HOW SUPPLIED

Tablets: 5mg and 10mg   Dispersible Tablet: 40mg
Oral Solution: 5mg/5ml and 10mg/ml
Oral Concentrated Solution: 10mg/ml
Injection: 10mg/ml 1ml ampules and 20ml vials
*Available by nonproprietary name

OVERVIEW

Methadone is a synthetic opioid analgesic used for relieving severe pain and for detoxification and maintenance treatment for heroin or other opiate dependence. Drowsiness, confusion, nausea, vomiting and miosis are the most common side effects. While it may produce less sedation and euphoria than morphine, it causes more respiratory depression and pulmonary edema which is a common cause of death in overdoses. Though used in detoxification, it too is highly addictive and though not as severe as morphine, withdrawal symptoms do occur.

INDICATIONS (NORMAL USE)

Methadone is indicated for the symptomatic relief of severe, chronic pain often seen with cancer or terminally ill patients. It is probably best known for its detoxification use and maintenance therapy for opiate dependence. Although methadone possesses the same actions as other opiate agonists, there are no other FDA approved uses.

PHARMACOLOGY

Methadone's action appears to be mediated through the stimulation of several types of opioid receptors throughout the CNS. The opioids possess some of the same properties which the naturally occurring peptides in the body, enkephalins, endorphins and dynorphins, can elicit to reduce pain and produce endogenous euphoria. Methadone effects the four main opioid receptors, (mu, kappa, delta and sigma) in such a way as to cause less sedation, constipation and euphoria than morphine, but more respiratory depression. As with all opioids, methadone is a CNS depressant.

ADVERSE REACTION AND OVERDOSE

The most common adverse effects are nausea, vomiting, drowsiness, confusion, miosis and facial flushing. Paradoxical effects include restlessness, muscle rigidity and mood changes. Due to opiates histamine-releasing effects, rash, itching and significant dermatitis has occurred. With overdoses, more serious adverse effects such as severe respiratory depression and pulmonary edema are accompanied with decreases in heart rate, blood pressure and body temperature with ensuing coma and death.

DRUG ABUSE AND DEPENDENCE

While methadone is used in detoxification treatment, physical dependence is a common finding. It does have a longer half-life (14-22 hours) and thus, it has a longer duration of action and a slower onset of withdrawal symptoms (24-48 hours). While less intense, the abstinence syndrome is more prolonged, possibly 6-16 days. Classic symptoms include yawning, mydriasis, muscle tremors, sweating, runny nose and watery eyes, diarrhea, nausea, vomiting and abdominal cramping. In contrast to an overdose, increases in heart rate, blood pressure, body temperature and respirations will occur. Insomnia and goose-flesh are also common findings.

∎

METHAMPHETAMINE (Desoxyn)
Drug Class: Cerebral Stimulant/Amphetamine

HOW SUPPLIED

Tablets: 5mg, 10mg and 15mg

OVERVIEW

Methamphetamine is not an isomer of amphetamine, but structurally, it is nearly identical and it is indicated in the short-term therapy (a few weeks) of exogenous obesity and attention deficit disorders. Common side effects include flushing, hyperexcitability, palpitations, nervousness, insomnia, tremors, mydriasis, increased blood pressure and heart rate and nausea and vomiting. Overdoses can result in death due to convulsions and coma which is frequently associated with a cerebral hemorrhage (stroke). Psychological addiction can occur, but withdrawal symptoms are not medically significant except that severe depression or suicidal ideation may appear.

INDICATIONS (NORMAL USE)

Methamphetamine is indicated as an adjunct to dietary measures in the short-term therapy of exogenous obesity and for attention deficit disorders (ADD or hyperactivity) in children.

PHARMACOLOGY

Methamphetamine is a sympathomimetic amine which has greater CNS stimulant activity than epinephrine and ephedrine. It appears to work by enhancing the release of norepinephrine which causes numerous effects including CNS and respiratory stimulation and increased blood pressure. The main site of action is the cerebral cortex and possibly the reticular-activating system which together account for increased motor activity, mental alertness and mild euphoria. Psychic stimulation and excitability over fatigue are also related to the drug's action on the CNS.

ADVERSE REACTION AND OVERDOSE

The most common adverse effects include excitability, nervousness, increased blood pressure and heart rate, as well as those listed in the Overview. Additional adverse effects are increased respiration and libido. Increased mental alertness can be hazardous because the individual is in a hyperexcitatory state and may use poor judgement or overreact. Continued use results in a loss of libido and mental alertness. Overdoses may be manifested initially by increased heart rate, blood pressure and respiration with subsequent cardiac arrhythmias, stroke, coma and death. Hallucinations, delirium, paranoia and combativeness may also be warning signs of an overdose.

DRUG ABUSE AND DEPENDENCE

Physical addiction to methamphetamine due to pharmacological action does not occur, but psychological addiction does. It is more potent than amphetamine and is the favored drug among habitual amphetamine abusers. It's stimulatory effects may persist for about 4-24 hours depending on dose and extended release form. Although true physical withdrawal symptoms do not occur, sleep disturbances, including insomnia and hypersomnia, and irritability, severe depression and suicidal ideation can necessitate careful supervision.

METHYLPHENIDATE (Ritalin)
Drug Class: Cerebral Stimulant

HOW SUPPLIED

Tablets: 5mg, 10mg, and 20mg
*Available by nonproprietary name

OVERVIEW

Methylphenidate is a stimulant structurally unrelated to amphetamines, but possessing similar properties. It is indicated in the treatment of attention deficit disorders (ADD or hyperactivity) and for narcolepsy. It is abused for it's stimulant activities. Common side effects include palpitation, nervousness, insomnia, tremors, mydriasis, increased blood pressure and heart rate and nausea and vomiting. Although overdoses can result in death due to convulsions and coma, the incidence is much less than seen with the amphetamines. Psychological addiction can occur, but withdrawal symptoms are not medically significant except that severe depression or suicidal ideation may appear.

INDICATIONS (NORMAL USE)

Methylphenidate is indicated in the treatment of attention deficit disorders (ADD or hyperactivity) in children and has also been used in the management of narcolepsy. NOTE: Methylphenidate and the amphetamines used for ADD appear to be a paradox since they all cause excitability. In actuality, the ADD child is thought to be under stimulated and he/she is channeling all energy to remain awake; therefore, a stimulant allows the child to redirect their energy towards normal daily tasks and studies.

PHARMACOLOGY

Methylphenidate is a piperidine-derivative stimulant with properties similar to amphetamines. The exact mechanism of action has not been determined, but the drug does cause CNS and respiratory stimulation and increased blood pressure. The main site of action is the cerebral cortex and possibly the thalamus which together account for increased motor activity, mental alertness, diminished sense of fatigue and mild euphoria. Psychic stimulation and excitability over fatigue are also related to the drug's action on the CNS.

ADVERSE REACTION AND OVERDOSE

The most common adverse effects include excitability, nervousness, increased blood pressure, respiration and heart rate, as well as those listed in the Overview. Overdoses may be manifested initially by increased heart rate, blood pressure and respiration with subsequent cardiac arrhythmias, stroke, coma and death, although all of these effects are less than observed with amphetamines. Hallucinations, delirium, paranoia and combativeness may also be warning signs of an overdose.

DRUG ABUSE AND DEPENDENCE

Physical addiction to methylphenidate due to pharmacological action does not occur, but psychological addiction does. It is known to be abused when diverted to the street. Methylphenidate's stimulatory effects may persist for about 3-8 hours depending on dose and extended release form. Although true physical withdrawal symptoms do not occur, sleep disturbances, including insomnia and hypersomnia, and irritability, severe depression and suicidal ideation can necessitate careful supervision.

METHYLTESTOSTERONE (Android/Oreton)
Drug Class: Androgen

HOW SUPPLIED

Tablets: 10mg and 25mg
Capsules: 10mg (Virilon)
Combination Tablets: Numerous combinations with estrogens
*Available by nonproprietary name

OVERVIEW

Methyltestosterone is a synthetic androgenic, anabolic steroid, hormone. It is primarily indicated for the management of hypogonadism to replace testosterone deficiency in males and to stimulate puberty in carefully selected males with delayed puberty. It is also used to treat inoperable breast cancer in women. Athletes, bodybuilders, weight lifters and physical laborers have used it to add muscle mass. It's most common side effects include increased hair growth and general masculinization, but it also leads to testicular atrophy, breast enlargement and premature baldness in men. It is known to increase aggression and antisocial behavior ("roid rage"). Liver damage or cancer and increased cardiovascular disease are possible. Though not physically addicting, there is some mood elevation. There is no known withdrawal.

INDICATIONS (NORMAL USE)

Methyltestosterone is indicated for the management of hypogonadism to replace testosterone deficiency in males and stimulate puberty when clinically necessary. It is used for inoperable breast cancer in women and sometimes for painful, postpartum breast engorgement and certain types of aggravating symptoms of menopause.

PHARMACOLOGY

Methyltestosterone is a synthetic androgenic hormone. The endogenous androgens are essential hormones that are responsible for normal growth and development of the male sex organs and for maintenance of secondary sex characteristics. Like testosterone, it causes retention of nitrogen, potassium, phosphorous and sodium which are subsequently used for protein anabolism; thus promoting an increase in muscle mass and edema (water weight gain). The androgens stimulate the closure of the epiphyseal growth plates and can cause premature termination of the growth process if used inappropriately in prepubertal children.

ADVERSE REACTION AND OVERDOSE

Hormones work by a biofeedback mechanism. If an individual is taking excessive doses of anabolic steroids, the body stops producing endogenous testosterone which after time, leads to male eunuchs with characteristics of testicular atrophy (a wasting or diminution of testicle size), aspermia which can cause male infertility, enlarged prostrate and the above mentioned. Serious hemolytic effects and cancer of the liver are possible with excess use. Inappropriate aggressive behavior has also been witnessed. Women will have irregular menstrual cycles, masculinization with excess hair growth, clitoral enlargement, acne and deepening of their voice, many of these changes are permanent.

DRUG ABUSE AND DEPENDENCE

While not physically addicting, some individuals experience a mood elevation. Initial excitation, including increased libido (which is later followed by impotence), may be appealing to the abuser and thus may contribute to continued use. Enhanced physical appearance may lead to narcissism (love of one's self) and this may account for a degree of psychological addiction. To attain the enhanced performance or physique the abuser desires, dosages of 10 to 1,000-fold that of therapeutic dosages are used. There is no known physical withdrawal.

METHYPRYLON (Noludar)
Drug Class: Sedative/Hypnotic

HOW SUPPLIED

Tablet: 200mg
Capsule: 300mg

OVERVIEW

Methyprylon is an hypnotic which has CNS depressant effects similar to barbiturates and glutethimide. It is primarily indicated for the short-term (one week) treatment of insomnia. Its effects are particularly enhanced by alcohol consumption. The most common side effects include excess sedation, blurred vision, mydriasis, nausea, vomiting, confusion, skin rashes, respiratory depression and ataxia. Overdoses can lead to further respiratory and cardiovascular depression, a fall in blood pressure, shock, coma and ensuing death. Methyprylon is addictive with prolonged use and withdrawal symptoms are very similar to those seen with barbiturate abstinence and may be life threatening.

PHARMACOLOGY

Methyprylon is indicated as an hypnotic in the short-term treatment of insomnia and sometimes as a sedative.

INDICATIONS (NORMAL USE)

Methyprylon is structurally related to glutethimide, both being a piperidinedione derivative. It's exact mechanism of action is unknown, but is most likely concerned with the arousal center and probably works by increasing it's threshold; therefore, having similar CNS depressant effects to those of barbiturates. It is capable of producing a progressive degree of CNS depression - from mild sedation to hypnosis to deep coma to death. It is similar to glutethimide in it's anticholinergic actions which are responsible for the mydriasis, dry mouth and urinary retention effects. Like barbiturates, the usual hypnotic doses of methyprylon significantly suppress rapid eye movement (REM) or dreaming stage of sleep.

ADVERSE REACTION AND OVERDOSE

The most common adverse effects are excess sedation, confusion, nausea, mydriasis, blurred vision, ataxia, respiratory depression and allergic skin reactions which may be serious. The more alarming effects of reduced blood pressure, body temperature, profound respiratory and cardiovascular depression can lead to coma and death. Paradoxical reactions include excitement, headache and vertigo.

DRUG ABUSE AND DEPENDENCE

Physical dependence to methyprylon is very similar to that of glutethimide and barbiturates. Withdrawal symptoms are also similar and usually begin in the first 12-24 hours. Methyprylon has a relatively short half-life of about 4 hours. Symptoms may not peak for several days and may be accompanied by REM rebound resulting in markedly increased dreaming or nightmares. Classic withdrawal symptoms include: weakness, apprehension, anxiety, nausea, vomiting, tremors, abdominal pains, insomnia and tachycardia. Hallucinations, delirium tremors and life-threatening convulsions are possible.

∎

MORPHINE

Drug Class: Opiate Agonist

HOW SUPPLIED

Tablets: 15mg and 30mg Soluble Tablets: 10mg, 15mg and 30mg
Extended Release Tablets: 15mg, 30mg, 60mg, and 100mg
Oral Solution: 10mg/5ml, 20mg/5ml and 100mg/5ml
Oral concentrated Solution: 4mg/ml and 20mg/ml
Suppositories: 5mg, 10mg, 20mg, and 30mg
Injection: 1mg/2mg/4mg/5mg/8mg/10mg and 15mg/ml syringes
*Available by nonproprietary name

OVERVIEW

Morphine is an opioid analgesic used for relieving moderate to severe pain. It is the principal alkaloid of opium, and is considered the prototype of the opiate agonists. Heroin, diacetylmorphine, is actually produced from morphine. Drowsiness, confusion, nausea, vomiting and miosis are the most common side effects. Decreased heart rate and blood pressure, along with respiratory depression can be life threatening. It's euphoric effects make morphine highly addictive and withdrawal symptoms can be severe.

INDICATIONS (NORMAL USE)

Morphine is indicated for the symptomatic relief of moderate to severe pain associated with cancer, heart attacks, surgeries and trauma. It has also been used to help treat anxiety and insomnia associated with pain, and in some cases, as a cough suppressant, an agent for diarrhea and to relieve the dyspnea associated with some types of heart failure and pulmonary edema.

PHARMACOLOGY

Morphine's action appears to be mediated through the stimulation of several types of opioid receptors throughout the CNS. The opioids possess some of the same properties which the naturally occurring peptides in the body, enkephalins, endorphins and dynorphins, can elicit to reduce pain and produce endogenous euphoria. There are four main opioid receptors, (mu, kappa, delta and sigma) which each activate various responses ranging from analgesia, sedation, miosis and respiratory depression to euphoria, hallucination and dependence. Although we refer to the stimulation of receptors, morphine, along with all opioids, is considered a CNS depressant.

ADVERSE REACTION AND OVERDOSE

The most common adverse effects are nausea, vomiting, drowsiness, confusion, miosis and facial flushing. Paradoxical effects include restlessness, muscle rigidity and mood changes. Due to opiates' histamine-releasing effects, rash, itching and significant dermatitis has occurred. With overdoses, more serious adverse effects, such as a decrease in heart rate, blood pressure, body temperature and respirations can lead to circulatory and respiratory failure with ensuing coma and death.

DRUG ABUSE AND DEPENDENCE

Physical dependence is a common finding with morphine and all related opiate agonists. Withdrawal symptoms usually begin within a few hours due to a short half-life (0.5-2 hours) and peak within 36-72 hours. Classic symptoms include yawning, mydriasis, muscle tremors, sweating, runny nose and watery eyes, diarrhea, nausea, vomiting and abdominal cramping. In contrast to an overdose, increases in heart rate, blood pressure, body temperature and respirations will occur. Insomnia and goose-flesh are also common findings.

▮

OXANDROLONE (Anavar/Oxandrin)
Drug Class: Androgen

HOW SUPPLIED

Tablets: 2.5mg

OVERVIEW

Oxandrolone is a synthetic androgenic, anabolic steroid, hormone. It is primarily indicated for the management of hypogonadism to replace testosterone deficiency in males and to stimulate puberty in carefully selected males with delayed puberty. Athletes, bodybuilders, weight lifters and physical laborers have used it to add muscle mass. It's most common side effects include increased hair growth and general masculinization, but it also leads to testicular atrophy, breast enlargement and premature baldness in men. It is known to increase aggression and antisocial behavior ("roid rage"). Liver damage or cancer and increased cardiovascular disease are possible. Though not physically addicting, there is some mood elevation. There is no known withdrawal.

INDICATIONS (NORMAL USE)

Oxandrolone is indicated for the management of hypogonadism to replace testosterone deficiency in males and stimulate puberty when clinically necessary.

PHARMACOLOGY

Oxandrolone is a synthetic androgenic hormone similar in structure to testosterone. The endogenous androgens are essential hormones that are responsible for normal growth and development of the male sex organs and for maintenance of secondary sex characteristics. Like testosterone, it causes retention of nitrogen, potassium, phosphorous and sodium which are subsequently used for protein anabolism; thus promoting an increase in muscle mass and edema (water weight gain). The androgens stimulate the closure of the epiphyseal growth plates and can cause premature termination of the growth process if used inappropriately in prepubertal children.

ADVERSE REACTION AND OVERDOSE

Hormones work by a biofeedback mechanism. If an individual is taking excessive does of anabolic steroids, the body stops producing endogenous testosterone which after time, leads to male eunuchs with characteristics of testicular atrophy (a wasting or diminution of testicle size), aspermia which can cause male infertility, enlarged prostrate and the above mentioned. Serious hemolytic effects and cancer of the liver are possible with excess use. Inappropriate aggressive behavior has also been witnessed. Women will have irregular menstrual cycles, masculinization with excess hair growth, clitoral enlargement, acne and deepening of their voice, many of these changes are permanent.

DRUG ABUSE AND DEPENDENCE

Oxandrolone is not physically addicting, but some individuals experience a mood elevation. Initial excitation, including increased libido (which is later followed by impotence), may be appealing to the abuser and thus may contribute to continued use. Enhanced physical appearance may lead to narcissism (love of one's self) and this may account for a degree of psychological addiction. To attain the enhanced performance or physique the abuser desires, dosages of 10 to 1,000-fold that of therapeutic dosages are used. As with all androgens, misuse is widespread with some estimates as high as 50%-80% of weight lifters and bodybuilders, 20% of college athletes and 7% of high school athletes admitting use of androgens. However, misuse and abuse is actually by individuals who never compete in sports. There is no known physical withdrawal.

OXAZEPAM (Serax)
Drug Class: Benzodiazepine

HOW SUPPLIED

Capsules: 10mg, 15mg, and 30mg
Tablet: 15mg
*Available by non proprietary name

OVERVIEW

Oxazepam is used for anxiety, anxiety-depressive disorder and acute alcohol withdrawal. Drowsiness, confusion, slurred speech and ataxia are common side effects, but paradoxically, anger and hostility has been witnessed. Allergic reactions including bronchial asthma may occur due to yellow dye in Serax 15mg tablets. Withdrawal leads to confusion, agitation, vomiting, sweating and possibly, seizures, rebound anxiety or psychotic symptoms.

INDICATIONS (NORMAL USE)

Oxazepam is indicated for the short-term relief of symptoms of anxiety or anxiety associated with depressive disorders. It has been used for the management of agitation associated with acute alcohol withdrawal.

PHARMACOLOGY

Oxazepam's action appears to be mediated through the inhibitory neurotransmitter gamma-aminobutyric acid (GABA) which, like all benzodiazepines, enhances the drug's affinity for certain sites within the limbic, thalamic and hypothalamic areas of the brain. It is this inhibition or blocking of the arousal components of these areas which produces the sedative and hypnotic activity. The anxiolytic and paradoxical CNS stimulatory effects are postulated to result from the release of previously suppressed responses (disinhibition) in much the same manner in which alcohol can effect an individual.

ADVERSE REACTION AND OVERDOSE

The most common adverse effects which can be visually observed are drowsiness, ataxia, fatigue, confusion, weakness and dizziness. Amnesia, blurred vision and slurred speech can occur. The 15mg Serax tablet contains the dye tartrazine (FD&C yellow No. 5) which can cause allergic reactions including bronchial asthma in susceptible individuals, particularly those sensitive to aspirin. Paradoxical CNS stimulation is not as common as seen with other benzodiazepines but can present as restlessness, hyperactivity, mania or possibly extreme anger and hostility. Acute overdose will generally result in somnolence or coma with respiratory depression. Concomitant ingestion of alcohol or other CNS depressants may aggravate symptoms.

DRUG ABUSE AND DEPENDENCE

Physical dependence can occur and due to oxazepam's short half-life, withdrawal symptoms may peak within 24-72 hours, much sooner than seen with diazepam (5-8 days). Confusion, agitation, rigidity of limbs, hallucinations and seizures are all possible after abrupt withdrawal. Less serious withdrawal symptoms include tremors, abdominal cramps, vomiting and sweating. As with all benzodiazepines, individuals using the drug for anxiety may experience a significant rebound in anxiety after the medication is discontinued which can be easily mistaken for drug withdrawal.

▮

OXYCODONE (Percocet, Percodan)
Drug Class: Opiate Agonist

HOW SUPPLIED

Tablet: 5mg (Roxicodone)
Oral Solution: 5mg/5mg and 20mg/ml (Roxicodone Intensol)
Combination Tablets: 2.44mg#, 4.88mg# and 5mg with acetaminophen (325-500mg) or aspirin (325mg)
Combination Capsules: 5mg with acetaminophen 500mg
Combination Solution: 5mg & 325mg acetaminophen/5ml
*Available by nonproprietary name and many other combinations
#A combination of two different salts of oxycodone

OVERVIEW

Oxycodone is a synthetic opioid analgesic used for relieving moderate to moderately severe pain. It is similar to hydrocodone but is more potent and has a greater abuse potential. Drowsiness, confusion, nausea, vomiting and miosis are the most common side effects. It can also decrease heart rate and blood pressure, along with respiratory depression, which can be life threatening. It too possesses euphoric effects which make it addictive and withdrawal symptoms can be severe.

INDICATIONS (NORMAL USE)

Oxycodone is indicated for the symptomatic relief of moderate to moderately severe pain associated with injuries, bursitis, dislocation, simple fractures and neuralgia. It is also used for postoperative and postpartum pain. It is usually used in combination with other analgesics such as acetaminophen and aspirin.

PHARMACOLOGY

Oxycodone's action appears to be mediated through the stimulation of the four main opioid receptors found in the CNS which activates responses ranging from analgesia to respiratory depression to euphoria. The opioids possess some of the same properties which the naturally occurring peptides in the body, enkephalins, endorphins and dynorphins, can elicit to reduce pain and produce endogenous euphoria. Oxycodone is considered a CNS depressant.

ADVERSE REACTION AND OVERDOSE

The most common adverse effects are nausea, vomiting, drowsiness, confusion, miosis and facial flushing. Paradoxical effects include ataxia and restlessness. Due to opiates' histamine-releasing effects, rash, itching and significant dermatitis has occurred. With overdoses, more serious adverse effects, such as decreases in heart rate, blood pressure, body temperature and respiration can lead to circulatory and respiratory failure with ensuing coma and death. Aspirin and acetaminophen overdoses in combination products can cause death due to an assortment of complications, including bleeding abnormalities and liver toxicity. Like meperidine, some oxycodone preparations contain a sulfite that may cause allergic reactions, including an asthmatic episode or even anaphylaxis.

DRUG ABUSE AND DEPENDENCE

Physical dependence does occur but is not as common a finding with oxycodone as morphine or related opiate agonists since it produces less euphoria. Withdrawal symptoms usually begin within a few hours due to a short half-life (3-4 hours) and peak within 36-72 hours. Classic symptoms include yawning, mydriasis, muscle tremors, sweating, runny nose and watery eyes, diarrhea, nausea, vomiting, abdominal cramping and other abstinence symptoms are similar to codeine or morphine.

▮

OXYMETHOLONE (Anadrol-50)
Drug Class: Androgen

HOW SUPPLIED
Tablets: 50mg

OVERVIEW
Oxymetholone is a synthetic androgenic, anabolic steroid, hormone. It is primarily indicated in the treatment of anemias caused by deficient red cell production. Athletes, bodybuilders, weight lifters and physical laborers have misused it to add muscle mass. It's most common side effects include increased hair growth and general masculinization, but is also leads to testicular atrophy, breast enlargement and premature baldness in men. It is known to increase aggression and antisocial behavior ("roid rage"). Liver damage or cancer and increased cardiovascular disease are possible. Though not physically addicting, there is some mood elevation. There is no known withdrawal.

INDICATIONS (NORMAL USE)
Oxymetholone is indicated in the treatment of anemias caused by deficient red cell productions such as aplastic anemia.

PHARMACOLOGY
Oxymetholone is a synthetic androgenic hormone similar in structure to testosterone. The endogenous androgens are essential hormones that are responsible for normal growth and development of the male sex organs and for maintenance of secondary sex characteristics. Like testosterone, it causes retention of nitrogen, potassium, phosphorous and sodium which are subsequently not only used for protein anabolism, but also for enhancing the production of erythropoietin in patients with anemias due to bone marrow failure and therefore, stimulate red cell synthesis. The androgens stimulate the closure of the epiphyseal growth plates and can cause premature termination of the growth process if used inappropriately in prepubertal children.

ADVERSE REACTION AND OVERDOSE
Hormones work by a biofeedback mechanism. If an individual is taking excessive doses of anabolic steroids, the body stops producing endogenous testosterone which after time, leads to male eunuchs with characteristics of testicular atrophy (a wasting or diminution of testicle size), aspermia which can cause male infertility, enlarged prostrate and the above mentioned. Serious hemolytic effects and cancer of the liver are possible with excess use. Inappropriate aggressive behavior has also been witnessed. Women will have irregular menstrual cycles, masculinization with excess hair growth, clitoral enlargement, acne and deepening of their voice, many of these changes are permanent.

DRUG ABUSE AND DEPENDENCE
Oxymetholone is not physically addicting, but some individuals experience a mood elevation. Initial excitation, including increased libido (which is later followed by impotence), may be appealing to the abuser and thus may contribute to continued use. Enhanced physical appearance may lead to narcissism (love of one's self) and this may account for a degree of psychological addiction. To attain the enhanced performance or physique the abuser desires, dosages of 10 to 1,000-fold that of therapeutic dosages are used. As with all androgens, misuse is widespread with some estimates as high as 50%-80% of weight lifters and bodybuilders, 20% of college athletes and 7% of high school athletes admitting use of androgens. However, misuse and abuse is actually by individuals who never compete in sports. There is no known physical withdrawal.

PEMOLINE (Cylert)
Drug Class: Cerebral Stimulant

HOW SUPPLIED
Tablets: 18.75mg, 37.5mg and 75mg

OVERVIEW
Pemoline is a stimulant structurally unrelated to amphetamines and methylphenidate, but possessing similar properties. It is indicated in the treatment of attention deficit disorders (ADD or hyperactivity). It has many unapproved uses in the medical field. It is abused for it's stimulant activities. Common side effects include palpitations, nervousness, insomnia, tremors, mydriasis, increased blood pressure and heart rate and nausea and vomiting. Although overdoses can result in death due to convulsions and coma, it is unlikely except in extreme cases. Psychological addiction can occur, but withdrawal symptoms are not medically significant except that severe depression or suicidal ideation may appear.

INDICATIONS (NORMAL USE)
Pemoline is indicated in the treatment of attention deficit disorders (ADD or hyperactivity) in children. Unapproved uses include the treatment of fatigue, mental depression and chronic schizophrenia, and as a mild stimulant for geriatric patients.

PHARMACOLOGY
Pemoline is an oxazolidione-derivative stimulant with properties similar to amphetamines. The exact mechanism of action, as well as it's sites of actions in the CNS have not been determined. However, the drug does cause CNS and respiratory stimulation and increased blood pressure. Pemoline also causes increased motor activity, mental alertness, diminished sense of fatigue and mild euphoria. Psychic stimulation and excitability over fatigue are also related to the drug's action on the CNS.

ADVERSE REACTION AND OVERDOSE
The most common adverse effects include excitability, nervousness, increased blood pressure, respiration and heart rate, as well as those listed in the Overview. Overdoses may be manifested initially by increased heart rate, blood pressure and respiration with subsequent cardiac arrhythmias, stroke, coma and death although all of these effects are less than observed with amphetamines. As found with all of the stimulants, drug-induced anorexia can result in unhealthy weight reduction. Pemoline also can cause liver toxicity which may be fatal. Hallucinations, delirium, paranoia and combativeness may also be warning signs of an overdose.

DRUG ABUSE AND DEPENDENCE
Physical addiction to pemoline due to pharmacological action does not occur, but psychological addiction does. It is known to be abused when diverted to the street. Pemoline's stimulatory effects may persist for about 4-8 hours depending on dose. Although true physical withdrawal symptoms do not occur, sleep disturbances, including insomnia and hypersomnia, and irritability, severe depression and suicidal ideation can necessitate careful supervision.

▮

PENTAZOCINE (Talwin)
Drug Class: Opiate Partial Agonist

HOW SUPPLIED

Injection: 30mg/ml syringes, ampules and multidose vials
Combination Tablets: 12.5mg with 325mg aspirin
25mg with 650mg acetaminophen

OVERVIEW

Pentazocine is a synthetic opioid partial agonist analgesic used for relieving moderate to severe pain. It is similar to morphine but is only one-half to one-sixth as potent. Drowsiness, dizziness, confusion, miosis and nausea are common side effects. Vomiting occurs less frequently than with morphine. It can also decrease blood pressure and respiration which can be life threatening. Paradoxically, increased heart rate, irritability and seizures have occurred. It is addictive and its use with an antihistamine, tripelennamine, comprise the street drug known as T's and Blues. Though less severe than morphine, withdrawal symptoms can occur.

INDICATIONS (NORMAL USE)

Pentazocine is indicated for the symptomatic relief of moderate to severe pain including postoperative pain, dental surgery, orthopedic, cancer and renal or colic pain. It is also used for preoperative sedation, as a supplement to anesthesia and for analgesia during labor.

PHARMACOLOGY

Pentazocine's action appears to be mediated through the stimulation of two of the four main opioid receptors found in the CNS which activates responses ranging from analgesia to respiratory depression to euphoria. It activates the kappa and sigma receptors, but is an antagonist to the mu receptor meaning it may interfere some with morphine's analgesic effect. The opioids possess some of the same properties which the naturally occurring peptides in the body, enkephalins, endorphins and dynorphins, can elicit to reduce pain and produce endogenous euphoria. Pentazocine is considered a CNS depressant.

ADVERSE REACTION AND OVERDOSE

The most common adverse effects are drowsiness, dizziness, confusion, miosis and nausea. Paradoxical effects include increased heart rate, muscle tremors and convulsions. Unlike most opiates, it has no histamine-releasing effects and is less likely to cause skin rashes. With overdoses, more serious adverse effects such as decreases in heart rate, blood pressure, body temperature and respirations can lead to circulatory and respiratory failure with ensuing coma and death. Like meperidine and oxycodone, pentazocine injections contain a sulfite that may cause allergic reactions including an asthmatic episode or even anaphylaxis. Toxic effects of aspirin and acetaminophen overdose may result with excess use.

DRUG ABUSE AND DEPENDENCE

Physical dependence does occur with pentazocine and is similar to morphine, but less pronounced. Withdrawal symptoms usually begin within a few hours due to a short half-life (4-5 hours) and peak within 36-72 hours. Classic symptoms include yawning, mydriasis, muscle tremors, sweating, runny nose and watery eyes, diarrhea, nausea, vomiting, abdominal cramping and other abstinence symptoms are similar to codeine or morphine. The use of pentazocine with tripelennamine tablets to make an IV mixture is used by opiate addicts and drug abusers since its effects are purported to be similar to IV heroin.

PENTAZOCINE/NALOXONE (Talwin Nx)
Drug Class: Opiate Partial Agonist

HOW SUPPLIED

Combination Tablets: 50mg with naloxone 0.5mg

OVERVIEW

Pentazocine is a synthetic opioid partial agonist analgesic used for relieving moderate to severe pain. It is similar to morphine but is only one-half to one-sixth as potent. Drowsiness, dizziness, confusion, miosis and nausea are common side effects. Vomiting occurs less frequently than with morphine. It can also decrease blood pressure and respiration which can be life threatening. Paradoxically, increased heart rate, irritability and seizures have occurred. It is addictive and before its reformulation with the opiate antagonist naloxone, it was mixed with an antihistamine, tripelennamine, to comprise the street drug known as T's and Blues, which was subsequently injected for its purported similarity to IV heroin. Though less severe than morphine, withdrawal symptoms can occur.

INDICATIONS (NORMAL USE)

Pentazocine/naloxone is indicated for the symptomatic relief of moderate to severe pain including postoperative pain, dental surgery, orthopedic, cancer and renal or colic pain.

PHARMACOLOGY

Pentazocine's action appears to be mediated through the stimulation of two of the four main opioid receptors found in the CNS which activates responses ranging from analgesia to respiratory depression to euphoria. It activates the kappa and sigma receptors, but is an antagonist to the mu receptor meaning it may interfere some with morphine's analgesic effect. The opioids possess some of the same properties which the naturally occurring peptides in the body, enkephalins, endorphins and dynorphins, can elicit to reduce pain and produce endogenous euphoria. Pentazocine is considered a CNS depressant.

ADVERSE REACTION AND OVERDOSE

The most common adverse effects are drowsiness, dizziness, confusion, miosis and nausea. Paradoxical effects include increased heart rate, muscle tremors and convulsions. Unlike most opiates, it has no histamine-releasing effects and is less likely to cause skin rashes. With overdoses, more serious adverse effects such as decreases in heart rate, blood pressure, body temperature and respirations can lead to circulatory and respiratory failure with ensuing coma and death.

DRUG ABUSE AND DEPENDENCE

Physical dependence can occur with Talwin Nx since the amount of oral naloxone is not adequate to antagonize the analgesic and euphoric effects of pentazocine. However, if the tablet is crushed and solubilized for injection, the naloxone by the IV route will precipitate withdrawal symptoms; therefore, these tablets are no longer misused to make T's and Blues. Withdrawal symptoms from oral use usually begin within a few hours due to a short half-life (4-5 hours) and peak within 36-72 hours. Classic symptoms include yawning, mydriasis, muscle tremors, sweating, runny nose and watery eyes, diarrhea, nausea, vomiting, abdominal cramping and other abstinence symptoms are similar to codeine or morphine.

PENTOBARBITAL (Nembutal)
Drug Class: Barbiturate

HOW SUPPLIED

Capsules: 50mg and 100mg
Oral Elixir: 18.2mg/5ml
Rectal Suppositories: 30mg, 60mg, 120mg and 200mg
Injection: 50mg/ml syringes
*Available by nonproprietary name

OVERVIEW

Pentobarbital is a barbiturate hypnotic primarily indicated for the short-term treatment of insomnia. Drowsiness may be preceded with a period of euphoria, excitement and confusion before its desired sedative actions take effect. Its effects have often been mistakenly attributed to alcohol consumption. The most common side effects include excess sedation, respiratory depression, confusion, ataxia and skin rashes. Overdoses can lead to further respiratory and cardiovascular depression, a fall in blood pressure, shock, coma and ensuing death. Pentobarbital is addictive and withdrawal symptoms are very similar to those seen with alcohol abstinence and may be life threatening.

INDICATIONS (NORMAL USE)

Pentobarbital is indicated for the short-term treatment of insomnia. It has been used preoperatively to control anxiety and provide sedation. At times it has been used to control certain types of acute seizure disorders and agitated behavior in psychoses. It has also been used to induce coma in brain injuries with the hope of reducing swelling and intracranial pressure.

PHARMACOLOGY

Pentobarbital is a substituted pyrimidine derivative. Like all barbiturates, the basic structure is barbituric acid. Pentobarbital acts throughout the CNS and reversibly depresses the activity of all excitable tissues. It is particularly active at the midbrain reticular formation which is specifically concerned with the arousal mechanism. All barbiturates are capable of producing a progressive degree of CNS depression - from mild sedation to hypnosis to deep coma to death. Pentobarbital has no analgesic effects and may actually increase the reaction to painful stimuli such as an injury.

ADVERSE REACTION AND OVERDOSE

The most common adverse effects are excess sedation, confusion, ataxia, respiratory depression and allergic skin reactions which may be serious. Neuralgic or arthralgic pain, nausea and vomiting are less common. Pupils are usually slightly constricted but may be dilated with severe overdoses. The more alarming effects of reduced blood pressure, body temperature, profound respiratory and cardiovascular depression can lead to coma and death. Paradoxical reactions include a period of euphoria, excitement and possible irritability prior to the time the desired sedative actions take effect.

DRUG ABUSE AND DEPENDENCE

Physical dependence to barbiturates like pentobarbital is more apt to occur than with other sedative hypnotics such as benzodiazepines. Withdrawal symptoms are similar to those of alcohol abstinence and will usually begin in the first 12-24 hours. Pentobarbital has a relatively long half-life of 21-42 hours and therefore, symptoms may not peak for several days. Classic symptoms include weakness, apprehension, anxiety, nausea, vomiting, tremors, abdominal pains, insomnia and tachycardia. Hallucinations, delirium tremors and life-threatening convulsions are possible.

PHENDIMETRAZINE (Prelu-2)
Drug Class: Cerebral Stimulant/Amphetamine

HOW SUPPLIED

Tablets: 35mg
Capsules: 35mg and 105mg
*Available by nonproprietary name

OVERVIEW

Phendimetrazine is an amphetamine congener which is indicated in the short-term therapy (a few weeks) of exogenous obesity. It is abused for it's stimulant activities, but is much less active than phenmetrazine, it's parent compound. The drug's anorexigenic effect appears to be related to CNS stimulation and not to increased metabolic effects or due to appetite suppression. Common side effects include flushing, hyperexcitability, palpitations, nervousness, insomnia, tremors, mydriasis, increased blood pressure and heart rate and nausea and vomiting. Overdoses can result in death due to convulsions and coma which is frequently associated with a cerebral hemorrhage (stroke). Psychological addiction can occur, but withdrawal symptoms are not medically significant except that severe depression or suicidal ideation may appear.

INDICATIONS (NORMAL USE)

Phendimetrazine is indicated as an adjunct to dietary measures in the short-term therapy of exogenous obesity.

PHARMACOLOGY

Phendimetrazine, like amphetamine, is a sympathomimetic amine which has greater CNS stimulant activity than epinephrine and ephedrine. It appears to work by enhancing the release of norepinephrine which causes numerous effects including CNS and respiratory stimulation and increased blood pressure; however, this pressure effect is much less potent than dextroamphetamine. The main site of action is the cerebral cortex and possibly the reticular-activating system which together account for increased motor activity, mental alertness and mild euphoria. Psychic stimulation and excitability over fatigue are also related to the drug's action on the CNS.

ADVERSE REACTION AND OVERDOSE

The most common adverse effects include excitability, nervousness, increased blood pressure and heart rate, as well as those listed in the Overview. Additional adverse effects are increased respiration and libido. Increased mental alertness can be hazardous because the individual is in a hyperexcitatory state and may use poor judgement or overreact. Overdoses may be manifested initially by increased heart rate, blood pressure and respiration with subsequent cardiac arrhythmias, stroke, coma and death. Hallucinations, delirium, paranoia and combativeness may also be warning signs of an overdose.

DRUG ABUSE ND DEPENDENCE

Physical addiction to phendimetrazine due to pharmacological action does not occur, but psychological addiction does. It is not as potent as dextroamphetamine or methamphetamine, but is known to be abused by patients and when diverted to the street. Phendimetrazine's stimulatory effects may persist for about 4-24 hours depending on dose and extended release form. Although true physical withdrawal symptoms do not occur, sleep disturbances, including insomnia and hypersomnia, and irritability, severe depression and suicidal ideation can necessitate careful supervision.

■

PHENMETRAZINE (Preludin)
Drug Class: Cerebral Stimulant/Amphetamine

HOW SUPPLIED
Tablets: 75mg

OVERVIEW
Phenmetrazine is an amphetamine congener which is indicated in the short-term therapy (a few weeks) of exogenous obesity. Although it is less active than amphetamine and it's isomers, it is one of the more potent congeners and has high abuse potential. The drug's anorexigenic effect appears to be related to CNS stimulation and not to increased metabolic effects or due to appetite suppression. Common side effects include flushing, hyperexcitability, palpitations, nervousness, insomnia, tremors, mydriasis, increased blood pressure and heart rate and nausea and vomiting. Overdoses can result in death due to convulsions and coma which is frequently associated with a cerebral hemorrhage (stroke). Psychological addiction can occur, but withdrawal symptoms are not medically significant except that severe depression or suicidal ideation may appear.

INDICATIONS (NORMAL USE)
Phenmetrazine is indicated as an adjunct to dietary measures in the short-term therapy of exogenous obesity.

PHARMACOLOGY
Phenmetrazine, like amphetamine, is a sympathomimetic amine which has greater CNS stimulant activity than epinephrine and ephedrine. It appears to work by enhancing the release of norepinephrine which causes numerous effects including CNS and respiratory stimulation and increased blood pressure; however, this pressure effect is much less potent than dextroamphetamine. The main site of action is the cerebral cortex and possibly the reticular-activating system which together account for increased motor activity, mental alertness and mild euphoria. Psychic stimulation and excitability over fatigue are also related to the drug's action on the CNS.

ADVERSE REACTION AND OVERDOSE
The most common adverse effects include excitability, nervousness, increased blood pressure and heart rate, as well as those listed in the Overview. Additional adverse effects are increased respiration and libido. Increased mental alertness can be hazardous because the individual is in a hyperexcitatory state and may use poor judgement or overreact. Overdoses may be manifested initially by increased heart rate, blood pressure and respiration with subsequent cardiac arrhythmias, stroke, coma and death. Hallucinations, delirium, paranoia and combativeness may also be warning signs of an overdose.

DRUG ABUSE AND DEPENDENCE
Physical addiction to phenmetrazine due to pharmacological action does not occur, but psychological addiction does. It is not as potent as dextroamphetamine or methamphetamine, but is known to be abused by patients and when diverted to the street. Phenmetrazine's stimulatory effects may persist for about 12-24 hours due to the extended release form. Although true physical withdrawal symptoms do not occur, sleep disturbances, including insomnia and hypersomnia, and irritability, severe depression and suicidal ideation can necessitate careful supervision.

▮

PHENOBARBITAL
Drug Class: Barbiturate

HOW SUPPLIED
Tablets: 15mg, 16mg, 30mg, 32mg, 60mg, 65mg and 100mg
Capsules: 16mg
Oral Elixir: 15mg/5ml and 20mg/5ml
Injection: 30mg/60mg/65mg and 130mg/ml ampules or syringes
*Available by nonproprietary name

OVERVIEW
Phenobarbital is a barbiturate hypnotic primarily indicated in the prophylactic management of epilepsy and to relieve anxiety and provide sedation preoperatively. Drowsiness may be preceded with a period of euphoria, excitement and confusion. Its effects have often been mistakenly attributed to alcohol consumption. The most common side effects include excess sedation, respiratory depression, confusion, ataxia and skin rashes. Overdoses can lead to further respiratory and cardiovascular depression, a fall in blood pressure, shock, coma and ensuing death. Phenobarbital is less addictive than other barbiturates, but can have withdrawal symptoms similar to those seen with alcohol abstinence. Because of its long half-life, it is frequently used to help manage withdrawal symptoms from other barbiturates and alcohol.

INDICATIONS (NORMAL USE)
Phenobarbital is indicated in the prophylactic management of epilepsy. It has also been used to relieve anxiety and provide sedation preoperatively. It is used to help control withdrawal symptoms associated with alcohol and other barbiturates at times. It is effective in preventing and treating hyperbilirubinemia in neonates.

PHARMACOLOGY
Phenobarbital is a substituted pyrimidine derivative. Like all barbiturates, the basic structure is barbituric acid. Unlike most of the other barbiturates, phenobarbital has anticonvulsant action at non-hypnotic doses. It acts throughout the CNS and reversibly depresses the activity of all excitable tissues. It is particularly active at the midbrain reticular formation which is specifically concerned with the arousal mechanism. All barbiturates are capable of producing a progressive degree of CNS depression - from mild sedation to hypnosis to deep coma to death. Phenobarbital has no analgesic effects and may actually increase the reaction to painful stimuli such as an injury.

ADVERSE REACTION AND OVERDOSE
The most common adverse effects are excess sedation, confusion, ataxia, respiratory depression and allergic skin reactions which may be serious. Neuralgic or arthralgic pain, nausea and vomiting are less common. Pupils are usually slightly constricted but may be dilated with severe overdoses. The more alarming effects of reduced blood pressure, body temperature, profound respiratory and cardiovascular depression can lead to coma and death. Paradoxical reactions include a period of euphoria, excitement and possibly, irritability prior to the time the desired sedative actions take effect.

DRUG ABUSE AND DEPENDENCE
Physical dependence to barbiturates like phenobarbital and mephobarbital is less likely to occur than with other barbiturates. Withdrawal symptoms are similar to those of alcohol abstinence and will usually begin in the first couple of days. Phenobarbital has a very long half-life of 48-120 hours and therefore, symptoms may not peak for several days. Classic symptoms include weakness, apprehension, anxiety, nausea, vomiting, tremors, abdominal pains, insomnia and tachycardia. Hallucinations, delirium tremors and life-threatening convulsions are possible.

▮

PHENTERMINE (Ionamin)

Drug Class: Cerebral Stimulant/Amphetamine

HOW SUPPLIED

Tablets: 8mg and 37.5mg
Capsules: 15mg, 18.75mg, 30mg and 37.5mg
*Available by nonproprietary name

OVERVIEW

Phentermine is an amphetamine congener which is indicated in the short-term therapy (a few weeks) of exogenous obesity. It is abused for it's stimulant activities, but is much less active than dextroamphetamine. The drug's anorexigenic effect appears to be related to CNS stimulation and not to increased metabolic effects or due to appetite suppression. Common side effects include flushing, hyperexcitability, palpitations, nervousness, insomnia, tremors, mydriasis, increased blood pressure and heart rate and nausea and vomiting. Overdoses can result in death due to convulsions and coma which is frequently associated with a cerebral hemorrhage (stroke). Psychological addiction can occur, but withdrawal symptoms are not medically significant except that severe depression or suicidal ideation may appear.

INDICATIONS (NORMAL USE)

Phentermine is indicated as an adjunct to dietary measures in the short-term therapy of exogenous obesity.

PHARMACOLOGY

Phentermine, like amphetamine, is a sympathomimetic amine which has greater CNS stimulant activity than epinephrine and ephedrine. It appears to work by enhancing the release of norepinephrine which causes numerous effects including CNS and respiratory stimulation and increased blood pressure; however, this pressure effect is much less potent than dextroamphetamine. The main site of action is the cerebral cortex and possibly the reticular-activating system which together account for increased motor activity, mental alertness and mild euphoria. Psychic stimulation and excitability over fatigue are also related to the drug's action on the CNS.

ADVERSE REACTION AND OVERDOSE

The most common adverse effects include excitability, nervousness, increased blood pressure and heart rate, as well as those listed in the Overview. Additional adverse effects are increased respiration and libido. Increased mental alertness can be hazardous because the individual is in a hyperexcitatory state and may use poor judgement or overreact. Overdoses may be manifested initially by increased heart rate, blood pressure and respiration with subsequent cardiac arrhythmias, stroke, coma and death. Hallucinations, delirium, paranoia and combativeness may also be warning signs of an overdose.

DRUG ABUSE AND DEPENDENCE

Physical addiction to phentermine due to pharmacological action does not occur, but psychological addiction does. It is not as potent as dextroamphetamine or methamphetamine, but is known to be abused by patients and when diverted to the street. Phendimetrazine's stimulatory effects may persist for about 4-24 hours depending on dose and extended release form. Although true physical withdrawal symptoms do not occur, sleep disturbances, including insomnia and hypersomnia, and irritability, severe depression and suicidal ideation can necessitate careful supervision.

PRAZEPAM (Centrax)
Drug Class: Benzodiazepine

HOW SUPPLIED

Capsules: 5mg, 10mg, and 20mg
Tablet: 10mg

OVERVIEW

Prazepam is used in the management of anxiety or for the short-term relief of symptoms of anxiety. Drowsiness, confusion, slurred speech and ataxia are possible side effects. Prazepam is very similar to halazepam except that on a mg per mg basis, it is more potent, i.e. dosing is approximately equivalent to diazepam. Not widely used, the side effect profile and paradoxical excitation seen with many benzodiazepines is not well documented. However, since prazepam shares similar chemical and therapeutic properties with diazepam, one would expect their actions to closely mimic one another.

INDICATIONS (NORMAL USE)

Prazepam is indicated for the management of anxiety disorders and the short-term relief of symptoms of anxiety.

PHARMACOLOGY

Prazepam's action appears to be mediated through the inhibitory neurotransmitter gamma-aminobutyric acid (GABA) which, like all benzodiazepines, enhances the drug's affinity for certain sites within the limbic, thalamic and hypothalamic areas of the brain. It is this inhibition or blocking of the arousal components of these areas which produces the sedative and hypnotic activity. The anxiolytic and paradoxical CNS stimulatory effects are postulated to result from the release of previously suppressed responses (disinhibition) in much the same manner in which alcohol can effect an individual.

ADVERSE REACTION AND OVERDOSE

The most common adverse effects which can be visually observed are drowsiness, ataxia, fatigue, confusion, weakness and dizziness. Amnesia, blurred vision and slurred speech can occur. Paradoxical CNS stimulation is not as common as seen with other benzodiazepines but can present as restlessness, hyperactivity, mania or possibly, extreme anger and hostility. Acute overdose will generally result in somnolence or coma with respiratory depression. Concomitant ingestion of alcohol or other CNS depressants may aggravate symptoms.

DRUG ABUSE AND DEPENDENCE

Physical dependence can occur and like diazepam, prazepam has a relatively long half-life. Withdrawal symptoms may not peak for 4-8 days. Confusion, agitation, rigidity of limbs, hallucinations and seizures are all possible after abrupt withdrawal. Less serious withdrawal symptoms include tremors, abdominal cramps, vomiting and sweating. As with all benzodiazepines, individuals using the drug for anxiety may experience a significant rebound in anxiety after the medication is discontinued, which can be easily mistaken for drug withdrawal.

▮

PROPOXYPHENE (Darvon, Darvocet N)
Drug Class: Opiate Agonist

HOW SUPPLIED
Tablet: 100mg (Darvon N)
Capsule: 65mg (Darvon)
Combination Tablets: 65mg and (50mg or 100mg N) with acetaminophen(325-650mg)
Combination Capsules: 65mg with 389mg aspirin and 32.4mg caffeine
*Available by nonproprietary name and many other combinations
(N is the napsylate salt, of which 100mg = 65mg of the HCL salt.)

OVERVIEW
Propoxyphene is a synthetic opioid analgesic structurally related to methadone, but is substantially less potent. It is used for relieving mild to moderate pain. It is more similar to codeine for relieving pain, but is a little less potent and causes less euphoria. Drowsiness, dizziness, visual disturbances, nausea, vomiting and miosis are the most common side effects. It can also decreases heart rate and blood pressure, along with respiratory depression which can be life threatening with a significant overdose. Although its euphoric effects are less than codeine, it can be addictive, but withdrawal symptoms are milder.

INDICATIONS (NORMAL USE)
Propoxyphene is indicated for the symptomatic relief of mild to moderate pain associated with injuries, simple fractures, neuralgia and numerous other types of pain including some headaches. It is also used as a supplemental agent during methadone detoxification of opiate-dependent individuals.

PHARMACOLOGY
Propoxyphene's action appears to be mediated through the stimulation of the four main opioid receptors found in the CNS which activates responses ranging from analgesia to respiratory depression to euphoria. (See morphine) The opioids possess some of the same properties which the naturally occurring peptides in the body, enkephalins, endorphins and dynorphins, can elicit to reduce pain and produce endogenous euphoria. Propoxyphene is considered a CNS depressant.

ADVERSE REACTION AND OVERDOSE
The most common adverse effects are nausea, vomiting, drowsiness, dizziness, visual disturbances and confusion. Paradoxical effects include restlessness, abdominal pain, headache, and insomnia. Due to opiates histamine-releasing effects, rash, itching, and significant dermatitis has occurred. With overdoses, more serious adverse effects, such as decreases in heart rate, blood pressure, body temperature, and respirations can lead to circulatory and respiratory failure with ensuing coma and death. Aspirin and acetaminophen overdoses in combination products can cause death due to an assortment of complications including bleeding abnormalities and liver toxicity.

DRUG ABUSE AND DEPENDENCE
Physical dependence does occur, but is not a common a finding with propoxyphene as codeine or related opiate agonists since it produces less euphoria. Withdrawal symptoms are usually delayed and are less severe since it has a longer half-life (six to twelve hours). Symptoms may not peak for three to five days. Classic symptoms include yawning, mydriasis, muscle tremors, sweating, runny noes and watery eyes, diarrhea, nausea, vomiting, abdominal cramping, and other abstinence symptoms which are similar to codeine. Capsule pellets have been willfully abused by dissolving them and injecting. Reports of digital gangrene requiring amputation have been reported.

QUAZEPAM (Doral)
Drug Class: Benzodiazepine

HOW SUPPLIED
Tablets: 7.5mg and 15mg

OVERVIEW
Quazepam is used as an hypnotic in the short-term management of insomnia. It is one of the newer additions to the benzodiazepine class of approved hypnotics. Drowsiness, confusion, slurred speech and ataxia are possible side effects. Paradoxical agitation, anger and hostility have been observed. Abrupt withdrawal is often characterized by rebound insomnia and anxiety. Dependency and withdrawal can occur.

INDICATIONS (NORMAL USE)
Quazepam is indicated as an hypnotic in the short-term management of insomnia.

PHARMACOLOGY
Quazepam's action appears to be mediated through the inhibitory neurotransmitter gamma-aminobutyric acid (GABA) which, like all benzodiazepines, enhances the drug's affinity for certain sites within the limbic, thalamic and hypothalamic areas of the brain. It is this inhibition or blocking of the arousal components of these areas which produces the sedative and hypnotic activity. The paradoxical CNS stimulatory effects are postulated to result from the release of previously suppressed responses (disinhibition) in much the same manner in which alcohol can effect an individual.

ADVERSE REACTION AND OVERDOSE
The most common adverse effects which can be visually observed are extreme drowsiness, ataxia, fatigue, confusion, weakness and dizziness. Amnesia, blurred vision and slurred speech can occur. Paradoxical CNS stimulation, agitation, restlessness and hyperactivity are all possible. Acute overdose will generally result in somnolence or coma with respiratory depression. Concomitant ingestion of alcohol or other CNS depressants may aggravate symptoms.

DRUG ABUSE AND DEPENDENCE
Physical dependence can occur and like flurazepam, quazepam has a long half-life; therefore, withdrawal symptoms may not peak for 3-5 days. Rebound insomnia and anxiety, agitation, confusion, rigidity of limbs, hallucinations and seizures are all possible after abrupt withdrawal. Less serious withdrawal symptoms include tremors, abdominal cramps, vomiting and sweating.

SECOBARBITAL (Seconal)
Drug Class: Barbiturate

HOW SUPPLIED

Capsules: 50mg and 100mg
Injection: 50mg/ml syringes
*Available in nonproprietary name

OVERVIEW

Secobarbital is a barbiturate hypnotic primarily indicated for the short-term treatment of insomnia. Drowsiness may be preceded with a period of euphoria, excitement and confusion before its desired sedative actions take effect. Its effects have often been mistakenly attributed to alcohol consumption. The most common side effects include excess sedation, respiratory depression, confusion, ataxia and skin rashes. Overdoses can lead to further respiratory and cardiovascular depression, a fall in blood pressure, shock, coma and ensuing death. Secobarbital is addictive and withdrawal symptoms are very similar to those seen with alcohol abstinence and may be life threatening.

INDICATIONS (NORMAL USE)

Secobarbital is indicated for the short-term treatment of insomnia. It has been used preoperatively to control anxiety and provide sedation. At times it has been used to control certain types of acute seizure disorders and agitated behavior in psychoses.

PHARMACOLOGY

Secobarbital is a substituted pyrimidine derivative. Like all barbiturates, the basic structure is barbituric acid. Secobarbital acts throughout the CNS and reversibly depresses the activity of all excitable tissues. It is particularly active at the midbrain reticular formation which is specifically concerned with the arousal mechanism. All barbiturates are capable of producing a progressive degree of CNS depression - from mild sedation to hypnosis to deep coma to death. Secobarbital has no analgesic effects and may actually increase the reaction to painful stimuli such as an injury.

ADVERSE REACTION AND OVERDOSE

The most common adverse effects are excess sedation, confusion, ataxia, respiratory depression and allergic skin reactions which may be serious. Neuralgic or arthralgic pain, nausea and vomiting are less common. Pupils are usually slightly constricted but may be dilated with severe overdoses. The more alarming effects of reduced blood pressure, body temperature, profound respiratory and cardiovascular depression can lead to coma and death. Paradoxical reactions include a period of euphoria, excitement and possibly, irritability prior to the time the desired sedative actions take effect.

DRUG ABUSE AND DEPENDENCE

Physical dependence to barbiturates like secobarbital is more apt to occur than with other sedative hypnotics such as benzodiazepines. Withdrawal symptoms are similar to those of alcohol abstinence and will usually begin in the first 12-24 hours. Secobarbital has a relatively long half-life of about 30 hours and therefore, symptoms may not peak for several days. Classic symptoms include weakness, apprehension, anxiety, nausea, vomiting, tremors, abdominal pains, insomnia and tachycardia. Hallucinations, delirium tremors and life-threatening convulsions are possible.

STANOZOLOL (Winstrol)
Drug Class: Androgen

HOW SUPPLIED

Tablets: 2mg

OVERVIEW

Stanozolol is a synthetic androgenic, anabolic steroid, hormone. It is primarily indicated prophylactically to decrease the frequency and severity of hereditary angioedema which causes swelling of the face, extremities and upper respiratory tract. Athletes, body-builders, weight lifters and physical laborers have misused it to add muscle mass. It's most common side effects include increased hair growth and general masculinization, but it also leads to testicular atrophy, breast enlargement and premature baldness in men. It is known to increase aggression and antisocial behavior ("roid rage"). Liver damage or cancer and increased cardiovascular disease are possible. Though not physically addicting, there is some mood elevation. There is no known withdrawal.

INDICATIONS (NORMAL USE)

Stanozolol is indicated for the prophylactic treatment of hereditary angioedema to decrease the frequency and severity. It has also been used by dentists in therapeutic doses to reduce swelling associated with dental extraction.

PHARMACOLOGY

Stanozolol is a synthetic androgenic hormone similar in structure to testosterone. The endogenous androgens are essential hormones that are responsible for normal growth and development of the male sex organs and for maintenance of secondary sex characteristics. Like testosterone, it causes retention of nitrogen, potassium, phosphorous and sodium which are subsequently used for protein anabolism. It also increases serum levels of an esterase which if deficient, can lead to episodes of angioedema. The androgens stimulate the closure of the epiphyseal growth plates and can cause premature termination of the growth process if used inappropriately in prepubertal children.

ADVERSE REACTION AND OVERDOSE

Hormones work by a biofeedback mechanism. If an individual is taking excessive doses of anabolic steroids, the body stops producing endogenous testosterone which after time, leads to male eunuchs with characteristics of testicular atrophy (a wasting or diminution of testicle size), aspermia which can cause male infertility, enlarged prostrate and the above mentioned. Serious hemolytic effects and cancer of the liver are possible with excess use. Inappropriate aggressive behavior has also been witnessed. Women will have irregular menstrual cycles, masculinization with excess hair growth, clitoral enlargement, acne and deepening of their voice, many of these changes are permanent.

DRUG ABUSE AND DEPENDENCE

Stanozolol, like all the synthetic androgens, is not physically addicting, but some individuals experience a mood elevation. Initial excitation, including increased libido (which is later followed by impotence), may be appealing to the abuser and thus may contribute to continued use. Enhanced physical appearance may lead to narcissism (love of one's self) and this may account for a degree of psychological addiction. To attain the enhanced performance or physique the abuser desires, dosages of 10 to 1,000-fold that of therapeutic dosages are used. Most misuse and abuse is actually by individuals who never compete in sports. There is no known physical withdrawal.

▮

TALBUTAL (Lotusate)
Drug Class: Barbiturate

HOW SUPPLIED

Tablets: 120mg

OVERVIEW

Talbutal is a barbiturate hypnotic primarily indicated for the short-term treatment of insomnia. Drowsiness may be preceded with a period of euphoria, excitement and confusion before its desired sedative actions take effect. Its effects have often been mistakenly attributed to alcohol consumption. The most common side effects include excess sedation, respiratory depression, confusion, ataxia and skin rashes. Overdoses can lead to further respiratory and cardiovascular depression, a fall in blood pressure, shock, coma and ensuing death. Talbutal is addictive and withdrawal symptoms are very similar to those seen with alcohol abstinence and may be life threatening.

INDICATIONS (NORMAL USE)

Talbutal is indicated for the short-term treatment of insomnia. In lower doses it has been used for its sedative action.

PHARMACOLOGY

Talbutal is a substituted pyrimidine derivative. Like all barbiturates, the basic structure is barbituric acid. Talbutal acts throughout the CNS and reversibly depresses the activity of all excitable tissues. It is particularly active at the midbrain reticular formation which is specifically concerned with the arousal mechanism. All barbiturates are capable of producing a progressive degree of CNS depression - from mild sedation to hypnosis to deep coma to death. Talbutal has no analgesic effects and may actually increase the reaction to painful stimuli such as an injury.

ADVERSE REACTION AND OVERDOSE

The most common adverse effects are excess sedation, confusion, ataxia, respiratory depression and allergic skin reactions which may be serious. Neuralgic or arthralgic pain, nausea and vomiting are less common. Pupils are usually slightly constricted but may be dilated with severe overdoses. The more alarming effects of reduced blood pressure, profound respiratory and cardiovascular depression can lead to coma and death. Paradoxical reactions include a period of euphoria, excitement and possibly, irritability prior to the time the desired sedative actions take effect.

DRUG ABUSE AND DEPENDENCE

Physical dependence to Talbutal can occur, but its use in the U.S. is extremely limited. Withdrawal symptoms are similar to those of alcohol abstinence and will usually begin in the first 12-24 hours. Symptoms may not peak for several days. The drug's half-life would be expected to be similar to pentobarbital since it has a fast onset and short duration of hypnotic activity. Classic symptoms include weakness, apprehension, anxiety, nausea, vomiting, tremors, abdominal pains, insomnia and tachycardia. Hallucinations, delirium tremors and life-threatening convulsions are possible.

TEMAZEPAM (Restoril)
Drug Class: Benzodiazepine

HOW SUPPLIED

Capsules: 7.5mg, 15mg, and 30mg
*Available by nonproprietary name

OVERVIEW

Temazepam is used as an hypnotic in the short-term management of insomnia. Drowsiness, confusion, slurred speech and ataxia are possible side effects. Paradoxical agitation, anger and hostility have been observed. Abrupt withdrawal is often characterized by rebound insomnia and anxiety. Dependency and withdrawal can occur.

INDICATIONS (NORMAL USE)

Temazepam is indicated as an hypnotic in the short-term management of insomnia.

PHARMACOLOGY

Temazepam's action appears to be mediated through the inhibitory neurotransmitter gamma-aminobutyric acid (GABA) which, like all benzodiazepines, enhances the drug's affinity for certain sites within the limbic, thalamic and hypothalamic areas of the brain. It is this inhibition or blocking of the arousal components of these areas which produces the sedative and hypnotic activity. The paradoxical CNS stimulatory effects are postulated to result from the release of previously suppressed responses (disinhibition) in much the same manner in which alcohol can effect an individual.

ADVERSE REACTION AND OVERDOSE

The most common adverse effects which can be visually observed are extreme drowsiness, ataxia, fatigue, confusion, weakness and dizziness. Amnesia, blurred vision and slurred speech can occur. Paradoxical CNS stimulation, agitation, restlessness and hyperactivity are less common than seen with triazolam. Acute overdose will generally result in somnolence or coma with respiratory depression. Concomitant ingestion of alcohol or other CNS depressants may aggravate symptoms.

DRUG ABUSE AND DEPENDENCE

Physical dependence can occur and withdrawal symptoms may not peak for 24-72 hours since Temazepam has an intermediate half-life. Rebound insomnia and anxiety, agitation, confusion, rigidity of limbs, hallucinations and seizures are all possible after abrupt withdrawal. Less serious withdrawal symptoms include tremors, abdominal cramps, vomiting and sweating.

▮

TRIAZOLAM (Halcion)
Drug Class: Benzodiazepine

HOW SUPPLIED

Tablets: 0.125mg and 0.250mg

OVERVIEW

Triazolam is used as an hypnotic in the short-term management of insomnia. Drowsiness, confusion, slurred speech and ataxia are possible side effects. Bizarre or abnormal behavior, agitation and hallucinations seem to occur more frequently with triazolam than the other hypnotic benzodiazepines. Abrupt withdrawal is often characterized by rebound insomnia and anxiety. Dependency and withdrawal can occur.

INDICATIONS (NORMAL USE)

Triazolam is used as an hypnotic in the management of insomnia.

PHARMACOLOGY

Triazolam's action appears to be mediated through the inhibitory neurotransmitter gamma-aminobutyric acid (GABA) which, like all benzodiazepines, enhances the drug's affinity for certain sites within the limbic, thalamic and hypothalamic areas of the brain. It is this inhibition or blocking to the arousal components of these areas which produces the sedative and hypnotic activity. The paradoxical CNS stimulatory effects are postulated to result from the release of previously suppressed responses (disinhibition) in much the same manner in which alcohol can effect an individual.

ADVERSE REACTION AND OVERDOSE

The most common adverse effects which can be visually observed are extreme drowsiness, ataxia, fatigue, confusion, weakness and dizziness. Amnesia, blurred vision and slurred speech can occur. Paradoxical CNS stimulation, agitation, restlessness and hyperactivity are more common with triazolam than other hypnotic benzodiazepines, as are hallucinations. Acute overdose will generally result in somnolence or coma with respiratory depression. Concomitant ingestion of alcohol or other CNS depressants may aggravate symptoms.

DRUG ABUSE AND DEPENDENCE

Physical dependence can occur despite the relatively short half-life. Withdrawal symptoms may peak within the first 24-36 hours. Rebound insomnia and anxiety, agitation, confusion, rigidity of limbs, hallucinations and seizures are all possible after abrupt withdrawal. Less serious withdrawal symptoms include tremors, abdominal cramps, vomiting and sweating. The elderly seem to be much more sensitive to the adverse effects of triazolam and withdrawal symptoms than younger users. While this would be expected with all the benzodiazepines, it appears to be even more noticeable with triazolam. ▮

ZOLPIDEM (Ambien)
Drug Class: Imidazopyridine-derivative

HOW SUPPLIED

Tablets: 5mg and 10mg

OVERVIEW

Zolpidem is used as an hypnotic in the short-term management of insomnia. Drowsiness, dizziness and diarrhea are the most common side effects. However, zolpidem possesses many of the same adverse effects seen with benzodiazepines though on a less frequent basis. Bizarre or abnormal behavior, agitation and hallucinations can occur along with amnesia, ataxia and confusion. Abrupt withdrawal can result in rebound insomnia and anxiety. Dependency and withdrawal are both possible.

INDICATIONS (NORMAL USE)

Zolpidem is used as an hypnotic in the management of insomnia.

PHARMACOLOGY

Although zolpidem is an imidazopyridine-derivative and not a benzodiazepine, it's action also appears to be mediated through the inhibitory neurotransmitter gamma-aminobutyric acid (GABA) which enhances the drug's affinity for certain sites within the limbic, thalamic and hypothalamic areas of the brain. It is this inhibition or blocking of the arousal components of these areas which produces the sedative and hypnotic activity. Unlike the benzodiazepines which bind nonselectively to many of the GABA receptors and thus produce multiple effects, zolpidem selectively binds to just one of the GABA receptors and thus has less anxiolytic, muscle relaxant and anticonvulsant activity than the benzodiazepines. This may also result in reduced abuse potential and dependency.

ADVERSE REACTION AND OVERDOSE

Possible adverse effects which can be visually observed are drowsiness, ataxia, fatigue, confusion, weakness and dizziness. Amnesia, blurred vision and slurred speech can occur. Paradoxical CNS stimulation, agitation, restlessness and hyperactivity are also possible and like triazolam are most apparent in the elderly who may have decreased liver function. This is frequently seen with alcoholics. Acute overdose will generally result in somnolence or coma with respiratory depression. Concomitant ingestion of alcohol or other CNS depressants may aggravate symptoms.

DRUG ABUSE AND DEPENDENCE

Physical dependence can occur despite the relatively short half-life. Withdrawal symptoms may peak within the first 24-36 hours. Rebound insomnia and anxiety, agitation, confusion, rigidity of limbs, hallucinations and seizures are all possible after abrupt withdrawal. Less serious withdrawal symptoms include tremors, abdominal cramps, vomiting and sweating.

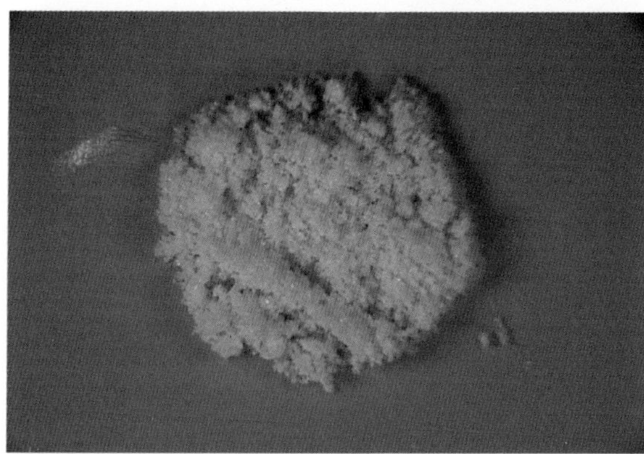

Kyle Hall

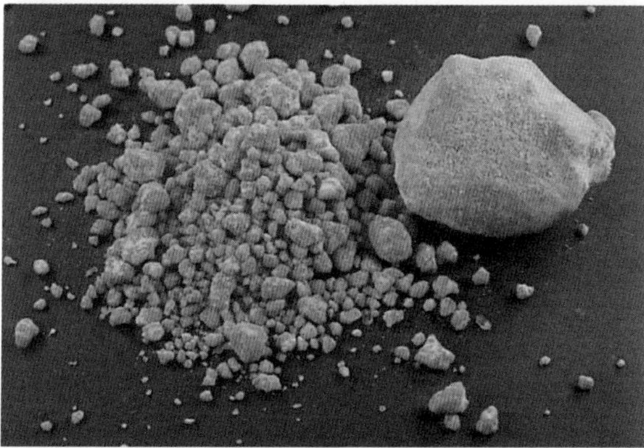

Amphetamine is a term used generically to refer to any member of a class of drugs that has an amphetamine base: amphetamine, dextroamphetamine, methamphetamine and dextromethamphetamine. In the illicit manufacture of these drugs, methamphetamine is the most common. Methamphetamine, commonly known as "meth", may be smoked (usually in a glass pipe), dissolved in water and injected, swallowed or snorted. Higher quality meth is usually an off-white fine powder (top photo). However, much of the meth on the street shows the results of sloppy manufacturing: dark yellow or brown in color, sticky consistency, or a very granular or even a solid-block appearance (bottom photos). Names for lower quality meth often refer to the drug's physical appearance: soapstone, peanut brittle, or peanut butter.

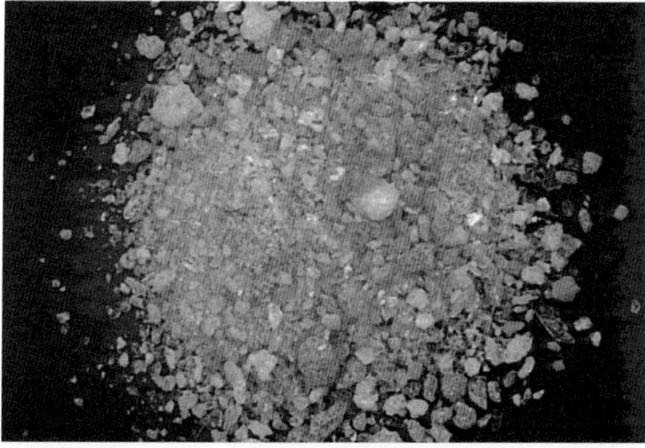

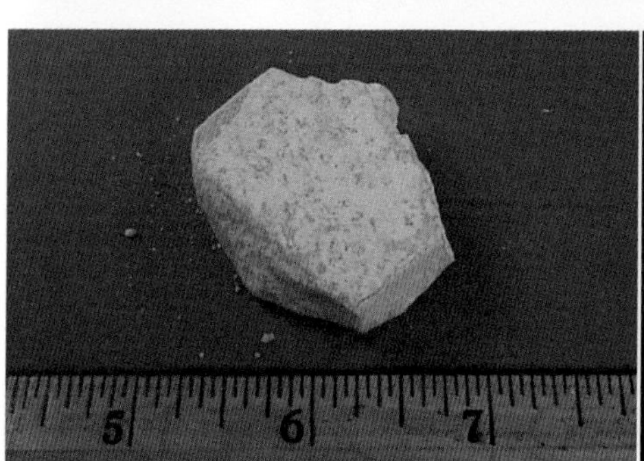

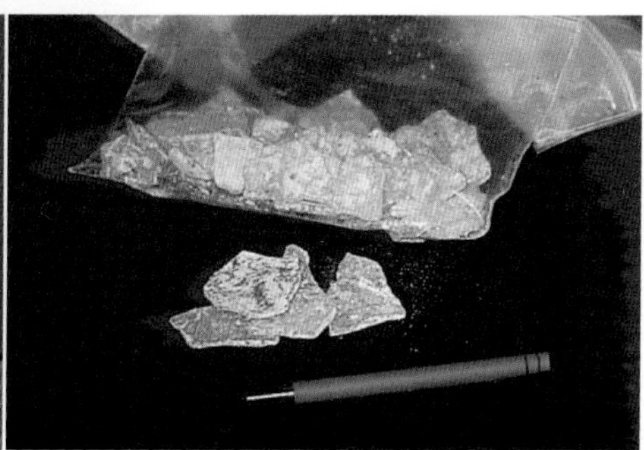

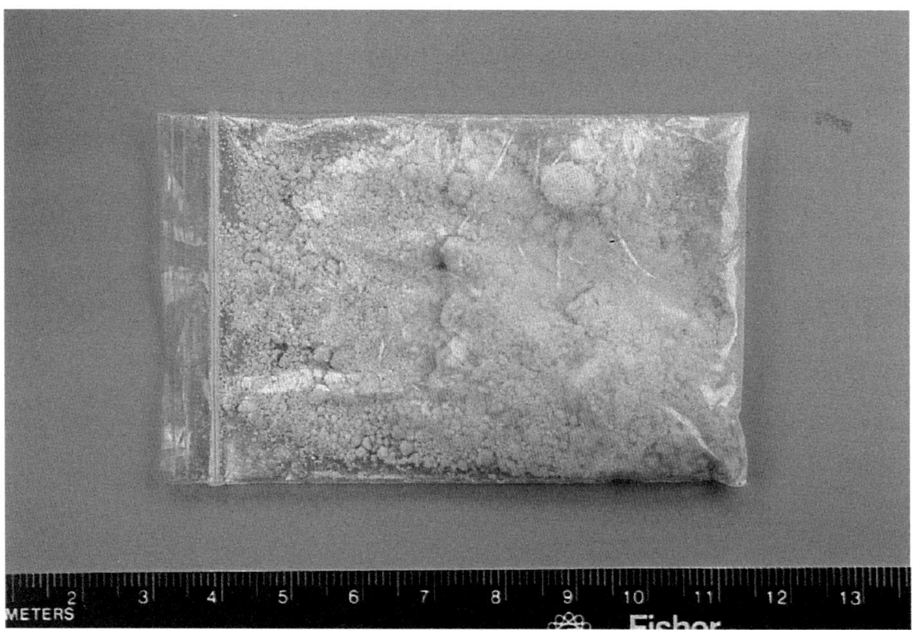

▲ Meth is often packaged in plastic bags, such as the small plastic ziplock bag shown. It is also, but less frequently, packaged in paper bindles and glass vials.

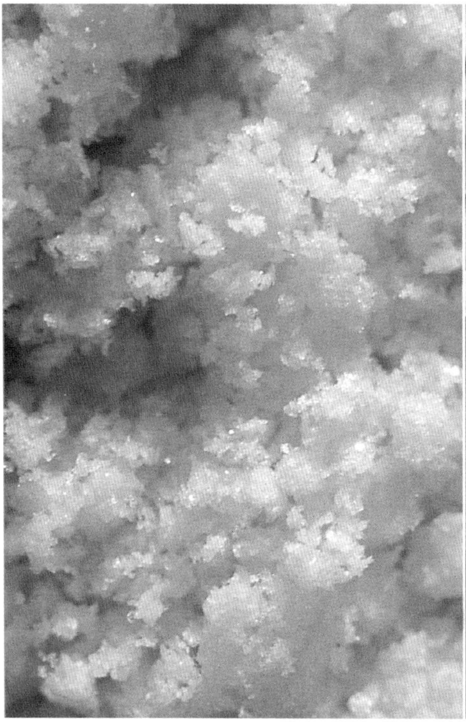

▲ Close-up of methamphetamine, a drug also commonly known as meth, crank, crystal, speed, crystal meth, and go-fast.

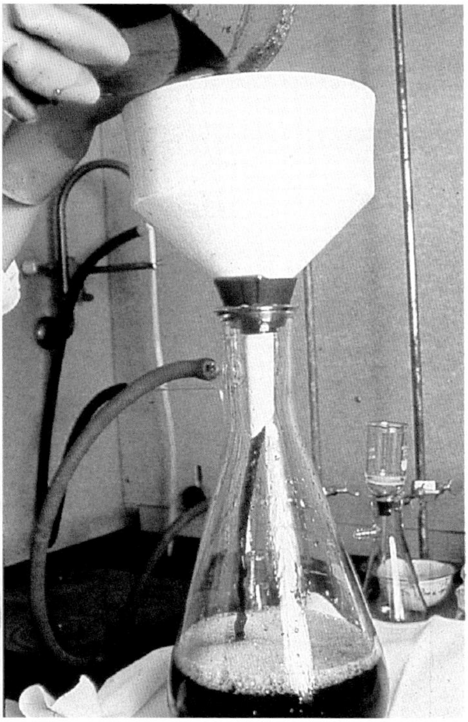

▲ Meth oil, an intermediate product in the manufacture of methamphetamine.

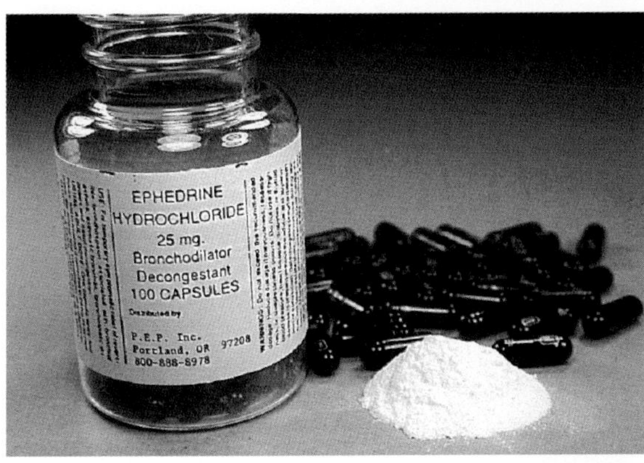

➤ Perhaps the most common starting material used in the manufacture of meth is ephedrine. Ephedrine is a legal substance which is readily available in tablet or capsule form and is sold as a decongestant. The tablets are boiled in water to separate the ephedrine from the fillers and other inert ingredients.

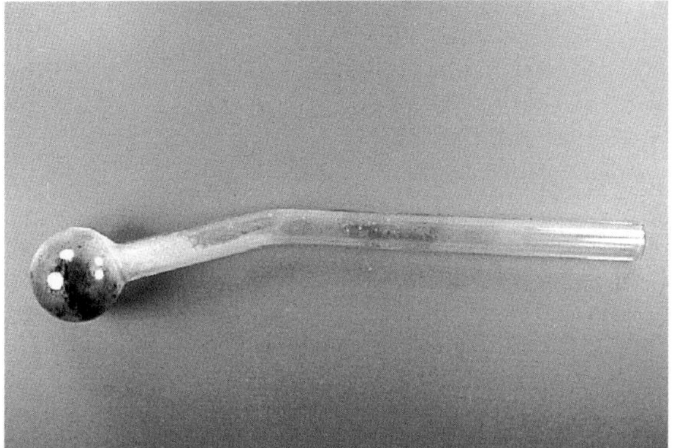

➤ A glass pipe of the type often used to smoke meth and ice. Unlike pipes used for other drugs, traditional meth pipes do not utilize metal screens; rather, the drug is placed loosely in the bottom of the pipe bowl.

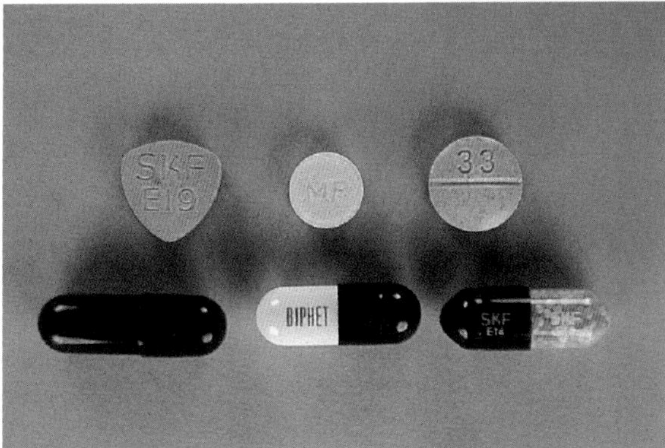

➤ Amphetamine, methamphetamine, dextroamphetamine, and combinations of these drugs are commonly prescribed for the treatment of attention deficit disorder, narcolepsy, and severe obesity. Pictured are various pharmaceutical amphetamine tablets and capsules.

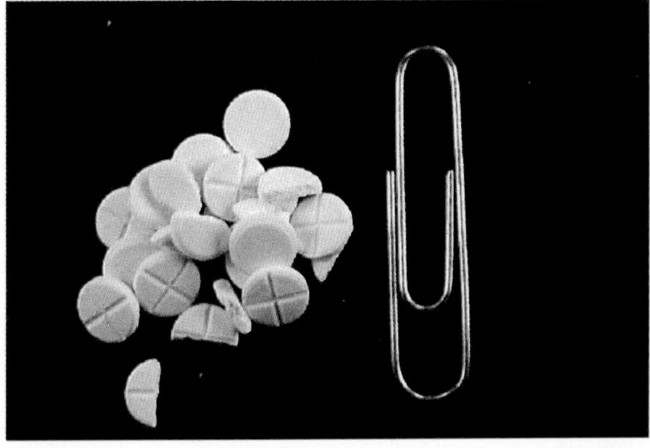

➤ Outdated illicit amphetamine tablets, commonly known as "white crosses". Virtually all tablets of this appearance in circulation today do not contain amphetamine. They are legally produced and contain substances such as caffeine or ephedrine, although they are still commonly referred to as white crosses.

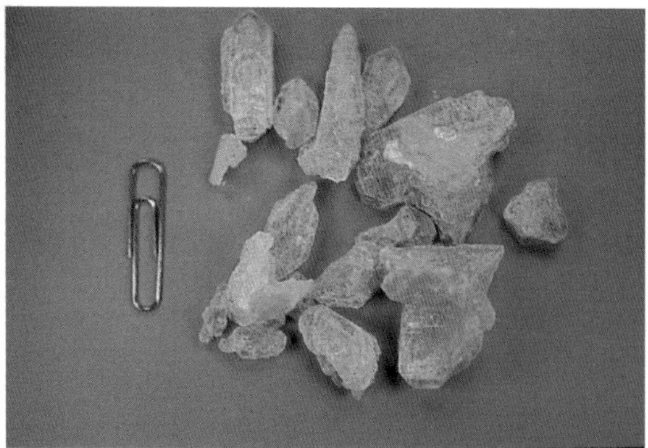

➤ "Ice" - a smokeable form of dextromethamphetamine. Its appearance is often described as that of broken glass or shattered ice. Other street names reflect the drug's physical appearance: "glass" and "crystal meth". Its purity is generally quite high.

➤ Close-up of an ice crystal. Ice is normally smoked in a glass pipe, such as that shown on the previous page. When heated, ice gives off potent vapors which can produce effects that last up to approximately fourteen hours. Ice has a hard texture and is odorless.

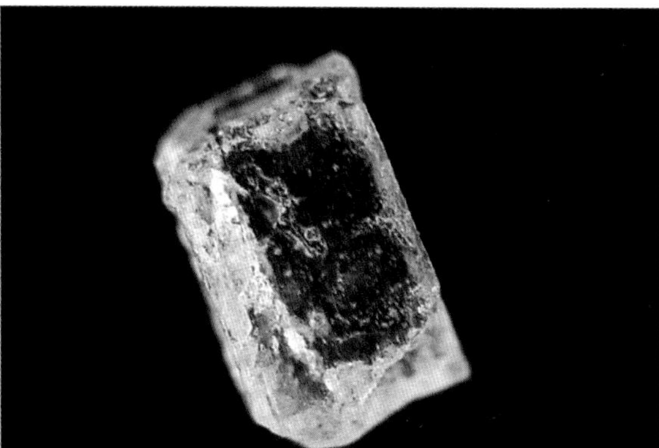

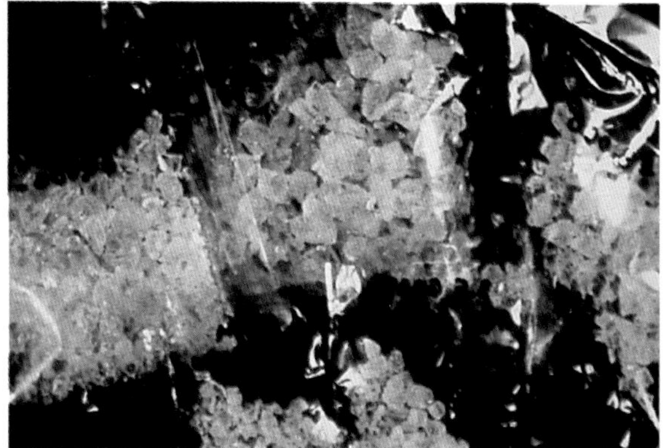

➤ Confiscated bulk packages of ice. Ice first appeared in Asia in 1985, and by 1988 its use was documented in Hawaii. Ice use remains concentrated in Hawaii and on the West Coast, with distribution being controlled by Asian gangs. The abuse of ice never quite reached the level predicted by the media, and confiscations are fairly rare.

➤ Methcathinone (cat) is a chemical analog of methamphetamine and thus shares many of the same effects. It is ingested in the same methods as is meth. It is new to the drug scene but is a Schedule I drug under the analog laws of the Controlled Substances Act. It normally appears as an off-white or yellowish powder.

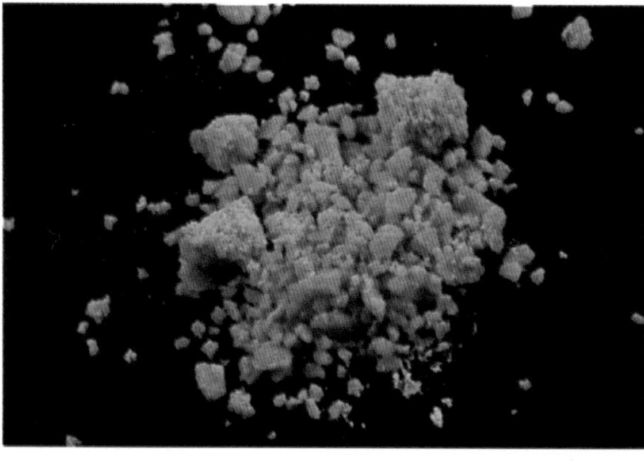

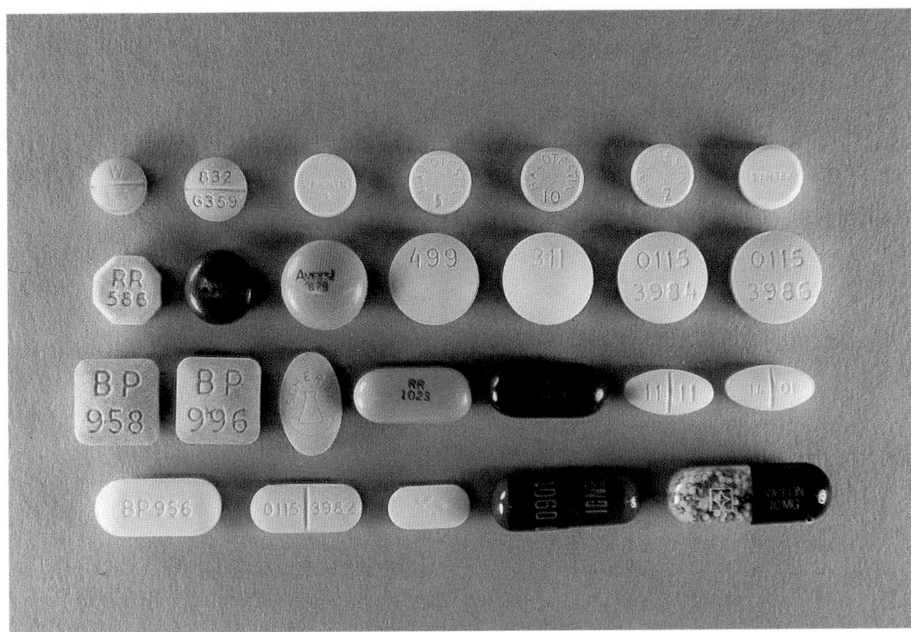

▲ Anabolic steroids were placed in Schedule III of the Controlled Substances Act in October 1990. They are unique among controlled drugs in that they are not psychoactive. Nonetheless, steroids have experienced a great deal of abuse and black market dealing. Pictured are twenty-six anabolic steroids available in tablet and capsule form.

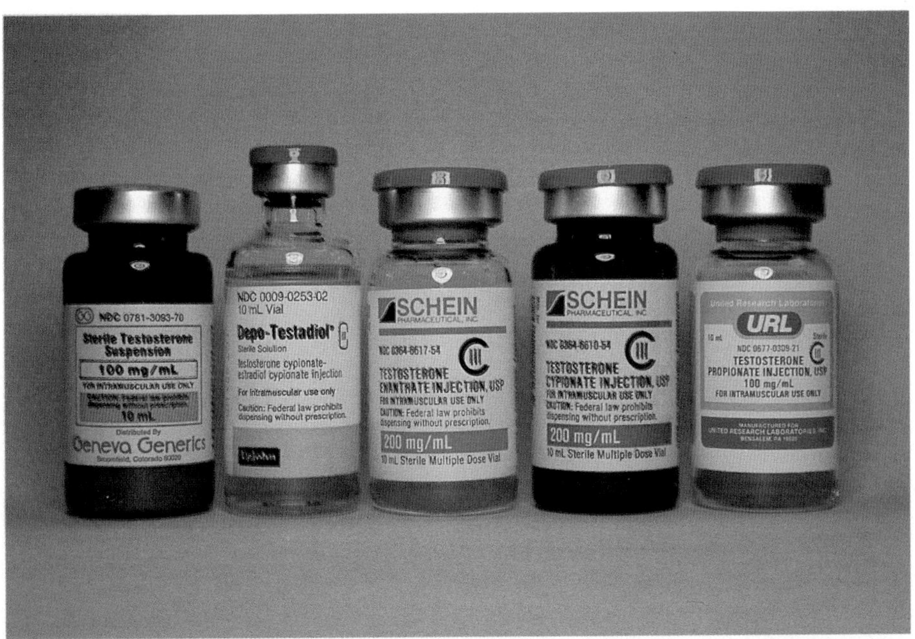

▲ A variety of injectable anabolic steroids. All are synthetic versions of the male hormone testosterone.

➤ Many unsuspecting American athletes are under the mistaken impression that Mexican pharmacies sell only real drugs like their American counterparts. Pictured at right are several illegally produced counterfeit steroids purchased at pharmacies in Tijuana, Mexico. All are professionally packaged and look real, but few, if any, contain an active ingredient.

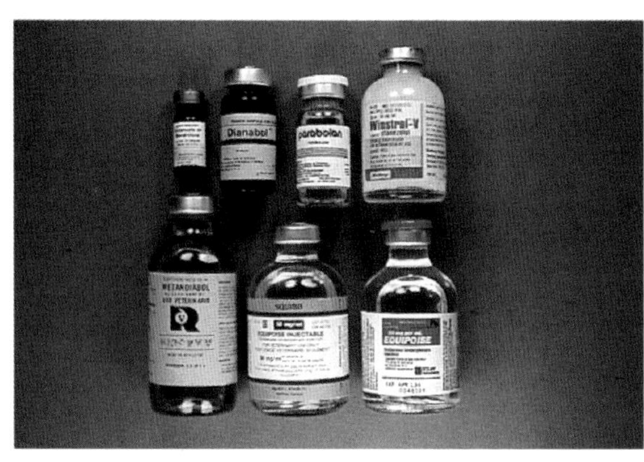

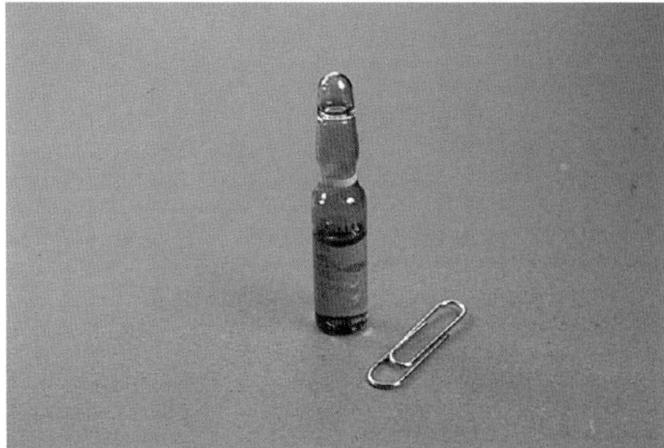

➤ Although steroids are commonly contained in ampules in other countries, this package is not commonly used in the United States. They are shaped similar to a bowling pin and are broken in two around the thin part of the neck by finger pressure, thereby allowing the contents to be drawn into a syringe.

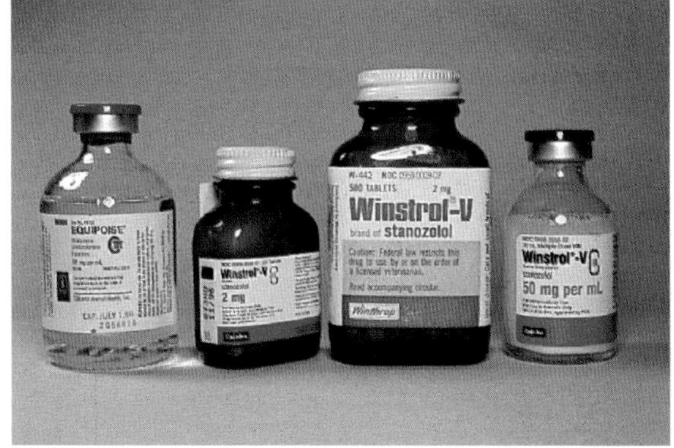

➤ Anabolic steroids designed for veterinary medicine are some of the more popular steroids used by athletes. Winstrol-V, a brand name for stanozolol, was the steroid Canadian sprinter Ben Johnson tested positive for during the 1988 Olympics.

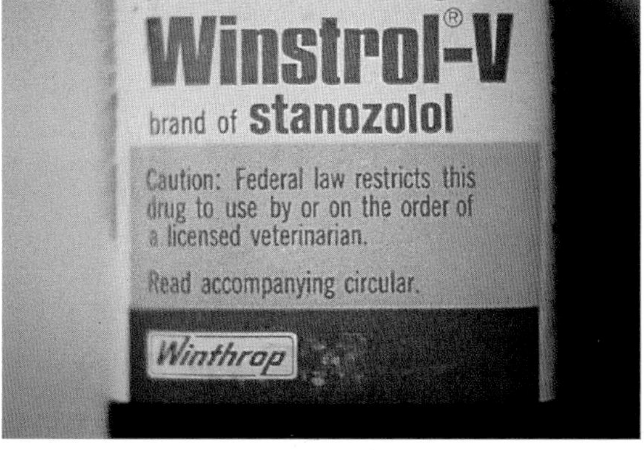

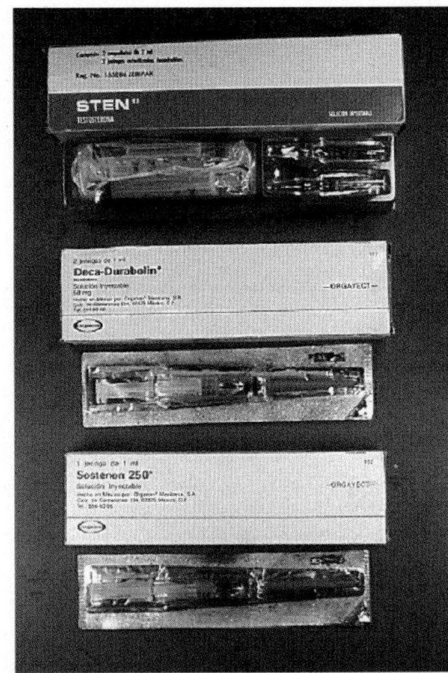

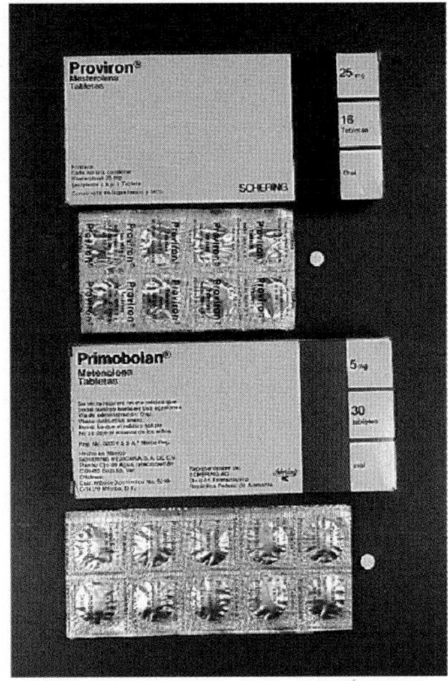

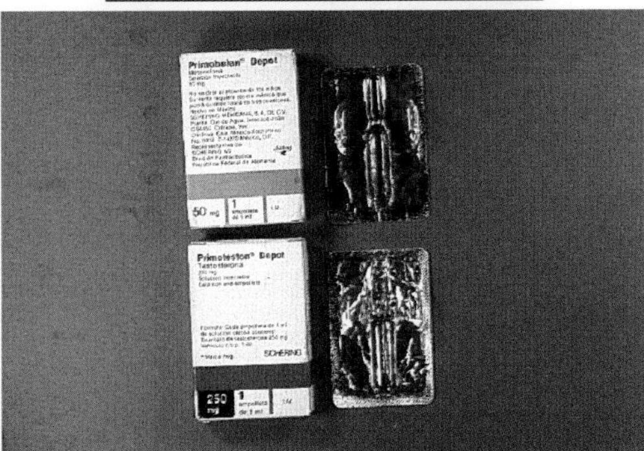

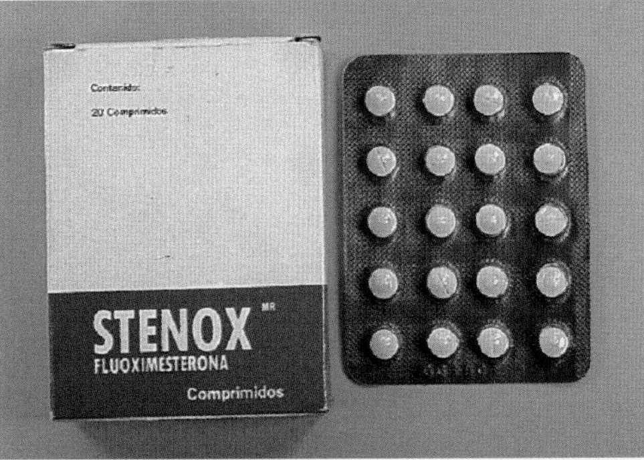

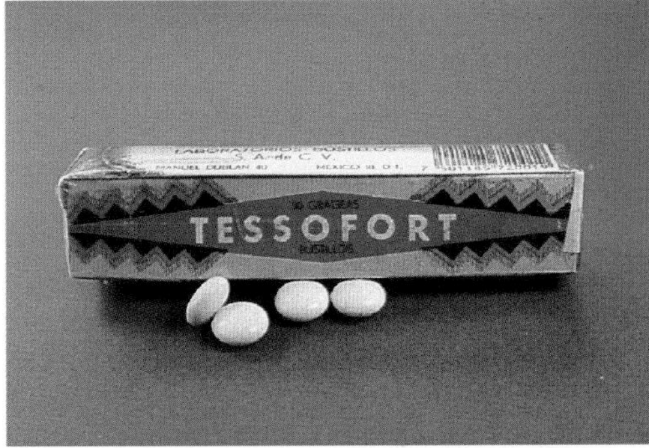

Due to over-the-counter sales in Mexico, a large percentage of the black market steroids sold in America originate from that country. Some estimates indicate that nearly 80% of all American steroid users include Mexican-made steroids in their repertoire. Pictured are five of the most popular injectable steroids available in Mexican pharmacies: Sten, a combination of three different types of testosterones packaged with a syringe and a couple of 2 ml ampules; Deca-Durabolin, brand name for nandrolone decanoate in a 1 ml preloaded syringe (Mexican Deca-Durabolin is possibly the most common legitimately made steroid on the American black market); Sostenon 250, a combination of four different types of testosterones packaged in a preloaded 1 ml syringe; Primobolan Depot, brand name for methenolone enanthate packaged in a 1 ml ampule; and Primoteston Depot, brand name for testosterone enanthate packaged in a 1 ml ampule. Popular oral steroids available in Mexican pharmacies include Stenox, brand name for fluoxymesterone; Tessofort, a combination of vitamins, minerals and methyltestosterone; Proviron, brand name for mesterolone; and Primobolan, brand name for methenolone.

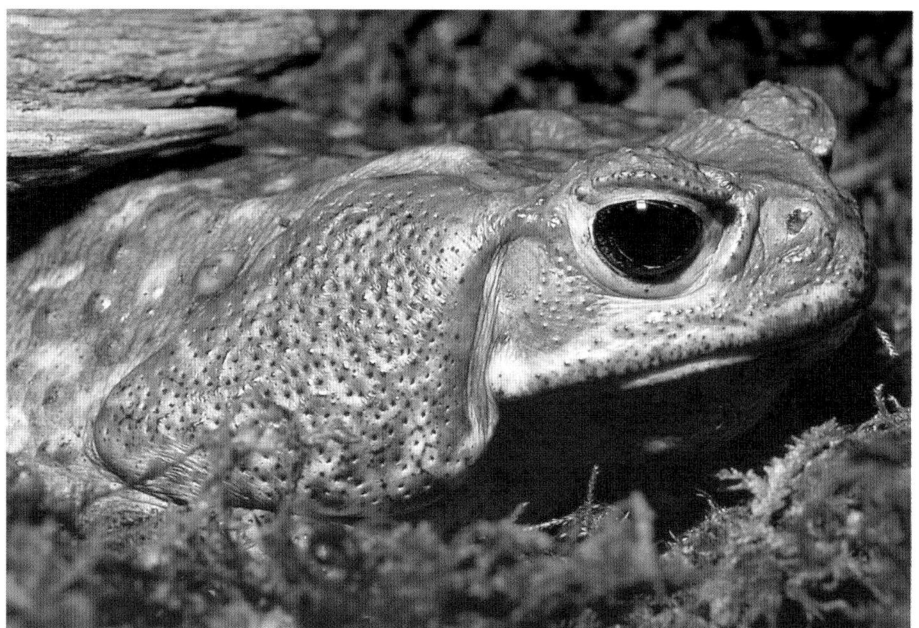

Stan Czolowski

▲ A toad of the species *bufo*, which excretes a venom from glands on its back as a defense against predators. Poisonous to many animals, the venom, closely related to the controlled drug bufotenine, can produce an LSD-like high when smoked. There are several dozen subspecies of the bufo toad in North America.

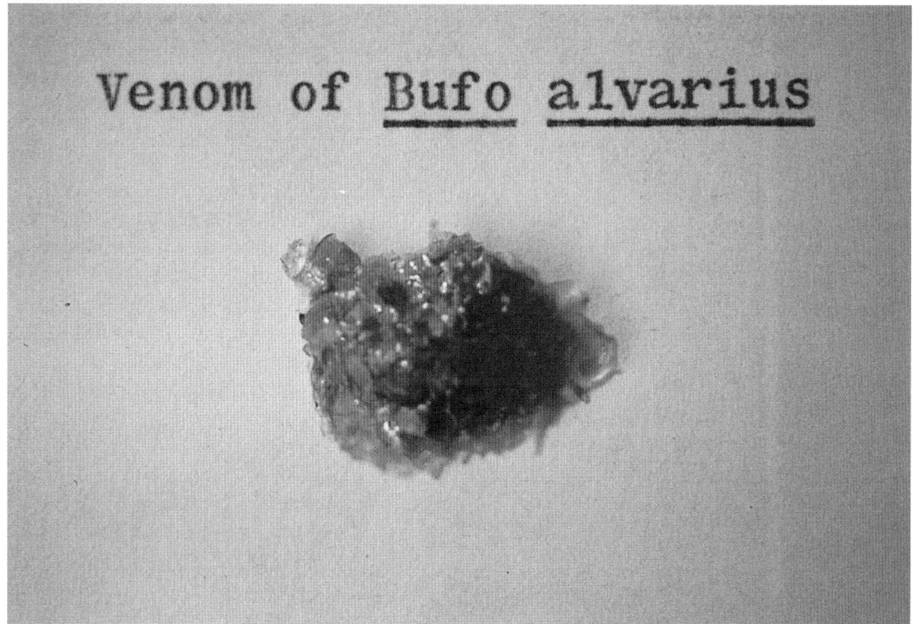

Jonathan Ott

▲ Venom of the bufo toad. The amber colored substance can be squeezed from glands on the back of the toad, collected, dried, and smoked in a pipe. Some users reportedly agitate the toad by shaking it and then lick the venom off the toad's back.

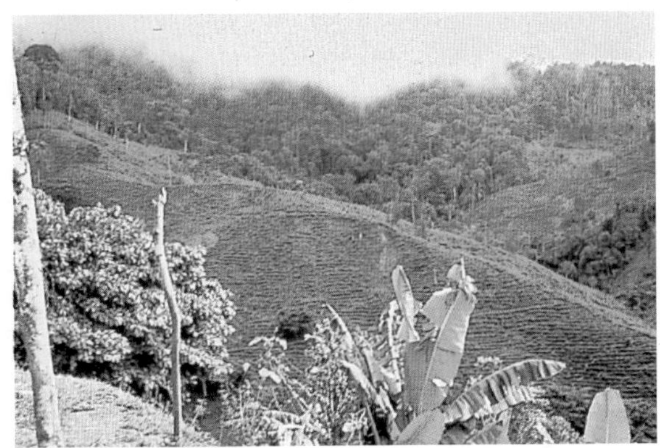

➤ Terraced coca field in southern Bolivia. Most of the world's supply of coca leaf is cultivated in the countries of Peru, Bolivia, and Colombia.

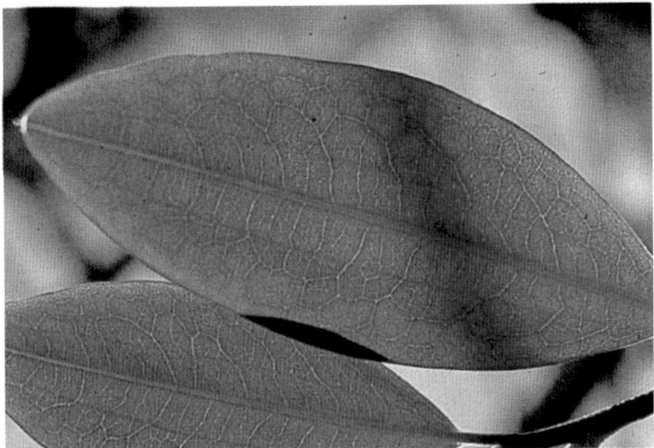

◄ Leaf of the erythroxylon coca plant, source of cocaine. South American Indians have chewed the coca leaf for centuries for social and religious occasions, for stamina, and to ward off hunger and fatigue. The cocaine content in the leaf is about 1% to 2%.

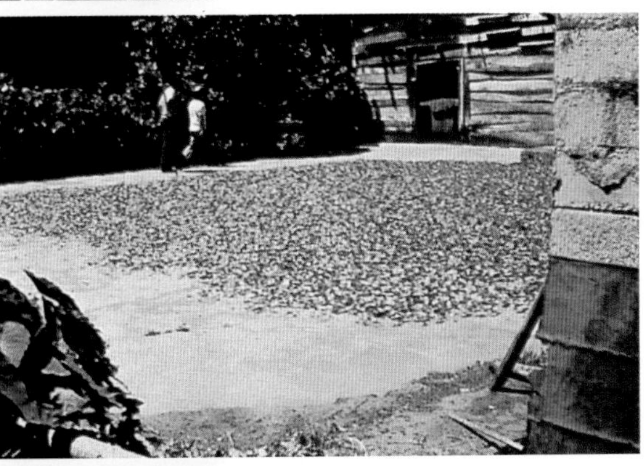

➤ Sun drying several hundred pounds of coca leaf in southern Bolivia in preparation for the extraction process. Two or three hundred pounds of leaves are generally required to produce one pound of the finished cocaine hydrochloride product.

Jose Azel/Aurora

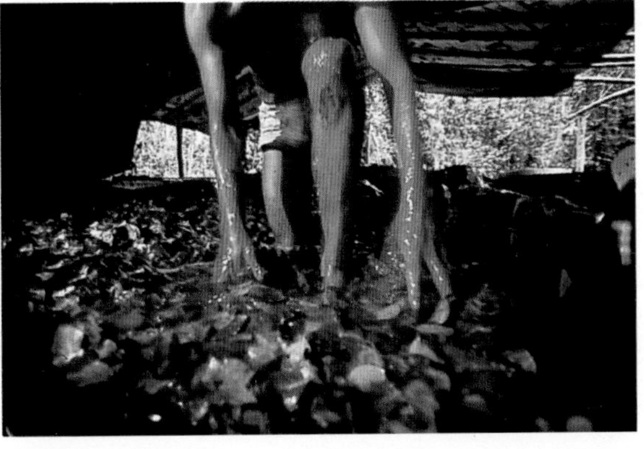

◄ After drying, the cocaine leaves are placed in a plastic-lined maceration pit containing water and a strong alkali such as lime. The mixture is left to soak for several days, breaking down the leaves and releasing the cocaine.

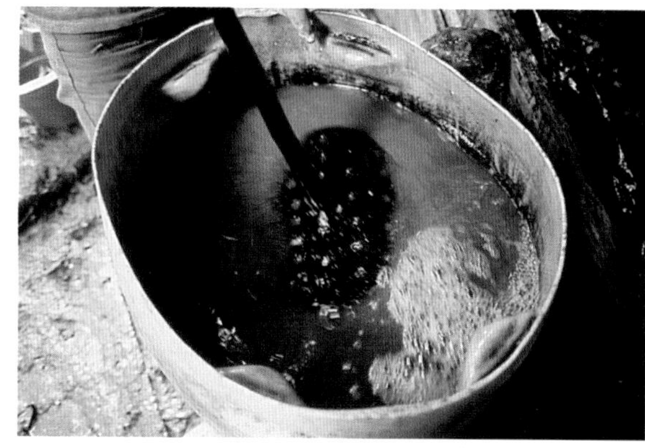

➤ Potassium permanganate being added to cocaine paste to remove impurities in a Colombian jungle "base" lab.

Jose Azel/Aurora

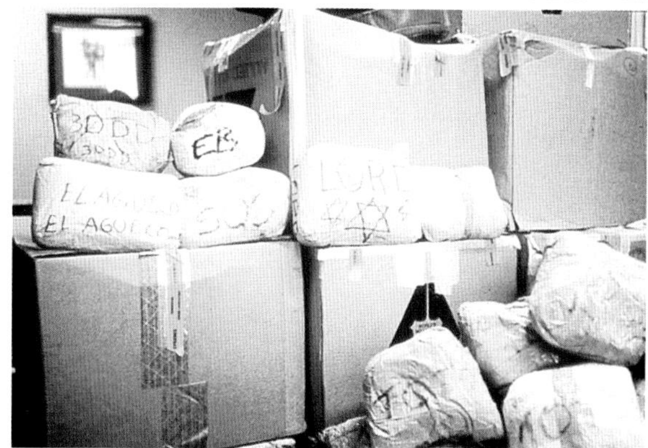

➤ A large cocaine shipment seized by the DEA. The various markings on the packages can designate either the producer or destination of the cocaine. It is estimated that the United States consumes 70% of all cocaine produced in South America.

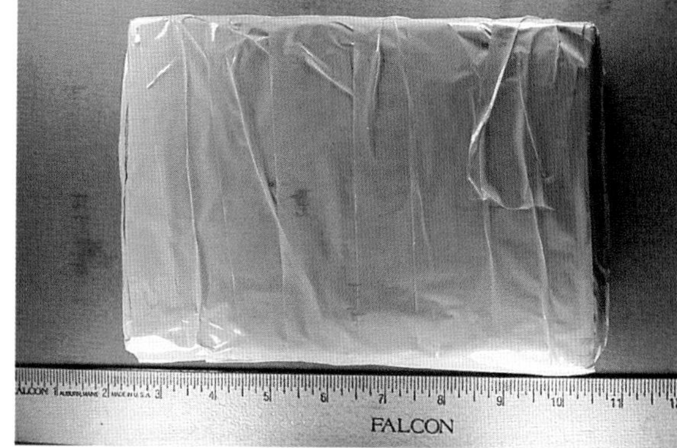

➤ A typical kilo (2.2 pounds) package of cocaine.

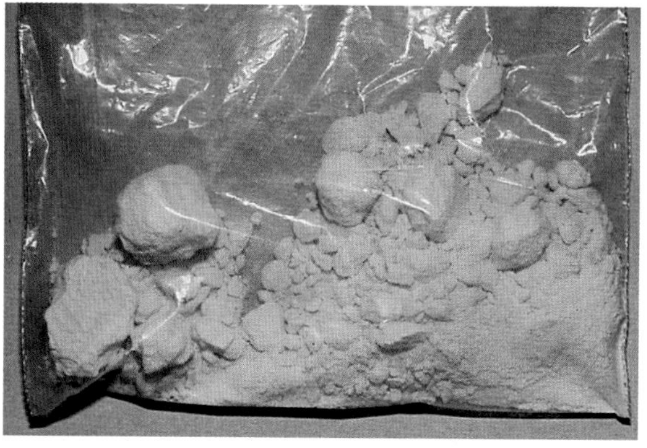

➤ As are many other drugs, cocaine is often packaged in plastic sandwich bags. The bag pictured contains 1 ounce of cocaine, consisting of both powder and rocks. The rocks are generally considered relatively pure as they cannot be easily cut without altering their physical appearance.

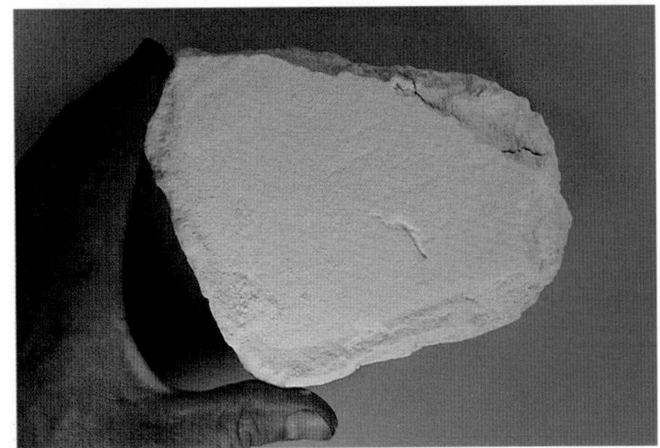

➤ One-half pound of 86% pure cocaine. If cut to the average purity level on the street of 60% and sold in gram quantities, the street value would be about $32,000.00.

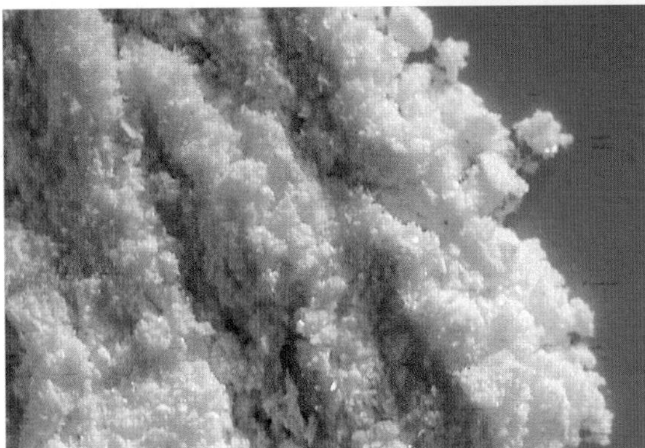

➤ Close-up of cocaine hydrochloride powder.

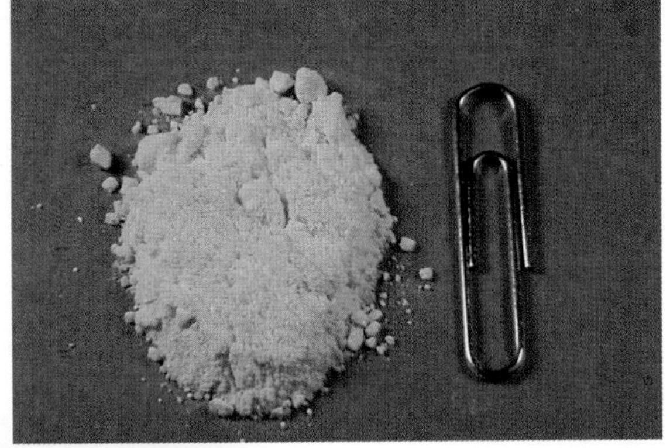

➤ One gram of cocaine, a typical street sale quantity, valued at about $100.00. One gram will produce about twenty to thirty snorting lines 1/8" wide and 1" to 2" long.

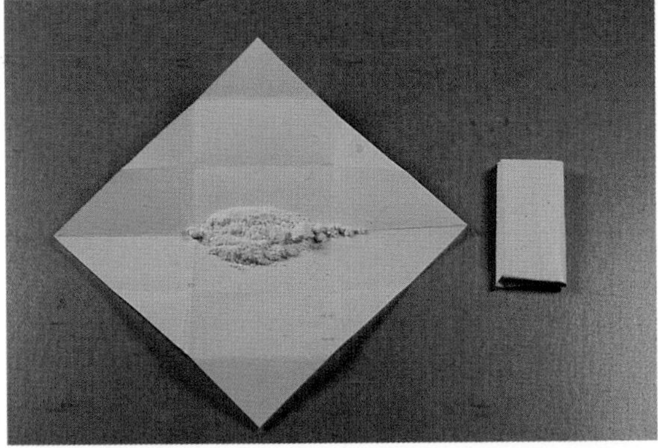

➤ A "bindle", or folded envelope of cocaine. Bindles vary in size and are often referred to as snow seals or locks. Perhaps the most commonly used material for bindles is glossy paper from magazines, although dark print can tint the cocaine.

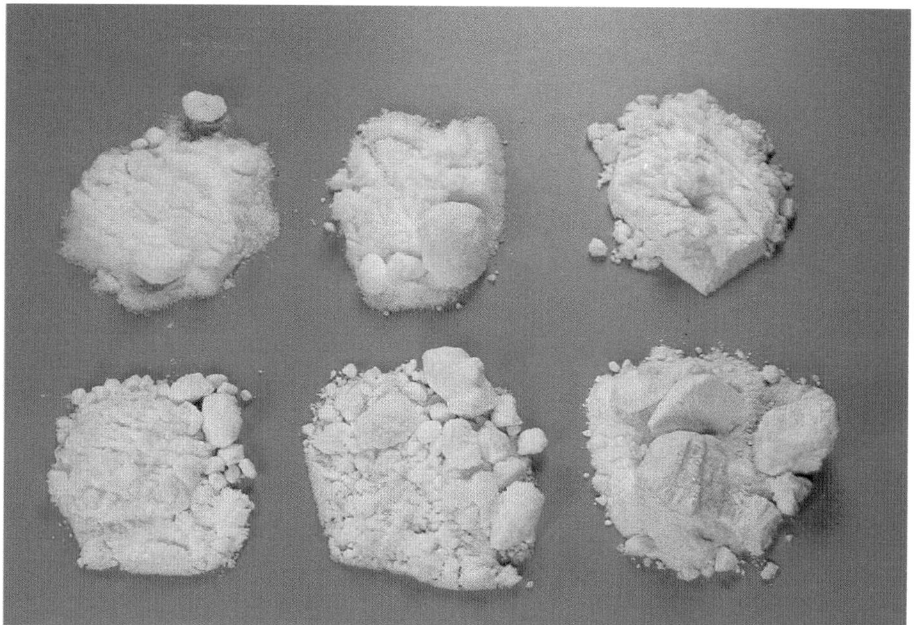

⮝ Many legal substances are used to cut or dilute cocaine to increase the seller's profits. Pictured are cocaine and commonly used cuts with a similar appearance. *Top row left to right:* mannitol, vitamin B, and lactose. *Bottom row left to right:* lidocaine, inositol, and cocaine.

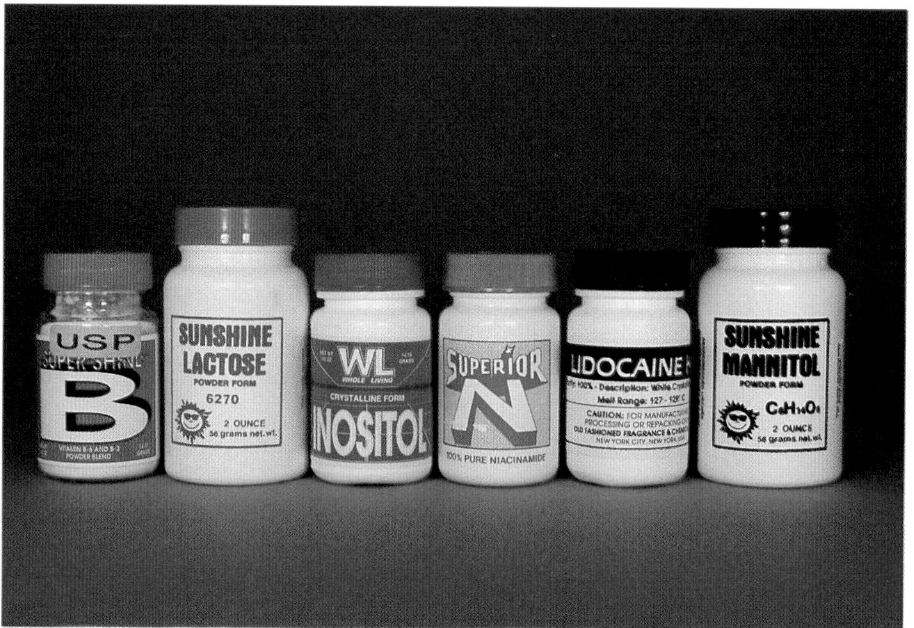

⮝ Most of the various cuts which are added to cocaine can be readily and legally purchased in paraphernalia shops, vitamin stores, and mail order outlets. The retail cost of the cuts pictured averaged less than $1.00 per gram, a fraction of the cost of a gram of cocaine.

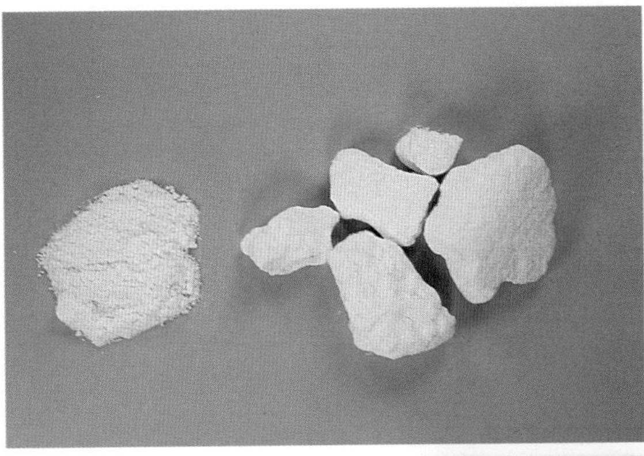

➤ As it moves down the distribution chain, dealers break larger rocks of cocaine into small rocks and powder to facilitate the addition of cuts or diluents. Some small rocks are generally left in street sale samples for cosmetic appeal.

➤ Close-up of flake cocaine. Flake cocaine is a high quality form of cocaine, which takes much more time and effort to produce than the powder form. Because the average cocaine consumer is satisfied with the lesser priced and lesser quality powder, relatively little flake is seen on the street.

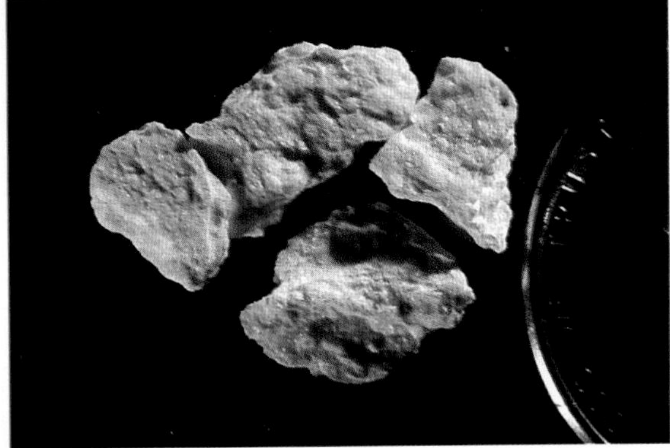

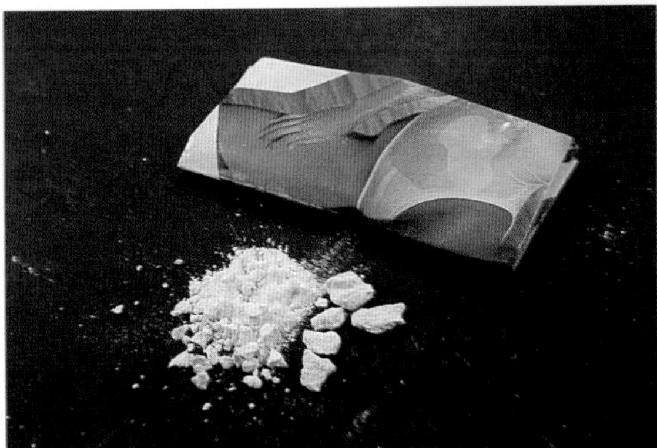

➤ Approximately 1/2 gram of flake cocaine and the bindle in which it was contained. Flake is generally considered the highest quality form of cocaine.

➤ Some cocaine users wash or purify their cocaine with a solvent, such as acetone or ether and then place it on filter paper to dry. The solvent removes many of the impurities left during the production process and results in a whiter cocaine. The photo at right is cocaine which has been washed in a solvent.

Bob Harris

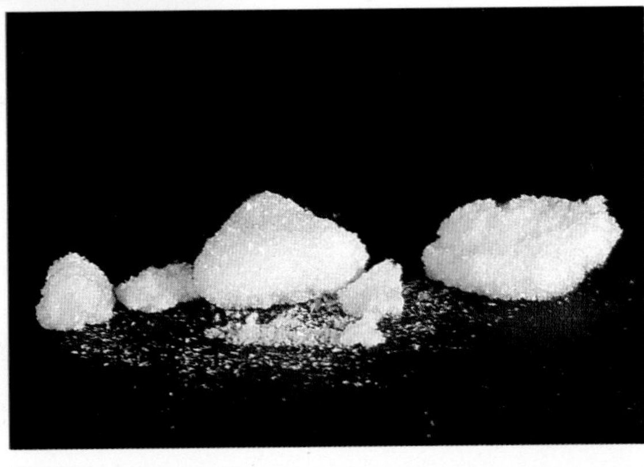

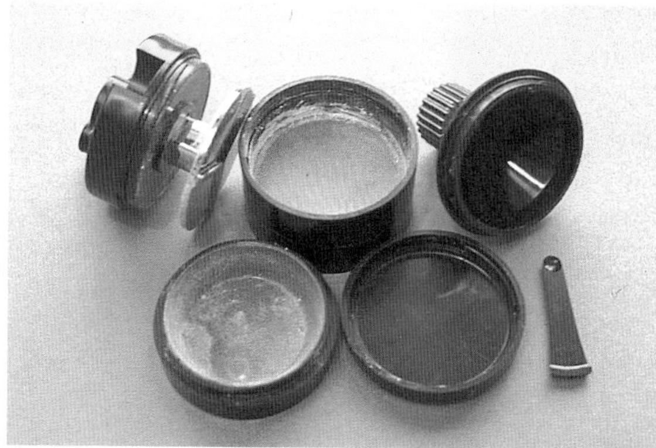

➤ In order to be snorted efficiently, cocaine must be a fine powder. Spice grinders may be used to grind chunks of cocaine into a fine powder. They also may be used to thoroughly mix cocaine with added cuts.

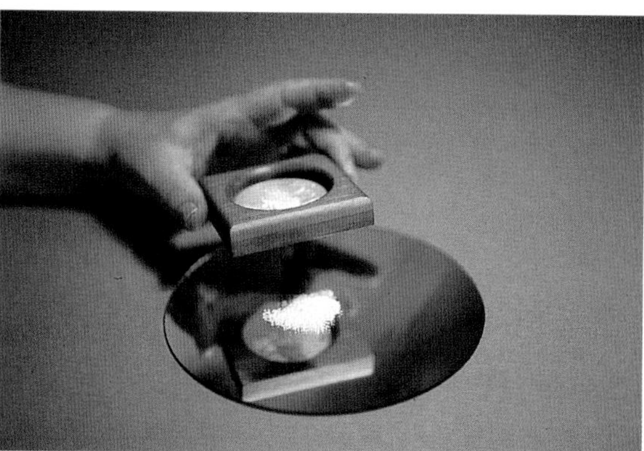

➤ Using a spice screen to sift fine cocaine powder from larger pieces for more efficient snorting.

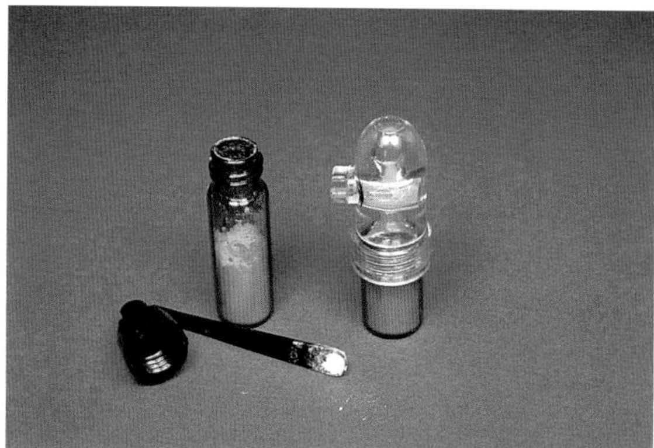

➤ Two types of cocaine vials. The vial on the left has a spoon affixed to the cap and is often referred to as a "flip top". The vial on the right has a snorting device, or "bullet" attached, which has an open/close valve on the side.

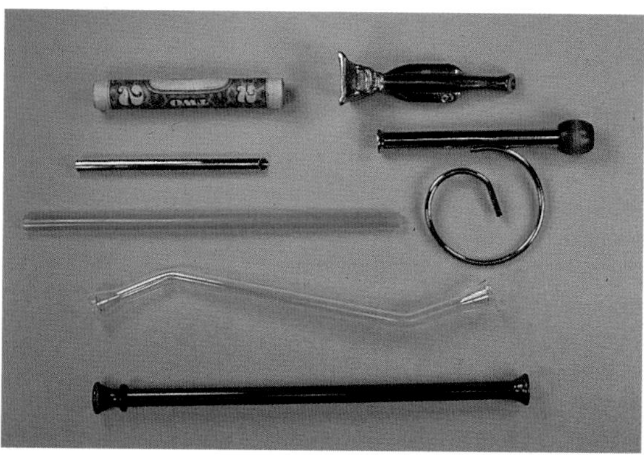

➤ A selection of tubular devices, or "tooters" used to snort lines of cocaine. These range from simple straws to rolled currency to commercially manufactured items which are available in paraphernalia stores.

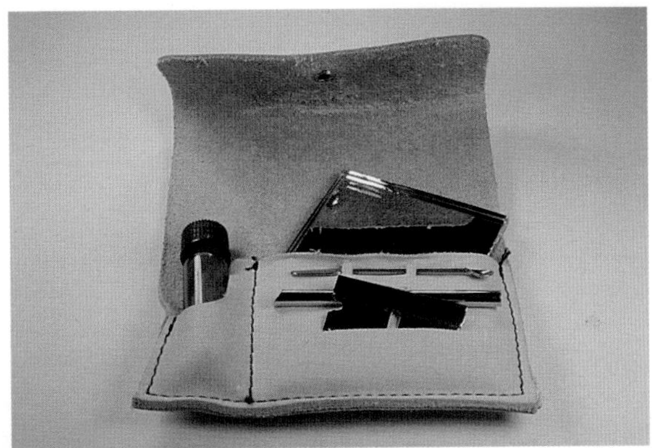

➤ A cocaine kit containing a glass vial for cocaine storage, a spoon for snorting, a mirror on which to place the cocaine, a razor blade to chop any larger pieces and form lines, and a snorting tube.

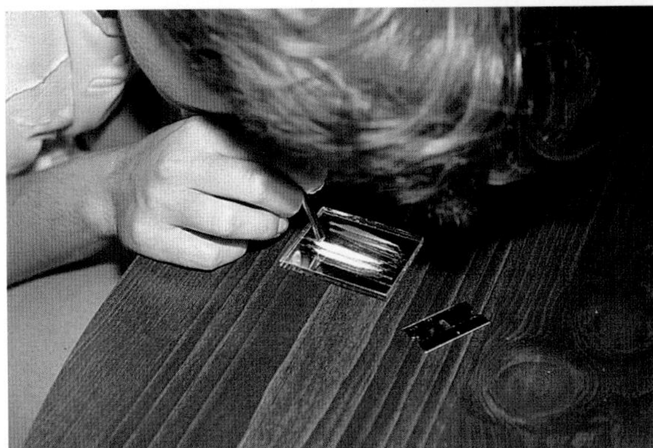

➤ Cocaine is usually ingested by placing it on a nonporous surface, chopping it into a fine powder with a razor blade, and forming it into thin lines which are snorted into the nose with a tubular device.

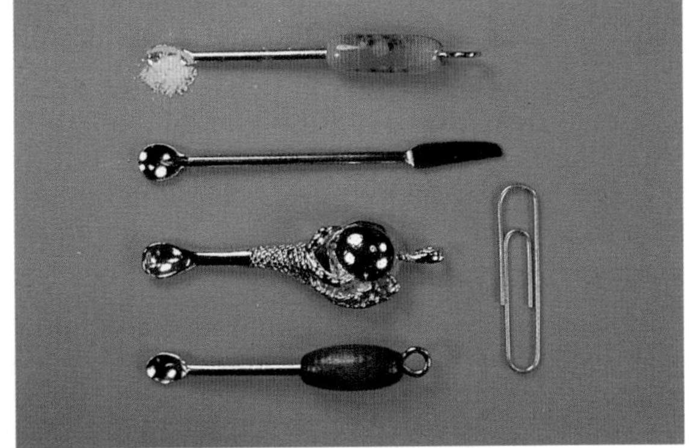

➤ A selection of coke spoons, which are used to hold a small amount of cocaine to the nostril for snorting. Coke spoons are sometimes made as jewelry, such as earrings and necklaces.

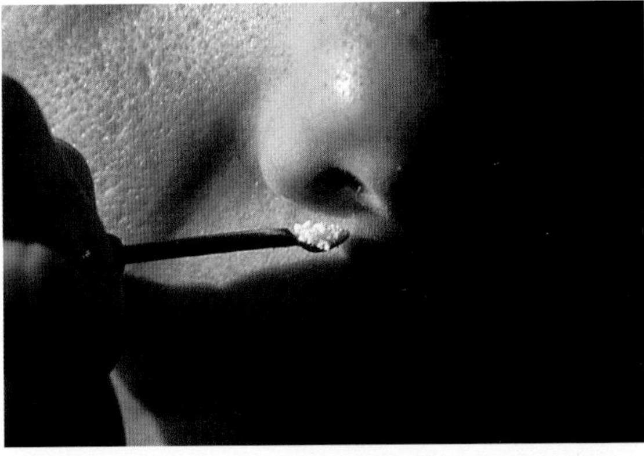

➤ Snorting cocaine with the use of a coke spoon. A typical coke spoon can hold approximately 1/25 of a gram. When snorted, the effects of cocaine are felt within three to five minutes, and the high usually lasts about sixty minutes.

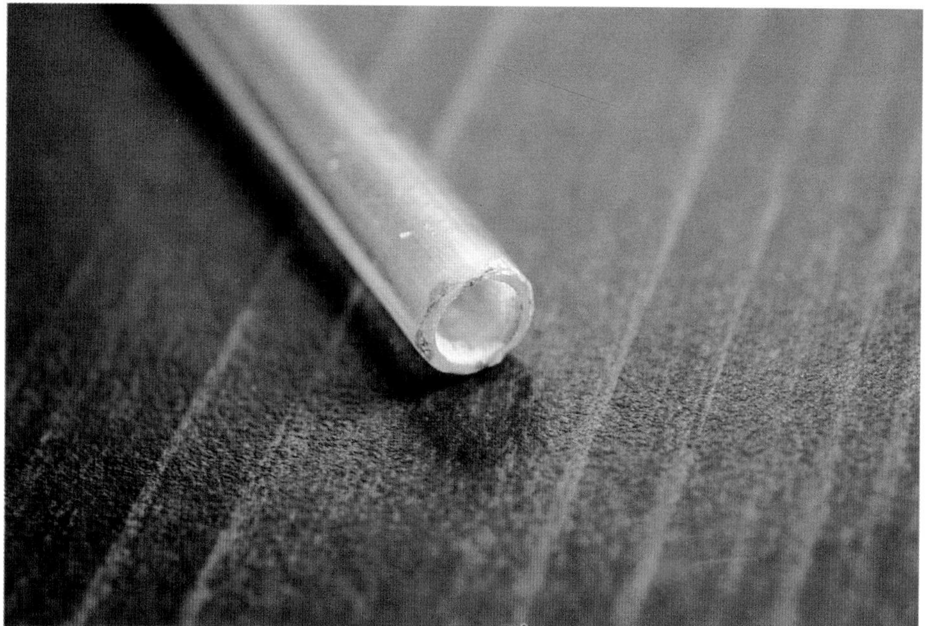

▲ An empty ball point pen casing used as a snorter for cocaine. A residual amount of cocaine can be seen on the inside of the tip.

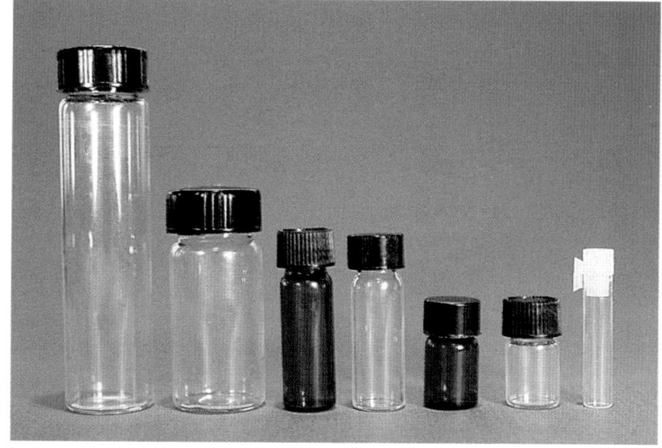

➤ An assortment of glass vials often used as containers for cocaine and other drugs. The capacity of these vials ranges from one gram to ten grams.

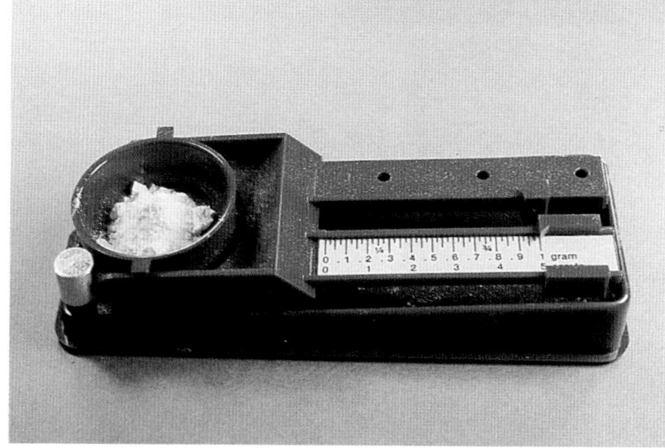

◄ Small gram scale, typical of the type often used to weigh cocaine. This particular scale measures amounts up to 4 grams, with an advertised accuracy to within 1/20 gram.

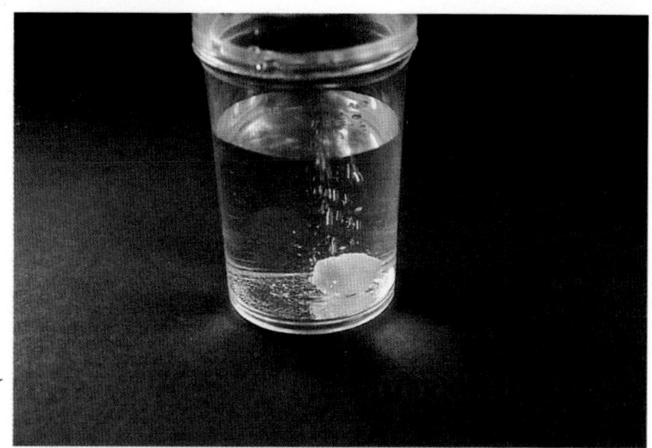

Many users of cocaine dissolve the drug in water so it can be injected. The high solubility of cocaine can be seen in this series of photographs: 1) A rock of cocaine about the size of a small marble is dropped into a container of tap water. Immediately upon contact with the water it begins to dissolve. 2) Within five seconds the rock has dissolved substantially. 3) Within fifteen seconds and with slight rotation of the container, virtually all of the cocaine has dissolved in the water. 4) About thirty seconds after placing the cocaine in the water, only a few insoluble particles remain. Like heroin addicts, users who inject cocaine normally use a spoon to prepare the cocaine. They may or may not heat the spoon from below with a flame as an aid to dissolve the drug. A small piece of cotton is usually placed in the liquid for use as a filter. The drug is drawn into a syringe through the cotton to remove any non-water soluble particles.

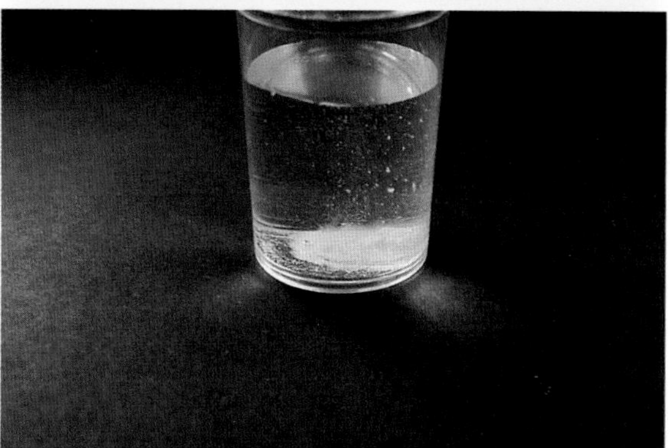

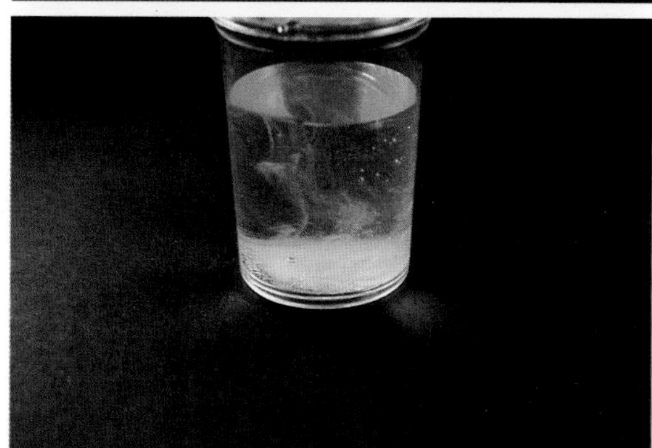

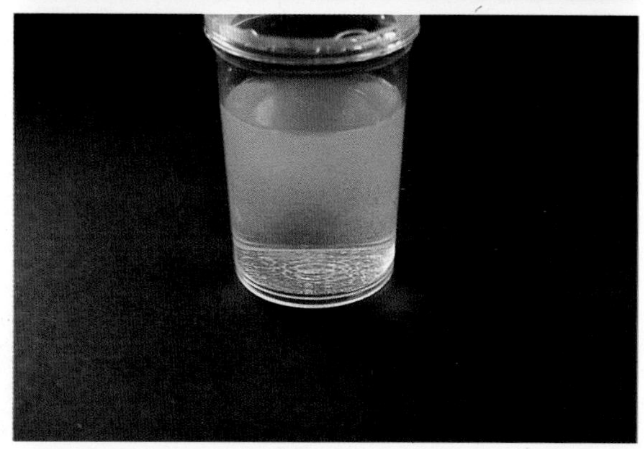

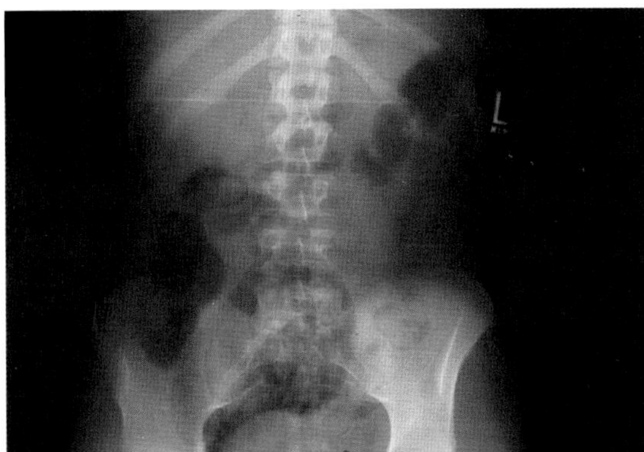

◄ An x-ray reveals packages swallowed by a body packer. Body packers may ingest several pounds of drugs packaged in condoms or balloons to avoid detection while smuggling. The packages are defecated once a safe haven has been reached.

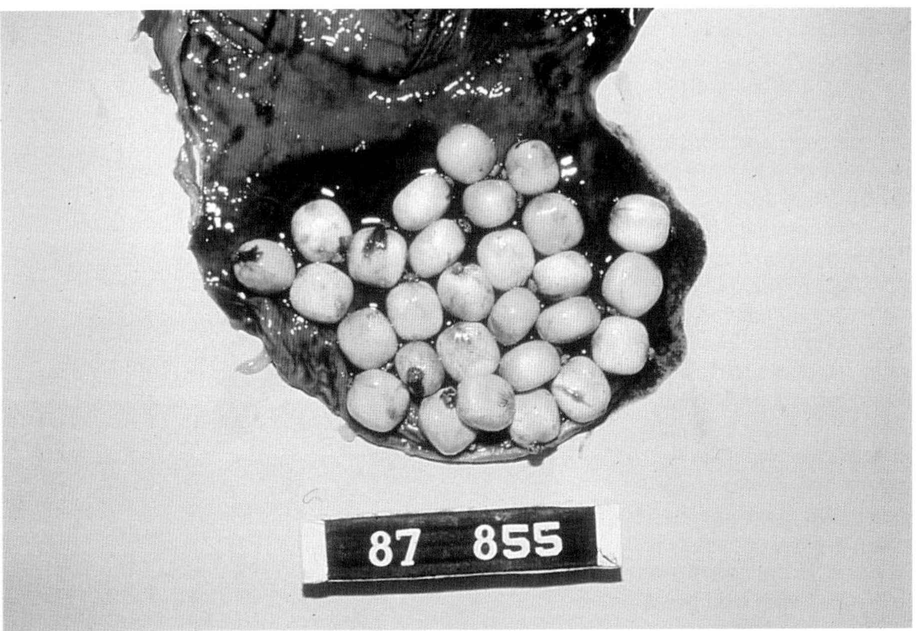

▲ The stomach contents of a body packer during an autopsy revealed about 1.5 pounds of cocaine packaged in condoms. In this case the cocaine permeated the package walls, causing a fatal overdose. It is reported that some South Americans receive the equivalent of a lifetime's worth of wages upon a single successful delivery of a large amount of cocaine.

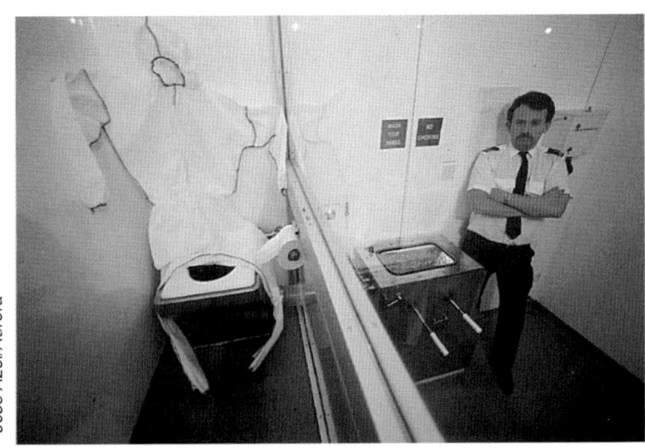

Jose Azel/Aurora

► Toilet used by British Customs to recover drug packages passed in fecal matter by body packers.

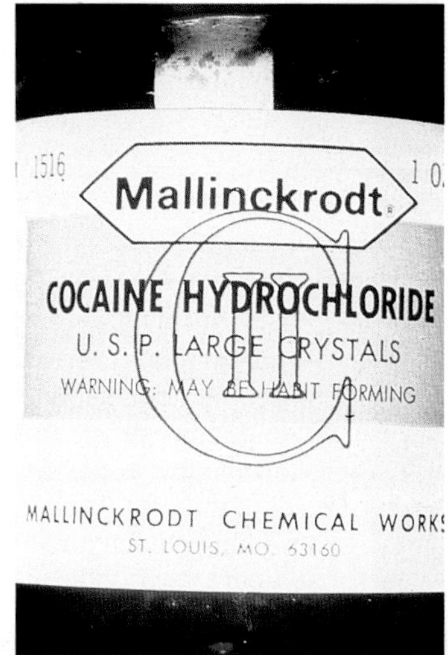

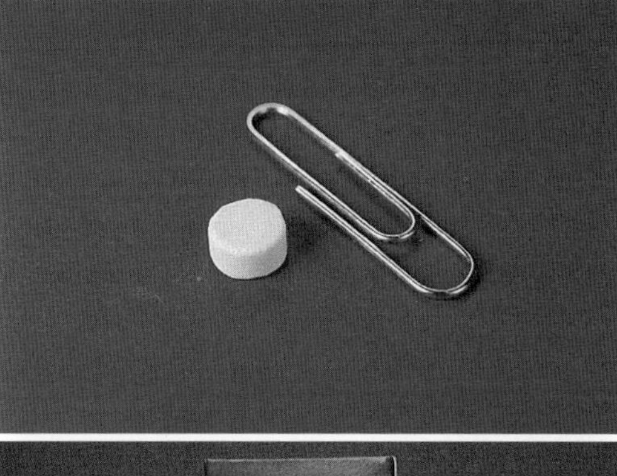

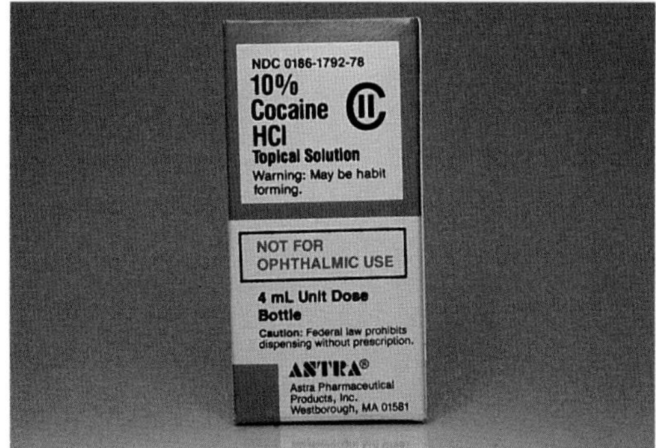

Cocaine has a legitimate medical use as a topical anesthetic, being used in over 200,000 ear, nose and throat surgeries in the United States every year. Anesthesia induced by cocaine lasts about two hours - twice as long as that of other topical anesthetics used for similar purposes. The cocaine is dissolved and diluted in distilled water, and is then applied with a cotton applicator or spray. Cocaine's vasoconstriction properties reduce bleeding as well. Cocaine is also used in a preparation called Brompton's Cocktail or Brompton's Mixture to control severe pain associated with cancer. This hospice or hospital prepared solution consists of cocaine mixed with a narcotic such as morphine or methadone in an alcoholic beverage. The stimulant effect of the cocaine counteracts the lethargy produced by the narcotic, allowing the patient to achieve some degree of physical and mental normalcy. The three forms of pharmaceutical cocaine are from top to bottom: cocaine powder and soluble tablet, both of which are dissolved in water, and a 10% liquid solution. Legally produced cocaine wholesales for about $60.00 per gram in the medical industry.

➤ One of the many cocaine-like products which have appeared on the retail market within the last several years. Pictured is an incense which has an appearance similar to that of cocaine.

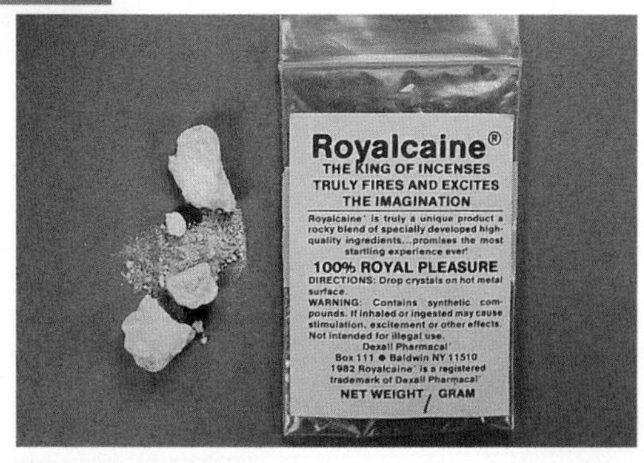

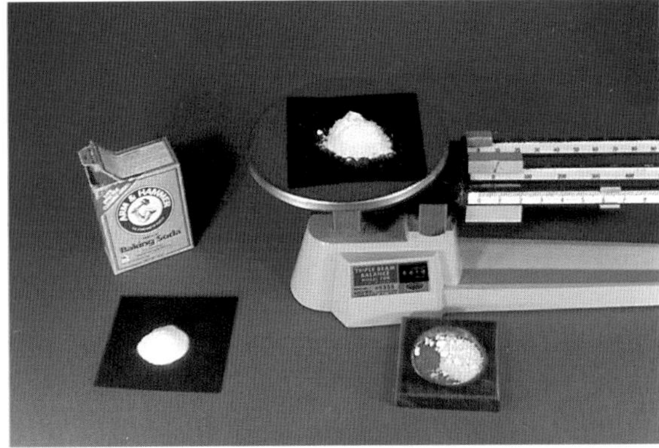

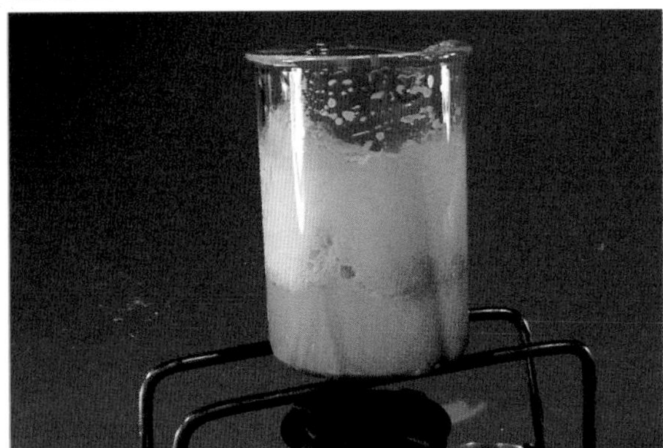

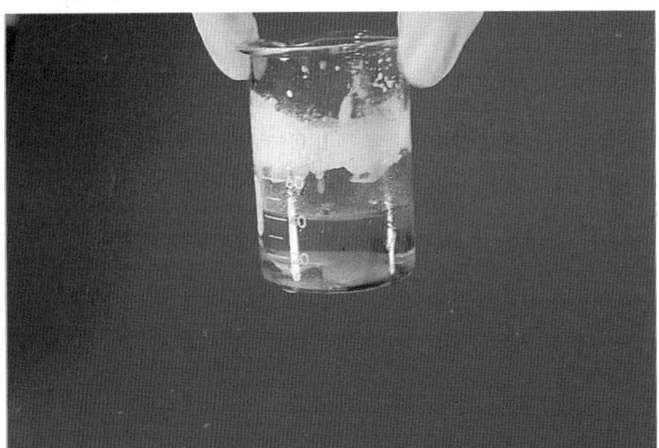

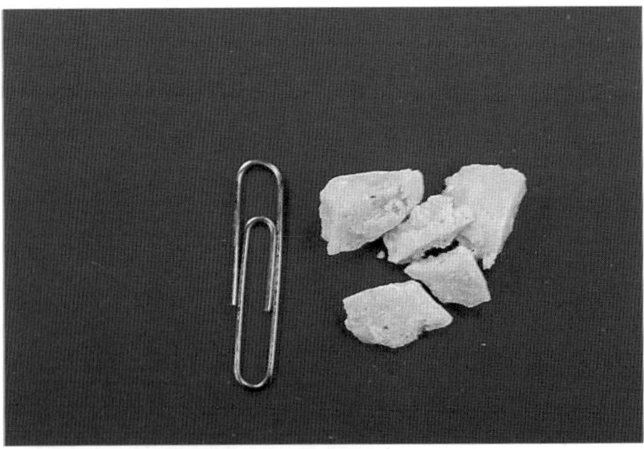

Although there are various street methods used to manufacture crack, the process shown in this series of photos is common. 1) Roughly equal amounts of cocaine and baking soda are thoroughly mixed together. 2) The mixture is placed in a container of water and then boiled to speed the chemical reaction. Some dealers place the mixture in a microwave oven rather than boiling it. 3) After boiling for a brief time, the container is removed and allowed to cool rapidly. The container may be placed in a refrigerator or a bowl of ice water. In this photo the crack almost immediately begins to coalesce into a solid mass at the bottom of the beaker. 4) The crack is removed from the beaker and dried. Crack is not a purified form of cocaine, as it contains virtually all of the impurities in the cocaine used in the preparation. No longer soluble in water, the crack must be smoked to be ingested. Snorting granulated pieces of crack would result in little more than the pieces lodging in the nose or rolling down the back of the throat.

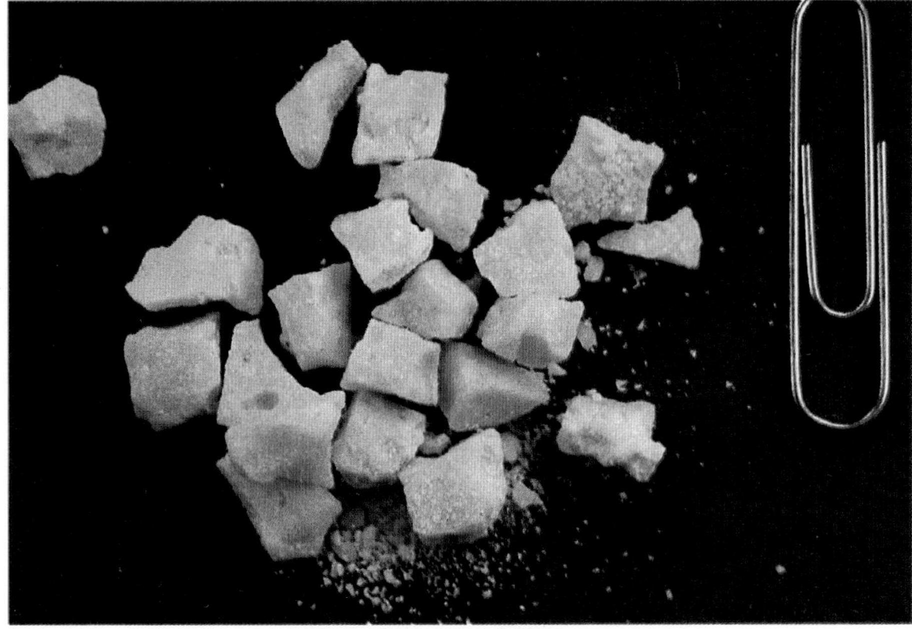

▲ Crack is almost always seen as an off-white or yellowish-white solid. It has often been described as looking like chunks of soap or plaster. Crack has reportedly been so named because of the crackling sound it makes when smoked.

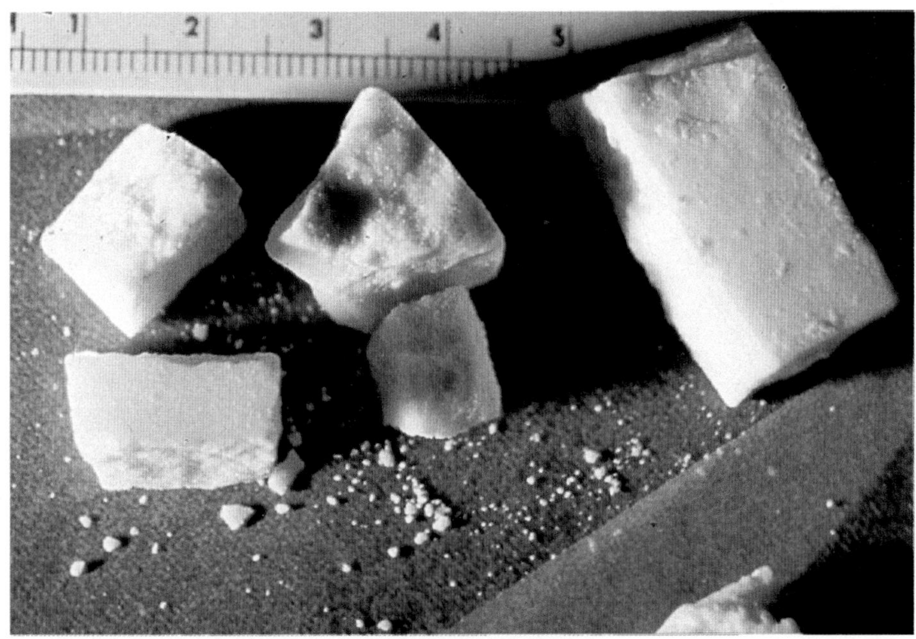

▲ The unusual appearance of the crack pictured above is the result of the production process. The mixture was placed in a cake pan and heated in a microwave oven for the chemical reaction to take place, and the resulting rectangular slab was then broken into small rocks.

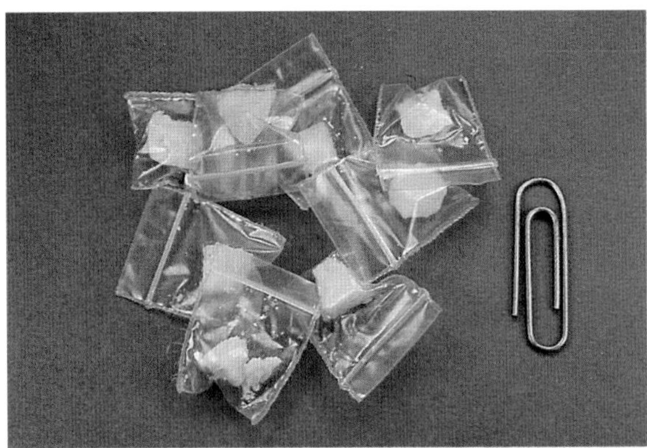

➤ Rock individually packaged in small ziplock plastic bags.

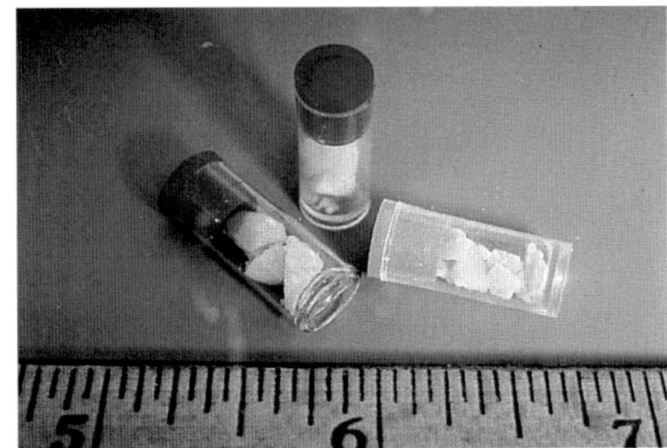

➤ Crack packaged in small vials. In most areas, plastic bags are a more popular packaging method in lieu of the small vials.

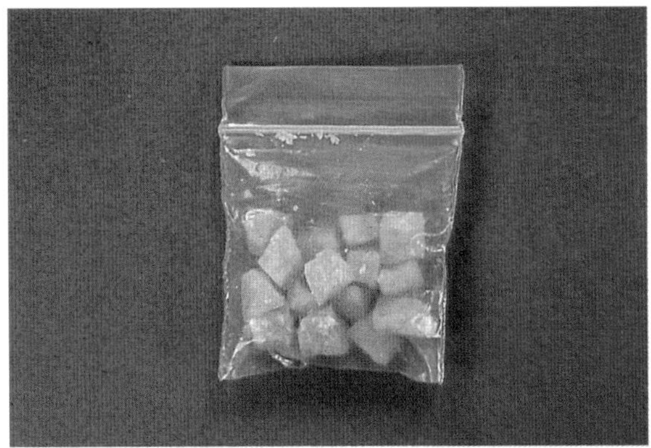

➤ A larger ziplock plastic bag containing several rocks.

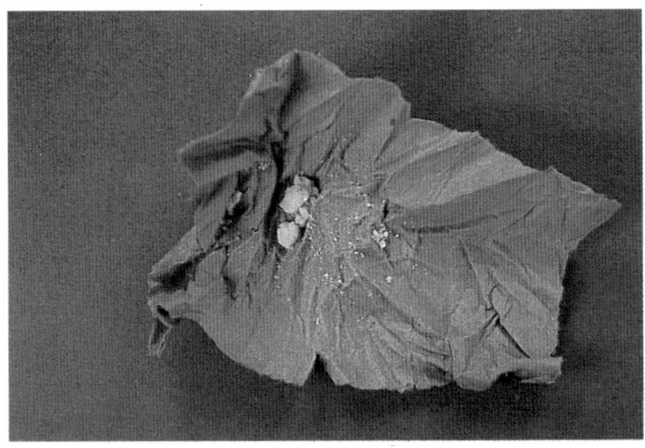

➤ Another method of packaging crack - a section of a paper lunch bag.

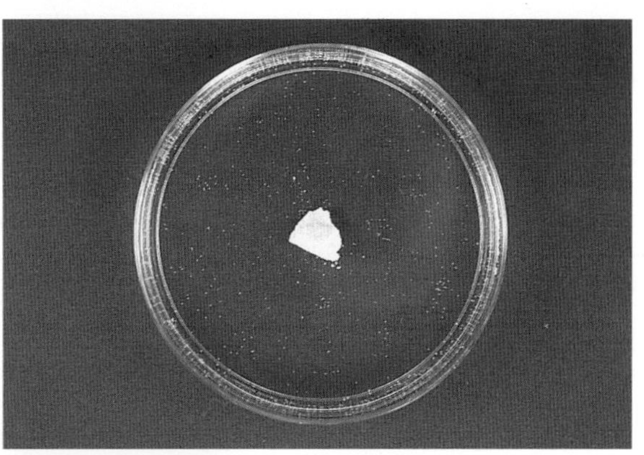

➤ Unlike the solubility of cocaine hydrochloride shown in a prior photo sequence, crack is not easily dissolved by water. This rock was placed in a container of water for thirty minutes with no dissolving action. For this reason crack cannot be snorted into the nostril and must be smoked for ingestion.

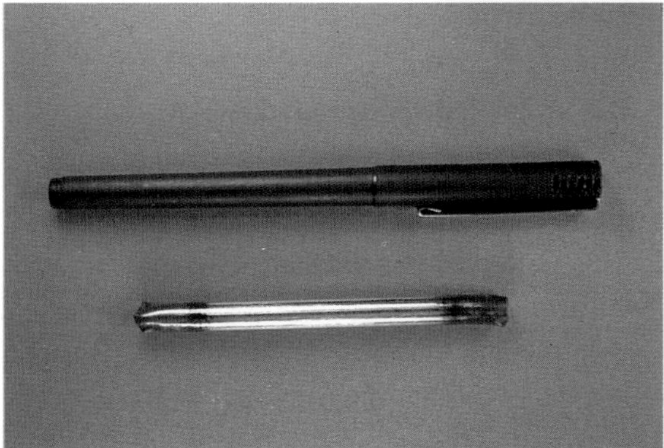

◄ With stringent paraphernalia laws in effect around the country, professionally made pipes are difficult to find. As a result, many users employ makeshift items to use drugs. In this case part of a hollow radio antenna is used as a crack pipe. A small amount of steel wool was placed in one end to hold the drug.

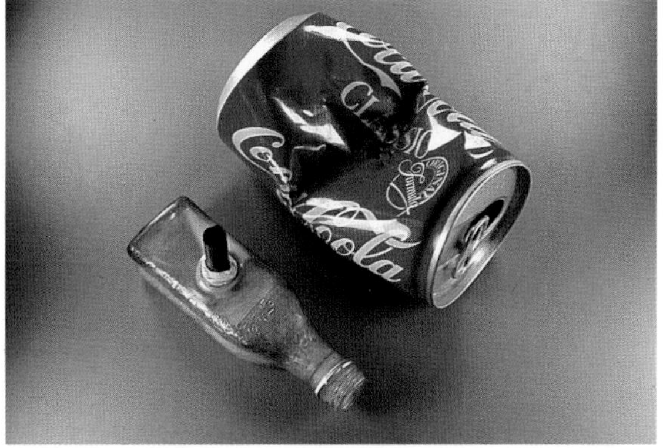

➤ Two makeshift pipes used to smoke crack. One is a small liquor bottle with a tubular piece of metal placed in one side. Steel wool was placed in the tip to hold the drug. The aluminum can with holes punched in one side to hold the drug is a very common method of smoking crack. The drug is heated and the vapors inhaled through the top of the can.

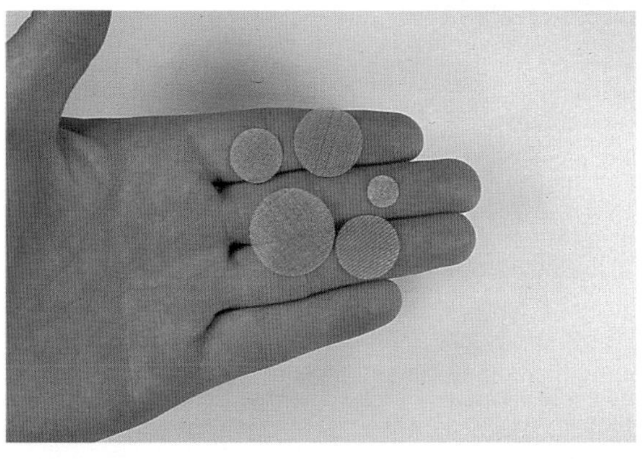

◄ Stainless steel screens, rather than brass screens, are often used in crack pipes because they have a finer mesh to hold the drug and withstand higher temperatures. Window screen and steel wool are also used to hold crack in pipes.

➤ Some users occasionally smoke small pieces of crack with marijuana rolled in a joint.

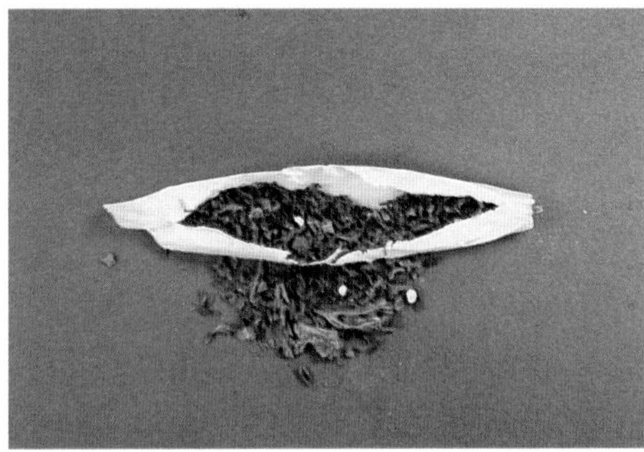

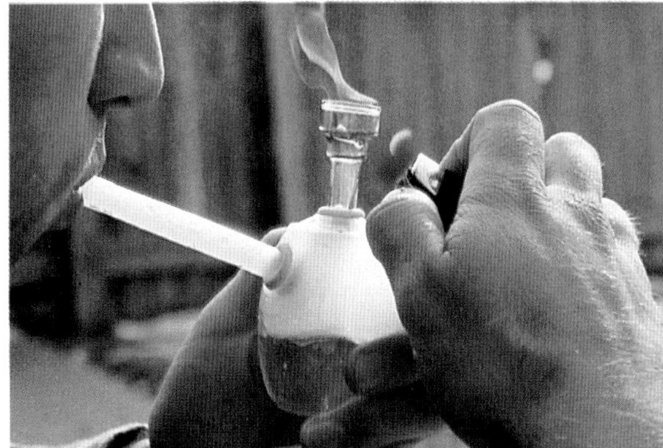

➤ Crack can be smoked in a glass pipe, in an empty aluminum can, or by any similar means where heat can be indirectly applied to vaporize the drug. The resulting fumes are inhaled, with effects appearing almost immediately. In this photo a glass water pipe is being used to cool the hot vapor as it is inhaled.

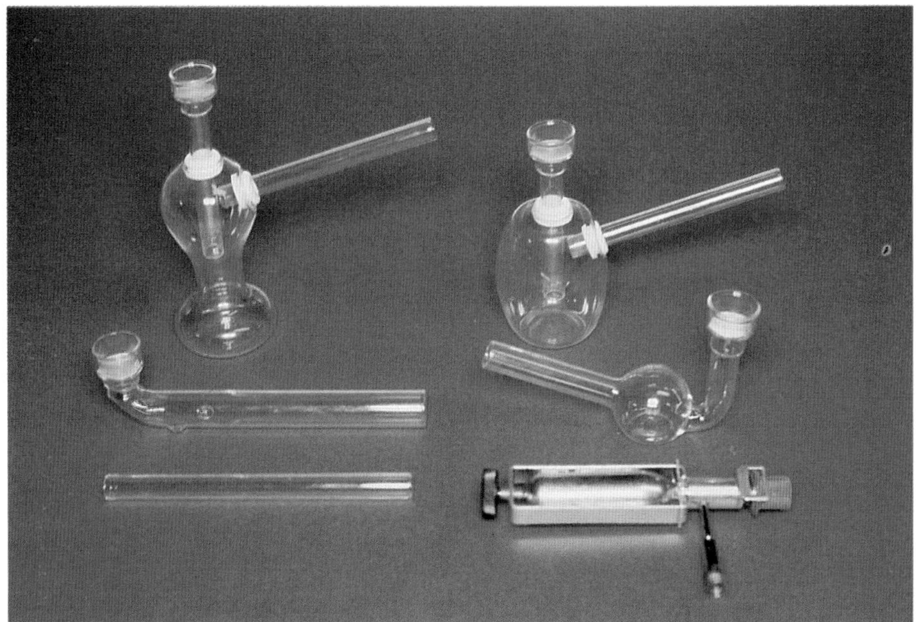

▲ An assortment of glass pipes used for smoking crack. Small butane torches, like the one pictured in the lower right hand corner are often used to heat the side of the pipe bowl to vaporize the drug. Some pipes may contain a water chamber through which the vapor passes and cools as it is inhaled.

➤ MDMA is also known as XTC, Ecstasy, Adam and Essence, and has a chemical name of 3,4-methylenedioxy-N-methylamphetamine. It is generally a white powder as shown but sometimes has a red or brownish tint or specks. It is routinely sold in gelatin capsules but is also pressed into tablets. Price for one dose ranges from $10.00 to $30.00.

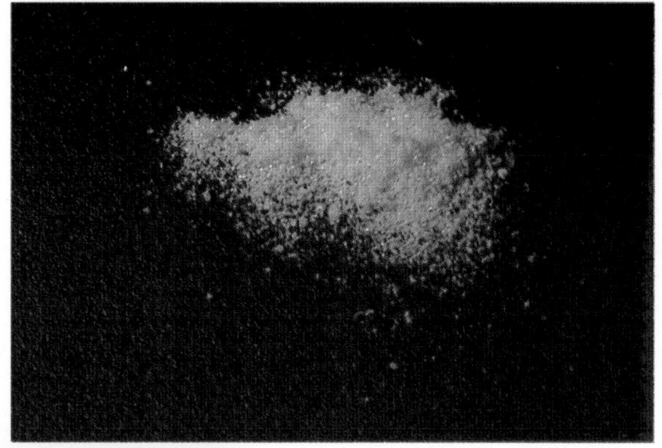

Bob Harris

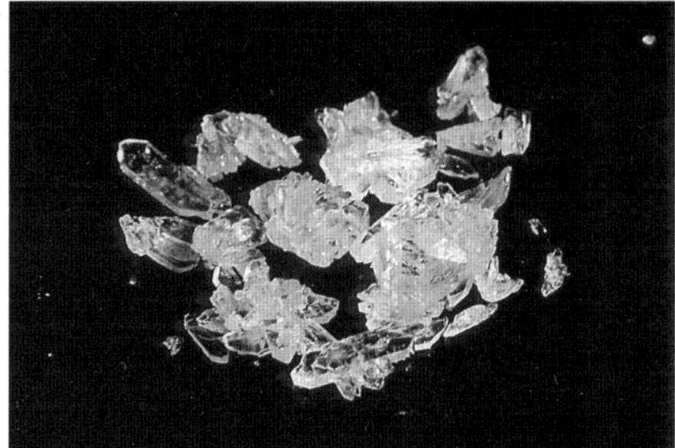

Jeremy Bigwood

➤ Large MDMA crystals. MDMA was developed in the earlier part of this century by a German pharmaceutical company, but it remained largely obscure until the early 1970s when the drug was reportedly first used by the counter culture. MDMA became a Schedule I drug in 1984.

➤ DMT, or N,N-dimethyl-tryptamine is a short duration hallucinogen. Its effects generally last about 1/2 hour. It occurs naturally in several West Indian and South American plants, but its most common form is synthetic. It is usually snorted or combined with vegetable matter and smoked. It is rarely injected. The powder form is usually tan or brown in color.

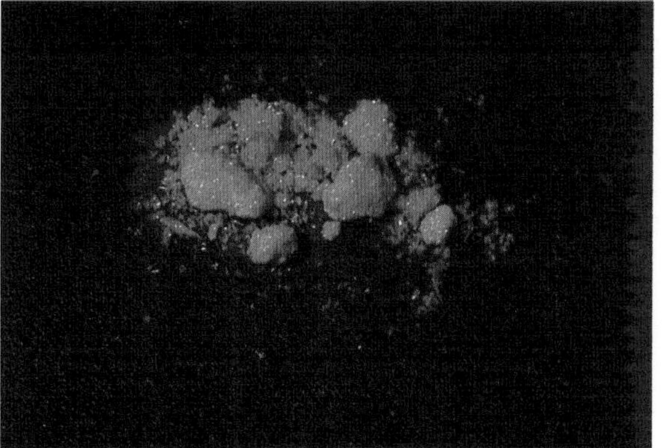

Bob Harris

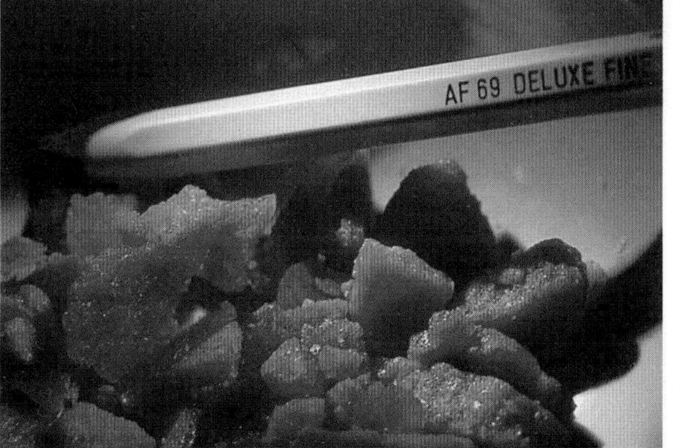

Paul Kroeger

➤ A crudely synthesized batch of DMT.

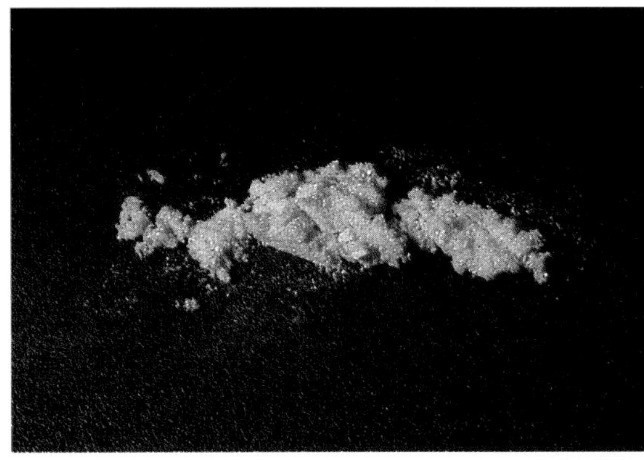

➤ Crystals of 2,5-dimethoxy-4-methyl-amphetamine, also known as DOM or STP. STP was introduced to the drug culture in 1967 and immediately developed a reputation as being an almost overpowering hallucinogen. The effects have been reported to last up to twenty-four hours.

Bob Harris

➤ DOB, or 2,5-dimethoxy-4-bromoamphetamine is one of the many amphetamine-like synthetic drugs available on the street. DOB is reportedly four hundred times more potent than mescaline. As with other drugs of this type, it is usually a white or off-white powder which may be tableted or encapsulated.

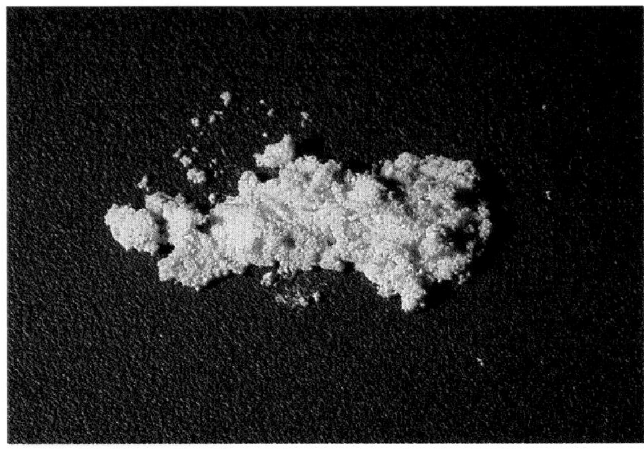

Bob Harris

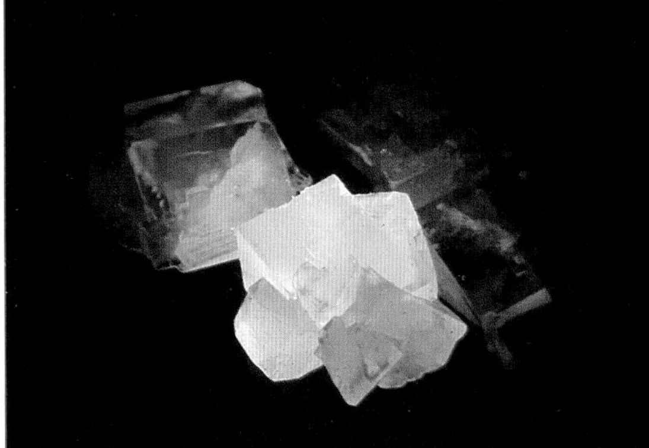

➤ MDA crystals. MDA, or 3,4-methylenedioxy-amphetamine, was first synthesized in the early part of this century and became a Schedule I drug in 1970. Like other drugs of this type, it can produce both hallucinogenic and stimulant effects.

Jeremy Bigwood

➤ Illicitly produced MDA tablets.

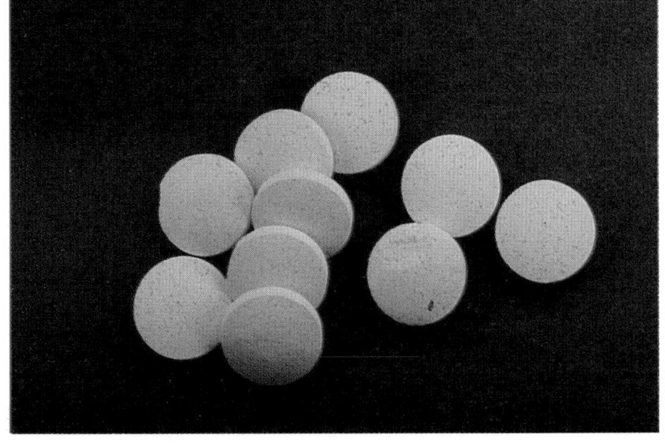

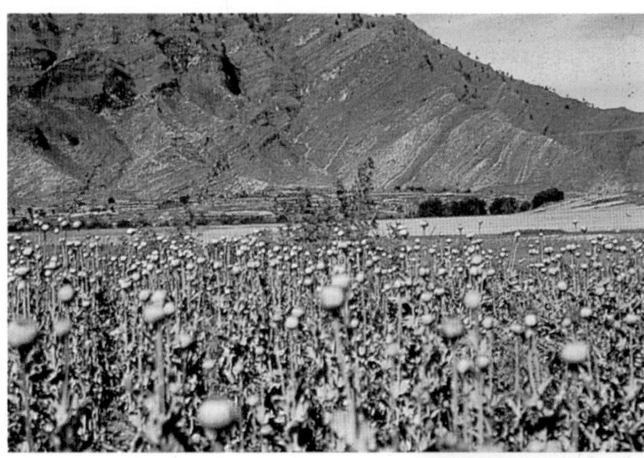

➤ Cultivated field of opium poppies. Most illicit opium is produced in two areas known as the Golden Triangle (Burma, Laos, and Thailand) and the Golden Crescent (Afghanistan, Pakistan, and Iran). Mexico and Colombia also are producing increasing amounts of illicit opium.

➤ Mature opium poppy pods prior to being incised. The poppy plant matures in about ninety days and grows to a height of about four feet. At maturity, the flower petals fall, exposing the green seed pod, which varies in size from 1 to 3 inches.

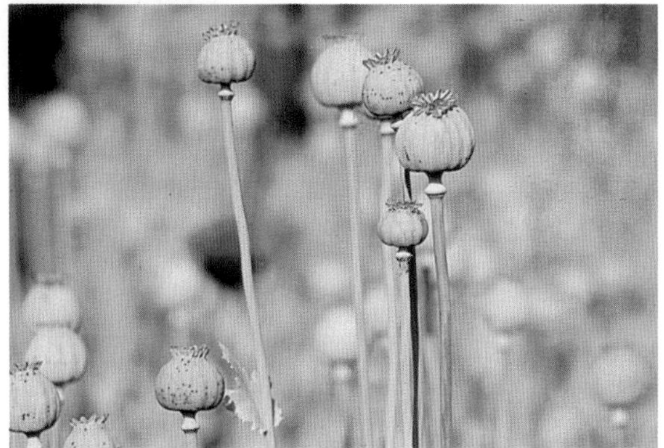

Stan Czolowski

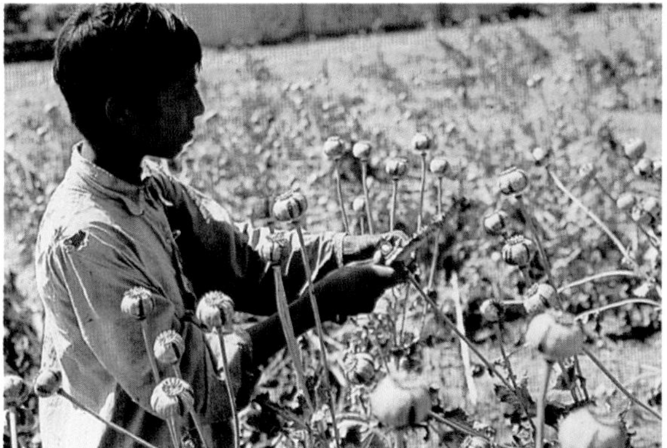

➤ A field worker scraping opium from incised pods. Most illicit opium producers are small farmers who work only a few acres of the labor-intensive crop, cutting and scraping the poppy by hand. Once collected, the opium is sold to a processor who extracts the morphine.

➤ Opium poppy seed of different varieties and maturation. Most mature opium seeds are black or dark gray in color. A single poppy pod may contain over 1,000 seeds.

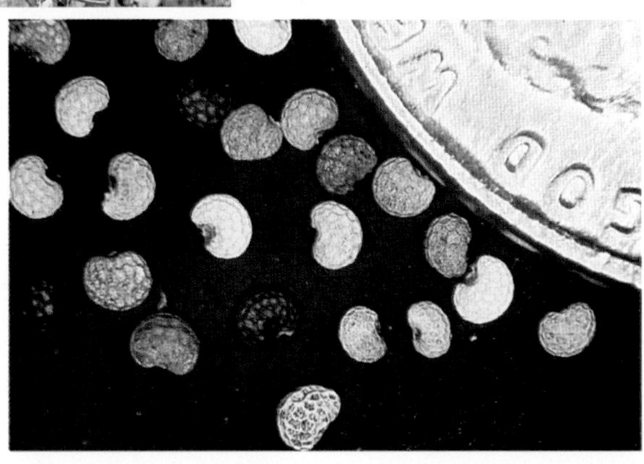

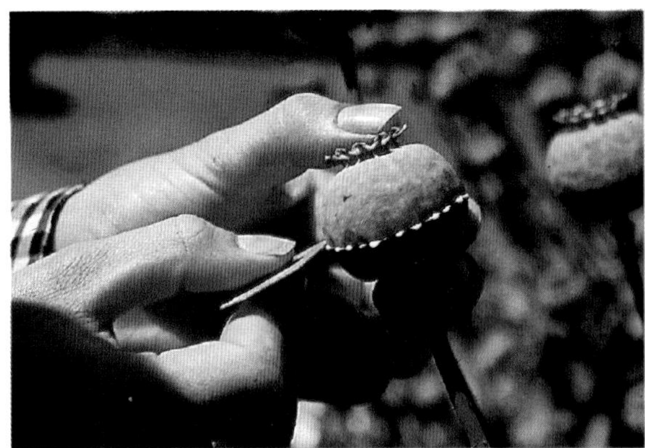

Stan Czolowski

➤ Incising the seed pod so the opium will ooze out and gather on the surface. The opium is initially white in color, but within 24 hours it dries and turns dark brown. Incisions may be either vertical or horizontal, depending on the particular local harvesting practices.

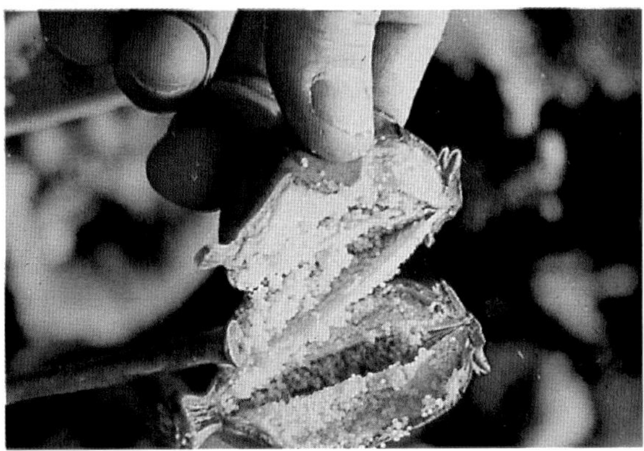

➤ A bisected opium poppy. The milky opium is concentrated in an outer layer of the capsule, very near the surface. It is not known why the poppy produces a potent substance like opium, but it is speculated that it may be a defense against animals and insects.

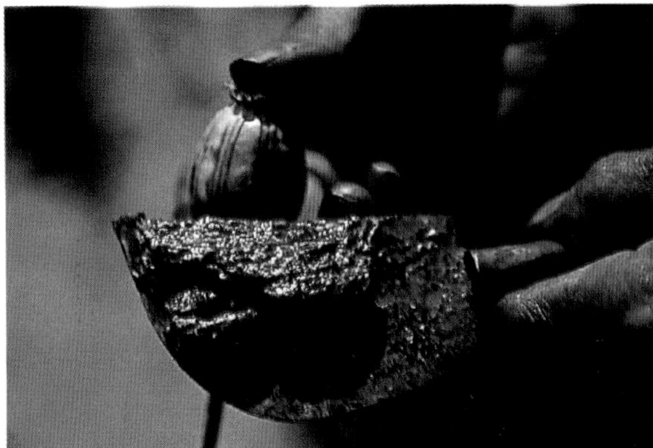

Steve Raymer/National Geographic

➤ A metal tool used to collect the opium from the pod. It takes about 1,000 poppies to produce 1 pound of opium.

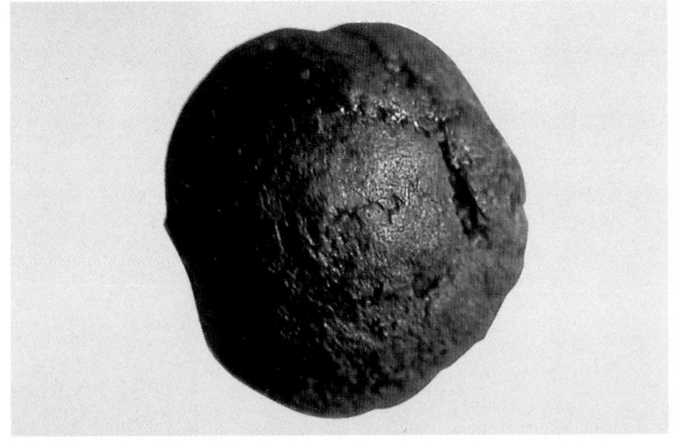

➤ Ball of opium. Heroin is produced by chemically extracting morphine from opium and then treating the morphine with acetic anhydride or acetic chloride and hydrochloric acid. Morphine is converted to heroin at a 1:1 ratio.

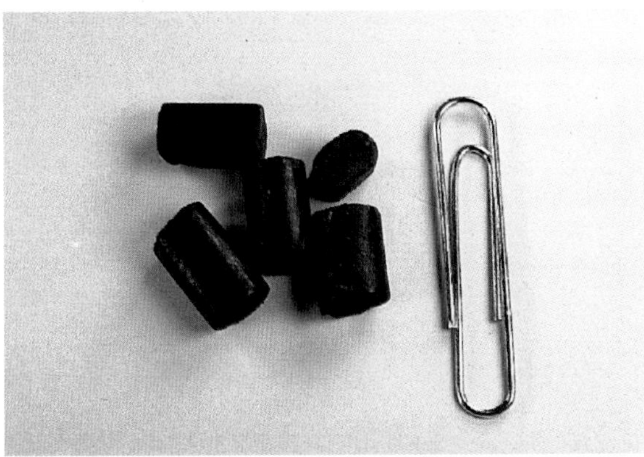

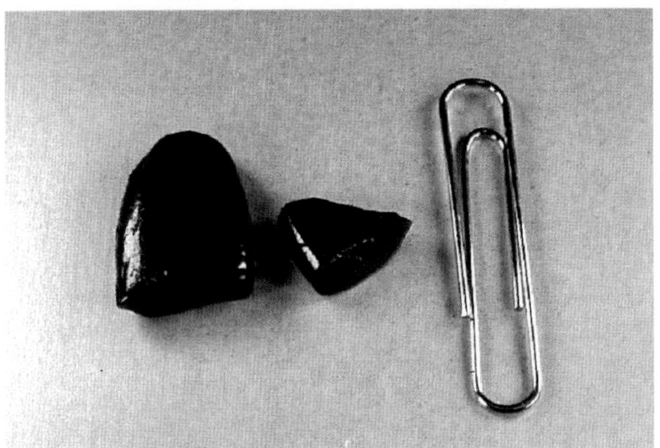

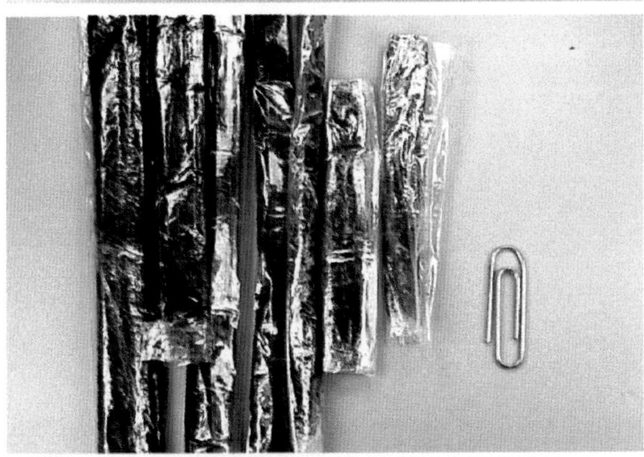

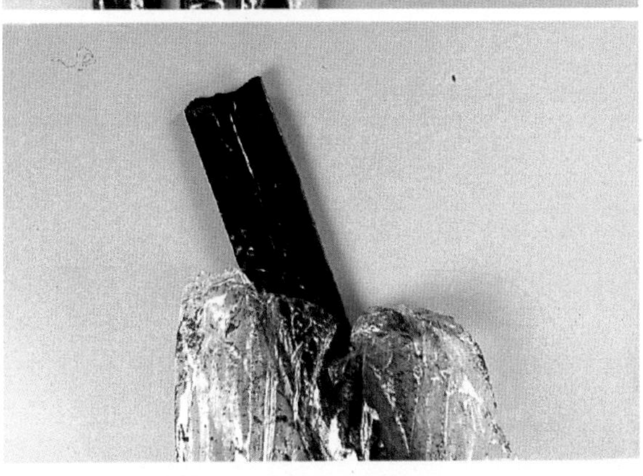

Various appearances of seized illicit opium. Although opium use is not as common as heroin, it does have a strong following among Asian groups. Opium can be placed on a sheet of aluminum foil and heated from below with an open flame, and the vapors inhaled (chasing the dragon), or it can be smoked in a pipe. Opium which is smoked is often called "hop". Opium is also added to water or alcoholic beverages and consumed orally. Injecting opium is generally more dangerous than injecting other drugs because it does not dissolve well in water and is a crude product which may contain many contaminants. As with other opiate drugs, being under the influence of opium causes a relaxed state often called the "nod", which refers to the head nodding down to the chest.

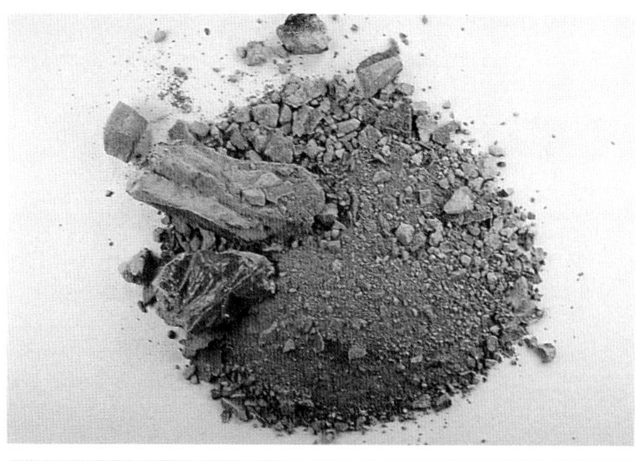

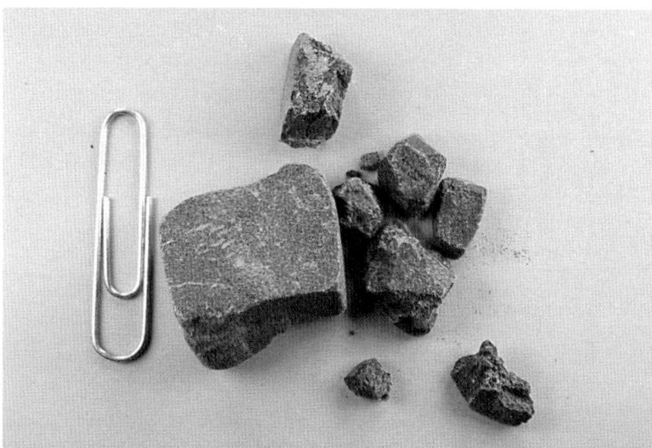

➤ As opium ages and dries, it turns from sticky and dark brown or black to hard and light brown. Pictured are two examples of aged opium.

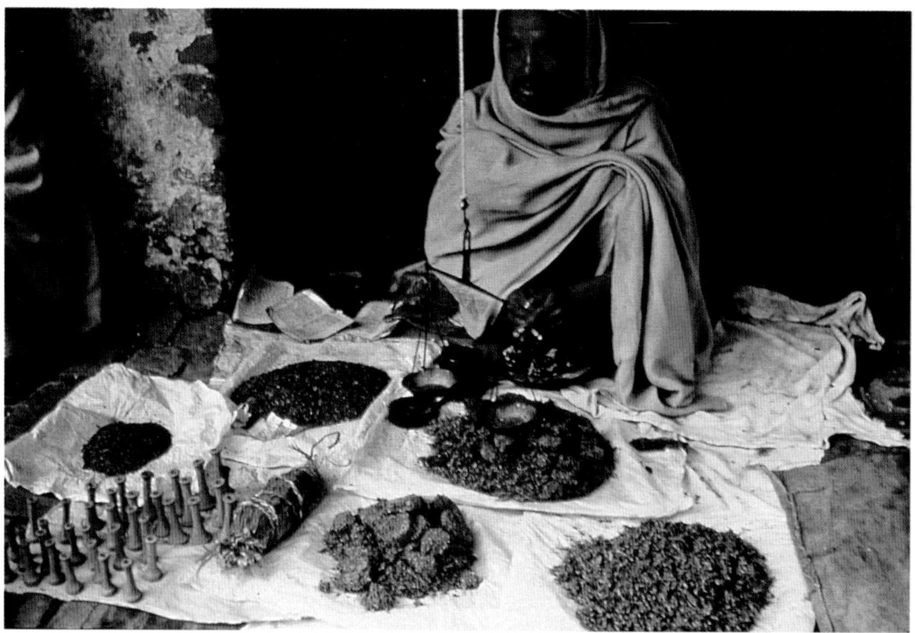

▲ An open-air market in Southwest Asia selling opium and hash. The objects in the bottom left corner of the photo are pipes called "chillums", used to smoke the drugs. Chillums are popular in parts of Europe, Asia, and Africa.

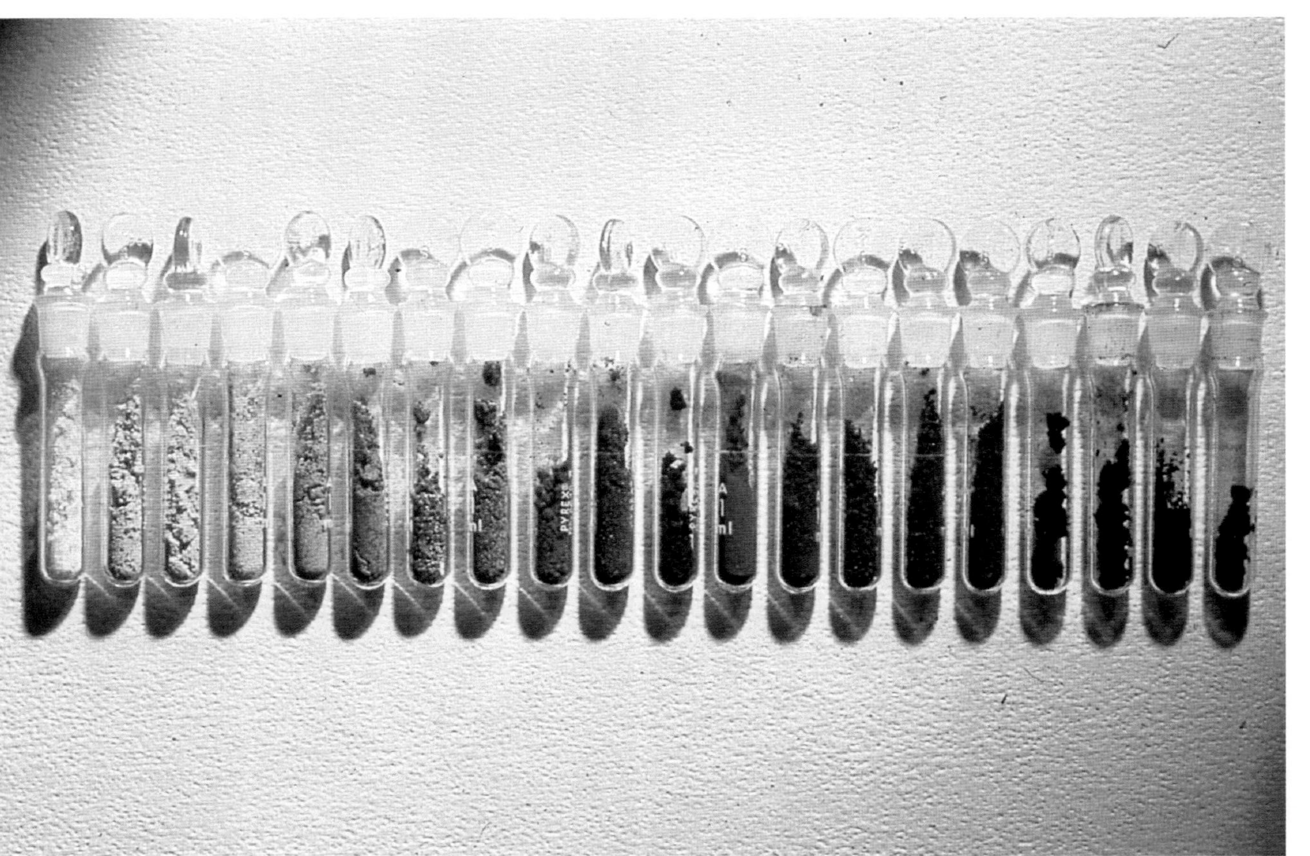

Numerous color and texture variations of heroin, ranging from China white, the most refined, to crude Mexican black tar.

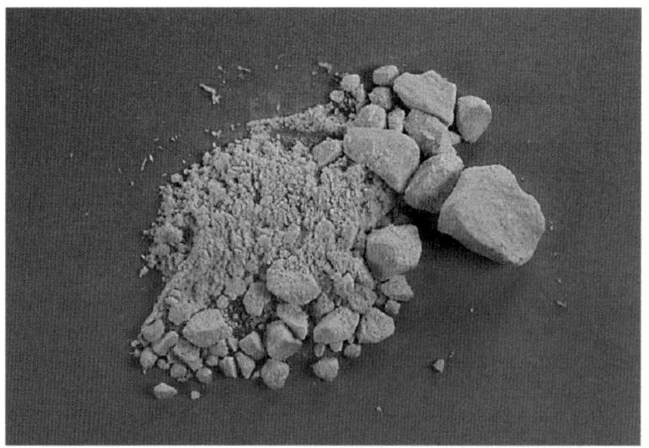

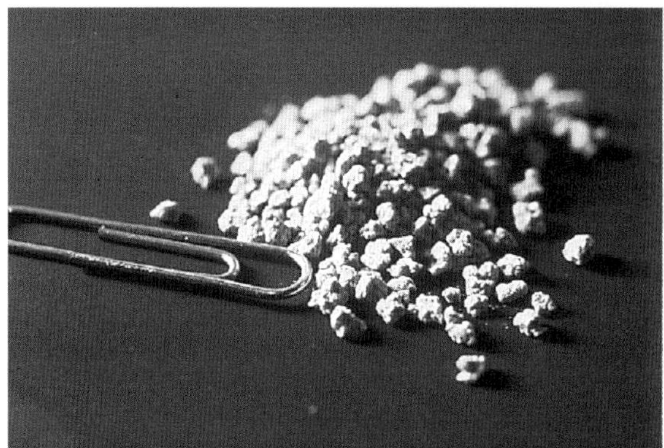

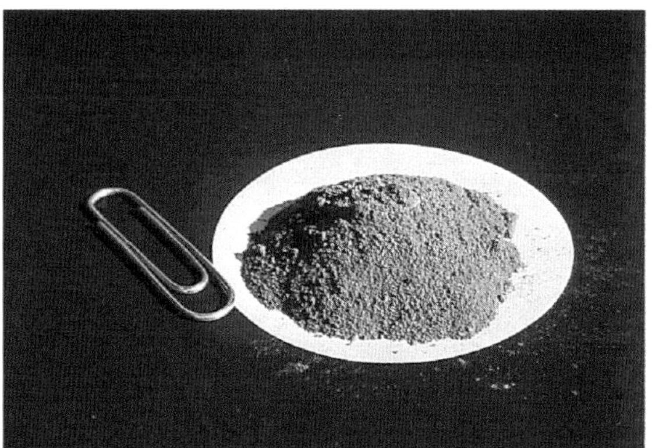

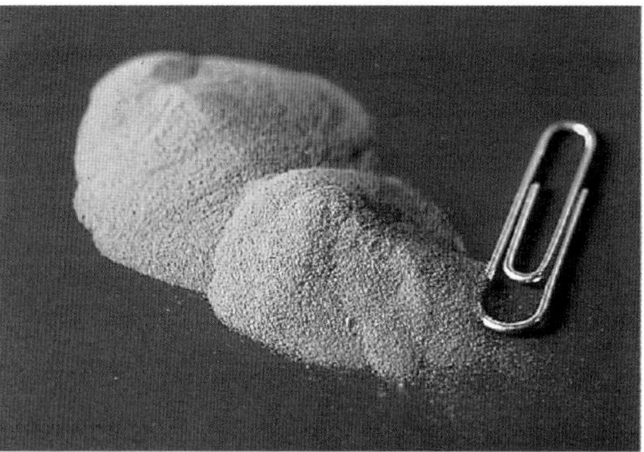

The color and texture of heroin vary widely based on the manufacturing process and the cuts or diluents added. In some cases, heroin has been so heavily cut that the heroin contained in the sample has little to do with the samples overall odor, texture, color, etc. Pictured are four samples of heroin, with color ranging from white to off-white to brown and texture ranging from a fine powder to coarse and granular.

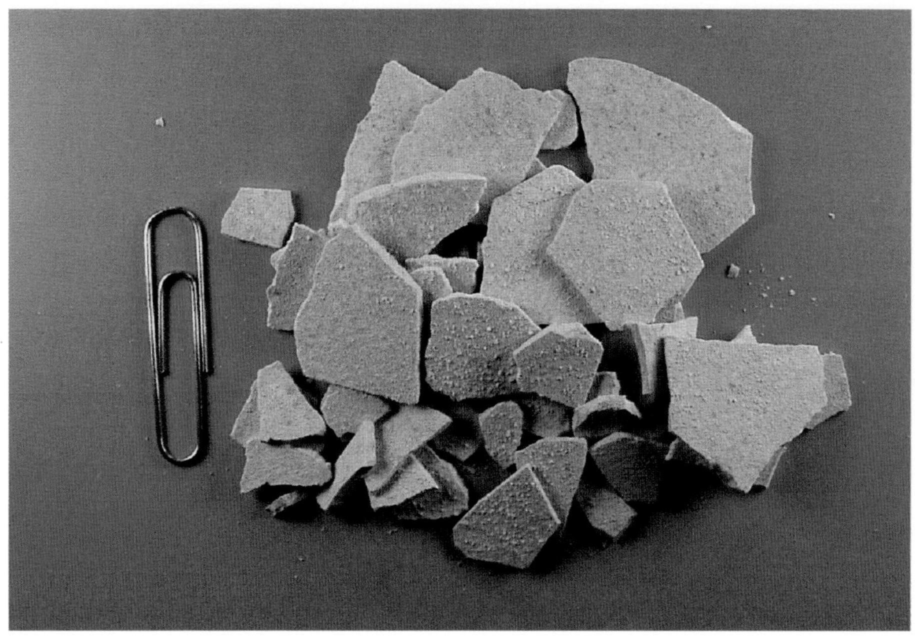

▲ Several grams of flake China white heroin. A variation in the manufacturing process results in a solid cake but still a refined heroin product. As with powdered heroin, the flake can be granulated and then mixed with water and injected, snorted, smoked, or taken orally.

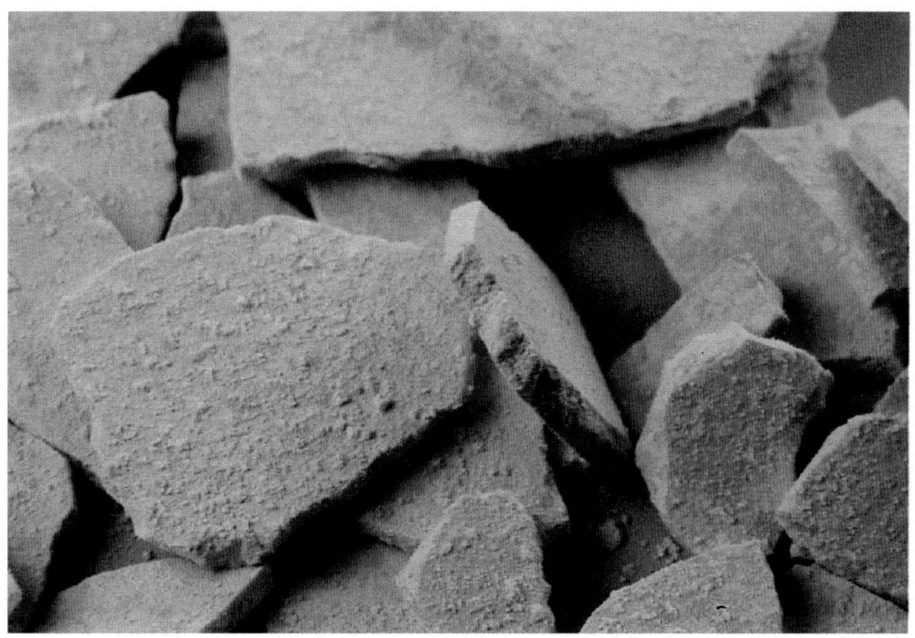

▲ Close-up of the above photo.

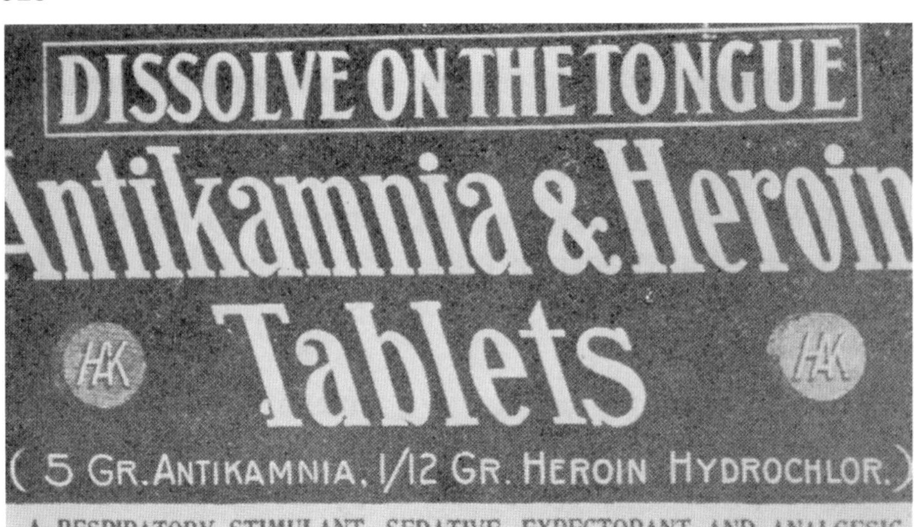

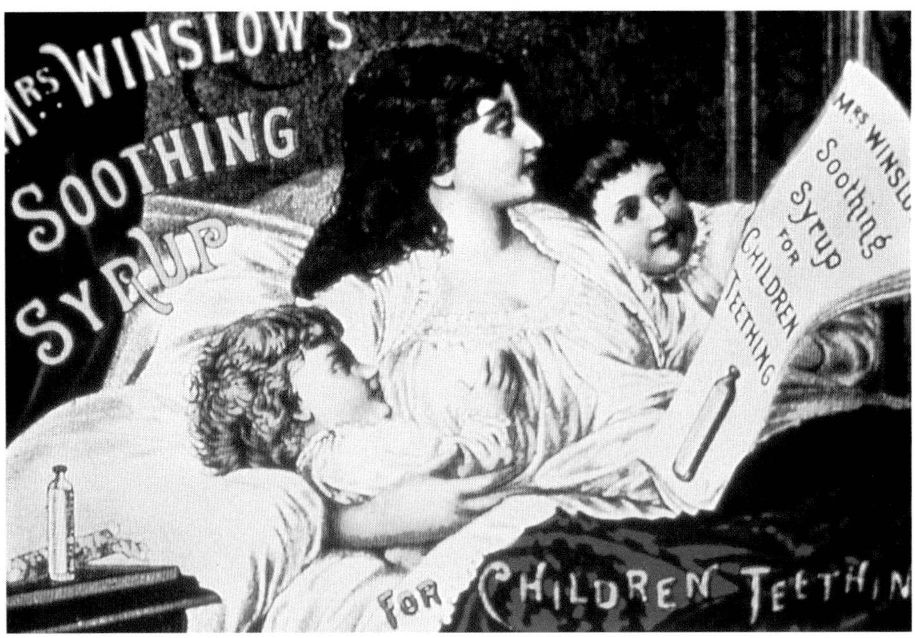

▲ Turn-of-the-century advertisements for medications containing heroin. In 1806 morphine was isolated from opium, and in 1874 heroin was synthesized from morphine. During the early 1900s, heroin was a common drug included in many over-the-counter medications. These medications included those to treat pain, diarrhea, insomnia, etc. Although illegal for any application in the United States since 1956, heroin is still used medically in many countries as a very effective but highly addictive treatment for pain.

➤ An assortment of balloons containing about 1/10 gram of heroin each. The heroin is funneled into the balloon, tied in a knot, and then the top is wrapped back over the bottom where the drug is held for extra protection. Balloons are often carried in the mouth, and if an arrest seems likely, they can be swallowed and later retrieved from the feces.

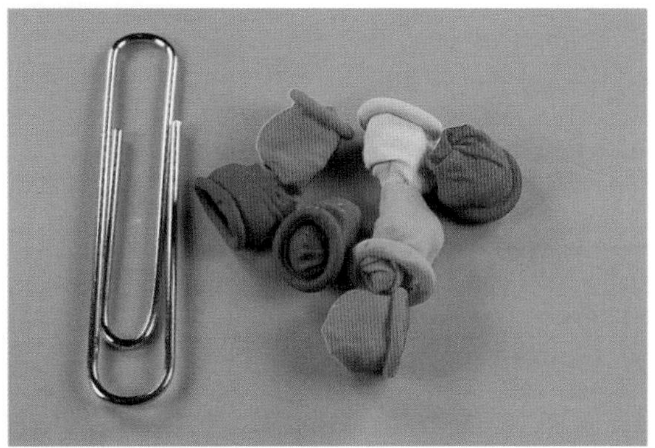

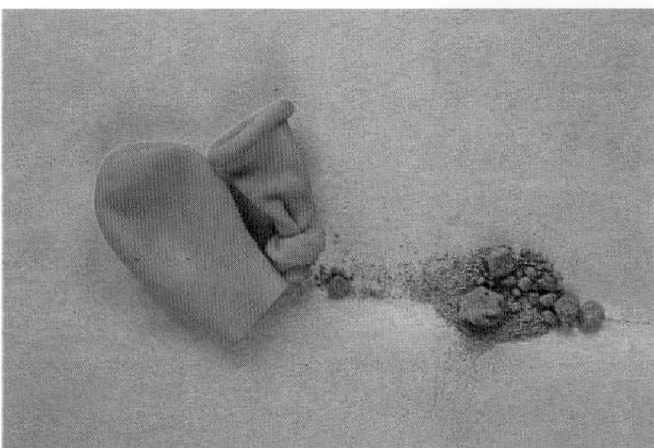

➤ A balloon opened to show the 1/10 gram of Mexican brown heroin it contained, valued at about $20.00. A heavy user of heroin may ingest the drug every four hours, using a total of about 1 gram each day.

➤ A folded sheet of aluminum foil used to hold a small amount of heroin, referred to in many areas as a "deck".

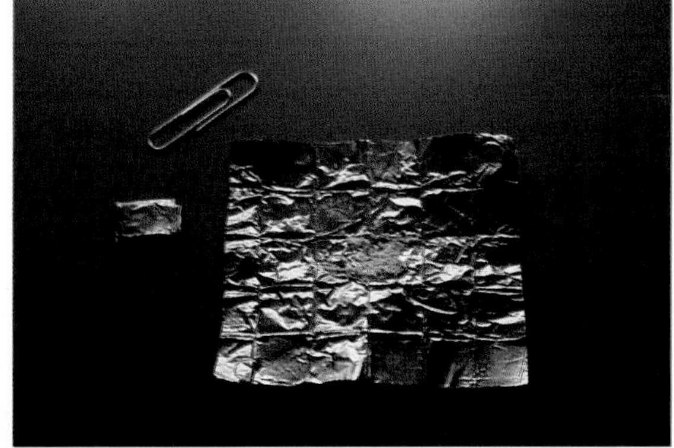

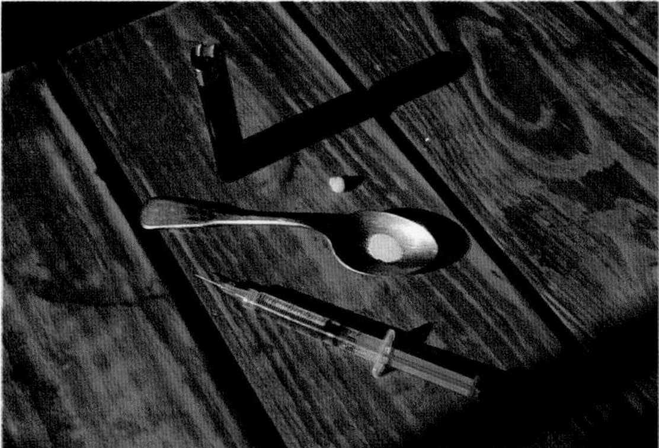

➤ Paraphernalia for injecting heroin. A spoon and lighter for cooking, a small piece of cotton for filtering the liquid solution, and a syringe for injection.

➤ Preparing heroin for injection into a vein first involves placing the drug in a spoon or other suitable metal container. An amount of water premeasured in the syringe is then added to the spoon to dissolve the heroin.

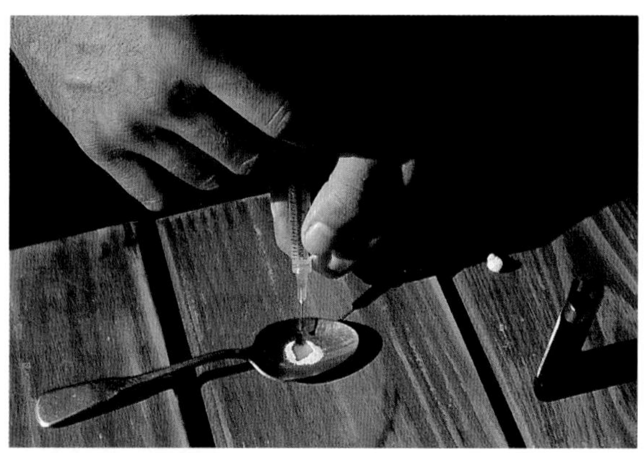

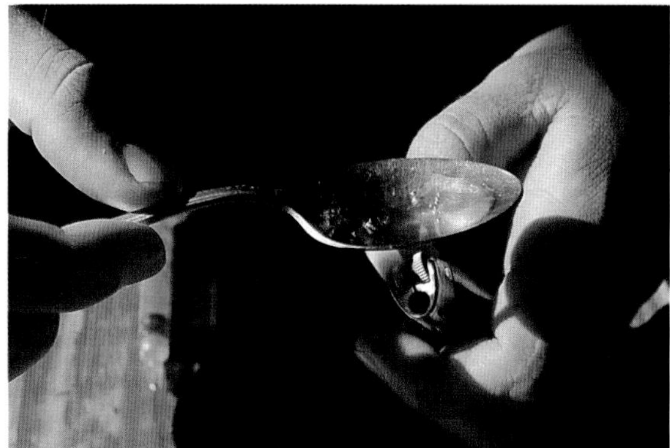

◄ The spoon is briefly held over an open flame, and the liquid is brought to a boil to help dissolve, or "cook" the heroin. Some users may add a small amount of lemon or lime juice to acidify the mixture, which aids in dissolving the heroin more readily.

➤ Because the heroin may contain insoluble cuts and impurities, most users filter the heroin as it is being drawn into the syringe. This is done by placing a small amount of cotton or a cigarette filter in the solution and filling the syringe by drawing the liquid through the cotton.

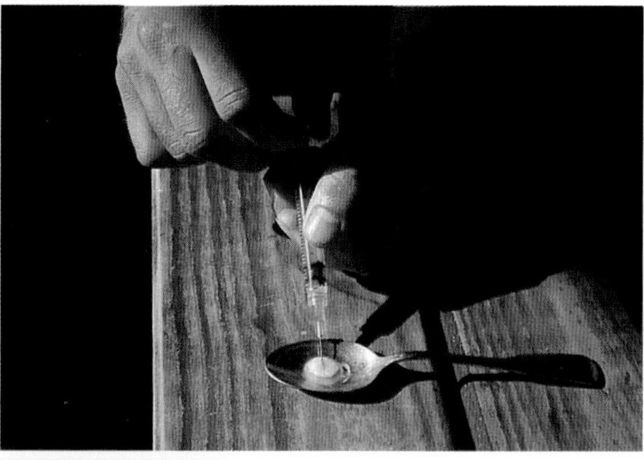

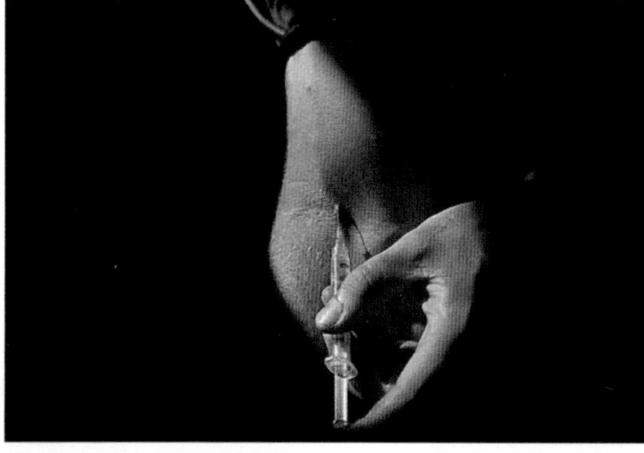

◄ Users generally inject into the major vein of the inner elbow. The needle is inserted into the vein, and a small amount of blood may be drawn back into the syringe to verify that the vein has been penetrated. The heroin is then usually injected in a series of small strokes to prolong the initial rush.

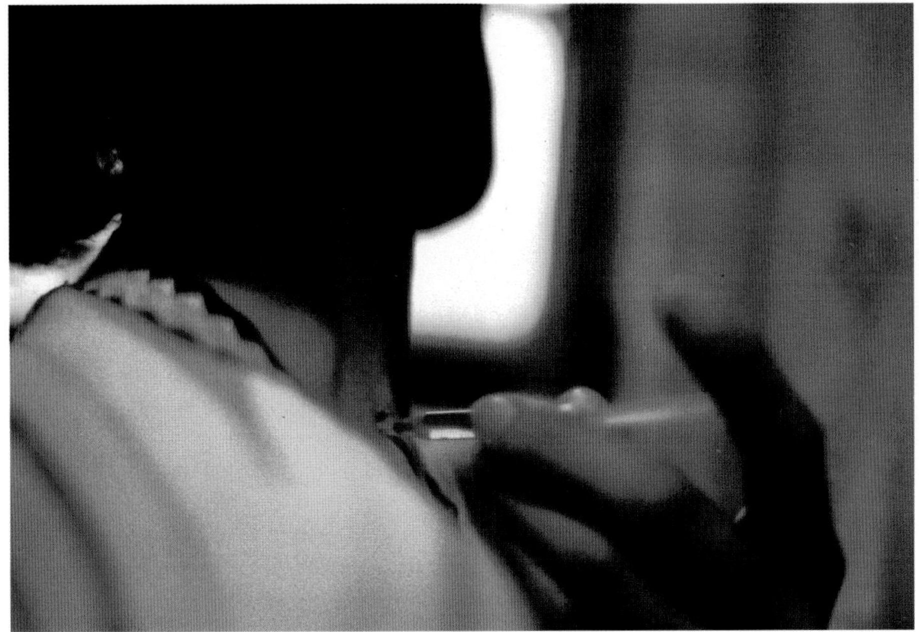

Steve Raymer/National Geographic

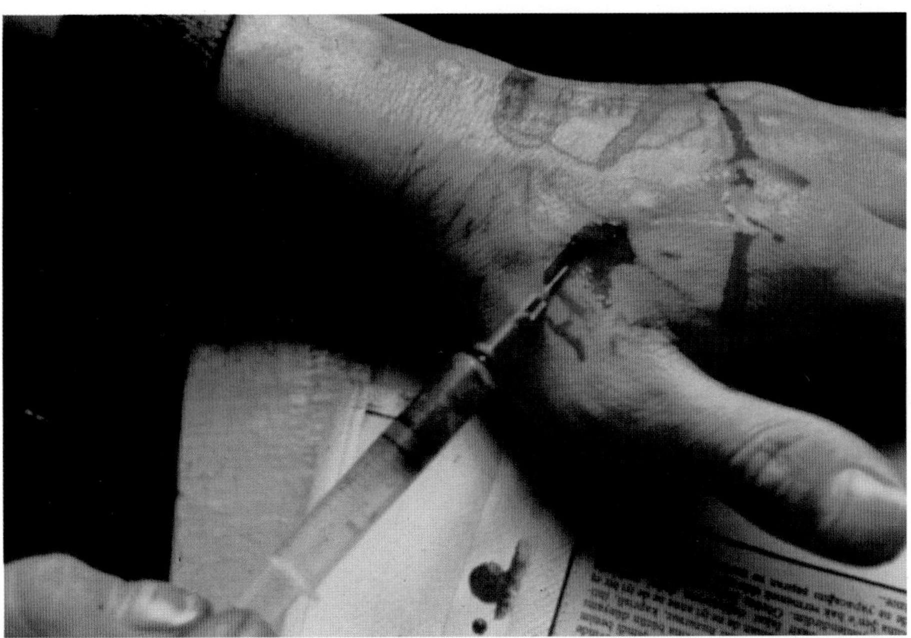

Laurence Cherniak

▲ After a vein is used repeatedly for injections, scar tissue develops, and the vein may harden or collapse, making injections difficult or impossible. As a result, addicts search the body for fresh veins into which their drug may be injected. Pictured are heroin addicts injecting into veins of the hand and the neck.

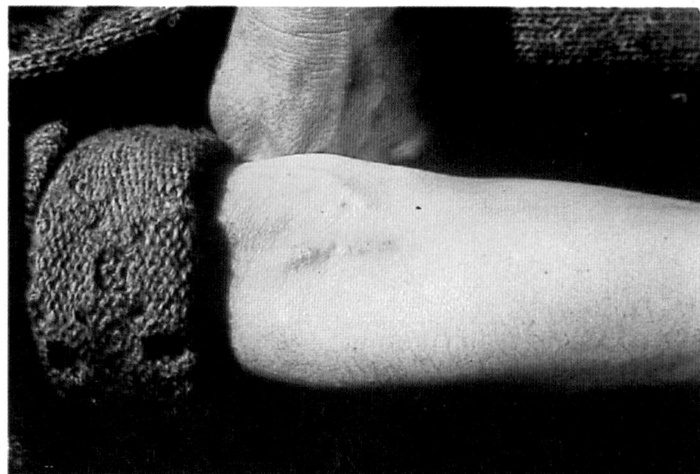

➤ Veins frequently used for injection develop scar tissue commonly known as tracks, turkey trots, marks, etc. To conceal injection marks, addicts often tattoo injection sites, wear long sleeved shirts, or use less noticeable veins, such as those of the legs, feet, groin, or other parts of the body.

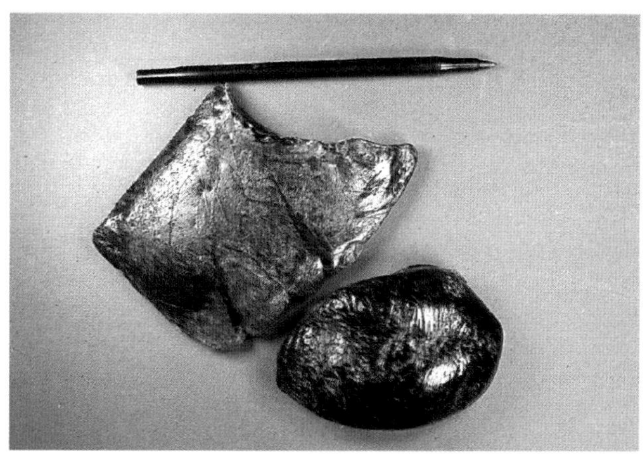

➤ Two pieces of Mexican tar heroin weighing 5 and 8 ounces. As the tar ages and is exposed to air, it turns from a very dark and shiny black to brown and from sticky and malleable to brittle. Tar heroin has a noticeable chemical odor similar to that of vinegar. If sold in gram quantities, the street value of these two pieces would be well in excess of $70,000.00 in most areas of the country.

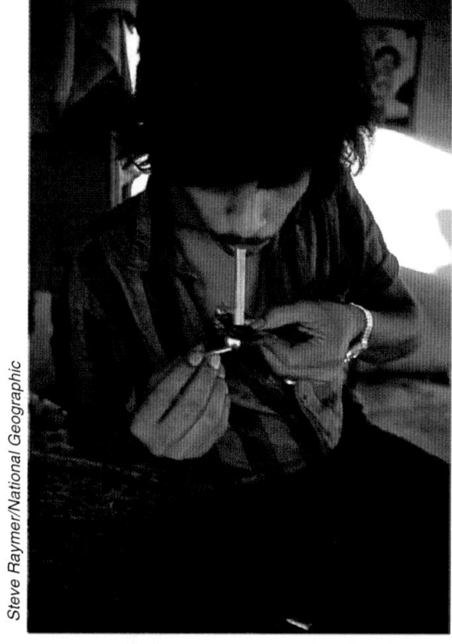

Steve Raymer/National Geographic

➤ An increasingly common method of ingesting heroin is by a method often referred to as "chasing the dragon". An amount of drug is placed on a sheet of aluminum foil and heated from below with an open flame. As the heroin vaporizes, the user inhales the fumes through a straw or similar device.

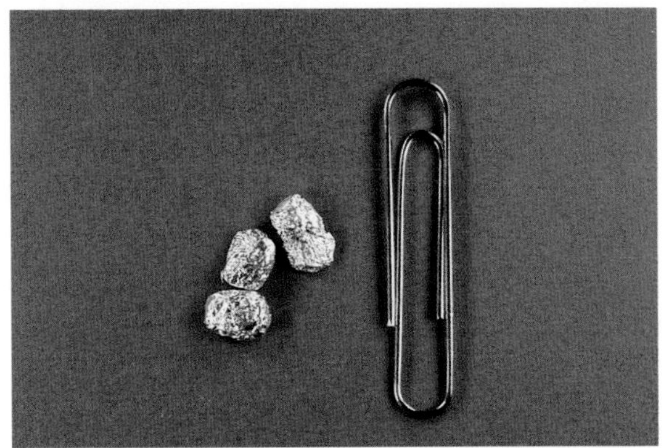

Due to the sticky consistency of most tar heroin samples, it is usually packaged in plastic or aluminum foil rather than paper. Pictured from top to bottom are small 1/10 gram quantities of tar wrapped in aluminum foil, a 1 gram piece of tar also wrapped in aluminum foil, and 1/10 gram pieces of tar wrapped in cellophane. At the bottom is tar heroin which has aged and the surface has discolored. Some of the chunks are broken, exposing the dark and shiny interior. Like other drugs, tar heroin is often cut to increase the sellers profits. Substances which have been used to dilute tar heroin have included brown sugar, cocoa mix, chocolate milk powder, coffee, and raisins. To add the cut, tar heroin can be warmed in an oven to make it soft and pliable, and the cut kneaded in.

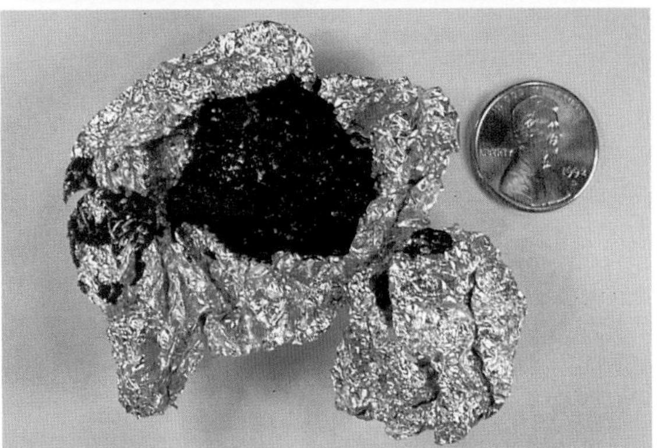

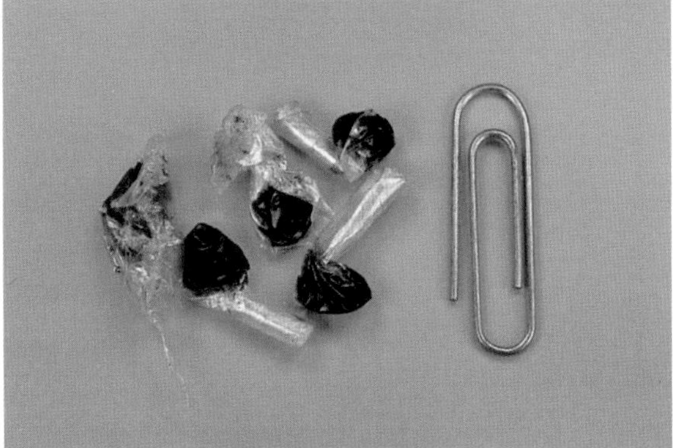

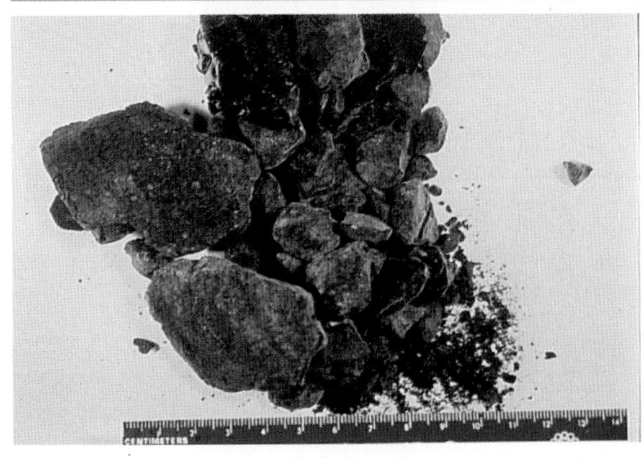

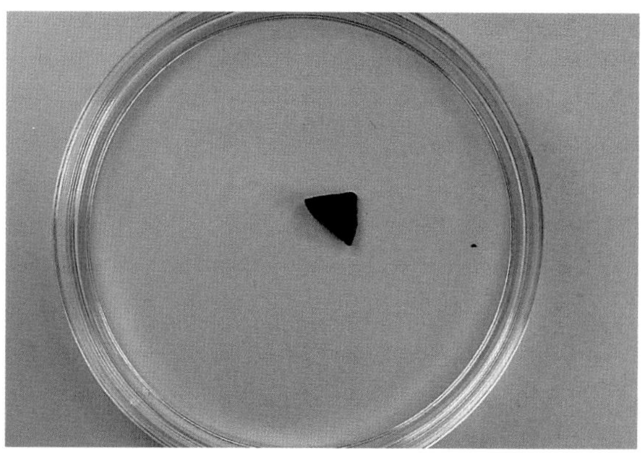

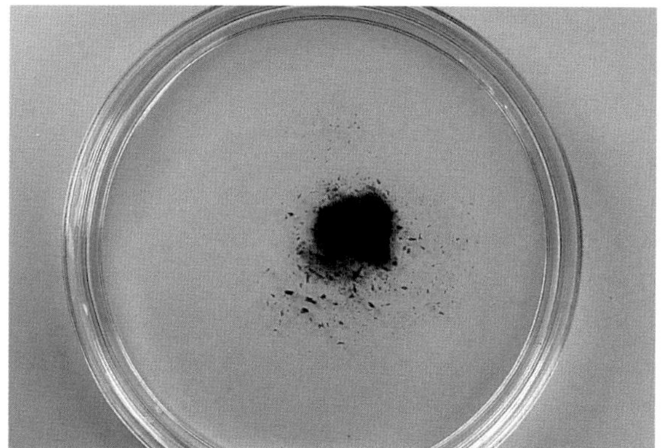

The most common manner of ingesting tar heroin is by dissolving it in water and injecting it in a vein. In this series of photos, a marble size piece of uncut tar heroin is placed into a dish of tap water. The heroin gradually dissolves, and with slight agitation totally dissolves in about five minutes. Like powder heroin, users of tar heroin also cook the drug in a spoon or similar device to help the drug dissolve in the water and filter out insoluble particles through cotton while drawing it into a syringe. Lemon or lime juice may also be added to acidify the solution and dissolve the heroin more readily.

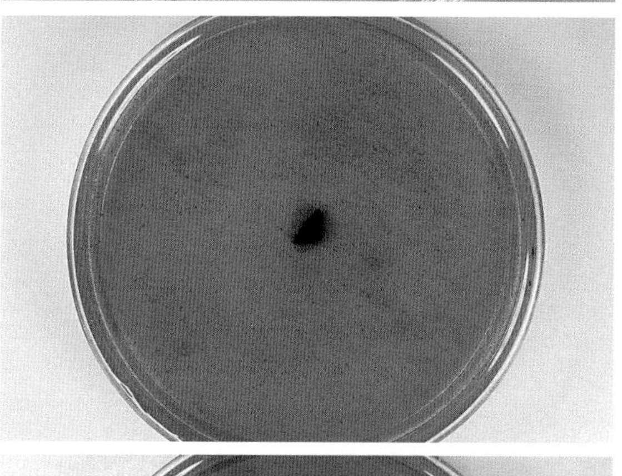

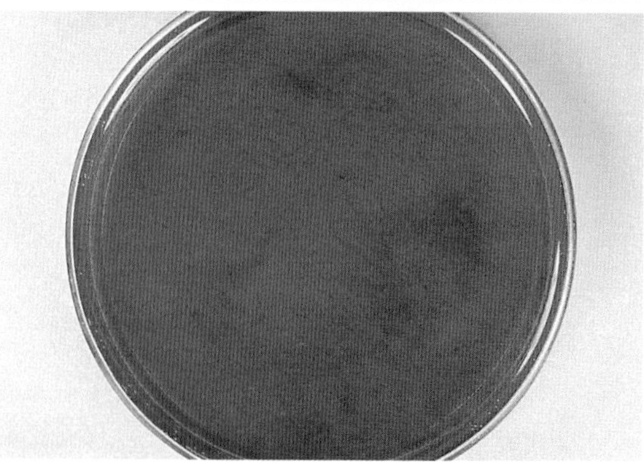

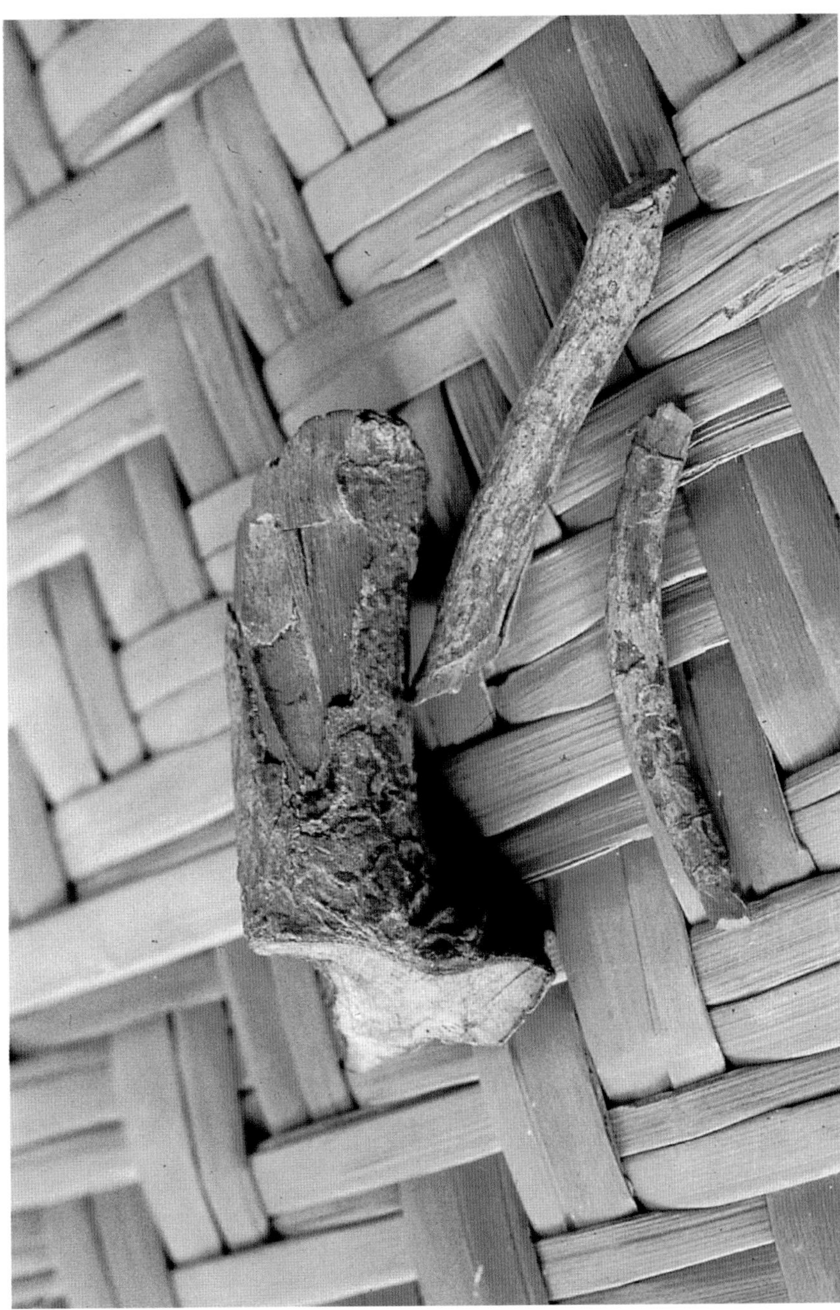

Jonathan Ott

Root sections of the Tabernanthe iboga bush, which grows in western equatorial Africa. The roots contain the alkaloid ibogaine, which is a powerful stimulant in smaller doses and a hallucinogen in larger doses. Although a Schedule I drug, ibogaine is currently being studied as a treatment for heroin addiction. Ibogaine is rarely seen on the illicit market.

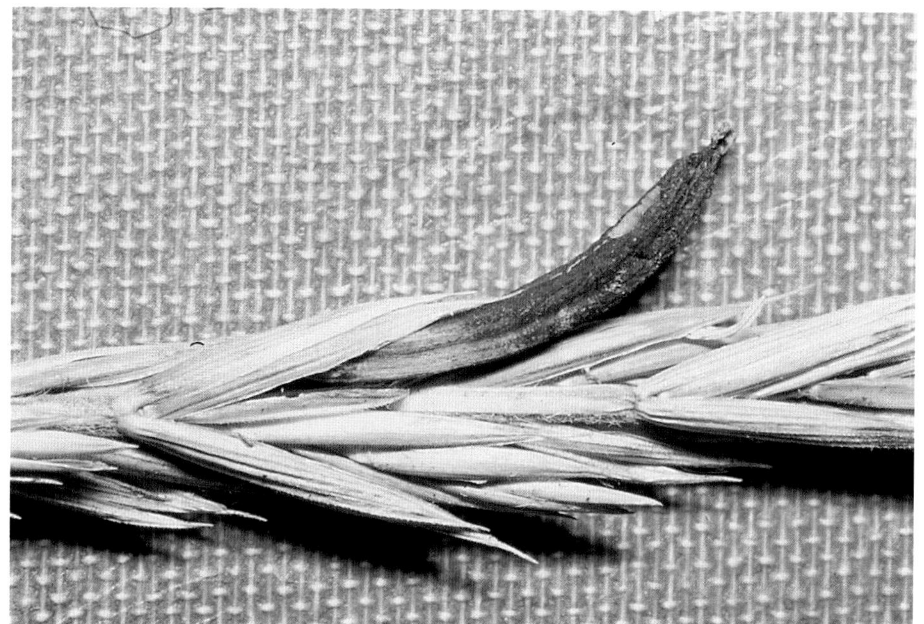

Stan Czolowski

▲ LSD was originally synthesized from lysergic acid obtained from the ergot of the fungus *claviceps purpurea*, the dark spur in this photograph. The fungus grows on grasses such as rye, wheat, and barley. Today the process is usually synthetic, utilizing such difficult-to-obtain chemicals as lysergic acid and ergotamine.

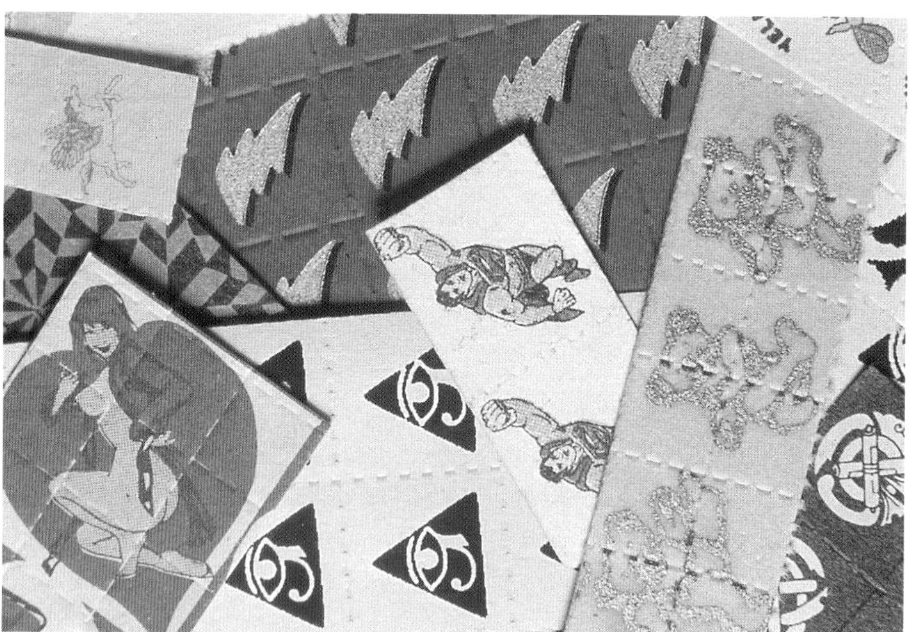

▲ Most LSD seen on the street is in the form of blotter (absorbent) paper. Blotter paper can be readily purchased at many art and office supply stores. Sheets are perforated into small squares and dipped into LSD which has been dissolved and diluted in ethyl alcohol. The blotter paper is often stamped with various designs, which are usually the trademark of the particular distributor.

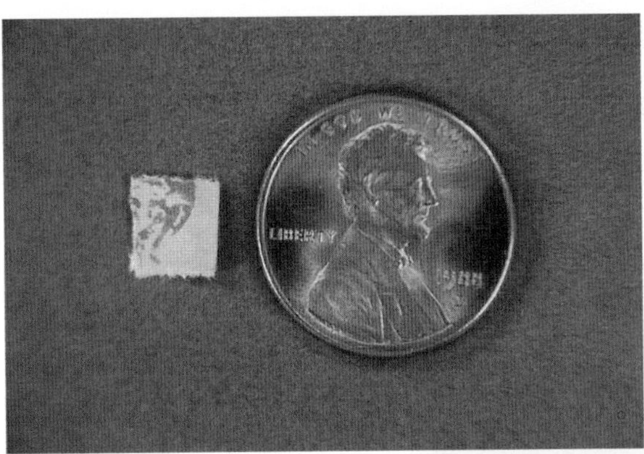

➤ A single dose or hit of LSD blotter. Most hits of blotter range in size from 1/4" to 1/2" and sell for anywhere between $1.00 to $10.00. On the street a "sheet" of blotter acid generally consists of 100 hits, and a "book" 1,000 hits.

➤ LSD is light and heat sensitive, and is often stored in a cool and dark environment. In this photo, a plastic bag containing about fifty hits of blotter acid sits beside the film cannister in which it was contained. Blotter paper is almost always found wrapped in plastic or cellophane.

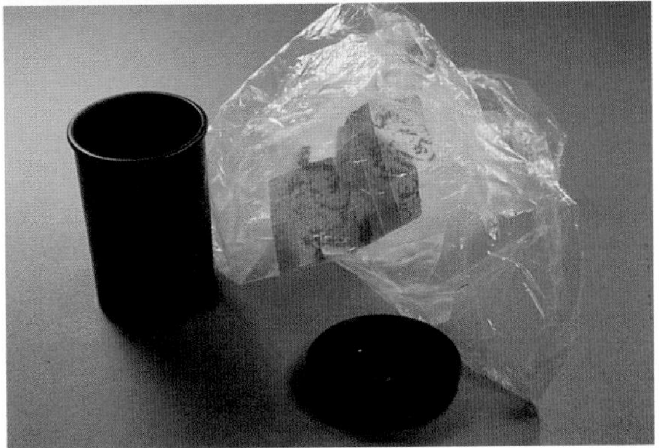

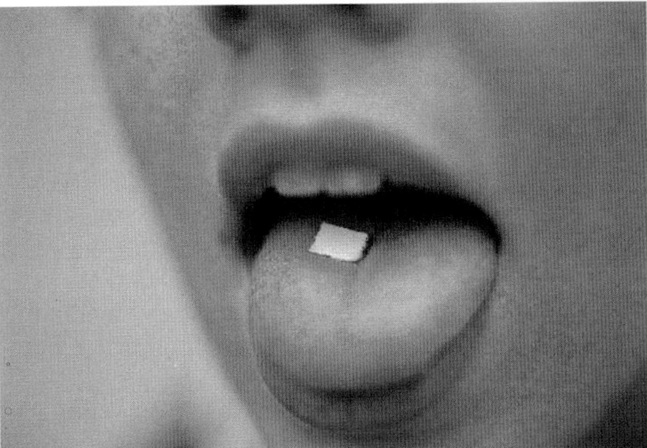

➤ LSD being ingested via blotter paper on the tongue. Absorption of LSD in this manner is very rapid, with an onset of effect within 30 to 60 minutes. The effects generally last about 5 to 12 hours. Although almost always taken by means of oral absorption, LSD can also be injected, absorbed through the skin or eye, or swallowed with food.

➤ LSD dissolved and diluted in ethyl alcohol or distilled water is sometimes kept in food coloring containers (green and blue seem to be the most popular) or small, dark colored glass vials. The liquid is usually placed on the tongue for absorption.

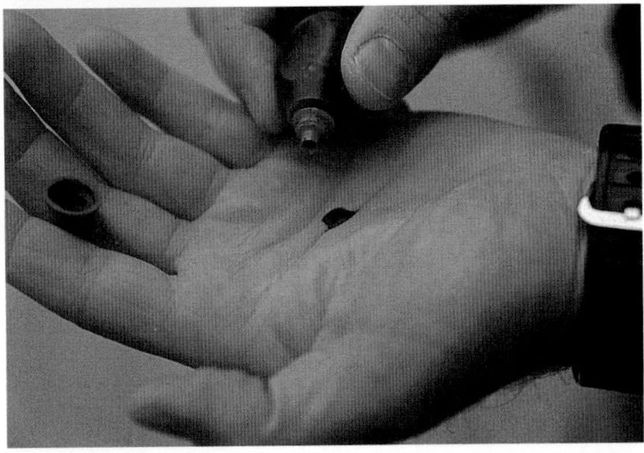

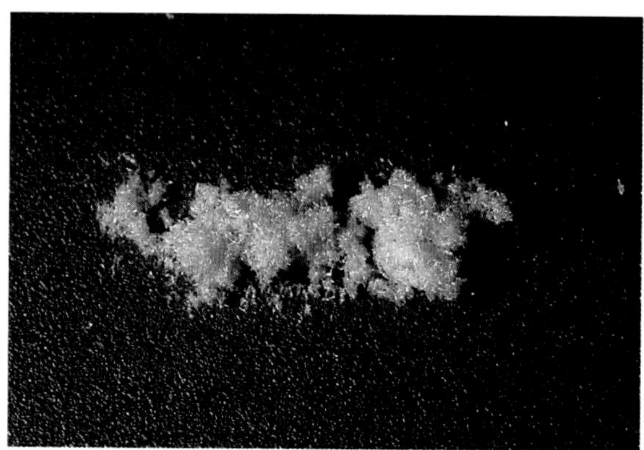

Bob Harris

➤ Crystalline LSD. In the crystalline form, a street dose of LSD is barely visible to the naked eye. An amount of pure LSD the weight of a penny could produce 567,000 hits of 50 micrograms each. Most LSD seen on the street has been dissolved and diluted in ethyl alcohol or distilled water and added to blotter paper.

➤ Currently, tablets are an infrequently encountered form of LSD. However, over the years tablets and capsules containing LSD have been produced in a multitude of sizes, shapes, and colors. LSD may be added to legitimately manufactured tablets such as vitamins or to an inert mixture which is then pressed into tablet form or encapsulated.

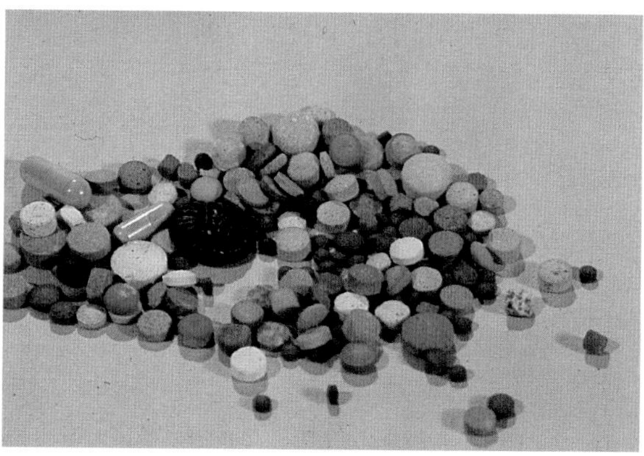

Miami Herald

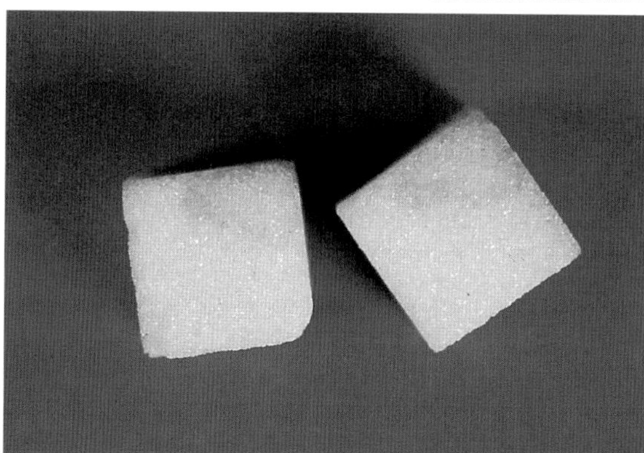

➤ As with the case of tablets and capsules, sugar cubes containing LSD are also not as common today as in years past but are still occasionally encountered. LSD can be placed on almost any medium, including cloth, toothpicks, etc.

➤ Samples of oral and injectable LSD-25 under the brand name Delysid, manufactured by Sandoz Laboratories of Switzerland. Sandoz was the original producer of LSD, but production was discontinued in 1965 when it became clear that LSD was being used more as a drug by the counterculture than as an investigative respiratory stimulant and psychiatric medicine.

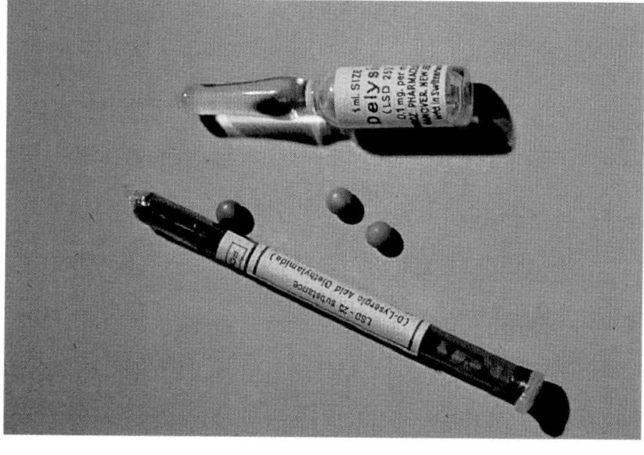

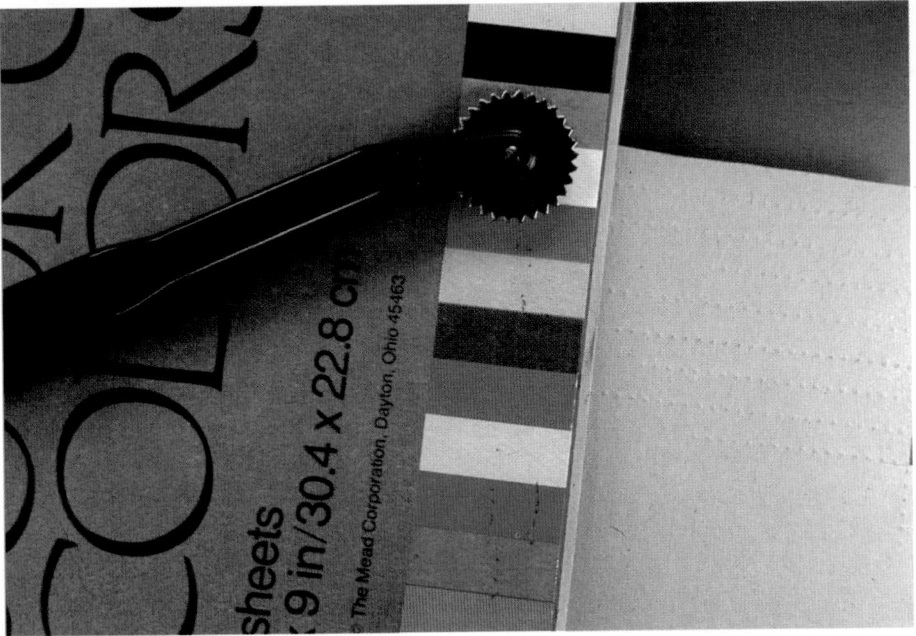

▲ A low level LSD distributor's tools of the trade: absorbent art paper, a simple perforating device, and a finished perforated sheet.

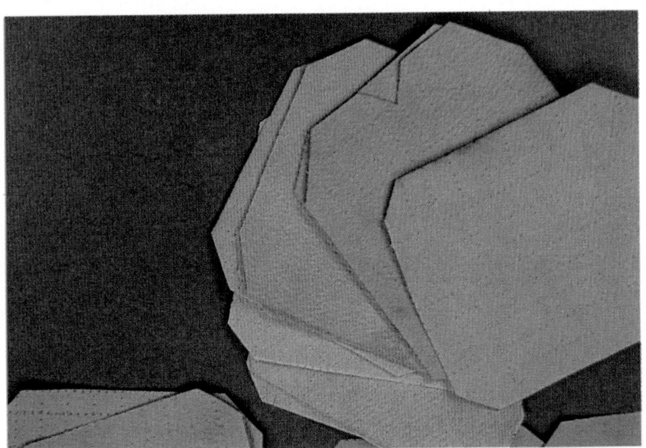

◄ Although most blotter acid samples display some sort of design, some, as in this photo, may be plain.

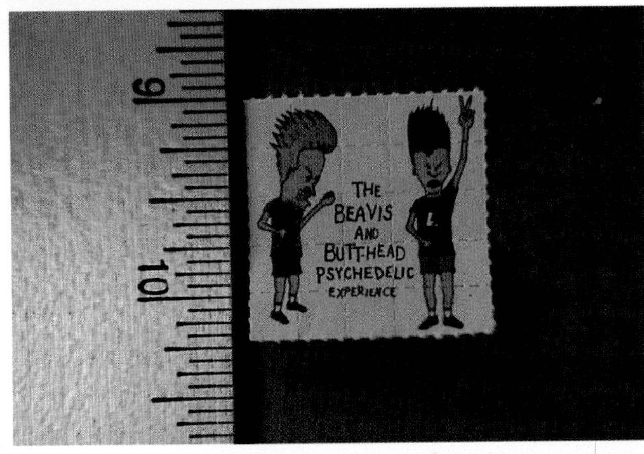

► Beavis and Butt-head, perhaps one of the most popular new designs seen on LSD blotter. Potency of Beavis and Butt-head LSD samples has varied widely.

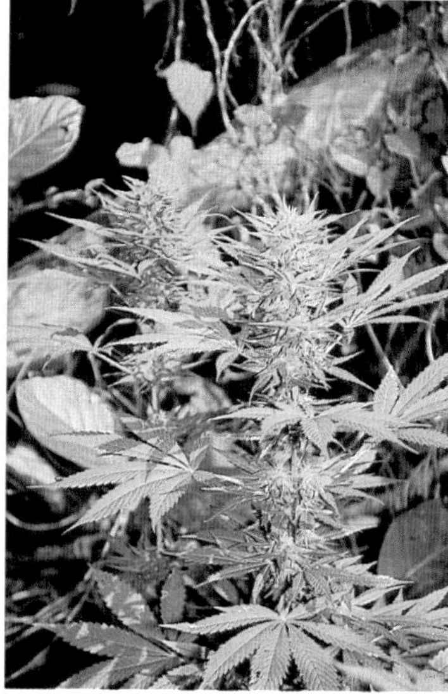

Brad Reynoso

◀ Marijuana, the most widely used and most familiar illicit drug, growing among other green foliage.

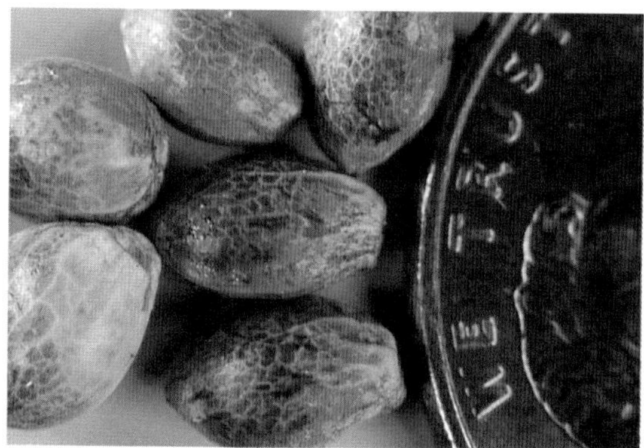

▲ Close-up of marijuana seeds showing their typical appearance. Most marijuana buds contain as many as several dozen seeds. The genetics of the seed is the single most important factor in determining the plants ultimate THC potency.

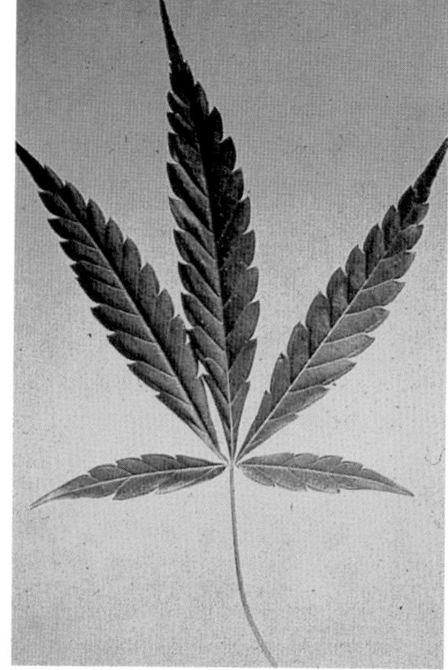

▲ The many varieties of marijuana produce leaves with their own unique characteristics. Typically, however, the leaves are slender and elongated with serrated edges, and normally have 3, 5, 7, 9 or 11 blades per leaf.

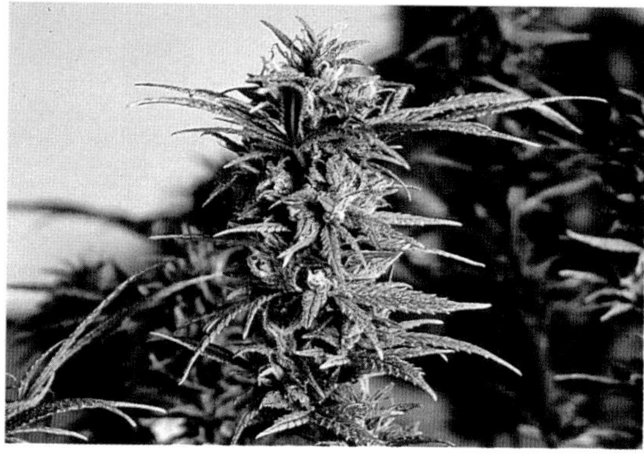

Paul Kroeger

▲ The flowering part of the marijuana plant, or bud, contains the highest amount of THC in the plant. Pictured is a "cola", or group of buds growing at the very top of the plant.

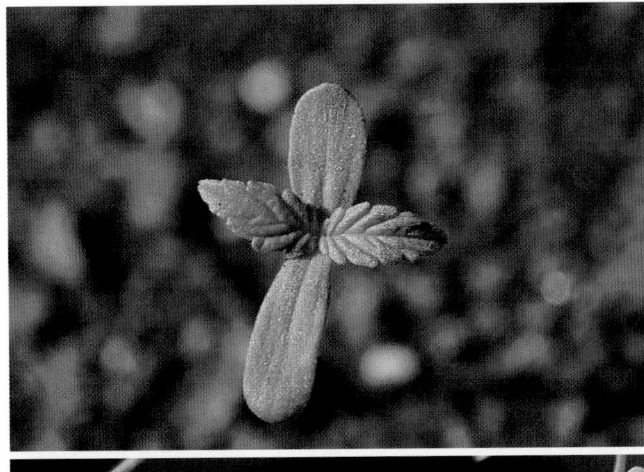

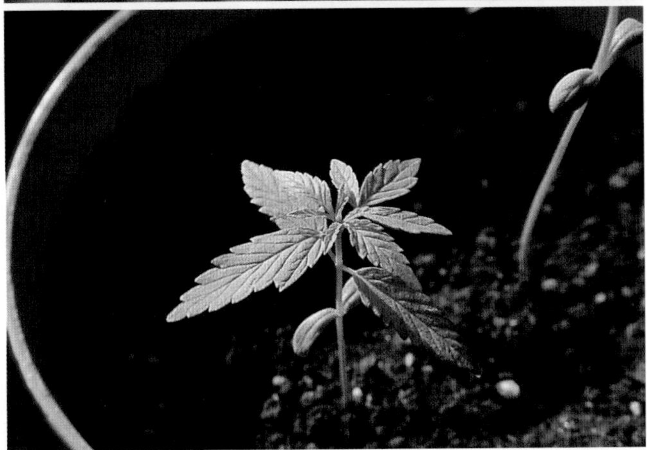

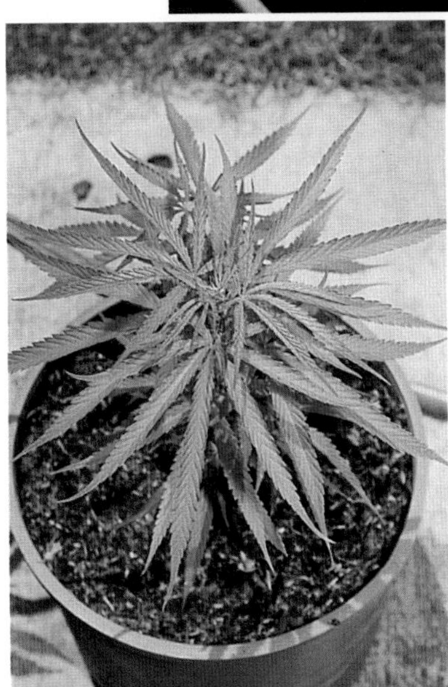

Brad Reynoso

➤ A backyard stash of marijuana plants.

◄ ▲ Photos showing the early stages of marijuana growth. After the seed sprouts, the plant has four leaves, two of which are serrated and two of which are round. As the plant grows, many more serrated leaves develop. Under ideal conditions a healthy marijuana plant may grow several inches every day.

Brad Reynoso

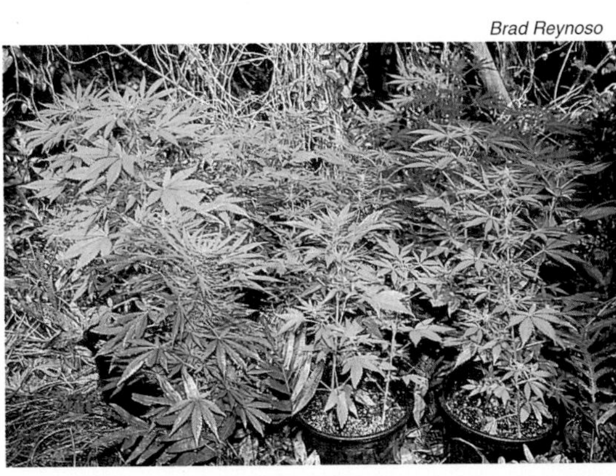

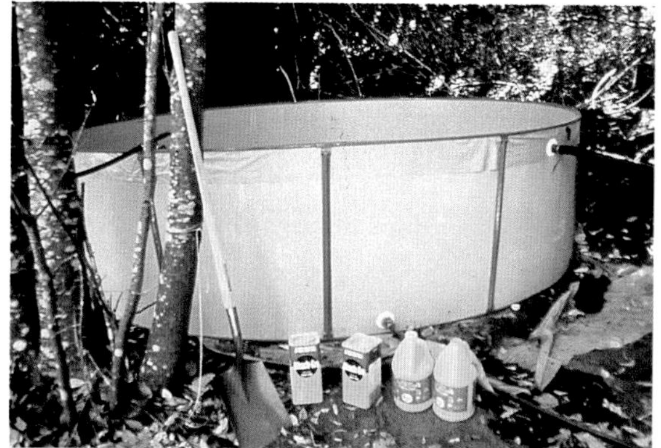

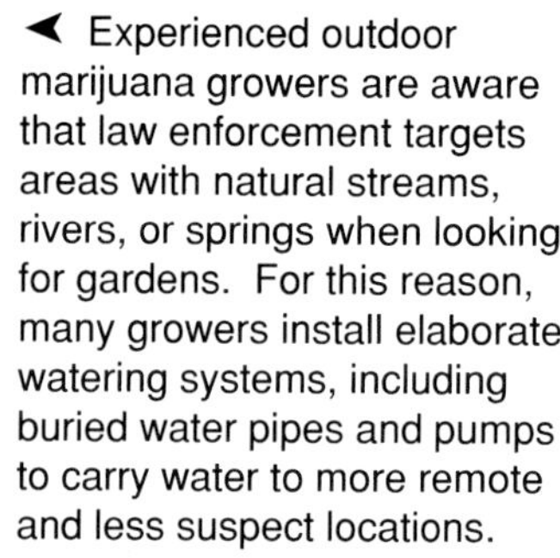

➤ Experienced outdoor marijuana growers are aware that law enforcement targets areas with natural streams, rivers, or springs when looking for gardens. For this reason, many growers install elaborate watering systems, including buried water pipes and pumps to carry water to more remote and less suspect locations.

Brad Reynoso

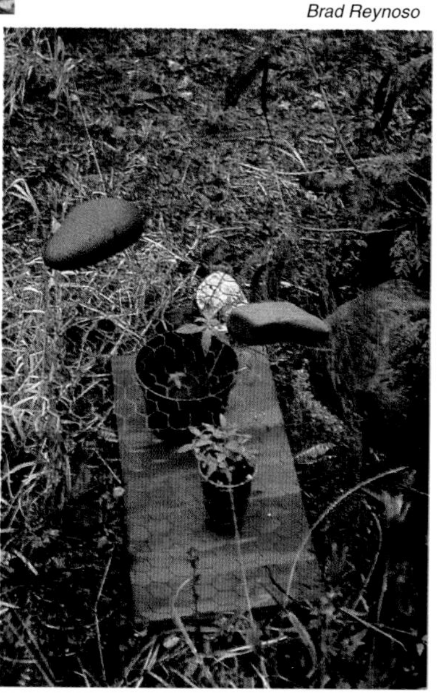

➤ Animals such as deer and rabbits find immature marijuana very edible. Marijuana plants grown outdoors are often covered with chicken wire or other protection to prevent such predation. Many growers also set up alarms or traps to prevent unwanted animal or human incursion.

Laurence Cherniak

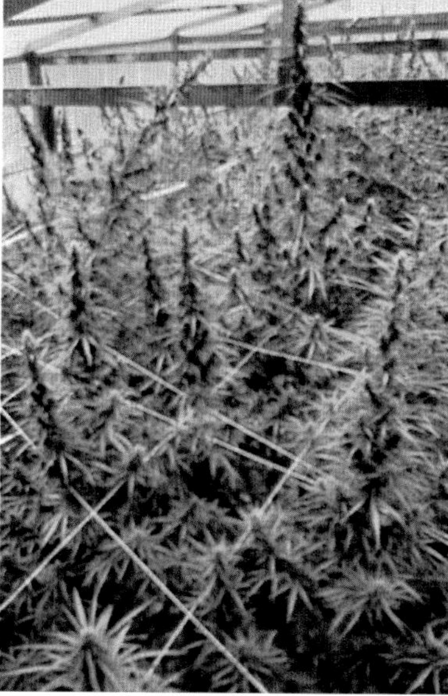

➤ Some of the most potent marijuana grown comes from indoor gardens. Growing marijuana indoors allows the grower to create a perfect atmosphere of light, temperature and nutrients, all factors which influence the plant's potency. Additionally, indoor growing allows for a level of security and year-round growing.

➤ Greenhouse marijuana plants with numerous well-developed buds along the branches. The buds are flower clusters and appear as dense clumps of green foliage. Several dozen buds may grow on a single plant, and each bud may be several inches long. String is used in this garden to support the plants upright under the heavy weight of the buds.

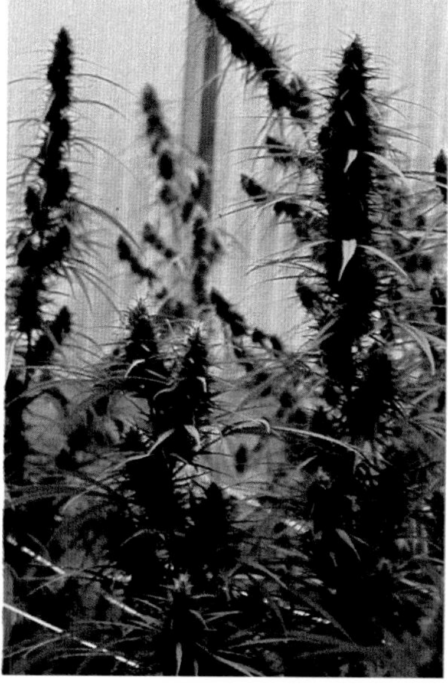

Laurence Cherniak

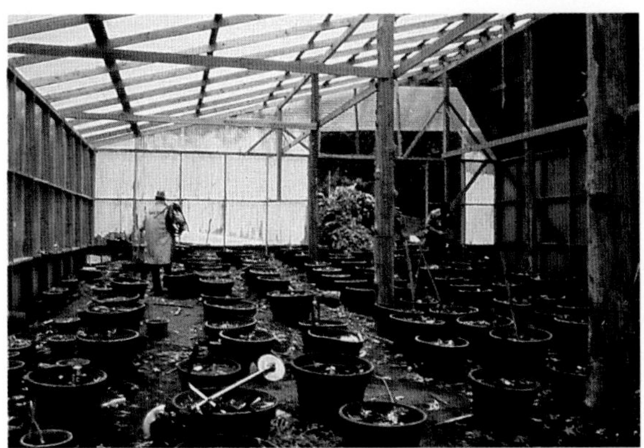

➤ A seized indoor marijuana garden which had been producing high quality sinsemilla. Note the size of the pots used to hold the plants and the size of the remaining stems, as well as the height of the ceiling. Some marijuana plants can grow to heights of over 20 feet. Larger indoor marijuana gardens can produce hundreds of pounds of buds every year.

Stan Czolowski

➤ Magnification of the resin glands which form on the outer surface of the marijuana plant. The resin contains the active substance in the marijuana plant, tetrahydrocannabinol (THC). The potency of the plant is related not only to the quantity of the resin produced, but also the quality, or THC content, of the resin as well.

➤ Resin buildup which has accumulated on the fingers from harvesting marijuana buds. Resin is a sticky sap-like substance which forms in glands on the outer surfaces of the marijuana plant. The THC content of the plant is concentrated in the resin glands.

Brad Reynoso

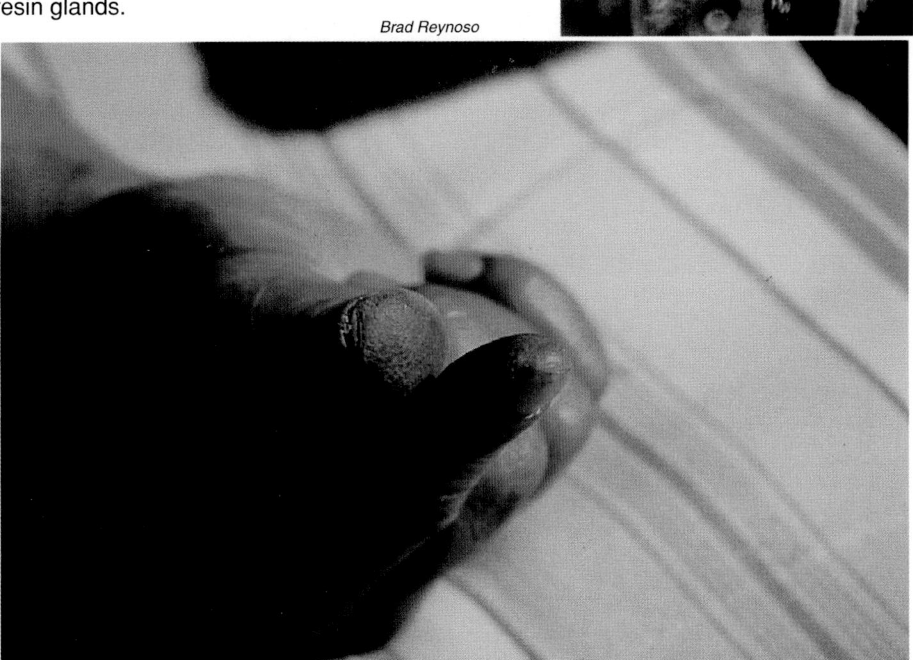

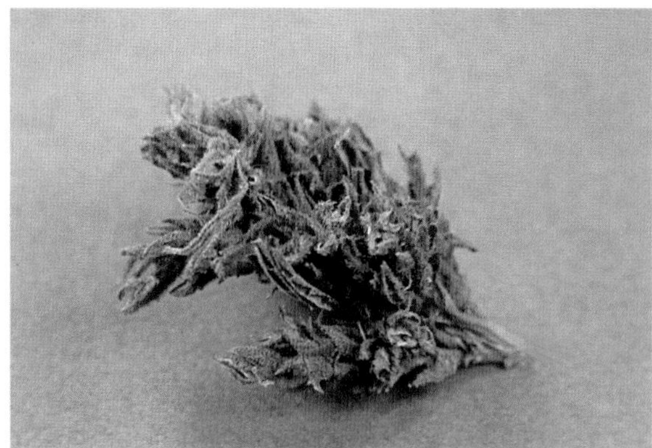

➤ A dried "sinsemilla" bud, which is Spanish for "without seed". Sinsemilla is a technique rather than a variety and involves separating female marijuana plants from the males so that they are not pollinated. An unpollinated female marijuana plant will continue to produce potent resin rather than divert its energies to producing seeds.

➤ A typical dried commercial marijuana bud. Commercial marijuana generally costs only half that of sinsemilla, generally due to a correspondingly lower THC level. Buds may appear green, brown, or gold in color, depending on the color of the plant when harvested, how it was stored, and its age.

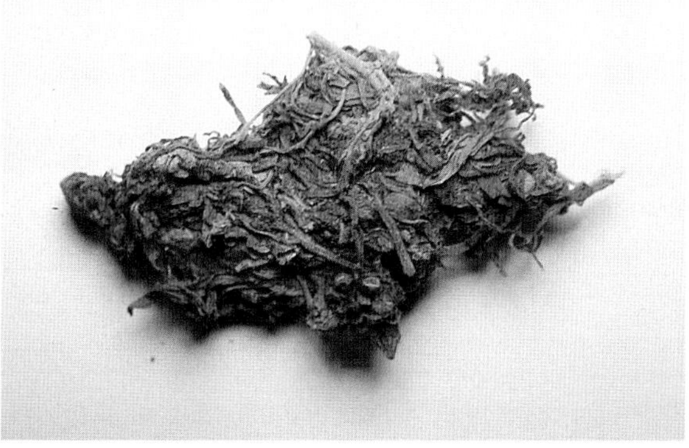

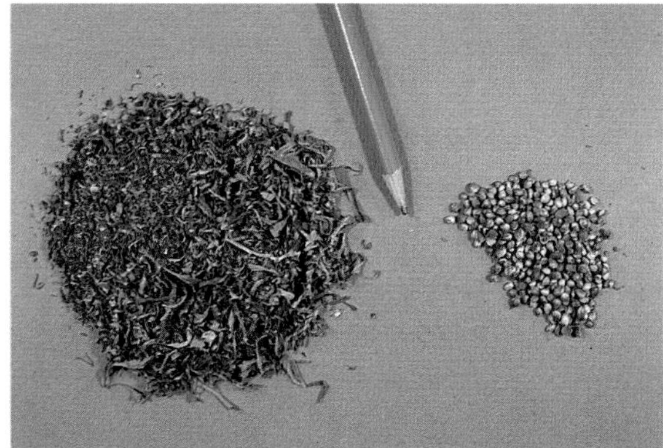

➤ Commercial marijuana normally has a high seed content. The sample pictured weighed 10 grams, 7 grams of which was plant material and 3 grams of which was seed. Because the seeds are not psychoactive and can pop when heated, most users remove the seeds before the marijuana is smoked.

➤ Marijuana is typically packaged in plastic bags in pound or ounce quantities, or fractions thereof. Pictured are pound, ounce, and half-ounce bags.

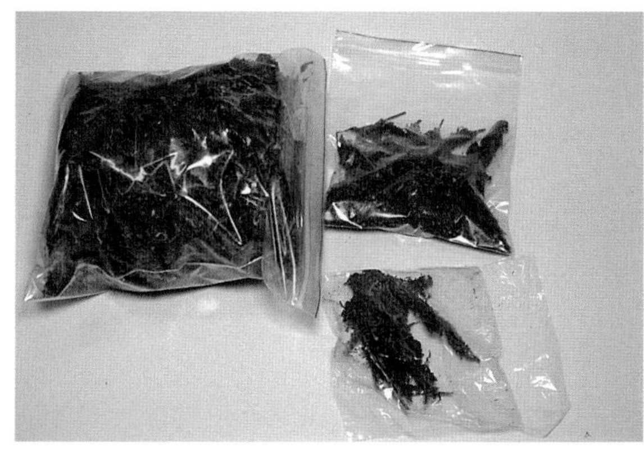

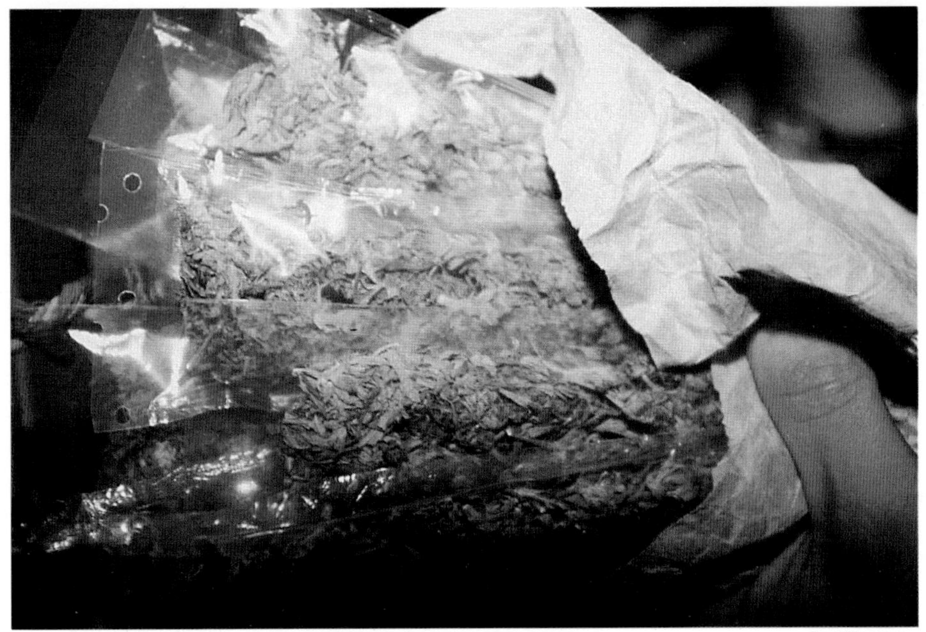

Brad Reynoso

▲ Large marijuana buds packaged individually in hermetically sealed plastic bags.

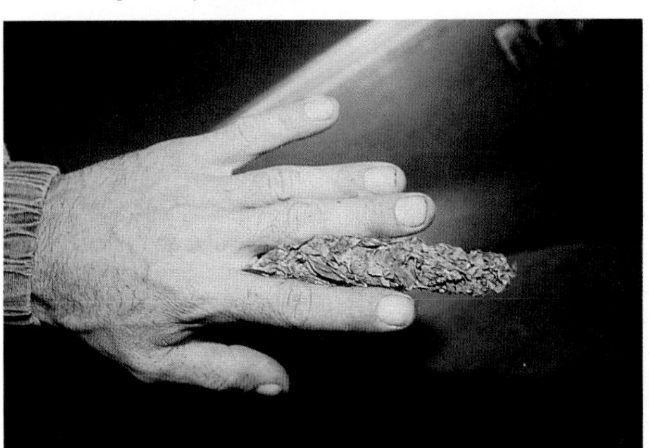

Brad Reynoso

◀ A rather large dried marijuana bud.

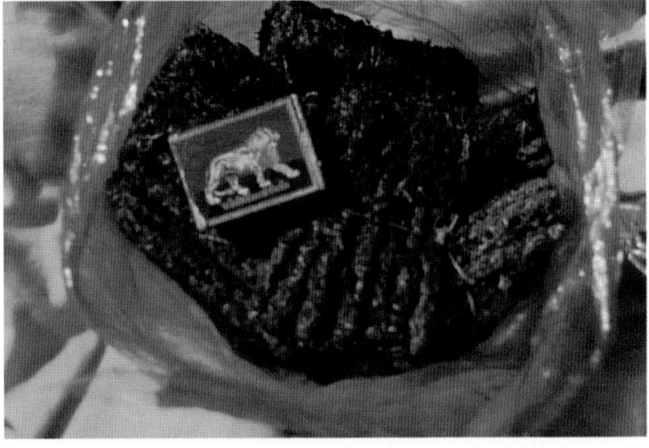

Laurence Cherniak

▶ Thai sticks consist of marijuana that has been cultivated in Thailand or its neighboring countries. The marijuana is wrapped around bamboo sticks ranging from about 5" to 10" in length. Although seldom seen in the United States, Thai sticks are considered to be of very high quality.

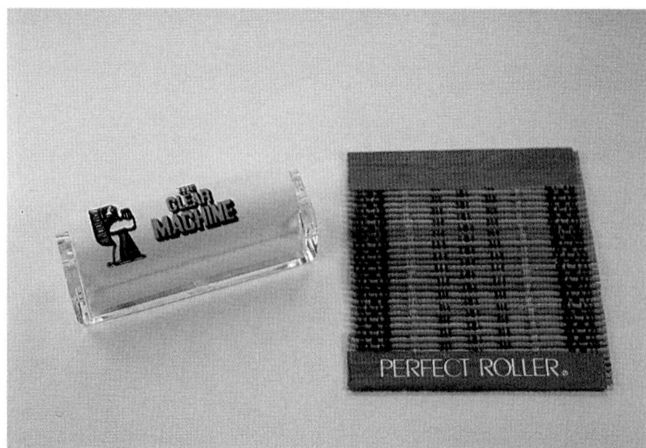

➤ Two types of cigarette rolling devices available in paraphernalia or smoke shops.

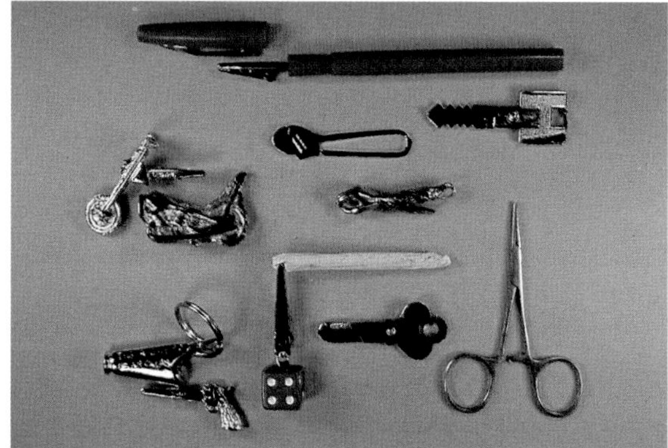

➤ A selection of roach clips, which are used to hold the butt end of a marijuana joint while it is being smoked. This allows the joint to be smoked almost completely without burning the lips or fingers.

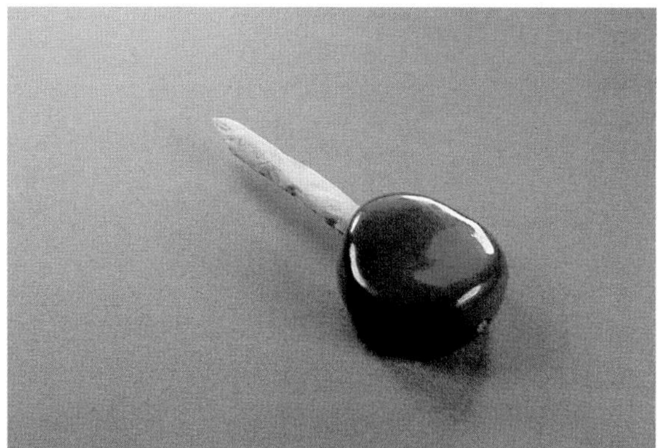

➤ A device used to hold and smoke a marijuana joint. Often called a "stone", it serves the same purpose as a roach clip.

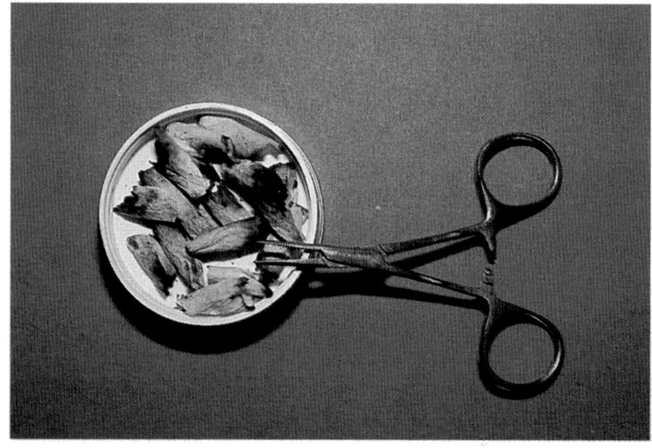

➤ As a joint is smoked, the unburned marijuana remaining in the butt end, or "roach", traps some of the THC. The roaches are saved and combined with others to roll new joints.

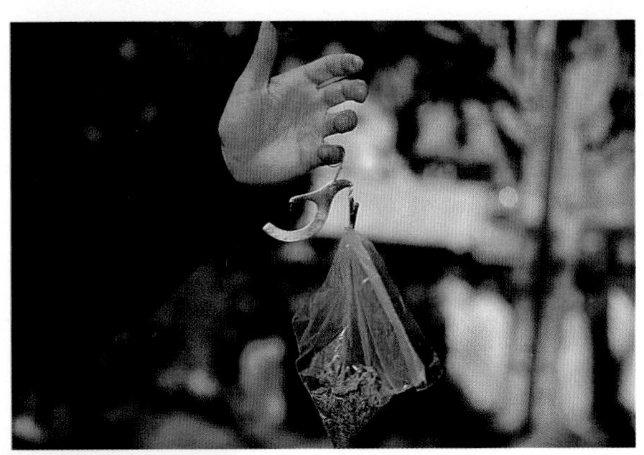

➤ Weighing out 1/2 ounce of marijuana with a postage scale, one of the most commonly used weighing devices in the marijuana trade. Cheap, easily concealed, and relatively accurate.

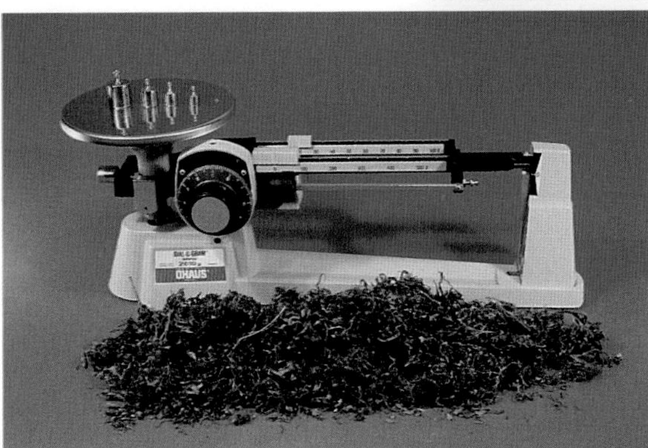

◄ A triple beam gram scale and 1/2 pound of marijuana. The triple beam scale is a common tool of many drug dealers, as it is extremely accurate and easy to use. Scale standards of 50 grams, 20 grams, 10 grams and 5 grams are also shown, and can be utilized by the buyer to ensure the accuracy of the dealer's scale.

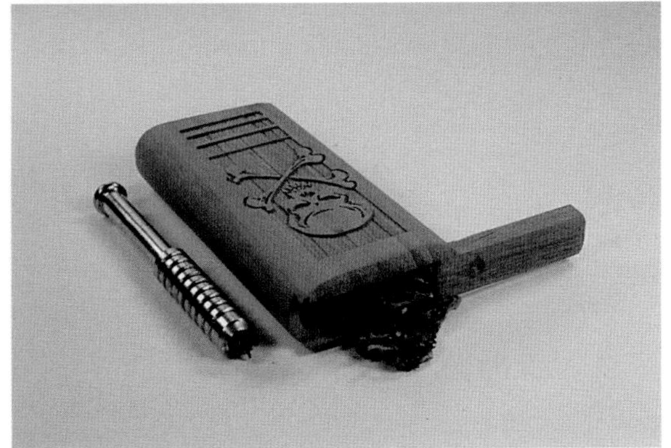

➤ A dugout is a decorative wooden carrying case with separate spaces for storing a small supply of marijuana and a small baseball bat shaped pipe.

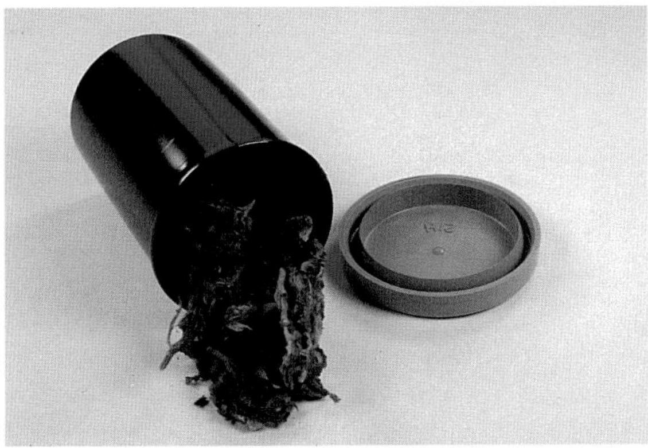

◄ For small quantities, 35mm film cannisters are often used to store marijuana. The cannisters protect the marijuana from loss of potency caused by air and light.

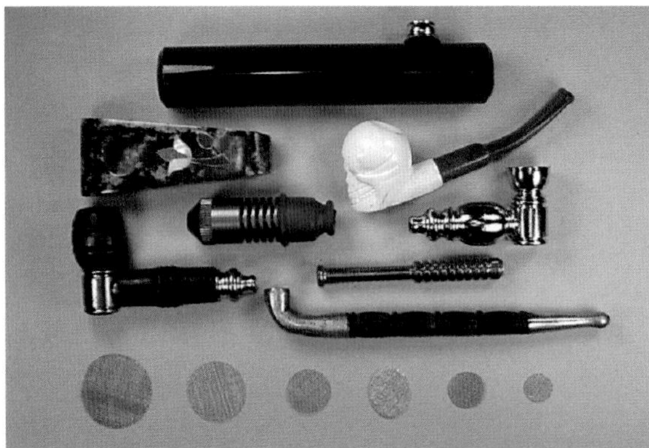

◄ A selection of marijuana pipes and the brass screens of various sizes that are placed in the bowls to hold the drug.

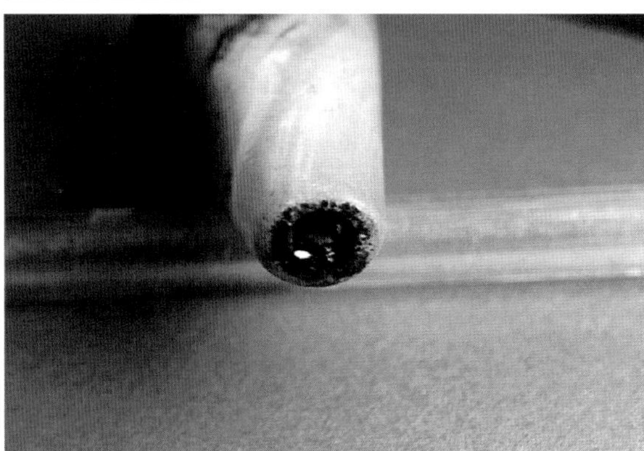

➤ Smoking marijuana produces a thick, shiny tar residue, some of which accumulates throughout the pipe.

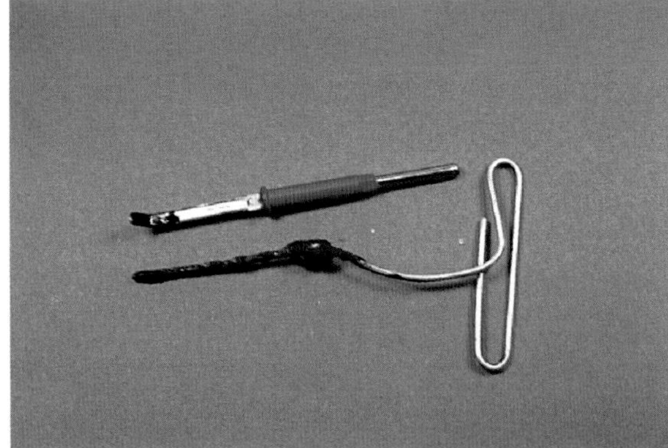

◄ Two homemade tools used to remove the thick tar accumulation from a marijuana pipe's bowl and stem.

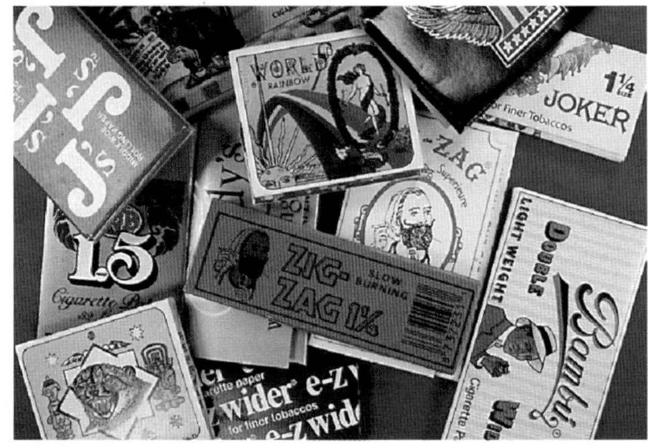

➤ Some of the many brands of cigarette rolling paper which may be used to roll marijuana joints.

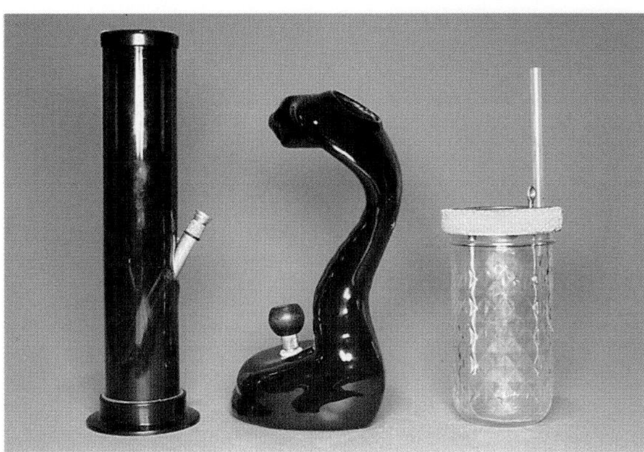

➤ Marijuana bongs, or water pipes, appear in an unlimited number of sizes and shapes. A small amount of water, through which the smoke passes, is placed in the bottom of the bong and cools the smoke as it is inhaled.

➤ Smoking marijuana with a bong. THC, the active substance in marijuana, is not water soluble and therefore passes through the water barrier. However, many of the harsh non-psychoactive chemicals in marijuana are water soluble and are trapped in the water.

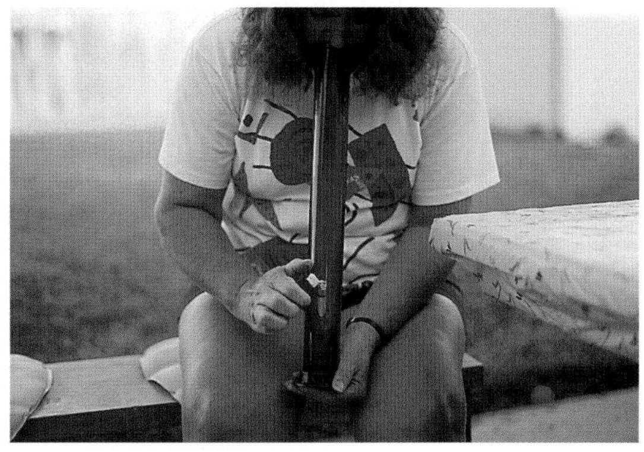

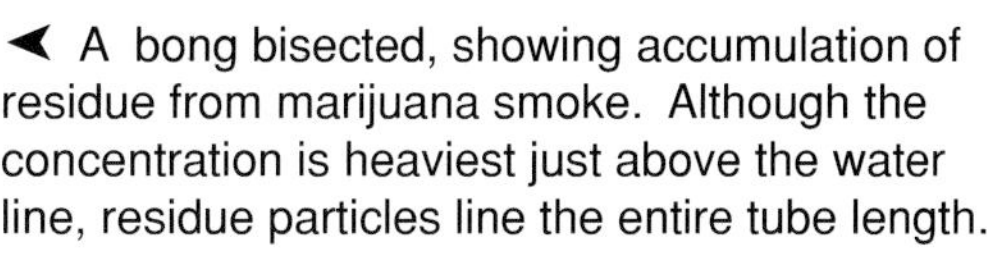

➤ A bong bisected, showing accumulation of residue from marijuana smoke. Although the concentration is heaviest just above the water line, residue particles line the entire tube length.

➤ Close-up of the residue from marijuana smoke deposited in the bong pictured above.

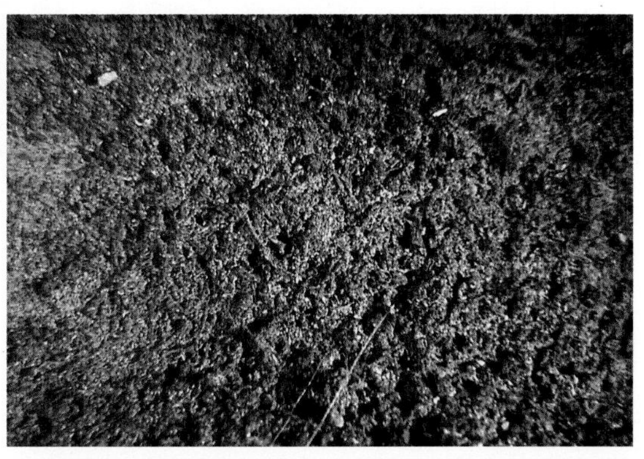

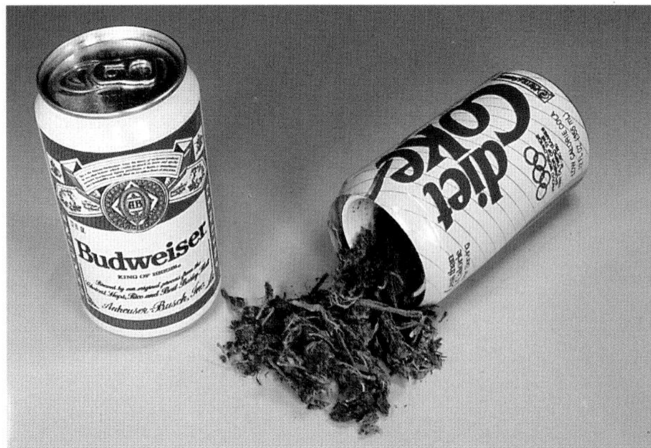

Two types of false containers with screw-on lids sold in paraphernalia stores. The containers are extremely accurate replicas of the real thing, including the weight.

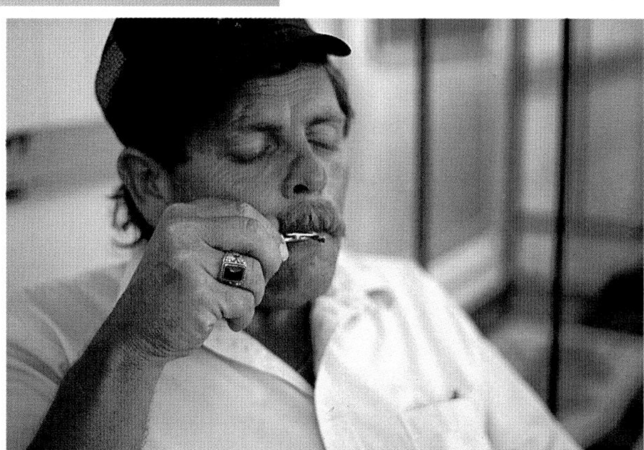

Using a roach clip to smoke a marijuana joint. The roach clip allows the joint to be smoked almost completely without burning the lips and fingers.

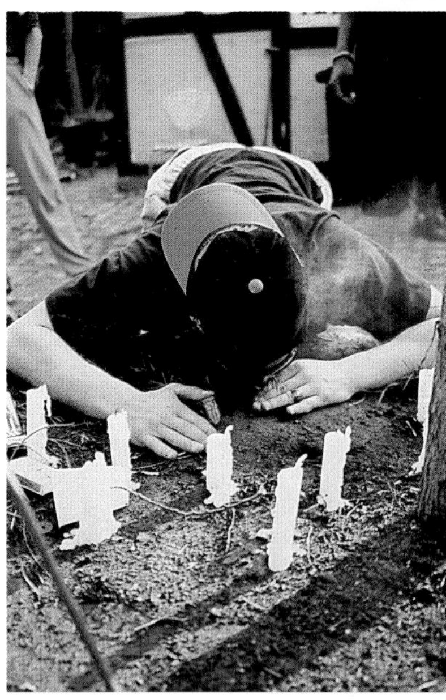

William Hurst

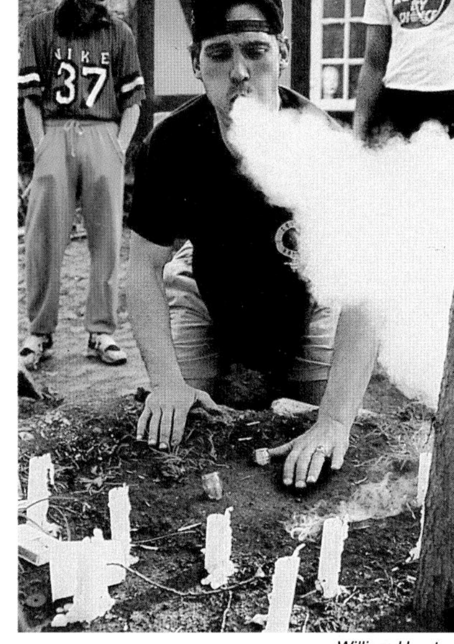

William Hurst

Smoking marijuana with an "earth pipe". An amount of marijuana and/or hash is lit and placed in a hole in the ground, to which the broken tops of two glass bottles and an aeration hole are connected. The marijuana is inhaled through the top of one of the bottles.

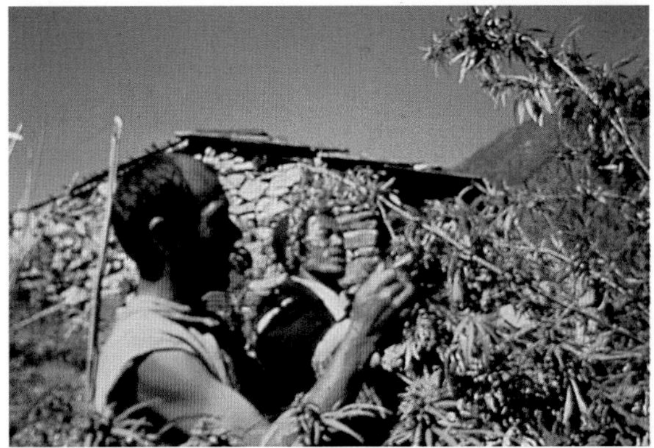

Laurence Cherniak

➤ The sticky resin of the marijuana plant is used to make hash. It can be collected by either thrashing the plants over cloth or plastic, and collecting the resin as it falls, or by simply rubbing the buds between the hands causing the resin to stick to them, as in this photo of Tibetan workers.

➤ Once the resin is collected, a small amount of water may be added and worked in to assure a uniform consistency. In this photo, the resin is being worked to form a very high quality hash product known as Royal Nepalese temple balls.

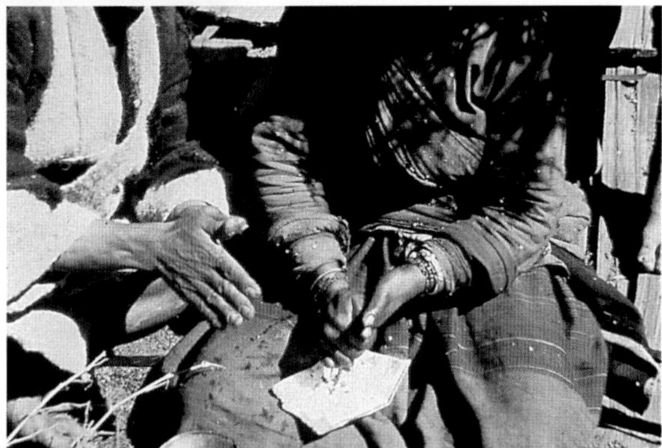

Laurence Cherniak

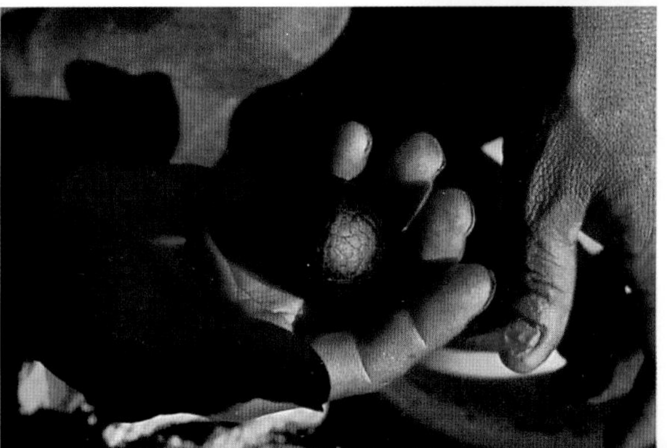

Laurence Cherniak

➤ A nearly completed Royal Nepalese temple ball. A few lines or cracks still appear on the surface. The ball will be worked until the surface is free of any such flaws.

➤ The finished Royal Nepalese temple balls, reputed to be some of the highest quality hash found anywhere. As a general rule, the darker the hash, the higher the quality.

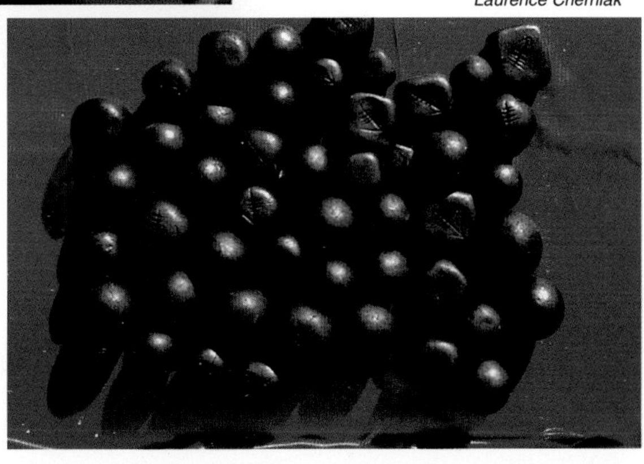

Laurence Cherniak

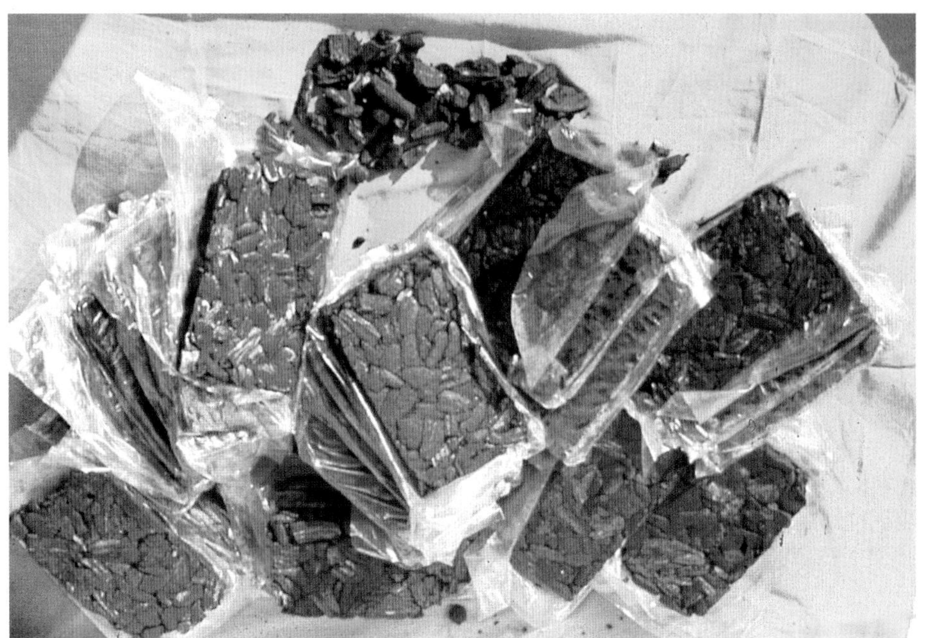

Laurence Cherniak

⮝ Thirty-five kilos (77 pounds) of Nepalese finger hash pressed into slabs. The physical shape of the hash is often used to describe it: finger, sole, ball, patty, etc.

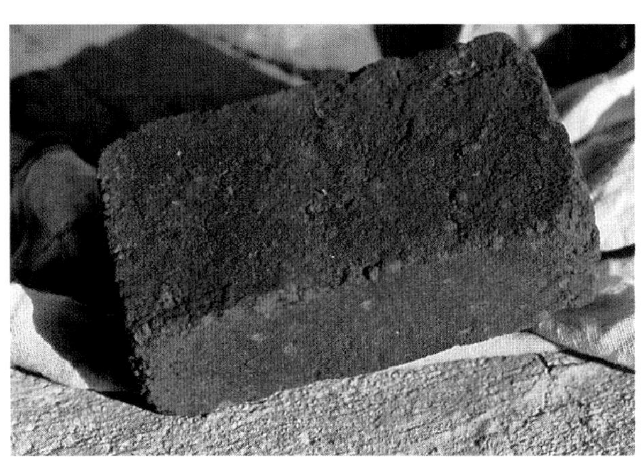

Laurence Cherniak

⮜ A six ounce piece of poor quality Mexican green hash.

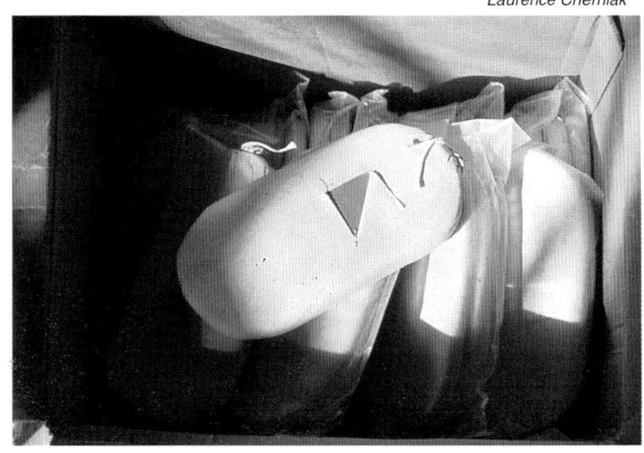

Laurence Cherniak

➤ A box containing 50 pounds of blonde Lebanese hash, packaged in cloth sacks and plastic bags. The color of Lebanese hash can vary from blonde to red.

➤ Pieces of hash, rolling papers and a pipe. Hash is smoked in the same various manners as marijuana, and the two are often consumed together.

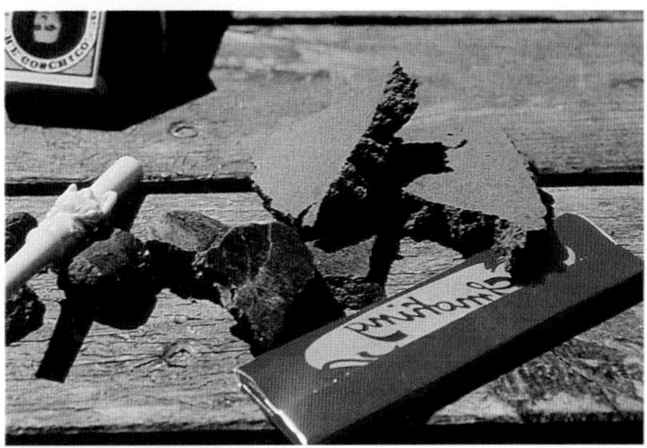

William Hurst

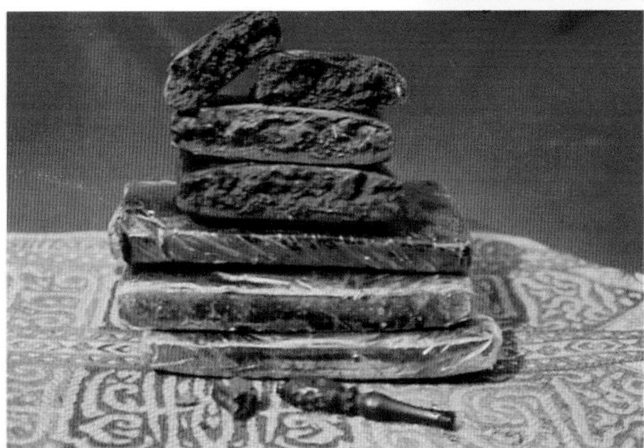

Laurence Cherniak

◄ Four and one-half pounds of high quality Afghani hash, showing a cross section of one of the slabs and a hash pipe in the foreground.

➤ A small block of high quality hash. The producer went to the trouble of pressing the hash into a custom and perhaps trademark type of mold.

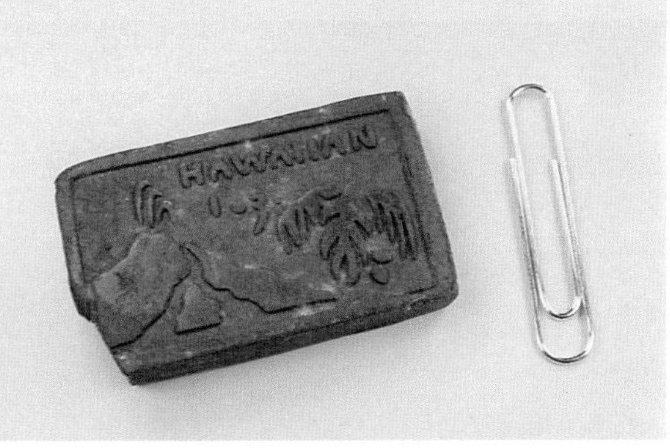

William Hurst

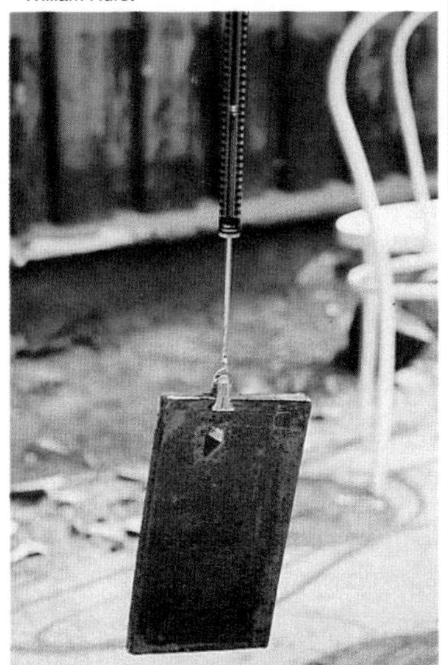

◄ Weighing a slab of hash of approximately 16 ounces.

➤ Hash oil is a refined oily extract of the marijuana plant that has a very high THC content, generally ranging from 20% to 60%. Because hash oil is light sensitive, it is normally packaged in dark colored glass vials.

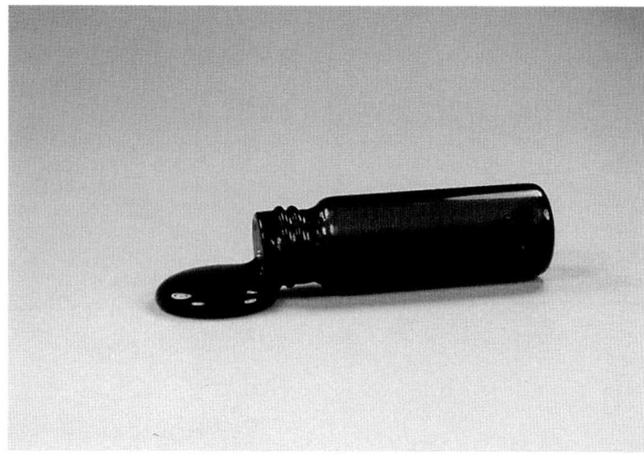

Bob Harris

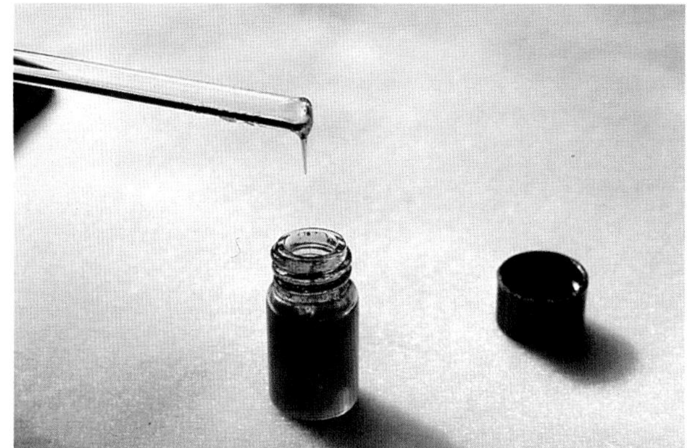

◄ Vial of red hash oil. Hash oil varies in color from a light honey, to red, to green, to brown, to coal black. Generally, lighter colors are indicative of more sophisticated refinement techniques and thus have a higher THC content than the darker varieties.

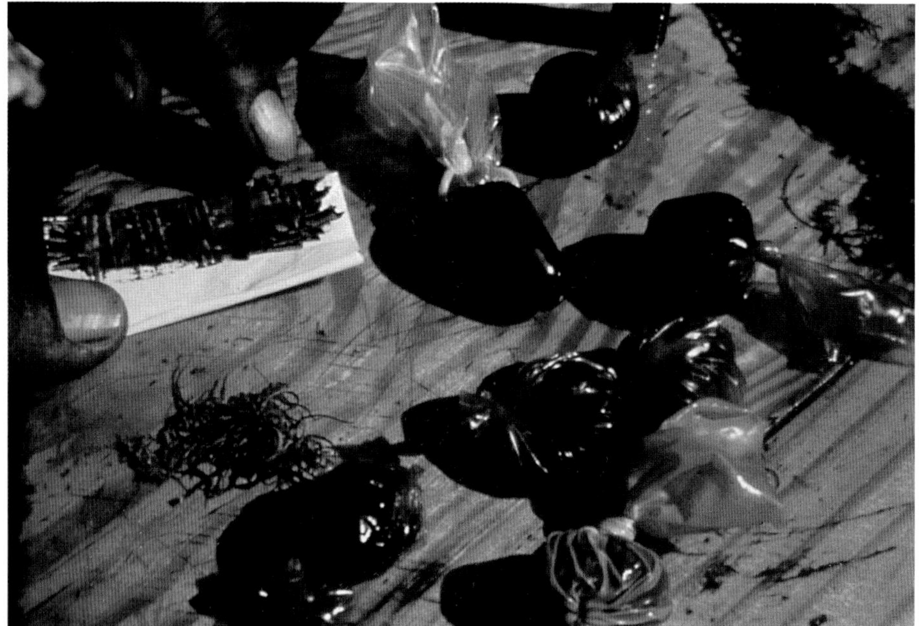

Laurence Cherniak

▲ Hash oil is typically added to marijuana to enhance its potency. In this photo hash oil contained in prophylactic packaging is being smeared onto the paper used to roll the joints. Hash oil is also sometimes vaporized by itself in pipes and smoked.

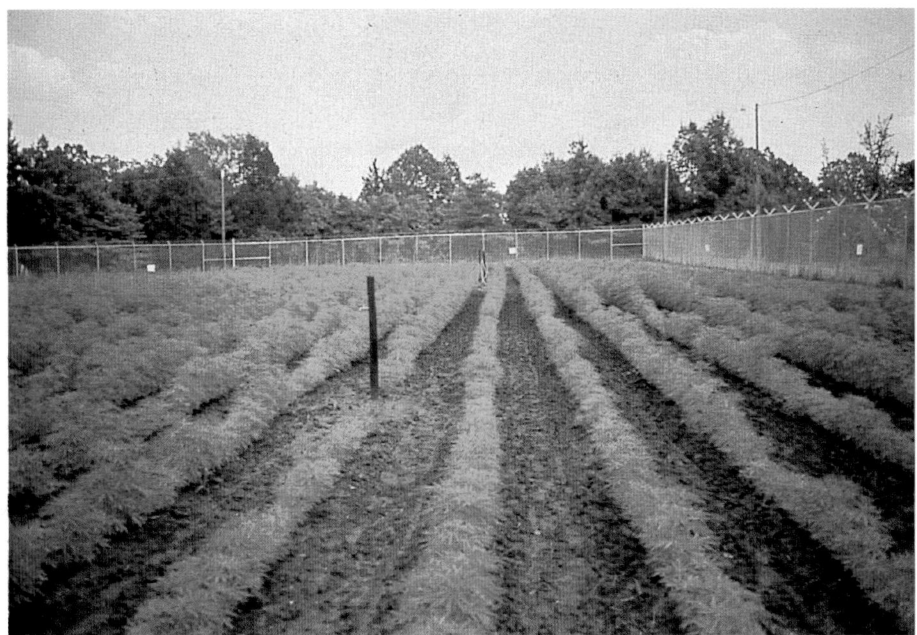

▲ A plot on the University of Mississippi's experimental marijuana farm. Some of the marijuana is currently supplied to eight individuals with serious illnesses under the FDA's Investigational New Drug Program. The IND program is not currently accepting any additional participants.

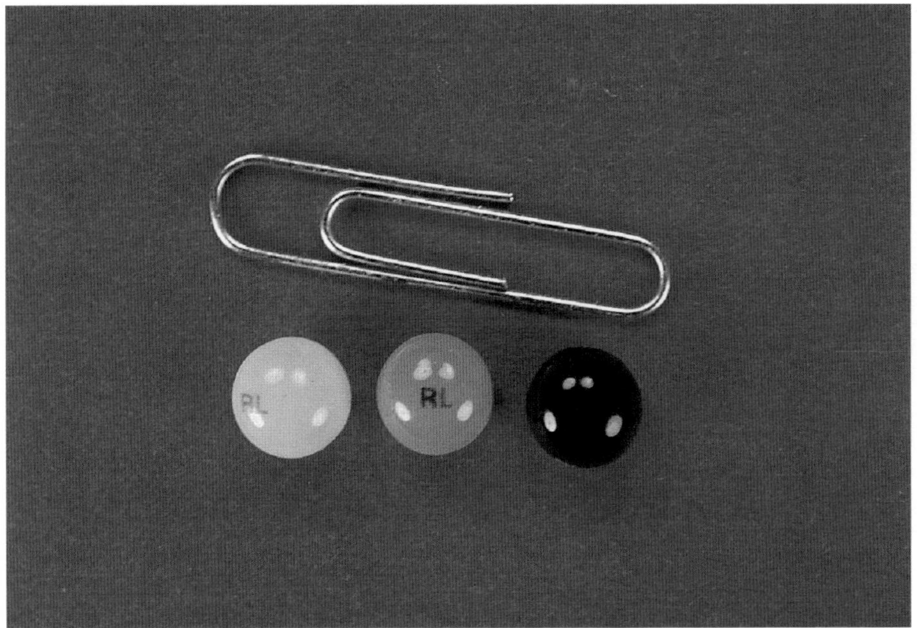

▲ A synthetic marijuana marketed as "Marinol" is available as a prescription drug in 2.5, 5, and 10 milligram capsules. It is used to control nausea in chemotherapy patients.

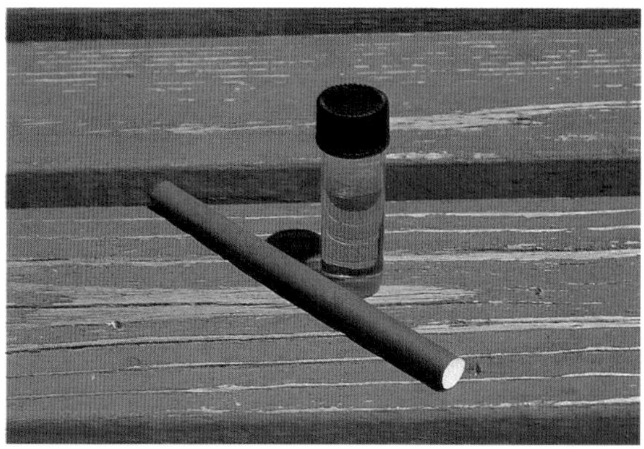

➤ A small glass vial containing about 3 cc's of liquid PCP. Dipping a cigarette into liquid PCP and then smoking it is the most common way of ingesting the drug. Sherman's brand of cigarettes (shown) is a perennial favorite of the PCP user, as the paper, which is thick and dark, withstands the saturation and helps conceal the fact that the cigarette has been dipped into a liquid.

➤ Part of a 22 gallon liquid PCP seizure made by the Los Angeles Police Department. The PCP was contained in one gallon glass apple juice jars. Assuming that the PCP would have been used to saturate commercial cigarettes (1cc of PCP to each cigarette), the estimated final retail street price could have reached two to five million dollars.

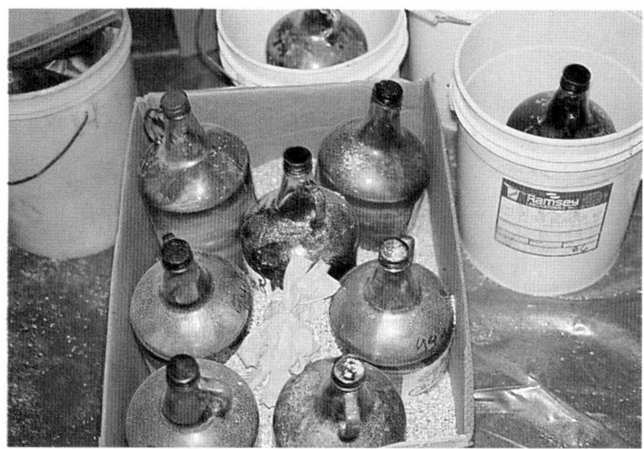

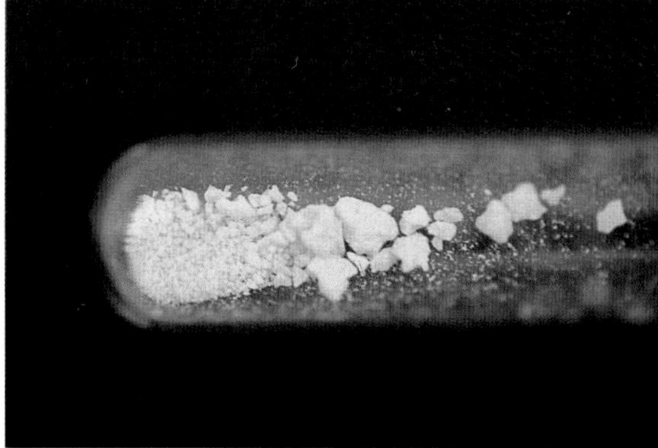

➤ Crystalline PCP in a small glass vial. This form is encountered less frequently than the liquid form of PCP and is usually much more expensive. Crystalline PCP may be snorted or added to vegetable matter, such as parsley, tobacco, or mint leaves and smoked.

➤ A chemical relative of PCP, Ketalar (brand name for ketamine hydrochloride) is used as a pre-operative general anesthetic. Although currently not controlled, the drug can produce hallucinations. It can be injected or allowed to evaporate and the remaining crystals snorted.

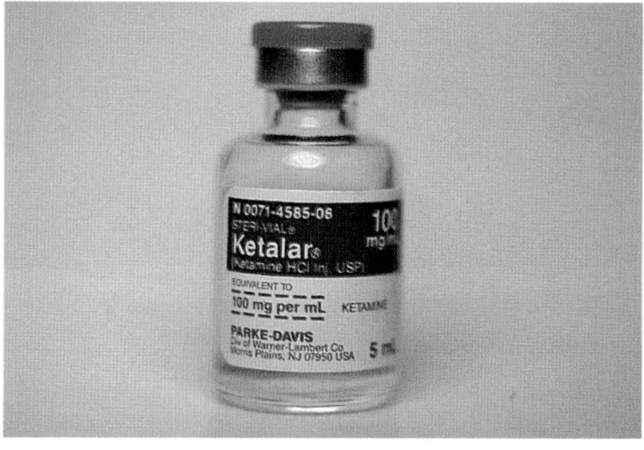

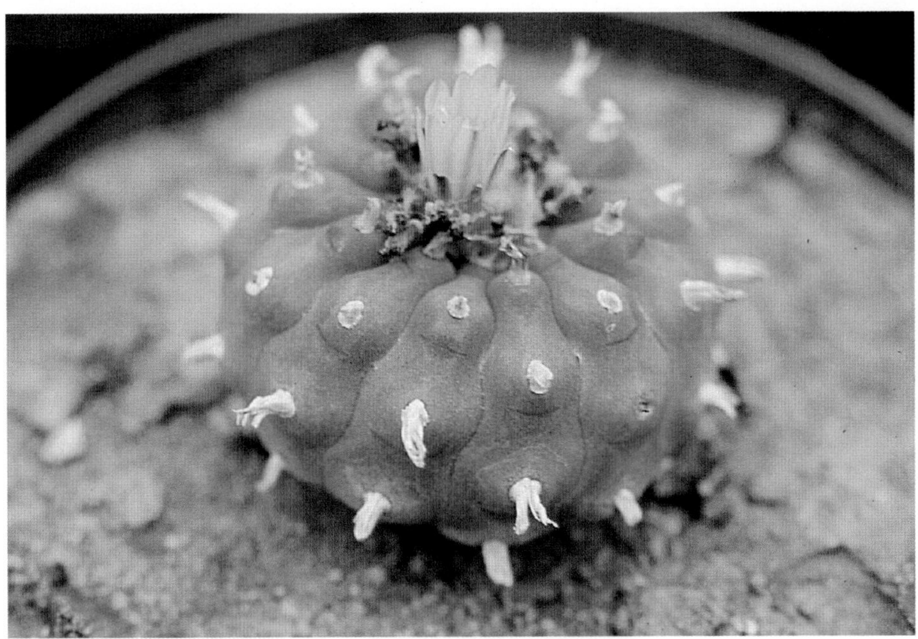

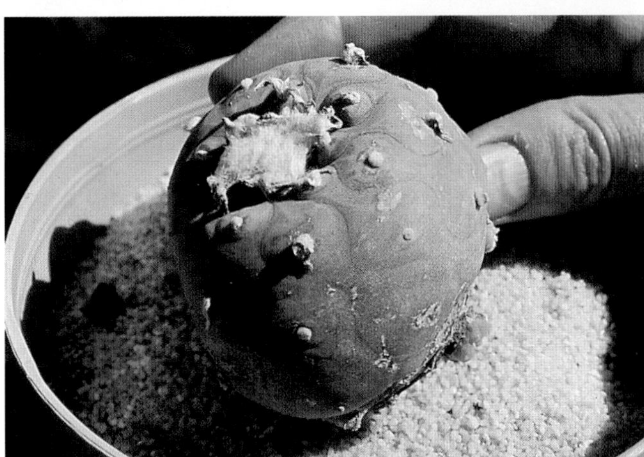

Paul Kroeger

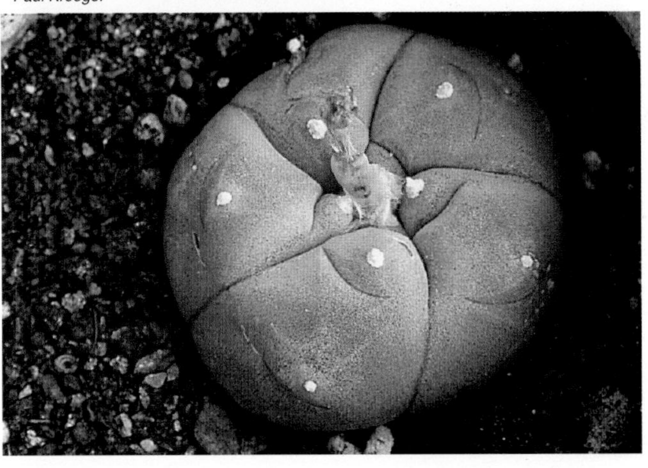

The peyote cactus is a small spineless cactus which grows wild only in north central Mexico and southern Texas, and contains the hallucinogenic substance mescaline. Ceremonial use of peyote by Indians of what is now Mexico predates recorded history. Although a Schedule I drug under the Controlled Substances Act, peyote is legally used by bona fide members of the Native American Church for religious purposes. Pictured are three specimens of peyote in different stages of development. Slow growing, it can take over a decade for a peyote cactus to grow to a diameter of only 3 inches. Once harvested, peyote buttons retain their potency for years.

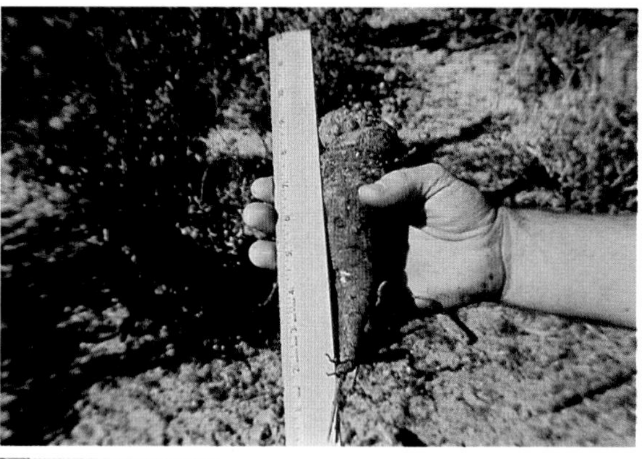

➤ The top of the peyote cactus, or "button", averages about 1" in diameter, although specimens may be as large as 4" or 5" in diameter. The relatively large and deep root contains only trace amounts of mescaline, and is normally left in place when the button is harvested. A new button or cluster of buttons will begin to develop on the root within three years.

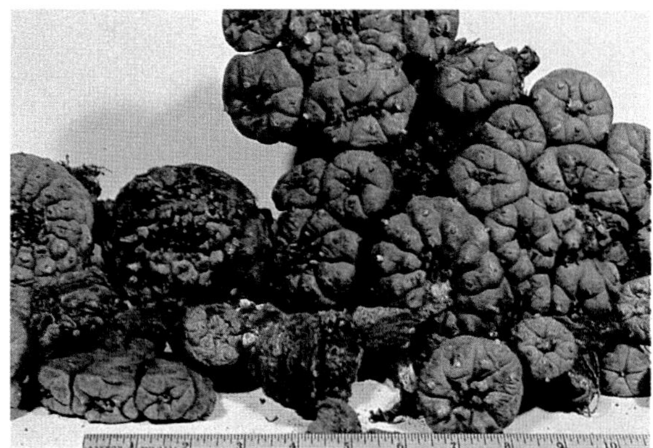

◄ Freshly harvested peyote buttons and button clusters. The Federal government and the state of Texas currently license 7 people to harvest peyote for sale to members of the Native American Church. Members of the Church may also harvest peyote after first providing proper documentation of their intent to the Texas Department of Public Safety.

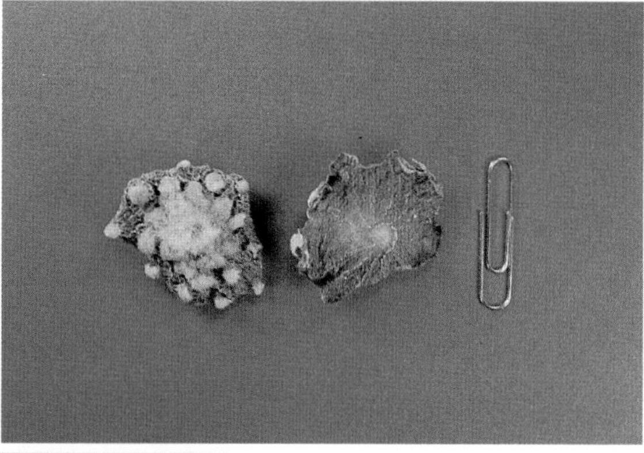

➤ Top and bottom view of dried peyote buttons about 1" in diameter. The street price for a single button generally ranges from $10.00 to $30.00. The texture of dried buttons is very hard and stiff and is without significant odor. The buttons may be chewed, encapsulated, or boiled to make a dark and somewhat thick tea.

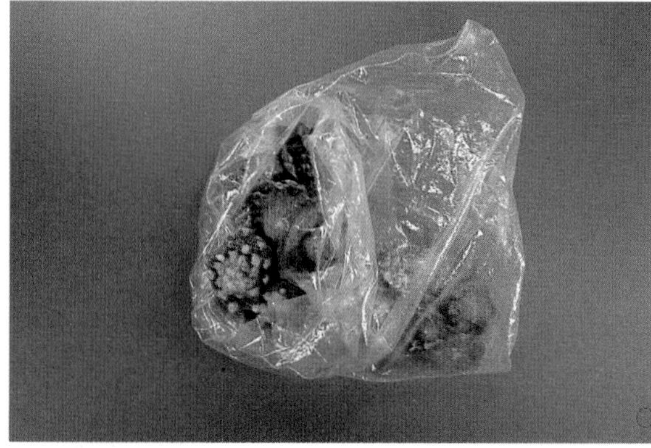

◄ A $200.00 bag of dried buttons packaged in a plastic sandwich bag. A typical dose usually consists of from three to twelve buttons, with an average button containing about 25 milligrams of mescaline. A mescaline high is reportedly very similar to an LSD high.

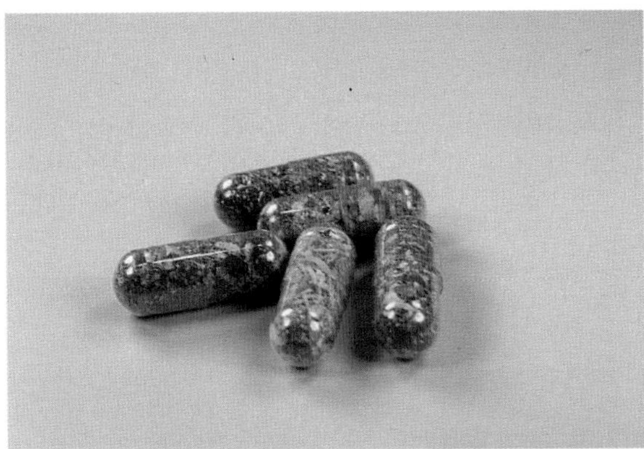

➤ Many users of peyote find the taste of the drug extremely bitter. For this reason they often grind the buttons with a mortar and pestle and then place the granulated buttons into oral gelatin capsules for consumption.

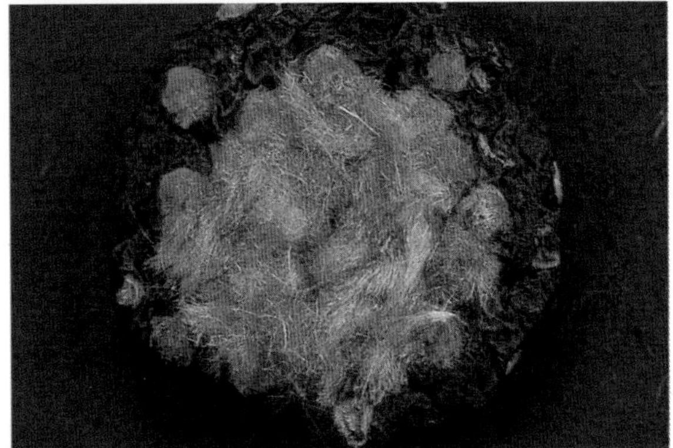

➤ Close-up of the top of a dried peyote button. The white hair in the center is often rumored to contain strychnine, but it is simply cellulose. No strychnine is contained in any part of the peyote cactus.

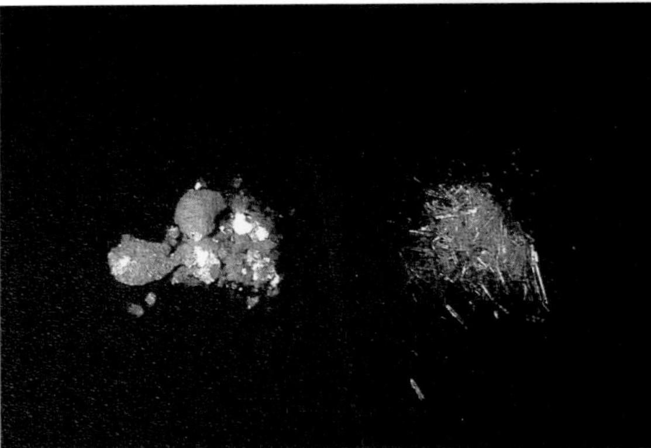

Bob Harris

➤ Two forms of mescaline, the main psychoactive substance in the peyote cactus. Mescaline may be extracted from the cactus or produced synthetically. On the left is mescaline hydrochloride, on the right mescaline sulfate. Most users of peyote do not possess the skills necessary to extract mescaline.

Jeremy Bigwood

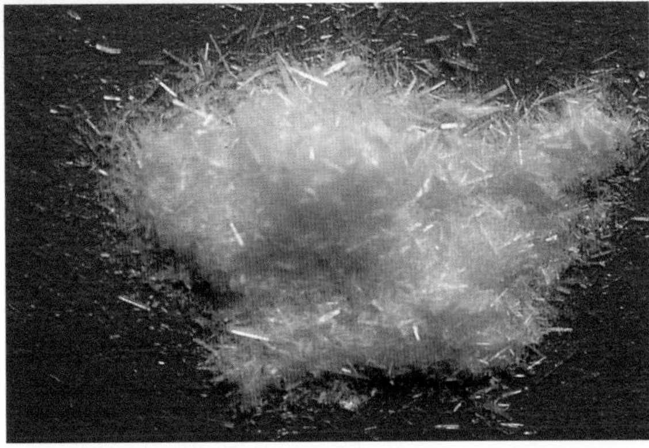

➤ Translucent, needle-shaped crystals of mescaline sulfate. The sulfate is reputed to be slightly more potent than the hydrochloride form.

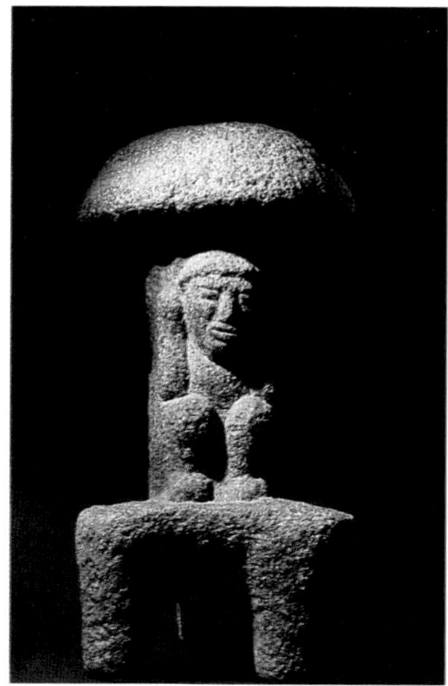

Stan Czolowski

◀ Stone artifact from the Mayan culture, dating back about 1,000 years. Psilocybin mushrooms have been used by Indian cultures of Mexico and Central America for at least 3,500 years.

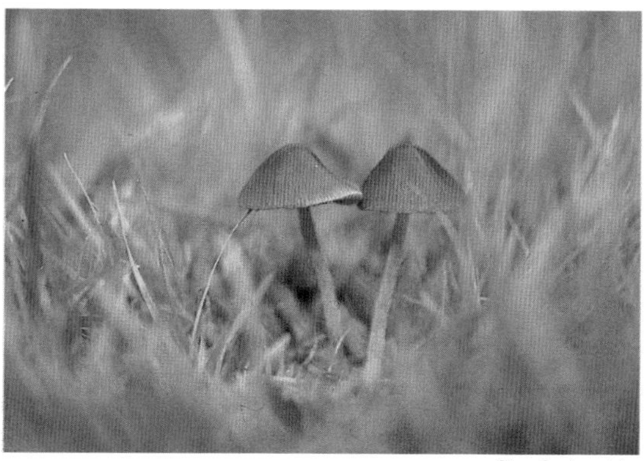

Stan Czolowski

▲ There are many species of mushrooms in North America which contain the hallucinogenic substances psilocybin and psilocin. Pictured are mushrooms of the conocybe cyanopus variety.

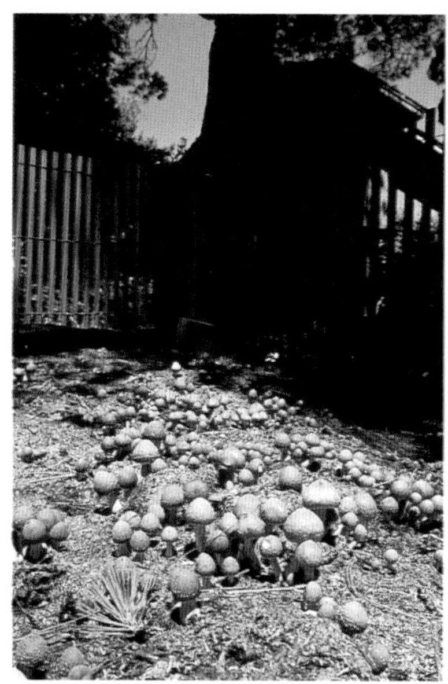

Bob Harris

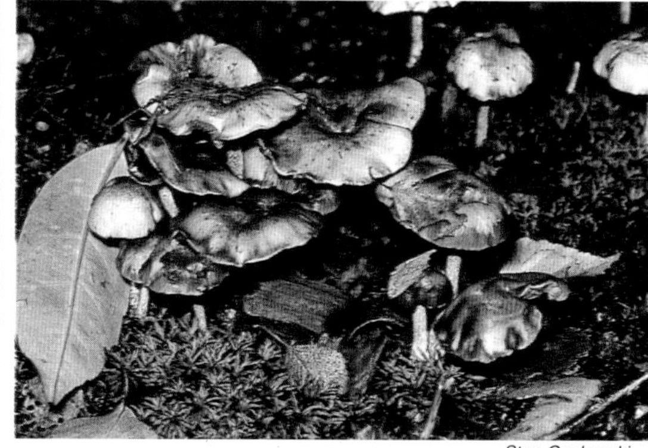

Stan Czolowski

▲ Outdoor cultivation of psilocybe cubensis mushrooms.

▲ Psilocybin mushrooms of the psilocybe baeocystis variety.

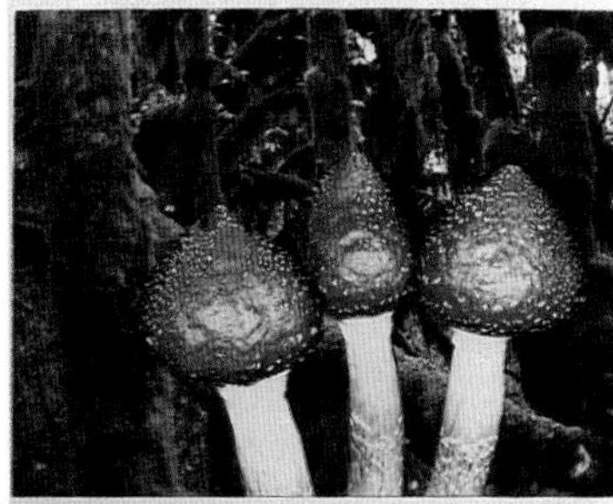

➤ Advertisement which regularly appears in *High Times* magazine. Although psilocybin mushrooms are a Schedule I drug, the spores, (a mushrooms equivalent of a seed) are not. Everything necessary to grow psilocybin mushrooms, including the spores, can be readily and legally purchased through a variety of sources.

➤ Indoor cultivation of psilocybe cubensis mushrooms. With street prices generally ranging from $100.00 to $200.00 per ounce, many indoor growing operations are quite large and profitable.

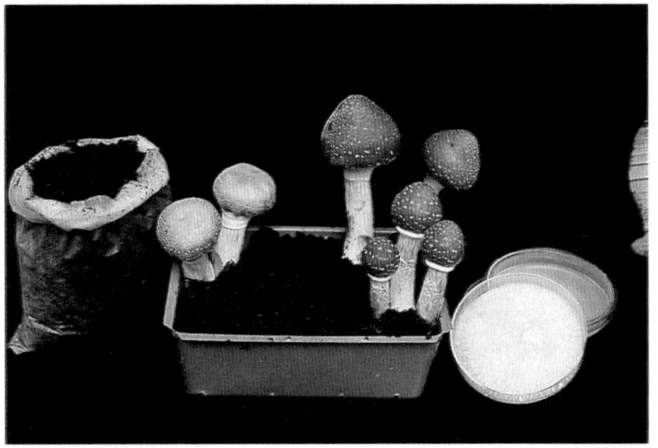

Bob Harris

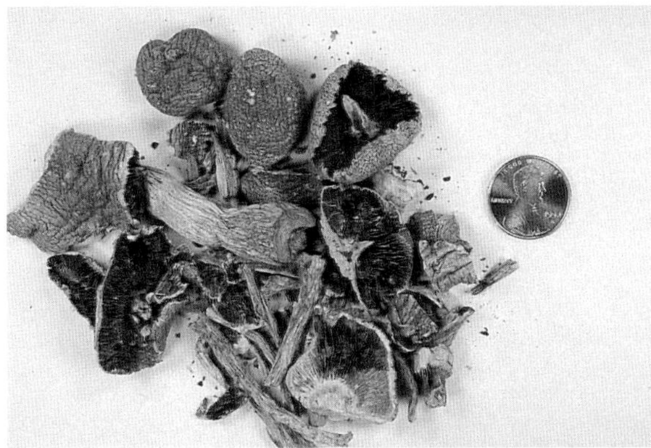

➤ One ounce of dried psilocybin mushrooms. Both the stem and cap are ingested, as both contain psilocybin.

➤ To prevent spoilage, psilocybin mushrooms are either air or low heat dried, and are normally packaged and distributed in plastic bags.

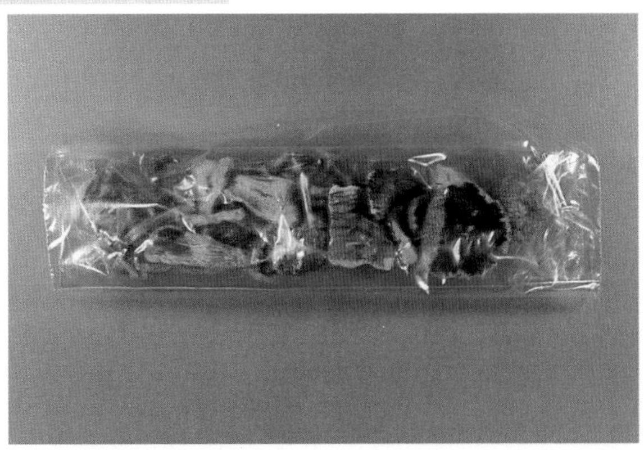

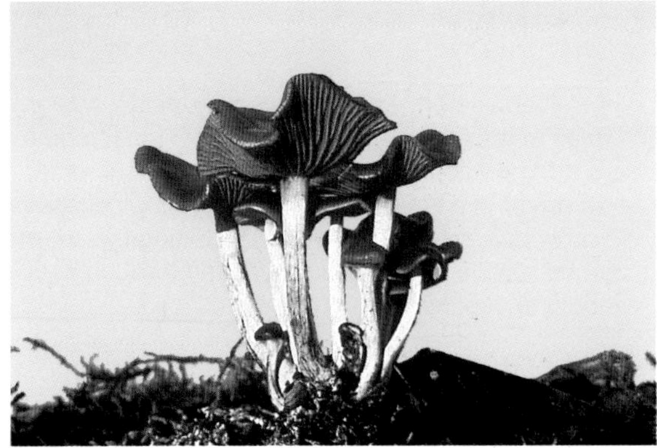

◄ Psilocybe cyanescens mushrooms, often called "wavy caps", reputed to be the most potent of the various psilocybin mushroom varieties.

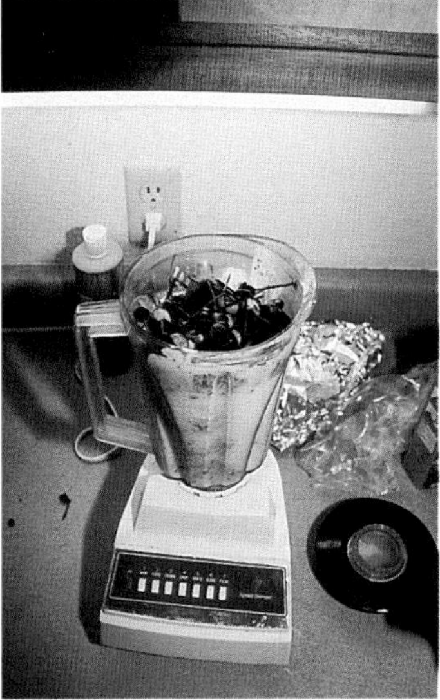

◄ Psilocybin mushrooms have a somewhat bitter taste, and many users opt to mix them with other foods or grind and place them in gelatin capsules. This user mixed the mushrooms with ice cream in a blender.

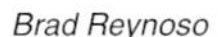

Brad Reynoso

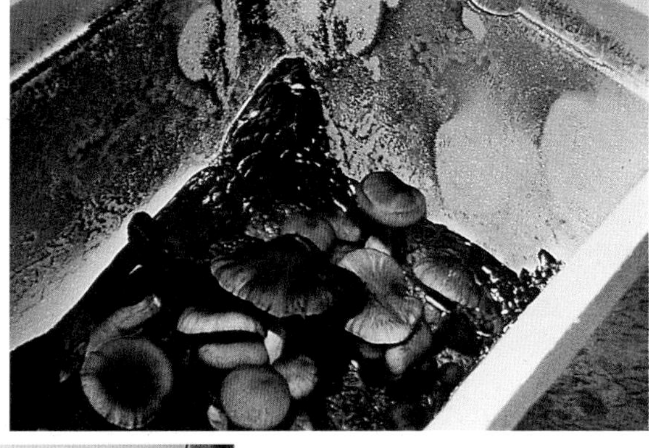

➤ Indoor cultivation of psilocybin mushrooms utilizing a large styrofoam cooler.

William Bartlett

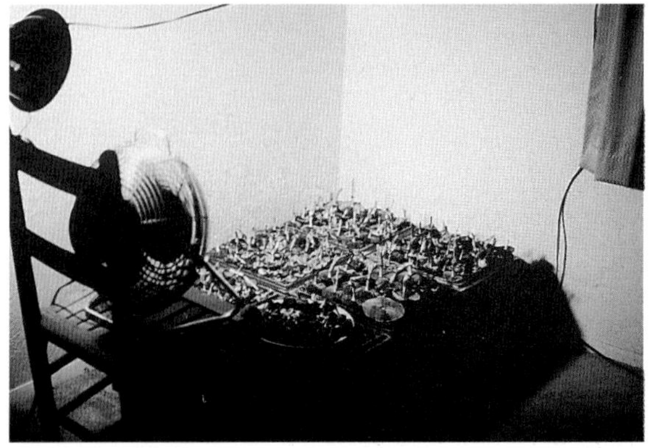

◄ Drying several dozen psilocybin mushrooms with the use of a fan and heat lamp. Other methods of drying mushrooms include placing them in an oven on low heat and sun drying.

AMPHETAMINES

CSA SCHEDULE: II

STREET NAMES: Batu, black beauties, chalk, copilots, crack meth, crank, cristy, crystal, dexies, drivers, glass, go, go fast, hanyak, Hawaiian salt, hearts, hiropon, ice, kaksonjae, L.A. turnarounds, leapers, meth, pep pills, quartz, shabu, speed, thrusters, ups, uppers, wake ups, wire, and zip.

PSYCHOPHYSICAL ACTION: Stimulant

STREET PRICES:

QUANTITY:	1990	1991	1992	1993
Pound	$6,000 - $20,000	$5,000 - $22,000	$5,000 - $25,0000	$4,000 - $20,000
Ounce	$500 - $2,500	$500 - $2,300	$300 - $2,500	$400 - $2,600
Gram	$50 - $150	$50 - $150	$30 - $200	$40 - $150

Source: Department of Justice

The term "amphetamine" is used generically to refer to any member of a class of drugs that have an amphetamine base, such as amphetamine, dextroamphetamine, and methamphetamine, and includes similar but less well known drugs. Most of the amphetamine or "speed" on the illicit market is methamphetamine. Amphetamines have many medical applications, and some of the more commonly used and prescribed are marketed under the registered names Dexedrine, Desoxyn and Ritalin.

HISTORY

Amphetamine was first synthesized in the 1880's, but its therapeutic possibilities were not investigated until 1927. The first medical product containing amphetamine, the Benzedrine inhaler, was marketed in 1932 to widen bronchial passages and help asthmatics breath. Soon after the product was introduced users found that not only did it dilate the bronchial passages, but it also relieved fatigue, increased energy levels, reduced the need for sleep and suppressed the appetite. Abuse of the drug started almost immediately.

Amphetamine became available in tablet form in 1937 and was used extensively during World War II by Japan, the United States, Great Britain and Germany. The drug was given to combat troops, and to civilians in some of the countries, to fight fatigue and maintain the alertness and energy levels required by combat and the war effort.

Medical use of amphetamines increased during the 1950's and they were routinely prescribed as antidepressants and diet pills. By 1962 legal production was estimated to be in excess of eight billion tablets annually. Use continued to increase and production peaked at an estimated twelve billion tablets in 1971, a substantial portion of which were diverted to the black market. The Controlled Substance Act of 1970 placed restrictions on the manufacture, distribution and use of amphetamines, and the 1972 production quota limited the amphetamine output to approximately 20% of the quantity manufactured in 1971. Amphetamine abuse has declined since the 1960's, but government estimates indicate that the drug is still used illegally by more than 1,750,000 Americans.

AMPHETAMINES

Percentage of Total DEA Laboratory Seizures by Drug (1992)

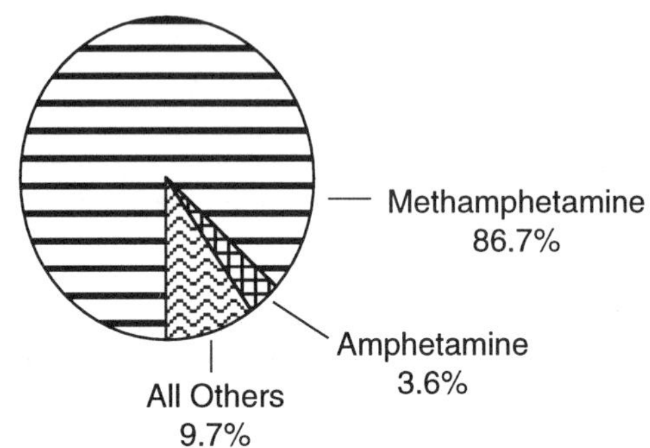

MANUFACTURE

Nearly all of the "amphetamine" on the street is methamphetamine, which is manufactured in illegal, or clandestine drug labs. Methamphetamine is the most prevalent clandestinely manufactured controlled substance in the U.S., with meth labs accounting for more than 80% of all illegal labs seized in recent years. The manufacture of methamphetamine requires little training, only a small amount of equipment, and chemicals that are relatively inexpensive. Most of the labs are located in the west and southwestern United States.

Nearly all of the illicit methamphetamine is produced by one of the following methods:

1. P2P Amalgam Method:
   For many years this was the most commonly used method. It uses phenyl-2-propanone (more commonly referred to as P2P) and methylamine as the primary precursors, along with mercuric chloride, hydrochloric acid, aluminum, isopropanol, and sodium hydroxide. In 1980, P2P was designated a Schedule II drug under the Controlled Substances Act. In order to use this method, operators must now manufacture their own P2P or obtain it on the black market.

2. Ephedrine Reduction:
   This method is now preferred over the P2P process. It is simpler and the end product is reportedly more potent because of a higher yield of the 'd' isomer in the methamphetamine. This process uses ephedrine, red phosphorous, hydriodic acid and aluminum. The key ingredient in this process is ephedrine, which is widely used in over-the-counter decongestants. Ephedrine is regulated under the Chemical Diversion and Trafficking Act, but is not subject to record keeping and reporting requirements when used in a drug product, even when it is the only active ingredient. Because of this loophole in the law, tablets consisting of 30% to 40% ephedrine are freely advertised and clandestine laboratory operators have a steady supply of chemicals needed to manufacture amphetamines.

AMPHETAMINES

The methamphetamine produced by the above methods is generally a white to tan powder. It is usually cut, or diluted to a purity of 40% to 50% by adding sodium bicarbonate, lidocaine, lactose, mannitol, procaine, or other similar substance.

The operator of a clandestine lab may be forced to use intermediate chemicals to produce a key chemical if it cannot be obtained through legal or black market channels. Because of this the chemicals used may vary from lab to lab. Listed below are the most common chemicals used by clandestine labs in the manufacture of amphetamines:

- Acetaldehyde
- Acetic acid
- Acetic anhydride
- Acetone
- Allyl chloride
- Allylbenzene
- Aluminum
- Ammonia
- Ammonium acetate
- Ammonium formate
- Ammonium hydroxid
- Benzaldehyde
- Benzene
- Benzyl chloride
- Chloroform
- Ephedrine
- Ethyl ether
- Formamide
- Freon
- Hexane
- Hydrochloric acid
- Hydrogen peroxide
- Hydroxylamine
- Iodine
- Isopropanol
- Lead acetate
- Lithium aluminum hydride
- Magnesium
- Mercuric chloride
- Methanol
- Methylamine
- Monomethylamine
- N-Methylformamide
- Nitroethane
- Norpseudoephedrine
- Palladium
- Phenyl-2-propanone
- Phenylacetic acid
- Phenylpropanolamine
- Phosphoric acid
- Propiophenone
- Pyridine
- Red phosphorous
- Sodium
- Sodium carbonate
- Sodium cyanide
- Sodium hydroxide
- Sulfuric acid
- Thionyl chloride
- Toluene

INGESTION

Amphetamines can be snorted, smoked, taken orally, or injected. Beginning or occasional users often snort the drug, but this method of ingestion is generally not used long term due to the irritation caused to the nasal lining. Ingesting amphetamine by smoking it in a glass pipe is becoming increasingly popular. Ice, a very pure crystal form of methamphetamine, is also usually smoked in a glass pipe.

Like heroin, amphetamines can be mixed with water and "cooked" in a metal spoon or similar device to prepare it for injection. Licit and illicit amphetamines are also manufactured in tablet and capsule form.

Regardless of the method of ingestion, the user can quickly develop a tolerance to the drug. Once a tolerance has developed, larger doses are required for the same high. Medical dosage of amphetamines seldom exceed 60 mg per day, but chronic abusers, or speed freaks, may ingest more than 5,000 mg every twenty four hours during a "speed run" lasting three to five days. After the end of the speed run, the abuser "crashes" and may sleep for one to two days. The abuser then experiences a state of depression, which may last for weeks unless amphetamines are taken, resulting in a repeat of the speed run - crash cycle.

AMPHETAMINES SURPASSED ONLY BY MARIJUANA IN PERCEIVED AVAILABILITY BY 1994 HIGH SCHOOL SENIORS

DRUG	% OF STUDENTS SAYING FAIRLY EASY OR VERY EASY TO GET
Marijuana	85.5
Amphetamines	62.0
LSD	50.8
Cocaine powder	43.7
Barbiturates	43.3
Steroids	42.9
Crack	40.5
Tranquilizers	39.2
Other opiates	38.0

Source: University of Michigan

ICE

Ice is a very pure, smokeable form of dextromethamphetamine hydrochloride. Ice first appeared in the Far East, and its manufacture and use is still centered in South Korea, Taiwan, and Hong Kong. However, ice has gained a user following in Hawaii and on the east and west coasts. Although ice received a substantial amount of media publicity, the drugs popularity has not lived up to expectations.

Ice is extremely powerful, having a purity which is generally in excess of 90%. It is usually smoked in a glass pipe. The physical and mental effects of smoking ice are very similar to those of crack, with one notable exception. The effects of crack wear off in ten to twenty minutes, while the effects of ice last for eight to sixteen hours.

Ice, as its name implies, has an appearance similar to broken pieces of ice or glass, but has also been seen with a clear yellowish color as well. It is usually packaged in plastic bags or paper bindles. Ice is one of the most expensive illicit drugs. The price for 1/10 gram ranges between $100.00 to $200.00, the gram price ranges between $600.00 to $1,000.00, and the ounce price from $9,000.00 to $16,000.00.

CAT

Cat is a common street name for methcathinone, a drug which is closely related to amphetamine. Cat first appeared on the American drug scene in Wisconsin in 1991, and its use steadily spread across America. Because of its high potential for abuse, methcathinone was placed in Schedule I of the CSA on May 1, 1992.

Manufacturing methcathinone is simple, and the chemicals used are inexpensive. As with methamphetamine, ephedrine is the key ingredient in manufacturing cat. The ephedrine is extracted from commercially available tablets and capsules, and is then oxidized by adding chromium salts such as sodium chromate or potassium dichromate. The final product is a off-white or yellowish powder. It is usually smoked or snorted, and its effects are similar to those of methamphetamine.

EFFECTS

Amphetamine is a central nervous system stimulant. It relieves fatigue, reduces the need for sleep, increases the energy and confidence level, and in general brings about a psychological and physical exhilaration. These effects are almost identical to those of cocaine. Individuals who use both cocaine and amphetamine often find it difficult to distinguish between the effects of the two drugs. There is one very important difference; the effects of cocaine lasts for only twenty to eighty minutes, but those of amphetamines are much more prolonged, lasting four to twelve hours.

Many individuals can handle an occasional amphetamine "pep pill" without any problems. The danger lies in the fact that psychological dependence can develop very easily, and this often leads to heavy and continual use.

Depending on the individual and the amount of the drug ingested, a high can last for four to twelve hours. As the effects begin to wear off, the heavy user is faced with the alternative of taking another dose or going through the "crash" and depression of withdrawal. Most users choose to "rehit" and the cycle of heavy use continues. Prolonged use of higher doses brings on many physical and mental problems. The most common conditions are:

Irritability
Mental confusion
Aggressiveness
Restlessness
Increased heartbeat and blood pressure
Increased respiration and body temperature
Weight loss
Anxiety and tension
Defective reasoning
Poor judgement
Dryness of lips and mouth

Long term high dosage users may experience the feeling that bugs or insects are "crawling" under their skin. This sensation is called formication, and the bugs are referred to as speed or crank bugs. Abusers experiencing this sensation can severely injure themselves by trying to dig or cut the "bugs" out of their skin. High level users may also experience a compulsion known as stereotypy, which causes the individual to repeatedly perform routine acts.

Chronic abusers of amphetamine may experience a psychosis called amphetamine delusional disorder or amphetamine psychosis. The individual may experience delusions, visual and auditory hallucinations, and can become violent. The psychosis is almost identical to that caused by cocaine.

Amphetamine withdrawal is very difficult for some individuals. It is generally agreed that amphetamine is not physically addictive, but it does have a very high degree of psychological addiction. For high dosage users, withdrawal symptoms start almost as soon as the high wears off. The individual may experience severe depression, a decrease in energy and activity levels, difficulty in sleeping, and a strong desire to again use the drug.

AMPHETAMINES

PHARMACOLOGY

Amphetamine is a sympathomimetic amine which has greater CNS stimulant activity than epinephrine (adrenaline) and ephedrine. It appears to work by enhancing the release of norepinephrine which causes numerous effects including CNS and respiratory stimulation and increased blood pressure. The main site of action is the cerebral cortex and possibly the reticular-activating system which together account for increased motor activity, mental alertness and euphoria. Psychic stimulation and excitability over fatigue are also related to the drug's action on the CNS. Hallucinations, delirium, paranoia and combativeness may be related to amphetamines action on neurotransmitters such as serotonin and dopamine in much the same way that hallucinogens, LSD and mescaline, act within the brain.

∎

ANABOLIC STEROIDS

CSA SCHEDULE: III

STREET NAMES: Anabolic steroids, androgens, hormones, juice, roids, steroids, vitamins, product.

STREET PRICES: $15.00 to $1,000.00 per bottle.

Stories of great strength have intrigued our imaginations for centuries. We have television series like "The Bionic Man", and "The Incredible Hulk", comic book heroes like Superman, biblical supermen like Samson, legendary strongmen like Hercules, that staple of carnivals, the sideshow strong man, professional wrestlers, and a long list of male movie stars who's muscular bodies are the main attraction for the ticket-buying public. Weight-lifting competitions are popular Olympic events. Bodybuilding contests attract large audiences. Children watching television cartoons aspire to the impossible-to-achieve muscularity of superheroes such as He-Man. Popeye's spinach eating produces the great strength that allows him to vanquish his comical opponent Brutus.

Clearly, there is something about muscular development and great strength that taps into something very basic to the male mentality. Sexual attractiveness is part of this. Men want to impress the women with their muscles. Some men feel that they cannot compete with the guy that has a great body. It is a real incentive for them to try to develop their own bodies as fast as possible. Steroids present the promise that such aspirations can be achieved quickly through chemistry.

HISTORY

In 1849, a German scientist demonstrated that the regression of a castrated roosters comb, wattles and behavior could be reversed by placing a testis in the roosters abdominal cavity. The testis returned necessary hormones to the blood supply of the rooster and restored its male characteristics. Related studies continued for several decades, and by the mid-1930's it was determined that the male body produced several compounds with hormone-like activity. These various compounds were given the name *androgens* (from the Greek, andro for male, and gen for produce).

The use of steroids in athletics is generally attributed to the Soviet weight lifting team in the early 1950's. In 1954, at the world weight lifting championships in Vienna, Dr. John Ziegler, the U.S. team physician, reportedly discovered that the Soviets were taking testosterone. Dr. Zeigler returned to the United States and experimented with testosterone on himself and other weight lifters, several of which quickly obtained championship status. In 1956, Dr. Ziegler, with the assistance of Ciba Labs, developed a very effective and perhaps the most well known anabolic steroid, Dianabol, brand name for methandrostenolone. Methandrostenolone no longer has FDA approval in the United States, but is smuggled from other countries where it is still legally manufactured.

Although steroid use among athletes was common for quite some time, it was not until the 1988 Olympics that the problem became so well known or publicized. During these Olympics, Canadian sprinter Ben Johnson posted the fastest time ever in the 100 meter dash, making him the fastest runner in history. Two days later, Johnson tested positive for the steroid stanozolol, and he was stripped of the gold medal. In response to the revelations of steroid use among athletes and teenagers, anabolic steroids were placed in Schedule III of the CSA in October, 1990.

ANABOLIC STEROIDS

STEROID TYPES

Although there are many different types of hormones (estrogens, progestins, thyroid, glucocorticoids, etc.), the androgens are the compounds which cause development of secondary male sex characteristics, such as facial hair, deepening of the voice, and muscle mass and strength. Androgens also promote aggression - a characteristically male trait, male pattern baldness, and growth during early puberty. The most active androgen is testosterone, which is produced mainly in the testicles.

An anabolic steroid is basically a synthetic version of the male hormone testosterone. Virtually all anabolic steroids are derived from substances found in the Mexican Sarsaparilla root. It is believed the primary force of testosterone and it's synthetic substitutes on the muscle is to increase the body's synthesis of protein, thereby allowing the muscles to become larger and stronger when subjected to strenuous exercise. Anabolic steroids are also believed to exert their influence by diminishing the effect of glucocorticoids - hormones which cause protein degradation and muscular atrophy. In current pharmaceutical literature, approximately twelve different anabolic/androgenic products have FDA approval in the United States. However, steroid users smuggle these drugs from all over the world, resulting in dozens of different types of steroids appearing on the black market.

Scientific studies of anabolic steroids in regards to building muscle and strength vary, probably due in large part to the variant amounts of steroids administered. For instance, researchers would not ethically administer the same high dose of a steroid to a test subject that an athlete would routinely administer to himself. Additionally, steroid abusers most often use more than one steroid at a time to saturate the steroid receptor sites of the body, referred to as "stacking". Also, certain individuals, due to genetic structure, posses exceptional ability to increase muscular strength and size as a result of steroid use. These individuals are the rare exception however, and most athletes do not respond considerably to steroids. In the words of the American College of Sports Medicine: *"The gains in muscular strength achieved through high intensity exercise and proper diet can be increased by the use of anabolic/androgenic steroids in some individuals."*

Anabolic steroids are manufactured in oral tablets and liquid injectables. The injectables are the more popular of the two forms. Injectable steroids are packaged in small glass vials which may contain 1cc, 2 cc's, 5 cc's, 10 cc's, 30 cc's, or 50 cc's each. Because most injectable steroids are contained in thick sesame or cottonseed oil, needles used for their injection are much larger than insulin type needles. And because the fatty tissues of the buttock is the most common injection site, the needles are usually one to two inches long. Steroids are also occasionally injected into the muscles of the biceps and legs. No steroids are injected intravenously.

Although some doctors would prescribe steroids for athletes in the recent past, the practice almost never occurs now, and steroid users have had to resort to the black market, which is estimated to involve hundreds of millions of dollars each year. The steroid black market is filled with a multitude of American and foreign made steroids, particularly from Mexico, where steroids can be purchased on an over-the-counter basis. These steroids are commonly diverted from legitimate medical and veterinary channels. The black market is also filled, perhaps in a majority sense, with fake or "counterfeit" steroids produced illegally in basements, garages, and makeshift laboratories. These counterfeits are often professionally packaged and look very much like the authentic steroids, but usually contain substantially less of the steroid than the label indicates, or contain only inert ingredients. Steroid sales activity is generally centered around local gyms, although substantial amounts of steroids are shipped through various package delivery services.

USE

When using steroids, athletes follow certain regimens. Oral steroids, because their effects dissipate rather quickly, are generally taken every day. Injectables are often used daily as well, but because they remain in the body longer, the user may only inject them every other day, every three days, once a week, etc. Some athletes take oral steroids exclusively, some only injectables, and some take both.

Most steroid users follow a regimen referred to as a "cycle". A cycle is a predetermined length of time that a steroid(s) is taken, followed by a period of time in which a different steroid(s) is taken, or a period of time in which no steroids are taken. Generally, a single cycle may last anywhere from six to twelve weeks. For instance, an athlete may take steroid A for three weeks, and then steroid B the following three weeks. Cycling is often used to minimize side effects caused by the steroids. Some athletes preparing for a sporting event may cycle steroids so that they benefit from a specific side effect, such as aggression, or to coincide peak effects of the steroids with an upcoming event.

A steroid user may reach what is called a "plateau", where his strength or muscle size has stopped progressing. To overcome the diminishing results, he may increase the amount of the steroid(s) he is currently taking, add another steroid to his regimen, change the steroid(s) he is taking altogether, or any combination of the above.

Although anabolic steroids are unique among controlled drugs in that they are not psychoactive or physically addicting, they can cause many serious and potentially life-threatening side effects. Some of the more serious and common side effects include cancer of the liver, prostate and kidney, blood filled liver cysts, cardiovascular problems due to high blood pressure and cholesterol imbalance, gynecomastia (male breast enlargement), jaundice, testicular atrophy, and stunted growth in teenagers. Severe acne, male pattern baldness, and depression are other common side effects caused by steroids. Body hair and a deepening voice are irreversible effects that may be experienced by women taking steroids.

▮

COCAINE

CSA SCHEDULE: II

STREET NAMES: Bernice, big C, blow, C, chick, coke, Corine, dust, flake, girl, happy dust, her, nieve, nose candy, nose stuff, snow, toot, uptown, white, and white girl. Freebase is variously known as base, hubba, roca, rock, crack, Roxane, and white pipe.

PSYCHOPHYSICAL ACTION: Stimulant

STREET PRICES:

QUANTITY	1990	1991	1992	1993
KILOGRAM	$11,000 - $40,000	$11,000 - $40,000	$11,000 - $42,000	$10,500 - $40,000
OUNCE	$500 - $2,500	$400 - $2,500	$350 - $2,200	$300 - $2,600
GRAM	$35 - $175	$35 - $175	$15 - $150	$15 - $200

Source: Department of Justice

To the user, it's coke, C, snow, blow, toot, and nose candy. To the chemist it's $C_{17}H_{21}NO_4$. To the physiologist, it is a powerful stimulant of the central nervous system. To the botanist, it is an alkaloid which is contained in the leaves of the coca plant.

To the economy, legally produced coca leaves and cocaine are important commercial products, particularly for the United States. By international agreement, coca leaves under government control are legally harvested in Bolivia and Peru. Under the same international agreement, cocaine is legally produced only in the United States and Peru. The International Narcotics Control Board estimated that the United States imported 660,000 pounds of coca leaves in 1993, and 619,000 pounds in 1994, primarily for the extraction of flavoring agents. Cocaine is obtained as a by-product of this extraction process. The Board estimated that the United States produced 880 pounds of cocaine in 1993 and 400 pounds in 1994 for medical application.

To the illicit drug industry, cocaine is a source of untold wealth. It is impossible to accurately determine the size of the illicit market, but it is huge even by the most conservative estimates. Based on the acreage devoted to production of coca leaves, government estimates place the annual potential for production as high as 2,600,000 pounds. Conservative estimates indicate that over 1,000,000 people are involved in growing and harvesting coca leaves and the production of cocaine in the countries of Peru, Bolivia, and Colombia. The Office of National Drug Control Policy estimates that in 1990, Americans spent eighteen billion dollars for illegal cocaine.

An estimated twenty two million Americans have used cocaine at some time in their life, and hundreds of thousands use it daily. A few inject it, many smoke it in the forms called freebase or crack, but most inhale it intranasally, or "snort" it.

HISTORY

For thousands of years the inhabitants of the Andes mountains of South America have chewed the leaves of the coca plant for the stimulating effect. The leaves of this plant are intertwined in the culture of these peoples, having been used in both civil and religious rituals for centuries. The Spanish conquerors considered leaf chewing paganistic, and

COCAINE

tried to ban this centuries old practice. They had a change of heart when they realized that the peasants worked harder if they chewed coca leaves, and the practice was allowed to continue and continues to this day. It is estimated that as many as 90% of the Indians living in the regions where coca is grown still chew the plants leaves. When the leaf is chewed, along with a small amount of lime, the cocaine is gradually released and absorbed by the body. The cocaine content of the leaf is small, about $^1/_2$% to 1% by weight, but the amount is sufficient to stave off fatigue and enable the user to work harder in the harsh environment.

Cocaine was first isolated from the other substances found in the coca leaf in 1860 by a German graduate student, Albert Nieman. Physicians in Europe and the United States began investigating medicinal applications for what many regarded as a wonder drug, a safe treatment for a whole spectrum of physical and psychological maladies. In 1884, Dr. Karl Koller discovered the local anesthetic properties of cocaine and began using it in eye surgery. At that time, cocaine was the only local anesthetic available, and its use was quickly extended to other types of surgery.

One of the most enthusiastic proponents of cocaine was Sigmund Freud. The Austrian psychoanalyst gave it to his patients, his colleagues, and his fiancee. He wrote and spoke extensively about its value in the treatment of depression, nervousness, alcohol and morphine dependence, and other ailments.

Reports of the drugs hazardous side effects - obsessive use, psychosis, convulsions, even death, began appearing in the medical literature near the end of the century. The first death as a result of a cocaine related cardiac arrest was reported in 1886. Freud, by then a long time habitual user himself, conceded in his final paper on the subject that cocaine causes rapid physical deterioration, as well as paranoia, hallucinations, and other severe psychiatric problems.

Around the turn of the century, cocaine was used in many medications, often in combination with alcohol and opium. Many of these medications contained a relatively high percentage of cocaine, and their use created addiction in many patients. Vin Mariani, a bordeaux wine containing six milligrams of cocaine per ounce, was used and endorsed by the leading political, religious, and literary figures of the day. Cocaine preparations were a popular treatment for asthma and hay fever. One of the most widely used medications for this purpose was Dr. Nathan Tucker's Asthma Specific, which contained 420 milligrams of cocaine per ounce and was applied directly to the nasal passages. Many soft drinks and soda fountain preparations contained cocaine, as did varieties of chewing gum and tea. Cigarettes and cigars containing cocaine were promoted by pharmaceutical companies as a medical cure for fatigue and as a source of increased vigor.

Eventually physicians and scientists built a solid case against the abuse of cocaine, and its use was restricted with the passage of the Pure Food and Drug Act of 1906. Cocaine was later labeled a narcotic under the Harrison Narcotic Act of 1914. Cocaine is still legally classified as a narcotic, although the common present day definition of a narcotic usually includes only those substances obtained from the opium poppy plant.

Cocaine is a Schedule II drug under the Controlled Substances Act, meaning it has legitimate medical uses, but also has a high potential for abuse. Today, cocaine is medically used primarily as a local anesthetic for ear, nose and throat surgery. The legal manufacture, distribution, and use of cocaine is tightly controlled and monitored.

COCAINE

ESTIMATED 1991 COCAINE PRODUCTION

COUNTRY	NET COCA CULTIVATION (ACRES)	COCA LEAF YIELD (TONS)	COCAINE HCl PRODUCTION (TONS)
PERU	298,376	244,970	710 - 759
BOLIVIA	118,313	86,240	275 - 462
COLOMBIA	92,625	33,000	66

Source: Department Of Justice

THE COCA PLANT

There are four varieties of the coca plant that produce leaves which are used for the production of cocaine: Erythroxylum coca, Erythroxylum ipadu, Erythroxylum novogratense, and Erythroxylum truxillense. Of these varieties, Erythroxylum coca is the most prevalent, accounting for perhaps 95% of the cocaine produced.

The coca plant grows almost exclusively in the Andean mountains of South America, and primarily in the countries of Peru, Bolivia and Colombia. It can grow to a height of thirty feet, but cultivated coca bushes are usually pruned down to about six feet for ease in harvesting the leaves. The coca plant yields abundant supplies of these leaves, which are typically harvested three times each year, and in some cases as many as six times.

Each coca bush will yield an average of four ounces of green leaves. After drying, the leaves lose at least 60% of their weight, so the average bush will yield about 1.6 ounces of dried leaves. Usually an acre will contain about 7,000 plants grown two or three feet apart. Therefore, the average yield of green leaves per acre is about 1,800 pounds. Since leaves are normally harvested three or four times a year, the grower usually produces about 5,400 pounds of green leaves per acre per year, or 2,160 pounds of dried leaves.

There are three markets for the coca leaf:

1) Traditional market. Purchased by local people primarily for chewing. Also used as tea and in a number of food preparations.
2) Legitimate market. Coca leaves are an important source of flavoring agents. Medically, cocaine is used as a local anesthetic for ear, nose and throat surgery.
3) Illicit cocaine market. The vast majority of the coca leaf production flows into this channel.

PRODUCTION

The production of cocaine hydrochloride begins with stripping the leaves off the coca plant. Once harvested, the leaves are dried and put through a chemical process to extract the cocaine as follows:

> The dried leaves are taken to a "pasta lab", which is generally located near the growing area. The leaves are shredded or

COCAINE

mashed and placed in drums or plastic lined pits called maceration pits. Depending on the size of the operation, the pit may be as long as forty feet.

Water and a strong alkali, such as lime, are added to breakdown the leaves and release the cocaine. The mixture is left to soak for several days. A solvent such as kerosene or gasoline is added to the mixture to dissolve the cocaine. The kerosene/cocaine solution is pumped or drained from the pit for further processing.

Sulfuric acid is added to the kerosene. An alkali is then added and an intermediate product, cocaine sulfate, precipitates out and is filtered from the kerosene/sulfuric acid mixture. The cocaine sulfate is then dried. This form of cocaine is known as "paste" or "pasta", and is relatively impure.

The paste is normally transported to Colombia for further processing in a "base lab". At the base lab the paste is dissolved in water and sulfuric acid, and potassium permanganate is then added to remove impurities. An alkali is added to precipitate the cocaine. The cocaine is then filtered out of the solution and dried. The product is cocaine base, which is not water soluble.

The cocaine base is then sent to a "crystal lab" for further processing. Most crystal labs are located in Colombia. There the cocaine is dissolved in acetone. Hydrochloric acid is added, which converts the cocaine base to cocaine hydrochloride. Ethanol is then added to the acetone/hydrochloric acid mixture to precipitate the cocaine hydrochloride. The solution is filtered to remove the cocaine hydrochloride, which is then dried. The dried cocaine hydrochloride has a purity of up to 90%. This form of cocaine is water soluble and can be snorted or dissolved in water and injected intravenously.

Quality control in these labs is unknown, and sometimes shortcuts are taken to speed up production, resulting in an off color, less pure product. Despite the primitive conditions, the production of the jungle laboratories is enormous. According to the U.S. Governments NNICC report for 1991, the potential cocaine production estimate for Peru, Bolivia and Colombia was approximately 2,600,000 pounds. How much was actually produced, and how much reached the streets of the United States is unknown. In 1991, over 134 tons of cocaine were seized in the United States, but supplies remained plentiful.

DISTRIBUTION

Once the cocaine hydrochloride is produced in the crystal labs of South America, it is ready for shipment to the world market. It is estimated that the United States consumes at least 70% of this production. Most of the cocaine is smuggled out of South America by private aircraft operating off of numerous unimproved airstrips. The cocaine is flown to distribution points in the Caribbean, Mexico, or Central America to be reshipped to the United States.

COCAINE

Cocaine Purity Data 1990 - 1993 National Range				
Quantity	1990	1991	1992	1993
Kilogram	80%	86%	83%	82%
Ounce	58%	72%	74%	70%
Gram	54%	59%	64%	63%

Source: Department Of Justice

Smugglers have proven to be very resourceful in attempting to get cocaine into the United States. More often than not they are successful. Smaller amounts may be smuggled through air freight or international mail shipments. Larger amounts may be flown in by private aircraft, boat, or by vehicle traffic from Mexico. Additionally, commercial flight passengers smuggle cocaine hidden in their luggage, in their clothing, taped to their bodies (body carrier), or even packaged in small balloons or condoms and swallowed. These "body packers", or "swallowers", as they are called, later defecate the rubber packages along with other fecal matter. Rupture of one of the packages while in the body would surely cause a massive overdose death. A swallower arrested at the Miami airport in 1990 was found to have swallowed 210 balloons containing a total of 3.16 pounds of cocaine.

A substantial portion of the cocaine reaching the United States arrives via smuggling routes that terminate in Southern California, Texas, Arizona, and Florida. Los Angeles, Phoenix, Houston, and Miami are the major staging areas and redistribution points for the United States. Shipments into these cities may weigh several hundred pounds or even several tons. The standard package for cocaine at this level is a kilogram (usually referred to as a kilo, kee, or k), the metric equivalent of 2.2 pounds.

CUTS

Most cocaine is "cut", "stepped on", or "stretched" three or more times with other substances before it reaches the user. A cut is a substance that has the same physical appearance as cocaine, but costs much less. The cut is added to artificially increase the weight and volume of the cocaine and thus increase the dealers profits. Because of the cuts, the purity of cocaine declines with each step in the distribution chain.

For example, the importer generally sells uncut cocaine in multi-kilo quantities to a limited number of large wholesalers. The large wholesalers in turn sell to a limited number of distributors in kilo quantities. The distributor cuts the cocaine he has purchased, and then sells to a large dealer in kilo or ounce quantities. The dealer also cuts the cocaine and sells to smaller dealers in ounce or less quantities. The smaller dealers add yet another cut and sell to the consumer in gram or fractional gram quantities.

Based on DEA statistics, cocaine purity drops from about 82% at the import level, to an average of about 63% at the gram or street level, but the purity of individual samples vary widely. Although many different substances have been used to cut cocaine, the more

COCAINE

commonly used cuts are listed below.

SUBSTANCE	NORMAL USE
Lidocaine	Local anesthetic
Ephedrine	Medicinal bronchodilator
Caffeine	An extract of coffee beans, tea leaves or kola nuts
Benzocaine	Local anesthetic
Phenylpropanolamine	Decongestant
Mannitol	A plant extract often used as a mild laxative
Lactose	Milk sugar; food additive
Dextrose (Glucose)	Corn sugar; food additive
Sucrose	Table sugar
Inositol	White powder form of vitamin B
Talc	Face powder, paint and plastic filler; toxic when inhaled
Flour	Ground and sifted grain
Corn starch	A carbohydrate obtained from corn; food additive
Procaine	Local anesthetic
Tetracaine	Local anesthetic
Amphetamine	A stimulant drug
PCP	An illicit drug
Quinine	A derivative of cinchona bark - treatment for malaria

If the street dealer were to purchase 1/8 ounce (3.5 grams) of cocaine, typically referred to as an "eight ball" for $350.00, and add 1.5 grams of mannitol, worth pennies, it would increase the weight to 5.0 grams. At the street level, this amount would sell for roughly $100.00 per gram, or a total selling price of $500.00. The street dealer would realize a profit of $150.00, all of which resulted from adding the cut.

Although many cuts are actually less toxic to the body than cocaine, some can be particularly dangerous to the user. When used for injection, cocaine is first dissolved in water. Many of the cuts are not water soluble, and the user attempts to filter those out by passing the cocaine/water solution through a piece of cotton as it is drawn into a syringe. If a harmful insoluble cut is not removed, it may kill or make the user seriously ill.

Cuts are present in varying levels in virtually all street cocaine samples. Novice or inexperienced users may simply rely on their dealer or "connection" for relatively pure cocaine, but experienced users employ various techniques to determine the purity of the cocaine they purchase:

APPEARANCE: The first observation made by the purchaser is the cocaine's appearance. Cocaine hydrochloride is seen in three basic forms: powder, flake, and rock (not to be confused with "rock" as it applies to crack). The flakes and rocks generally indicate a purer cocaine because they are difficult to cut without altering their physical appearance. The powdered form, called "duff", is easily cut because of the ease in adding adulterants with a similar appearance.

COCAINE

TASTE: Many users "taste" the cocaine before it is purchased. They place a very small amount of the powder on their tongue to see how it tastes, and how quickly it numbs the tongue. Many of the local anesthetic cuts that are used cause an immediate numbing effect, unlike the comparatively slow numbing caused by cocaine.

FEEL: The buyer rubs a small amount of cocaine between the thumb and forefinger to determine the consistency and how readily it dissolves.

SNORTING: Many users snort a sample of the cocaine in an effort to determine its purity.

FOIL OR FLAME TEST: A small amount of cocaine is placed on a sheet of aluminum foil and held over a flame, causing the cocaine to melt and vaporize. Depending on the purity, the cocaine will usually leave an amber colored residue, or no residue at all. Any cuts will leave various colored residues on the aluminum foil.

CLOROX, WATER AND METHANOL TESTS: Cocaine is placed in a glass containing clorox, water, or methanol. The buyer can determine the purity of cocaine and the presence of cuts by the manner in which it dissolves in these liquids.

MELTING POINT TEST: Cocaine and the cuts that may have been added to it melt at different temperatures. Determining the melting point of the sample aids the buyer in estimating the purity of the cocaine.

FREEBASE

Prior to the mid-1970's, the only form of cocaine available on the street was cocaine hydrochloride. The temperatures required to vaporize cocaine hydrochloride for smoking destroy much of its potency, so it is usually either snorted or dissolved in water and injected. During the mid-1970's, a new form of cocaine appeared on the street called "freebase". Unlike the hydrochloride form, freebase could be smoked without destroying its potency. Freebase melts at 98°C, whereas cocaine hydrochloride melts at 187°C. Freebasing converts cocaine hydrochloride to a base, in essence freeing the cocaine molecule from the hydrochloric acid. Although the process for converting cocaine hydrochloride into freebase can vary, the following process is typical:

> A quantity of cocaine hydrochloride is placed into a vial containing a small amount of water. The mixture is vigorously shaken to dissolve the cocaine. A few drops of ammonium hydroxide or other alkali is added to the mixture and again shaken. The addition of ammonium hydroxide "frees" the cocaine from the hydrochloric acid.
>
> Ether is added to the solution, and the container is again vigorously shaken. The freebase cocaine dissolves in the ether. The ether is separated from the solution and placed in a dish and allowed to evaporate. The freebase cocaine crystals remain in the dish after

COCAINE

> the ether evaporates, and are ready to be smoked. Ether is extremely flammable and it's use in this manner has resulted in a number of highly publicized injuries.

Because many of the cuts that are present in cocaine hydrochloride are removed by this process, freebase is a purified form of cocaine. This form of freebase remained popular until the early 1980's, when another form of freebase appeared on the street called "crack".

CRACK

Crack is also a form of freebase cocaine, but it is produced in a different manner which does not involve the use of highly flammable chemicals. Unlike freebase cocaine, which is usually prepared by the user, crack is generally prepared by the dealer. Crack is not a purified form of cocaine. Crack contains many of the cuts and other impurities that were present in the cocaine hydrochloride used in it's preparation. Although there are variations in the crack manufacturing process, the following process is typical:

> Cocaine hydrochloride is placed into a small container of water and mixed thoroughly. Baking soda is added to the solution and mixed thoroughly. The addition of baking soda "frees" the cocaine from the hydrochloric acid. The container is then either placed into a boiling pot of water or in a microwave oven to increase the speed of the chemical reaction between the baking soda and the cocaine hydrochloride. After removal from the heat source the crack, along with any insoluble cuts, settles to the bottom and solidifies. The liquid is poured off leaving the crack to dry. The dried material is then broken into small pieces called rocks, which are units of sale.
>
> The melting point of crack is approximately the same as freebase produced by the ether method. It can be readily smoked, but is no longer water soluble and cannot be dissolved and injected or pulverized and snorted.

IDENTIFICATION AND PACKAGING

Cocaine hydrochloride is usually seen on the street in the form of a fine white powder, flakes, small chunks or rocks, or a combination of these forms. The powder is often called "duff". Users generally view cocaine that has some rocks or chunks in the sample as being relatively pure, because it is difficult to add a cut without first reducing the cocaine to powder form. Flake is generally considered to be the highest quality cocaine available, but is seldom seen on the street.

The appearance of crack has often been described as looking like chunks of white soap or plaster. These chunks, or "rocks" as they are usually called, may vary in size but are usually no larger than a small marble. Crack is a solid and is odorless. It reportedly received its name from the sound it makes when smoked.

There is nothing unique about cocaine packaging. Small glass vials, paper bindles, and plastic bags are the most common. Crack is often packaged in plastic bags, clear plastic vials, and 35 mm film cannisters.

COCAINE

METHODS OF INGESTION

The most common method of ingesting cocaine is by inhaling or snorting it into the nostrils. Cocaine is prepared for snorting by placing the drug on a smooth surface such as a mirror. A razor blade, credit card, or other edged object is used to chop the cocaine into a fine powder. The powder is then formed into thin lines about 1/8" wide and approximately 1" to 2" in length. These are called "lines" or "rails". The cocaine is snorted by holding a straw, rolled paper currency, or other tubular device to one nostril and sniffing as the tube is moved along the line.

Cocaine can also be snorted by using a "coke spoon". The spoon is held immediately below the nostril and the cocaine is sniffed into the nose. Another commonly used device is called an "inhaler" or "bullet". It is a bullet shaped vial which has a valve on one end. When the user wishes to snort cocaine, he opens the valve, places the inhaler to one nostril and inhales.

When snorted, a portion of the cocaine moves through the nasal passages and particles flow down through the throat, but the majority of the drug is trapped in the mucous linings of the nasal passages. The moisture in the nasal passages dissolve the cocaine, enabling it to pass through the mucous membrane and enter the blood stream. Other portions of the cocaine become lodged in the hairs of the nose, and if permitted to remain there for any length of time, tend to irritate the membrane causing sores and bleeding. Continued snorting can cause a perforation or hole in the cartilage and mucous membrane separating the nostrils.

Another method by which cocaine hydrochloride is ingested is by injection. The cocaine is placed in a common metal spoon, and a small amount of water is added to dissolve it. Unlike heroin, cocaine readily dissolves in water, so users generally do not heat or "cook" the solution. Because there may be insoluble cuts in the cocaine, the liquid is often filtered through a piece of cotton as it is drawn into the syringe. The user then injects the cocaine into a major vein.

Crack and freebase are usually smoked in glass pipes. These pipes may be simple straight pyrex tubes, or more sophisticated glass water pipes. The crack or freebase is placed in a pipe, and a small butane torch or cigarette lighter is used to apply heat to the outside of the pipe where the cocaine is located. The heat vaporizes the drug and the fumes are inhaled. Crack is also placed into empty pop cans, heated from below, and the fumes inhaled through the top of the can.

Cocaine can be used in conjunction with other drugs for a combined effect. The combination of cocaine and heroin is called a "speedball". Additionally, there have been reports of cocaine and crack being used in conjunction with other drugs, such as marijuana, tar heroin, etc.

EFFECTS

The initial effect of cocaine is a feeling of euphoria - an extremely pleasurable sensation. The user experiences increased alertness and intellectual functioning, greater confi-dence, more energy, release of social inhibitions, and an overall feeling of power and confidence. This is a drug induced euphoria and it disappears quickly as the cocaine level in the blood drops, usually with thirty to sixty minutes. After the high has worn off, dysphoria sets in; anxiety, apathy, insomnia, along with a general sense of negative feelings, plus a craving for more cocaine. The user is prompted to again use cocaine so these feelings can be dispelled and replaced by the euphoric high. The individual now runs the risk of being caught in a cycle of repeated use.

Cocaine is a fast acting stimulant, but with a short duration. When smoked, cocaine quickly enters the blood stream through the lungs, and the effects are felt almost immediately. This very intense "rush" lasts for only about ten minutes. When snorted, the effects are felt within three to five minutes, and the high lasts up to sixty minutes. When injected, the cocaine causes an intense rush within fifteen to thirty seconds, and the high lasts about thirty minutes.

The effects of cocaine include an increase in the pulse rate, blood pressure, and body temperature. Pupils become noticeably dilated. Fatigue and appetite disappear. The user may be hyperactive, full of energy, very talkative, and experience a feeling of euphoria. The user feels there are no problems, and he has a sense of increased physical and mental abilities.

After the high has worn off, the user experiences what is often called the "cocaine crash". The stimulating effects experienced during the high shift to depressant effects as the drug wears off. Pulse rate and blood pressure drop to a point lower than normal. The user is often depressed, has a lack of energy and desire, and a craving to again experience the high.

Cocaine abusers experience various side effects. Weight loss, insomnia, fatigue, headaches, nasal infections, sexual dysfunction and paranoia are common. Many experience hallucinations known as "coke bugs" or "snow bugs"; the user believes he has bugs crawling under the skin. In extreme cases, the user may try and dig the bugs out with a knife or tweezers.

Excessive doses of cocaine may cause seizures and death from convulsions, respiratory failure, or heart failure. The amount of cocaine required to cause an overdose is unpredictable, and varies from individual to individual. A dose which would have little effect on a regular user may cause an overdose for a first time user.

PHARMACOLOGY

Cocaine's stimulating and addicting effects are due to its interference with the normal reuptake of norepinephrine and dopamine at nerve terminals in the brain. Cocaine's CNS stimulant effects are comparable to amphetamines and produces hyperstimulation lasting about thirty minutes. Cocaine's addicting qualities appear to focus around the so-called "pleasure centers" of the brain where basic instinctive drives such as hunger, thirst and sexual desires are reinforced. These "drives", mediated by dopamine, are replaced with the drive to obtain more cocaine which blocks dopamine's normal reuptake and continues the CNS stimulation at the expense of natural occurring dopamine which is severely depleted.

▮

DESIGNER DRUGS

CSA SCHEDULE: I

STREET NAMES: MDMA: Adam, clarity, doctor, E, ecstasy, essence, hug drug, love drug, M, M and M, MDM, presence, X, XTC. MDE: Eve. 2C-B: Bromo, U4EUH. MDA, DOB, BOB, STP. Fentanyl analogs: Synthetic heroin, AMF, China white, Persian white.

PSYCHOPHYSICAL ACTION: Phenethylamines: Hallucinogen
Fentanyl analogs: Narcotic analgesic

STREET PRICE: Phenethylamines: $10 to $30 per dose
Fentanyl analogs: Comparable to heroin

"Designer drug" is a term used to describe any drug produced by making a slight change in the molecular structure of a controlled psychoactive drug. Chemically, the newly designed drug is an analog of the original drug. Often times the objective of the chemist is to "design" a new chemical compound, which is at least temporarily legal, that closely resembles the original drug and retains its psychoactive properties. In other cases the chemist is after a better or more powerful psychoactive drug. Hundreds of designer drugs have been produced, but only a few have the unique combination of physical and psychoactive effects that have made them popular with the drug culture.

Designer drugs seen on the street generally fall into two categories: the fentanyl analogs, which are sold as synthetic substitutes for heroin, and those related to the amphetamine family of drugs. This latter group is often referred to as methylated amphetamines, hallucinogenic amphetamines, or phenethylamines.

FENTANYL ANALOGS

Fentanyl, marketed under the trade name Sublimaze, is a quick acting powerful synthetic narcotic which is used as a surgical anesthetic. It was introduced to the medical community in 1968, and by 1979 its first illicit analog appeared on the street. The chemical name of this analog was alpha-methylfentanyl, but it was sold on the street under the names China White and synthetic heroin. A number of deaths were attributed to this drug during the period 1979-1981, and it was placed into Schedule I of the Controlled Substances Act effective September 22, 1981.

An even more powerful analog appeared in late 1983. The chemical name of this drug was 3-methyl fentanyl. It is extremely powerful, and an effective dose is less than 0.05 milligram. A number of deaths were attributed to this drug, and it was placed into Schedule I of the Controlled Substances Act effective April 25, 1985.

Because the cuts that are typically added to heroin (quinine, lactose, etc.) are also added to the fentanyl analogs, and generally make up the majority of the sample, the two drugs cannot usually be distinguished from each other by visual inspection. The color and texture of the analogs are very close to heroin. The psychoactive effects are nearly identical to heroin and experienced users reportedly cannot tell the difference between the two. The analog acts on the brain in a manner very similar to heroin.

DESIGNER DRUGS

There is one very important difference between synthetic heroin and the real product. All of the synthetics on the street are many times stronger than heroin. If the fentanyl analog is not diluted heavily enough, the user may overdose on an unexpectedly potent dose.

Despite the dangers associated with the use of fentanyl analogs, they are still sold on the street, and they are still killing. In February of 1991, several hundred users of fentanyl analogs were hospitalized for overdoses in the New York - New Jersey - Connecticut area, and a number of deaths were reported.

PHENETHYLAMINES

This large chemical family consists of hundreds of psychoactive compounds. They differ widely in the speed of the onset, length of the effect, and the intensity of the mood modification. The following are the most frequently encountered compounds in this group:

Symbol	Chemical Name
MDMA	3,4-methylenedioxy-n-methylamphetamine
MDA	3,4-methylenedioxyamphetamine
MMDA	3-methoxy-4,5-methylenedioxyamphetamine
DOM	2,5-dimethoxy-4-methylamphetamine
TMA	3,4,5-trimethoxyamphetamine
2C-B	4-bromo-2,5-dimethoxyphenethylamine
MDE	3,4-methylenedioxy-n-ethylamphetamine

In pure form, almost all of the hundreds of phenethylamines are a white powder, but the color may vary due to impurities resulting from make-shift manufacturing. The powder can be snorted, mixed with a liquid, tableted, or encapsulated for ingestion. These drugs are rarely injected.

The psychophysical action of the phenethylamines varies from drug to drug. Some produce warm personal feelings at low dosage levels (the Love Drug effect), while others produce pseudo-hallucinations (those which the user knows are not real, but are a product of the drug). The effects are felt within thirty to sixty minutes and last from four to twenty four hours, depending on the particular drug. At lower dosage levels, many produce nausea, sweating, fatigue, jaw tightening, and increased blood pressure.

Because most of the phenethylamines have a similar appearance, they are subject to misidentification. Each successive handler often relies on information provided by the person the drug was purchased from. Misidentification of these drugs could result in an overdose illness or death, as some phenethylamines are many times more potent than others.

MDMA

MDMA is the most common of the phenethylamines in use on the street. Although its illicit use in the United States goes back to about 1970, it was not until 1985 that it became classified as a Schedule I drug under the CSA. This scheduling was in response to mushrooming street use, as well as animal studies which showed that MDMA reduced serotonin levels.

DESIGNER DRUGS

Many legitimate researchers objected to MDMA being placed into the Schedule I category. These researchers felt that MDMA may be a key to a further understanding of the human mind and a possible aid in the treatment of certain mental illnesses. These researchers, along with other interested parties, continued to lobby for further testing. In July of 1992 the Food and Drug Administration, along with the National Institute on Drug Abuse, granted permission for authorized psychiatrists to use MDMA on research subjects.

MDMA is sold on the street under the names XTC, Ecstasy, and Adam. In its purest form it is a white crystalline powder, but often times there is a reddish or brownish color as a result of impurities.

Ingestion of low doses of MDMA brings on feelings of relaxation, euphoria, enhanced mental clarity, increased ability to solve problems and emotional warmth. Researchers maintain that defenses and communication barriers are removed, enabling users to more openly communicate with one another.

Despite the fact that MDMA was transferred to Schedule I in 1985, clandestine laboratories have continued production. Reports seem to indicate that it is readily available in many parts of the country, and prices are quoted regularly in High Times magazine.

PHARMACOLOGY

Designer drugs are divided into two principle types: 1) phenethylamines which have properties in common with both amphetamines and mescaline and 2) fentanyl analogs which are synthetic, high-potency heroin products with the same basic pharmacology of fentanyl or heroin. (See heroin pharmacology)

The phenethylamine derivatives possess stimulatory effects related to sympathomimetic activity on the CNS which is nearly identical to amphetamine's action. The main site of action is the cerebral cortex and reticular-activating system which accounts for increased motor activity, mental alertness and euphoria. The psychic and hallucinatory effects of this class of designer drugs appears to result from stimulation of both dopamine and serotonin neurotransmitters in much the same way that LSD and PCP act, but not nearly to the same degree of mental distortion.

∎

HEROIN

CSA SCHEDULE: I

ACTIVE SUBSTANCE: Diacetylmorphine

STREET NAMES: Antifreeze, big daddy, big H, big Harry, boy, brown, brown heroin, brown stuff, brown sugar, caballo, carga, China man, crap, doje, downtown, dyno, estuffa, garbage, globo, H, hard stuff, Harry, him, hombre, horse, junk, lemon dope, mierda, Persian, rufus, scag, schmeck, shit, skag, smack, smeck, stoffa, stuff, white stuff. Mexican tar heroin is variously known as tar, ball, black heroin, black tar, chapapote, chiva, chocolate, goma, gomero, gum, gumball, Mexican mud, mud, pedazo, tar, and tootsie roll.

PSYCHOPHYSICAL ACTION: Narcotic analgesic

STREET PRICES:

QUANTITY	SOURCE	1990	1991	1992	1993
Kilogram	Mexican	$65,000 - $180,000	$50,000 - $200,000	$50,000 - $150,000	$50,000 - $250,000
	Southeast Asian	$70,000 - $260,000	$90,000 - $260,000	$90,000 - $250,000	$150,000 - $250,000
	Southwest Asian	$70,000 - $200,000	$80,000 - $220,000	$80,000 - $200,000	$70,000 - $200,000
Ounce	——	$1,000 - $13,000	$900 - $14,000	$1,000 - $12,000	$1,000 - $13,000
Gram	Powder	$50 - $450	$40 - $450	$100 - $600	$90 - $600
	Black Tar	$100 - $460	$110 - $500	$100 - $500	$50 - $600

Source: Department of Justice

Heroin is the epitome of hard drugs, conjuring up such thoughts as city slums, prostitution, syringes, AIDS, and violent crime. The Department of Justice places the number of heroin addicts in the United States between 500,000 and 750,000. One of the primary concerns of heroin addiction is the need for the addict to commit crimes to support his habit. Although it is not accurately known how much the average addict spends on heroin, a recent estimate indicates about $60.00 per day, or a total annual cost of 11 to 15 billion dollars. It is further estimated that about 60% of this 11 to 15 billion dollars per year is obtained by consensual crimes, such as prostitution and drug sales, and also welfare payments and occasional work. Most of the remaining 4 to 6 billion dollars comes from the commission of property crimes, such as burglary and shoplifting. Stolen merchandise that is sold on the street sells for perhaps 25% of the true value. This means that approximately 16 to 24 billion dollars worth of merchandise is stolen and resold each year to supply the 4 to 6 billion dollars needed by the heroin addicts.

HEROIN

Society ultimately pays an even greater cost because of the high rate of HIV infection and AIDS among intravenous drug users. A number of illicit drugs can be injected, but heroin is involved in the vast majority of IV drug cases. HIV infection can be transmitted by all shared equipment: needles, cookers (spoons, bottle caps, etc.), cotton filters, syringes, etc. According to the Center for Disease Control, as of June 30, 1994, 401,749 cases of AIDS have been reported since record keeping began. Intravenous drug use was the only known route of infection in 24.5%, or 98,367 cases. Another 6.3%, or 25,447 cases, involved men who had sex with men and injected drugs, and 3.5%, 14,239 cases, involved individuals who had sex with an injecting drug user.

Unless there is a medical breakthrough, individuals with HIV infection will eventually develop AIDS. The U.S. Department of Health and Human Services estimates that 1,000,000 people in the United States are infected with HIV. Based on statistics from the Center for Disease Control, 245,000 of these cases are probably the result of injecting drug use, 63,000 involve men who had sex with men and injected drugs, and 35,000 individuals infected through sex with an injecting drug user. When these estimated HIV figures are added to the known AIDS totals, the human tragedy is staggering.

Heroin is a semisynthetic drug that is produced by treating morphine with acetic anhydride. Morphine in turn, is the prevalent alkaloid found in opium. Although heroin is the most notorious product of opium, there are many drugs derived from opium that are cumulatively referred to as "opiates". There are also several synthetic, or man made drugs called "opioids", which produce the same effects as the opiates. The opiates and opioids are both classified as narcotics, from the Greek word “narkitos”, meaning numbing. Medically, the opiates and opioids are used as cough suppressants, to control diarrhea, and to relieve moderate to severe pain. Illicitly, they are used for their euphoric depressant effects.

OPIATES **(natural or semisynthetic)**	**OPIOIDS** **(synthetic opiates)**
Heroin	Meperidine (Demerol)
Morphine (MS Contin)	Levorphanol (Levo-Dromoran)
Codeine (Tylenol w/codeine)	Methadone (Dolophine)
Hydromorphone (Dilaudid)	Propoxyphene (Darvon)
Oxycodone (Percodan)	Fentanyl (Sublimaze)
Oxymorphone (Numorphan)	Pentazocine (Talwin)

HISTORY

Opium was used for medicinal purposes by the Assyrians over 9,000 years ago. In 4,000 B.C., the Sumerians were cultivating opium poppies in what is now Iraq. Written records indicate that opium was used by the Greeks around the third century B.C. Its medicinal and recreational use eventually spread to Asia, Africa, and Europe.

In 1803, a German pharmacist, F.W. Serturner, isolated the main active substance in opium. He named this newly discovered alkaloid morphium, after the Greek god of dreams, Morphius. The name morphium was later changed to morphine. Morphine, it was discovered, was about ten times more powerful than opium.

During the 1800's, opium and morphine were popular medications in the United States, and were widely and legally available on an over-the-counter basis. In this setting, they were used as relaxants, to treat alcoholism, diarrhea, cough, teething pain, physical discomfort, and a host of other conditions. Examples of medications of this type were The Keeley Cure, Mrs. Winslow's Soothing Syrup, Watkin's Cough Remedy, Eilert's Diarrhea Remedy, Dr. H.A. Ingham's Pain Extractor, and Dover Powder. Most of these preparations were liquids that contained opium or morphine. One preparation that was commonly used was laudanum, a drink consisting of opium and spices dissolved in wine. This concoction had been formulated in 1520 and remained popular until outlawed in 1906 by the Pure Food and Drug Act.

During the middle 1800's, opium smoking was introduced into the United States by immigrant Chinese laborers. Smoked opium provided a much more pleasurable and quicker effect than it did when swallowed, because the drug entered the bloodstream directly from the lungs rather than through the digestive process.

The introduction of the syringe in 1853, although a medical breakthrough, was to forever change the opiate drug scene. With this method of ingestion, morphine could be injected directly into the bloodstream. The first widespread use of injected morphine was during the American Civil War (1861 - 1865). During this time, morphine was used indiscriminately on injured soldiers. After the War, so many soldiers were addicted to morphine that addiction to the drug was often known as the "soldiers illness" or "army disease".

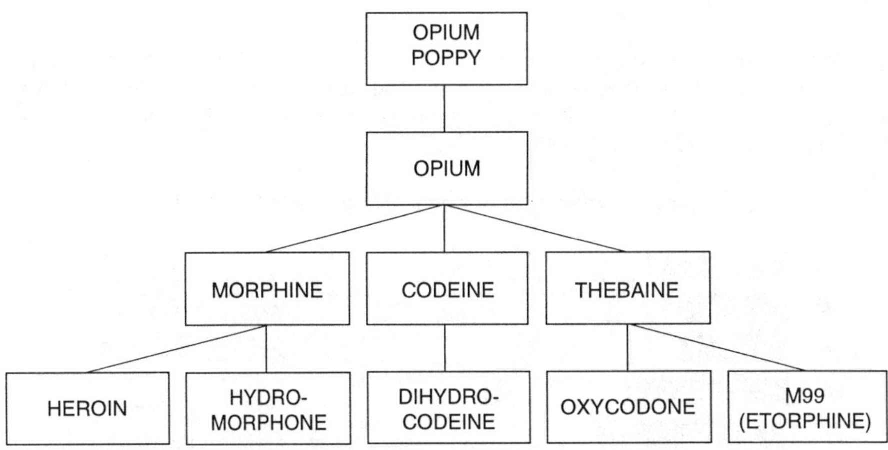

In 1874, an English chemist, Alder Wright, synthesized diacetylmorphine (heroin) from morphine, by treating morphine with acetic anhydride. However, diacetylmorphine remained somewhat obscure until 1898, when the Bayer Chemical Company of Germany introduced it as a medicine and named it "heroin". (From the German word "heroisch", meaning large or powerful). As was the case with opium and morphine before it, heroin quickly became an ingredient in numerous tonics and medications.

By 1900, it was estimated that 250,000 to 400,000 Americans were dependent on narcotics. The abuse of the opiate drugs, and their association with crime finally hit home by the early 1900's, and a series of laws were passed to deal with the problem:

HEROIN

1906 - The Pure Food and Drug Act ended over-the-counter sales of medications containing heroin and other opiates.
1914 - The Harrison Narcotics Act regulates heroin manufacturing and distribution.
1922 - Medical doctors were no longer permitted to continue the common practice of providing heroin and other opiates to addicts.
1924 - Heroin production in the United States is outlawed.
1942 - Opium poppy cultivation in the United States is outlawed.
1956 - Heroin is outlawed, all remaining stocks of heroin were required to be surrendered to the Federal Government.

Opium and morphine are still used extensively in modern medicine. The International Narcotics Control Board estimates that the United States used 1,600,000 pounds of opium in 1994, primarily for the production of morphine, codeine, hydrocodone and other opiate based medicines. This figure represents over 50% of the worldwide legal opium use of 3,100,000 pounds for the same year.

Medicinal use of heroin has continued to decline since the 1930's. Today, licit heroin is manufactured and used primarily in England, with limited use in Canada, Iceland, Netherlands, Switzerland and Belgium. The International Narcotics Control Board estimated the 1994 licit world use at 693 pounds, with 660 pounds of that total being used in England.

SUPPLY SOURCES

Opium is the source of all opiate drugs (heroin, codeine, morphine, etc.), and is obtained from the opium poppy plant, Papaver somniferum. The word "papaver" is from Greek meaning "poppy", while "somniferum" is from Latin, and means "dream" or "induce sleep". Thus, we have the poppy that produces sleep.

Heroin Availability In The U.S. By Area Of Origin

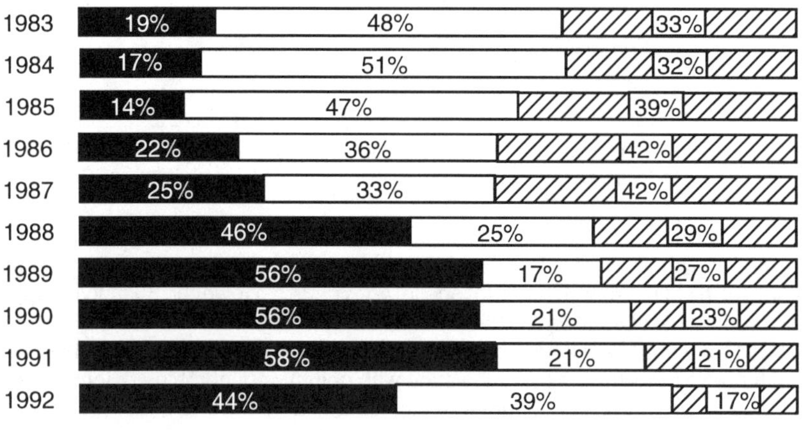

Southeast Asia | Southwest Asia | Mexico

Source: Department Of Justice

HEROIN

	COUNTRY	ESTIMATED 1992 ILLICIT OPIUM PRODUCTION
Golden Triangle	Burma	2,553 tons
	Laos	258 tons
	Thailand	27 tons
Golden Crescent	Pakistan	196 tons
	Afghanistan	717 tons
	Iran	336 tons
	Mexico	45 tons

There are hundreds of species of poppy plants, but only Papaver somniferum produces opium. Papaver pavonium, the typical American poppy plant with large orange flowers and a black center does not produce opium, nor does the California poppy. The opium poppy grows from one to five feet high, and the opium content varies widely from region to region. Its flowers may be white, pink, red, purple, crimson, or a combination of any of these colors.

Prior to the Opium Poppy Control Act of 1942, opium poppies were cultivated across America for supplies of opium for medicinal drugs, as well as for it's edible seed. The opium poppy seed is the same seed that is commonly found on many foods. The seeds contain trace amounts of morphine and codeine, and although huge amounts would have to be consumed for a high, ingestion of as little as a teaspoon can reportedly cause a positive morphine urine test.

Although the opium poppy grows wild in many parts of the world, its illicit cultivation is mainly in areas which provide the best climatic and legal or politically tolerant environments. The vast majority of heroin that makes its way to the United States originates from either Mexico or from two areas known as the "Golden Triangle", and the "Golden Crescent". There has been a sharp increase in the heroin production in Colombia, and some authorities expect this country to become a major supplier of opium to the U.S.

India is the sole supplier of licit raw opium to the world market. The production and export of raw opium by India has been steadily declining since 1978 due to increasing use of "poppy straw" as an alternate source of opium. Poppies are grown in Australia, Turkey, France and Spain for the extraction of alkaloids. The entire plant (poppy straw) is harvested and processed into an intermediate product known as concentrate of poppy straw. This concentrate is then used in the production of opiates for medicinal use.

In the spring or fall, the illicit opium farmer plants his crop. About three months later, the plants have matured and brightly colored flowers appear. After fertilization, the petals drop from the flower, exposing the seed pod. The seed pod is usually about the size of a large walnut. Opium is produced in the root system and distributed to all parts of the plant, with the majority collecting in the seed pod. To release the opium, the farmer makes a series of shallow vertical or horizontal incisions across one or two sides of the seed pod with a small cutting tool. Milky opium slowly bleeds from the incisions, turning from white to brown as it dries. The following day, the farmer scrapes and collects the dried opium from the surface of the pod. The pods may be incised up to five or six times before the

HEROIN

Heroin Purity Data 1990 - 1993 National Range/Seized Samples				
Quantity	1990	1991	1992	1993
Gram	44%	44%	49%	59%
Ounce	59%	56%	64%	68%
Kilogram	78%	73%	75%	73%

Source: Department of Justice

opium is depleted. Both the quantity and quality of the opium produced by the plants varies from region to region, depending on soil, water, and other environmental conditions.

Because the incising and harvesting of opium is very labor intensive, hired labor is not economical. Most opium poppy is grown by small family type farmers, who usually plant no more than 1/3 to 1 acre of poppy, usually along with several acres of a legitimate crop. The typical opium field will have 25,000 to 50,000 plants per acre, with a total of 50,000 to 120,000 opium producing seed pods.

Once the opium is collected, the farmer sells it to a processor who extracts the morphine base. Ten pounds of opium will generally yield one pound of morphine. The morphine is then synthesized into heroin at roughly a 1:1 ratio. Often, the operators of the clandestine laboratories that produce heroin are not skilled chemists. Consequently, due to their lack of expertise, the heroin they produce may be of low quality, and yields are relatively low. However, many knowledgeable operators succeed in producing very high quality heroin. Virtually all of the world's heroin production is in the illicit market. According to the International Narcotics Control Board, the legal production of heroin in 1992 was approximately 760 pounds. The International Narcotics Control Strategy Report estimated that illicit production of heroin in 1992 was 826,000 pounds and possibly as high as 940,000 pounds. Worldwide heroin seizures in 1992 totaled only 35,000 pounds. It is clear that the vast majority of illicitly produced heroin is successfully smuggled throughout the world, and local markets have a plentiful supply.

Based on chemical make up, purity and physical characteristics, illicit heroin is placed in the following four categories for purposes of identification and discussion:

Heroin #1. This is the first product obtained in the process of converting opium to heroin. Heroin #1 is not actually heroin, but is crude morphine base. It may be smoked, but is generally used in the production of heroin #2.

Heroin #2. This is heroin base, or crude heroin, obtained by treating the morphine base (heroin #1) with acetic anhydride. It is not readily soluble in water, but can be smoked. Most heroin #2 is used in the production of the more refined heroin #3 and #4.

Heroin #3. Heroin base is treated with hydrochloric acid, producing heroin hydrochloride,

HEROIN

or heroin #3. This form of heroin is designed for smoking. The drug is heated and fumes are inhaled through a straw or similar device.

Heroin #4. This is similar to heroin #3, but is more highly refined. Heroin #4 is the type most commonly used by abusers who inject the drug, but it can also be smoked or snorted.

DISTRIBUTION

Heroin traffickers use any number of means to transport heroin into the United States. Air freight, international mail shipments, containerized ocean freight and marine vessels are all utilized. Additionally, commercial flight passengers smuggle the drug in luggage, in clothing, taped to their bodies, and even swallowed in balloons or condoms (swallowers), which are later defecated. One swallower was found to have consumed 227 balloons containing 2.9 pounds of heroin.

Much of the heroin which originates in Asia is smuggled into New York, where existing chains of distribution are well established. Over one half of all DEA heroin seizures occur in the New York City metro area. Chains of distribution for Mexican heroin are centered in the southwest part of the United States, particularly Los Angeles. As heroin moves down the chain of distribution, each handler has the opportunity to add a diluent, or "cut" to the drug to increase his profits. Competition caused by a glut of opium has resulted in the increased purity of heroin sold at the street level. The average purity of heroin sold in gram quantities in 1993 was 58%.

There are many substances that are used to cut heroin. Quinine, starch, powdered milk, powdered vitamins, caffeine, phenobarbital, lactose, glucose, mannitol, sucrose and procaine are often used to dilute powdered heroin that is white in color. Coffee, chocolate milk powder, cocoa mix, and brown sugar are often used to dilute powdered heroin which is tan or brown in color.

Because of its hard texture, tar heroin can be difficult to cut. One method used is to heat the tar in an oven on low temperature until it becomes soft and gummy. A cut is added and the tar kneaded until there is a uniform consistency. Cuts added to tar heroin have included starch, molasses, cocoa mix, coffee, and brown sugar.

IDENTIFICATION AND PACKAGING

Heroin is usually seen in powder form, with color varying from white, to tan, to red, to dark brown, depending on the production methods used and any cuts that have been added. White heroin is considered the most refined and most potent. Like cocaine, heroin samples may also consist of a mixture of powder and chunks. The powder may be fine or granular. Mexican tar heroin may be gummy, hard, or a powder, and vary in color from brown to black, again depending on manufacturing methods and cuts.

Heroin is generally packaged in paper bindles, glassine envelopes, and small balloons. The heroin is funneled into the bottom of the balloon which is then securely tied. The tied end containing the heroin is folded back into the mouth of the balloon for added protection. Tar heroin is commonly packaged in cellophane and aluminum foil.

HEROIN

METHODS OF INGESTION

Despite the risk of AIDS and other infections, the most common method of ingesting both powder and tar heroin is by injecting it into a vein. The heroin is first prepared by "cooking it up". Cooking heroin involves placing a small amount of the heroin in a metal spoon, mixing it with water, and heating the spoon from below very briefly with a cigarette lighter to help dissolve the mixture. A small amount of lemon juice is often added to the water, as its acidity helps dissolve the heroin. A piece of cotton is often placed in the liquid solution to act as a filter to remove some of the impurities in the heroin as it is drawn into the syringe. The used cotton is usually saved after use because it retains a small amount of the drug, which can be extracted if the user is unable to obtain additional drugs. The needle is then inserted into a vein. A small amount of blood (called a flag) is drawn back into the syringe to ensure that the vein has been penetrated. The heroin is then pumped into the vein in a series of short strokes.

Most heroin users begin injecting into the vein on the inside of the elbow. After repeated injections, the vein begins to scar and harden, making injections difficult, and also advertises to others that the individual is an addict. The addict often resorts to injecting in veins in other parts of the body, such as the legs, hands, groin, neck, and elsewhere.

Although much less effective than when injected, ingesting heroin by snorting it is becoming more popular. Heroin is also smoked. In a method often referred to as "chasing the dragon", the heroin is placed on aluminum foil and heated from below with a match or cigarette lighter, and the resulting fumes inhaled.

Heroin is often used in conjunction with other drugs. A combination known as a "speedball" or "fireball", is heroin mixed with either cocaine or amphetamine. Heroin has also reportedly been mixed with marijuana and smoked in joints. A combination of crack and heroin is often called "hot rocks". Smoking a combination of heroin and freebase cocaine is often called "chasing and basing".

EFFECTS

Heroin is used as a legitimate medicine in various parts of the world; it relieves both cough and diarrhea, and is an effective pain killer and tranquilizer. From the standpoint of the heroin abuser, heroin provides a soothing sense of relaxation and well being. The abuser will try to repeatedly experience the euphoria, and will soon find it very difficult to stop taking the drug. The life style of the heroin addict is typified by malnutrition and crime, collapsed veins and disease. Sharing needles is common in the heroin subculture, resulting in AIDS, meningitis, hepatitis, and other diseases.

The effects of heroin generally last about four to six hours. The table below lists several observations which may be seen in an individual under the influence of heroin.

- Pinpoint pupils
- Loss of coordination
- Lowered sensation of pain
- Lowered pulse and respiration rate
- Slow, slurred speech
- Disorientation
- Itchy nose and skin
- Lowered blood pressure
- Constipation
- Sweating
- Drooping eyelids and the head nodding forward. (Heroin intoxication is often referred to as "on the nod".)

HEROIN

Like other street drugs, the heroin user can never be certain of the potency of the drug he is taking. Although two different samples may have similar appearances, one may contain a very small percentage of heroin, and the other may contain a very high percentage. Purity levels on some heroin samples exceed 90%, thus the user is constantly at risk of overdosing on an unexpectedly pure fix.

If a sufficiently high dose is taken, respiratory depression, coma, and death may occur. In the event of overdose, the narcotic antagonist naloxone (Narcan) is often used to help the victim recover. Naloxone removes the opiate/opioid molecules from their receptor sites in the brain within minutes, thus removing their effects. A person who is comatose one moment, may be up and walking a few minutes after an injection of naloxone. Naloxone does not produce addiction, nor is it psychoactive, and its effects are limited only to the opiates/opioids.

WITHDRAWAL

If the heroin addict is unable to obtain a dose of heroin known as a "fix" or "treat", withdrawal symptoms will usually appear within six to twelve hours of the last dose. Although withdrawal symptoms are not life threatening, they can be very painful, and are often compared to a bad flu. These symptoms usually peak at about 24 to 72 hours after the last dose, and then gradually subside and disappear within seven to ten days. The table below shows common signs of heroin withdrawal.

- Agitation and restlessness
- Stomach and muscle cramps
- Dilated pupils
- Yawning
- Sneezing
- Increased pulse rate and blood pressure
- Runny nose
- Goose bumps
- Watery eyes
- Insomnia
- Diarrhea
- Alternating chills and sweating
- Depression

Although withdrawal symptoms can be quite easily managed, it is very difficult to keep an addict who has gone through withdrawal from again reverting to heroin use. Most heroin addicts who are imprisoned for several years may go through withdrawal symptoms within the first few days of imprisonment, but promptly return to heroin use upon their release.

METHADONE

The most widely accepted treatment for heroin addiction is methadone. Methadone is an opioid that was first produced in Germany to supplement the limited supply of morphine during World War II. Methadone is also used as a medication to relieve severe pain.

Methadone is significant in the treatment of heroin addiction because the two drugs are pharmacologically similar. As such, methadone 1) prevents heroin withdrawal symptoms, 2) fulfills the addicts physical need for heroin, 3) at sufficiently high doses it blocks the effects of heroin through cross-tolerance, thus a fix of street heroin while undergoing methadone treatment will probably give no pleasurable effect, 4) it is a longer acting drug than heroin, the average dose lasting about 24 hours, thus making it more convenient to administer, 5) it is effective orally, thus breaking the reliance on the ritual of injection, and 6) it can be dispensed at a treatment center.

HEROIN

Another drug that is sometimes used to treat heroin addiction is naltrexone (Trexan). At the proper dosage level, naltrexone blocks the effects of the opiates/opioid drugs for approximately three days. During this time, no effects would be experienced if heroin were consumed. The problem with naltrexone is that it cannot be given to an addict unless he has been drug free for at least seven to ten days, or the drug will cause almost immediate withdrawal symptoms.

The ultimate goal is to wean addicts from heroin and the heroin life-style and allow them to adjust to a new life-style through which they can withdraw from methadone and live drug free. Methadone treatment is somewhat controversial. Critics argue that because methadone is also addictive, heroin addicts are simply changing one drug for another. In fact, methadone is the drug of choice for many people, and it has generated an active street market. Further, estimates indicate that at best, only 20% of methadone patients remain off heroin.

However, methadone has proven itself to be somewhat effective. For instance, in one program where the addicts averaged two arrests per year before admission, the overall arrest rate of those who entered and remained in the program was reduced to about one fifth of the previous rate.

PHARMACOLOGY

Heroin's action appears to be mediated through the stimulation of several types of opioid receptors throughout the CNS. The opioids possess some of the same properties which the naturally occurring peptides in the body, enkephalins, endorphins and dynorphins, can elicit to reduce pain and produce endogenous euphoria. Of the four main opioid receptors, (mu, kappa, delta and sigma), heroin possesses a high degree of "mu" and "sigma" activities and it is the euphoric and hallucinogenic qualities of these receptors which attracts the heroin addict. Other responses ranging from analgesia, sedation, miosis and respiratory depression are also actions associated with the opioid receptors.

∎

LSD

CSA SCHEDULE: I

ACTIVE SUBSTANCE: d-lysergic acid diethylamide

STREET NAMES: Acid, big D, blotter, blotter acid, blue heaven, California sunshine, cube, D, dose, dot, L, microdot, paper acid, royal blue, Sandoz, sheet acid, sid, spots, sunshine, ticket, window pane.

PSYCHOPHYSICAL ACTION: Hallucinogen

STREET PRICES:

Year	1990	1991	1992	1993
Retail (1 hit)	$1 - $10	$1 - $15	$1 - $15	$1 - $10
Wholesale (1,000 hits)	$0.30 - $3.50	$0.25 - $4.00	$0.30 - $5	$0.30 - $5

Source: Department of Justice

HISTORY

LSD was first produced in 1938 by the Swiss scientist Albert Hofmann. Hofmann was working in the laboratories of the Sandoz Company, investigating derivatives of the alkaloids of the ergot of claviceps purpurea, a fungus which grows on cereal grasses, particularly rye. Several medical drugs had already been produced from the alkaloids of the ergot. It was hoped that the 25th derivative to be studied, lysergic acid diethylamide, or LSD-25, would prove to be a circulatory stimulant. The drug did not appear to have any medical applications and was set aside for five years. While again working with LSD-25 in 1943, a small amount of the solution came in contact with Hofmann's skin, and somehow entered his system. Within a short time, Hofmann experienced hallucinations which he attributed to the LSD.

Hofmann carefully documented his hallucinogenic experience but was not certain that LSD was responsible. To verify this, he took a subsequent dose of 250 micrograms. As he would later learn, this was a relatively large dose of LSD, and shortly after the ingestion Hofmann again experienced the hallucinogenic effects of the drug. Reports on initial studies were released in 1947, and shortly thereafter it was being investigated by members of the scientific community. A number of psychologists and psychiatrists felt that LSD held the key to a greater understanding of the mind and was a possible treatment for certain types of emotional illness. The U.S. military was interested in its possible application to mind control, and conducted studies from the early 1950's thru the mid 1960's. LSD failed to live up to the scientists expectations and serious investigation gradually gave way to society's abuse of the drug.

Many noted scientists, actors, musicians and educators openly praised the mind-expanding properties of LSD and encouraged its use. One of the most outspoken proponents of LSD was the Harvard psychologist Timothy Leary. Leary encouraged the generation of the 1960's to "turn on - tune in - drop out". LSD became the drug of choice not only for the "acid heads", but also for many of the middle-class and others whose life style embraced the counterculture of the time. Abuse of the drug continued to spread, and it's nonmedical use was outlawed in 1966.

LSD

MANUFACTURING AND DISTRIBUTION

One ounce of pure LSD is enough for 567,000 hits of fifty micrograms each; one pound is enough for 9,072,000 hits. It is relatively easy to conceal a major LSD laboratory because of the small quantities of raw material and finished product. The lab does not have to produce on a continual basis; one batch can supply the market needs for several months or more. It is believed that a small group of individuals, perhaps as few as ten to fifty people, manufacture nearly all of the LSD produced in the U.S. It appears that most LSD is manufactured in northern California, with San Francisco serving as the central distribution point. For nearly twenty years, law enforcement has been largely unsuccessful in penetrating this organization because arrested distributors either did not know their contacts or refused to cooperate.

Lysergic acid is the key ingredient in the manufacture of LSD. Lysergic acid can be produced by using commercially available ergotamine, or by processing alkaloids obtained from the ergot of the fungus claviceps purpurea. The chemical process to produce LSD is complicated and involves the use of a number of dangerous chemicals. The end product of the process is pure crystals of LSD, which are white, odorless, tasteless, and water soluble.

The manufacturers usually sell the LSD crystals to a limited number of multi-gram dealers, who in turn sell to gram dealers. The gram dealers convert the crystals to a liquid form, which is then placed on blotter paper, or in other retail sales forms, and sell to local wholesalers in quantities of 100 to 1000 doses. The local wholesaler in turn sells to retailers, generally in doses of 100 or less.

Many of the transactions between the gram dealers, wholesalers, and retailers are handled thru the mail. The LSD is included in parcels sent to a post office box or temporary address established by the recipient. This process tends to insulate the manufacturer and multi-gram distributors from detection by law enforcement agencies.

At the retail level, LSD is generally available in liquid doses, on sugar cubes, toothpicks, very small tablets ("microdots"), thin gelatin squares ("window pane"), and blotter paper. Nearly all retail sales of LSD are in the blotter paper form. The LSD is diluted in ethyl alcohol, and the blotter paper is dipped into the solution. Generally, the blotter paper is perforated into small squares called "tickets", and is stamped with unique pictures, designs or characters as a trademark of the distributor. These may range from the signs of the zodiac to cartoon characters. A "sheet" normally consists of 100 perforated squares, and a "book" 1,000.

USE

LSD is normally taken by placing a square or ticket of blotter paper on the tongue. The LSD is dissolved by the saliva and absorbed through the mucous membrane. This method of ingestion produces the most rapid effects. LSD can be mixed with liquids, consumed with foods, and added to pills or sugar cubes. Although LSD can be absorbed through the skin, it would require prolonged contact with a potent dose. LSD is not ingested by smoking.

LSD is a powerful semisynthetic hallucinogenic drug. It is so potent that doses are measured in micrograms (a microgram is one millionth of a gram). For comparison, a one cent penny weighs about 2.8 grams. An equivalent weight of pure LSD would contain about 56,000 doses of fifty micrograms each. A dose or hit of only twenty micrograms will affect the body. Doses of fifty to seventy five micrograms produce a euphoric state, while doses above that level can result in a "trip". In the early 1960's to late 1970's, the strength of doses sold on the street ranged from 100 to 300 micrograms. Since the mid 1980's street doses have contained about twenty to eighty micrograms.

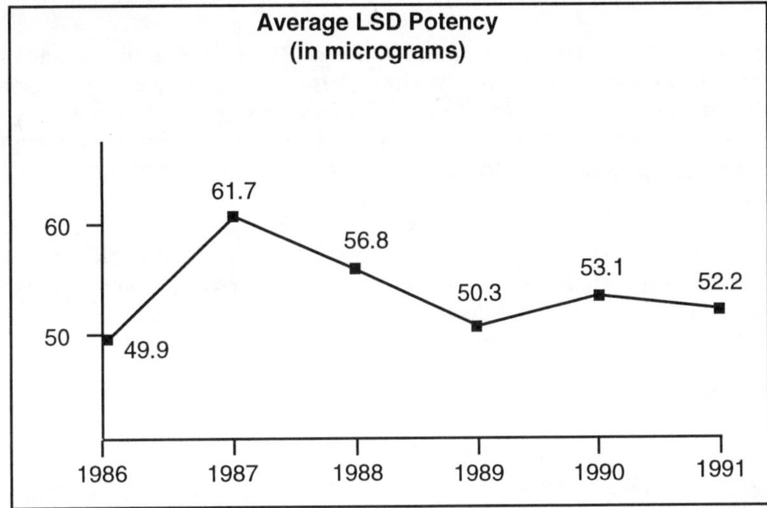

Source: Department of Justice

The highest use of LSD occurred during the period 1965 thru 1968. Use of the drug dropped during the 1970's, but began to increase in the 1980's. The 1990 National Institute on Drug Abuse survey indicated that 10,500,000 Americans have used LSD at least once. This figure represents 5.3% of the U.S. household population over age twelve, and reflects a substantial increase over the 1985 survey figure of 4.4%. The 1994 University of Michigan survey of high school seniors indicated that 10.5% has used LSD at least once.

EFFECTS

Approximately thirty to sixty minutes after ingestion the user feels the initial effects of LSD. It may take up to twelve hours for the effects of the drug to wear off. The effects of an equivalent dose varies from person to person, and even from dose to dose for the same individual. An individuals mental state (set), surroundings (setting), and dosage strength all play a role in the intensity of the high, and whether or not it will be a good trip or a "bummer" or "bad trip".

Ingestion of LSD brings about physical changes in the body, but the most profound changes occur in the mind. Physically, there is an increase in blood pressure, pulse rate, temperature and respiration. The pupils dilate and there is an increase in salivation. Mentally, there is a distortion of sensory perception, along with impaired judgement. The user may experience vivid hallucinations. Visual perception is often distorted as well as the user's sense of distance and time.

Often times there is a sharp increase in the perception of sound and color. These two senses can become crossed to the point where color is "heard" and sound is "seen". This effect is known as synesthesia and is common in trips resulting from the ingestion of higher doses of LSD.

LSD

If the trip is a "bummer", the user can experience extreme fear, anxiety and paranoia. The individual is at risk of physical injury by reacting in a state of panic. The usual treatment for a bad trip is to "talk down" the individual. They are placed in a quiet, nonthreatening surrounding and constantly reassured that they are safe, that the effects of the drug will wear off shortly, and they will return to normal.

Flashbacks are a phenomenon experienced by some LSD users. They occur after the effects of the drug have worn off, and the user has returned to normal. They are a spontaneous and fragmentary recurrence of a previous LSD trip, and may occur weeks, months, or years after the last usage. The flashbacks may last for only a few seconds, or for a much longer period of time, and may be pleasurable or frightening. The exact cause of the flashback phenomenon is unknown.

There is no evidence that LSD is physically addictive. As with other hallucinogenic drugs, the body quickly develops a tolerance to LSD, generally within three to six days of continued use. Further use of LSD will have little effect on the user until the tolerance has been reduced by an abstinence of three to seven days.

BLUE STAR HOAX

A false rumor which is believed to have originated in 1981 warns parents that LSD is being sold in the form of children's washable transfer tattoos. This rumor, which is usually referred to as the "Blue Star Hoax", warns parents that the LSD can be absorbed through the skin. Warning letters supposedly sponsored by police officials or parents' groups have appeared often; however, no LSD-laden "tattoo" has been recorded, though hundreds of incidents of the "Blue Star Hoax" have been documented.

PHARMACOLOGY

LSD is an indolealkylamine which is known to act on multiple sites of the CNS. It appears to bind to areas in the brain known as the hippocampus, corpus striatum, cerebral cortex and cerebellum where it is postulated to prevent the inhibition or displacement of the neurotransmitter, serotonin, also known as 5-hydroxytryptamine (5-HT). It is this inhibition of serotonin that results in certain sensory neurons to go "unchecked" and increase their electrical firing, thus causing the perceptual and thought distortions which are the basis for hallucinations. This stimulation leads to distorted visual perception, hypersensitivity to sounds, depersonalization, warped thoughts and time sense and psychosis associated with panic anxiety which is the classic "bad trip". "Flashbacks" can occur months, even years later and have been speculated to be a type of "visual seizure" or an atypical memory disorder.

∎

MARIJUANA

CSA SCHEDULE: I

ACTIVE SUBSTANCE: There are hundreds of chemical substances in marijuana, but a series of compounds called cannabinoids are the most important. Of these, delta-9-tetrahydrocannabinol, commonly known as delta 9-THC, or just THC, accounts for virtually all of the psychoactive effect.

STREET NAMES: Astro turf, bhang, bush, cannabis, charas, daga, ditch weed, dope, duby, ganja, grass, green, grifa, hay, hemp, herb, hierba, home grown, indica, j, jay, jane, Juanita, junk weed, kali, kif, kush, leaf, marijuana, Mary, Mary Jane, M.J., mota, northern light, pakalolo, punta roja, ragweed, reefer, roach, sativa, sens, sins, sinsemilla, smoke, stink weed, tea, Texas tea, THC, wacky weed, weed, and zacate. Other names such as Colombian, Oaxacan, Maui Wowie, Acapulco gold, Afghani, African black, Canadian black, Panama gold, Panama red, Kona gold, and Jamaican indicate the geographical origin and color hues that the marijuana may have.

PSYCHOPHYSICAL ACTION: Variable

STREET PRICES (1993):

	Gram	Ounce	Pound
Commercial	-	$25 - $450	$300 - $5,000
Sinsemilla	-	$75 - $1,000	$1,000 - $9,500
Hash	$6 - $20	$80 - $1,200	$1,000 - $2,500
Hash Oil	$35 - $55	$150 - $300	$2,500 - $4,000

Marijuana is the most widely used and most familiar illicit drug. Despite its near universal contraband status, it is found in nearly all sectors of the globe, and its use is deeply ingrained in the cultures of many countries such as India, Jamaica, Morocco, and Nepal.

As with any illicit drug, it is nearly impossible to compile accurate information on the number of users and the amount of marijuana used, but there are a number of generally accepted guidelines. In the 1993 National Household Survey on Drug Abuse, 18,600,000 Americans reported using marijuana at least once within the past year. Other estimates place the number of users much higher, some as high as 28,000,000. It is generally agreed that marijuana is the highest dollar value crop grown in America. Estimates place the value of domestic marijuana production between twenty and twenty eight billion dollars, well ahead of the next most valuable crop, which is corn. This twenty billion dollar domestic production supplies only 35% of the estimated fifty seven billion dollars worth of marijuana consumed annually in the United States. Why the popularity? Peer pressure, curiosity, less fear about side effects, anti-establishment symbolism, and abundant availability are all involved to a degree. But certainly the most important factor is the intoxicating and altered sense effect that the drug produces.

MARIJUANA

HISTORY

Cannabis is a plant that has been used throughout history. Perhaps as early as 6,000 years ago, peoples of India and Asia used the quality fiber obtained from the stalks of the plant to make rope and clothing, and its seeds were a source of food and oil.

Marijuana has also been used as a medicine since antiquity. As early as 3000 B.C., marijuana was used in China and India as an anesthetic, to improve appetite, and as a treatment for a variety of other conditions. Scientist in the Middle East recently exhumed the body of a woman who died during childbirth 1,600 years ago. Along with the body, they also found marijuana, which had apparently been used to ease the pain of childbirth. Marijuana was accepted into professional Western medicine around 1839, and enjoyed medical status for over 100 years. During this time, several major pharmaceutical companies marketed about three dozen different preparations containing marijuana as a treatment for a host of ills, from insomnia to menstrual cramps.

Cannabis is not native to North America. Its introduction here is attributed to the early settlers, who brought seeds with them from Europe and began harvesting the plant for its fiber around the year 1600. In this setting, hemp fiber was used for cloth and rope, and in certain areas laws required that it be grown. Hemp production flourished in many states, and for many years its production was exceeded only by cotton. The invention of the cotton gin and competition from cheap imported hemp in the late 1800's reduced the amount of hemp cultivated in the United States.

By 1935, certain federal government agencies were becoming concerned about the abuse of marijuana. This resulted in the passage of the Marijuana Tax Act of 1937. The Act did not outlaw marijuana, but imposed heavy excise and transfer taxes, which effectively eliminated the sale of marijuana for legitimate uses. Marijuana products became more difficult to obtain and were prescribed less frequently. In 1941, marijuana was dropped from the two official compendia of drugs in the United States, the U.S. Pharmacopeia, and the National Formulary.

Government policy on the growing of marijuana was quickly reversed when Japan cut off the United States supply of hemp fiber from the Philippine Islands in 1942. This fiber was vital to the war effort, and the government promptly arranged for a seed crop to be planted in 1942, with the objective of having 350,000 acres of marijuana under cultivation by 1943. American farmers continued to grow marijuana through 1945.

Cannabis is a weed, and as such it can grow in a wide variety of soil and climatic conditions, and has spread from its once cultivated fields. It is estimated that wild cannabis is scattered over several hundred thousand acres throughout the United States, particularly in the mid-west. Predecessors of this wild cannabis were varieties grown for the fiber and it has little or no THC content.

Until recently, growing cannabis was illegal in nearly every country in Europe and the Americas. Cannabis is a valuable source of pulp and fiber, which can be used in making paper, textiles, rope, etc. As more and more emphasis is placed on preserving forests and protecting the environment, an increasing number of countries have legalized the growing of cannabis as an alternate source of fiber and pulp. Cannabis with a very low THC content is now grown in France, Italy and Yugoslavia. England and Canada have also approved limited growing of agricultural cannabis.

MARIJUANA

Although marijuana has probably been used as a psychoactive drug in America for at least 200 years, like many drugs, it wasn't until the late 1960's that its use became widespread. It is estimated that in the early 1960's, only about 3% of the American population between the ages of 18 and 25 had used marijuana. By the early 70's, it had been used by about 40% of the population in that age group. By the early 80's, it is estimated that it had been used by roughly 70% of all people in America between the ages of 18 and 25.

THE PLANT

Cannabis, marijuana, and hemp are all terms that are commonly used interchangeably, but there is generally some technical distinction. Cannabis is the botanical genus of these plants. Marijuana is a term used to describe marijuana plants, or products of these plants, that have a high THC content and are used as a drug. Hemp on the other hand, is commonly used to describe cannabis plants which have a low THC content, and which are cultivated for fiber and seed.

There has been a long standing controversy as to whether there exists a single species of the genus cannabis, or several. Cannabis sativa, Cannabis indica, and Cannabis ruderalis have been considered distinct species by many botanists, but the consensus among most experts is that there exists only one species, Cannabis sativa. The other varieties, or strains, have distinct characteristics, but are within the same species. Because cannabis is dioecious, which means it has both male and female plants, selective breeding between varieties has resulted in literally hundreds of strains.

The potency of the marijuana plant is related to both the amount and quality of the resin it produces. Resin is a sticky sap-like substance which is formed on the outer surfaces of the plant by very small glands. The resin contains the active substance of the marijuana plant, THC. The THC content in marijuana varies from plant to plant, and depends on the available nutrients, climate, and the genetics of the plant. Some marijuana plants may have little or no THC, while the content of others may be as high as 30%.

The typical marijuana plant, grown outdoors in the U.S., will reach a height of six to twelve feet and produce one to five pounds of dried buds and smokeable leaves. Plants mature between the end of July and early October, depending on the latitude in which they are grown and the genetics of the plants. Growers continue to crossbreed different varieties to develop plants that require a shorter growing period and produce more buds with a higher percentage of the psychoactive cannabinoid, THC. In 1970, the average THC content of commercial marijuana was 1.5%; today it is almost 4%.

THC is produced by and stored in the plants resin glands. The resin glands are located on all parts of the plant, but the heaviest concentration, and the largest glands, are located on the buds and surrounding small leaves. The percentage of THC in the resin varies from plant to plant.

VARIETIES OF MARIJUANA

As discussed earlier, there exists only one species of cannabis, Cannabis sativa, but there are literally hundreds of varieties. Geographical variations include Colombian gold, Maui wowie, Mexican, Kona gold, Canadian black, Thai, etc. Marijuana from any of these varieties may be "commercial" quality, which is either from the male plant or seeded female plant, or "sinsemilla", which is from the seedless, or unpollinated female plant.

MARIJUANA PRODUCTS

COMMERCIAL

The term "commercial" is generally used to describe all dried marijuana on the market, with the exception of sinsemilla. Most commercial marijuana consists of heavily seeded female buds. The average THC content of commercial marijuana is about 3.6% to 4.0%.

SINSEMILLA

Marijuana consists of both male and female plants, with the female generally being considered the more potent of the two. During late fall, the male plants release pollen to fertilize the female plants. Once a female plant is fertilized, it devotes much of its energy to the production of seeds. However, if the female plant is not fertilized, it uses its energy to produce additional flowers. By removing the male plants from a garden (which typically consists of 50% female and 50% male plants) before pollination begins, the grower can produce a garden which consists of very potent, unfertilized female plants. This growing technique, commonly called "sinsemilla" (pronounced seen-suh-mee-yuh), which is Spanish for "without seed", produces some of the most potent marijuana available. The THC content of sinsemilla averages 6% to 7%, nearly double the average THC content of commercial marijuana. Sinsemilla samples with a THC content in excess of 10% are common. The most potent sinsemilla tested was grown in Cooper Center, Alaska, and reportedly had a THC content of 29.86%, nearly eight times stronger than commercial marijuana.

HASH

Hash is the dried and pressed resin of the marijuana plant. Hash has been a popular drug in parts of Asia and the Middle East for hundreds of years, but it has not gained a large following in the United States. This is due to the Americans preference for marijuana, as well as general unfamiliarity with the drug.

Hash is produced by collecting the sticky resin from the leaves and buds of the marijuana plant. This is often done by simply rubbing the plant between the hands, and gathering the resin that collects on them by scraping or rubbing it off. Another method is to shake the cut plant over cloth or plastic which collects the powdery resin as it falls. A small amount of water is added to the resin, which is then rolled or pressed into a variety of forms, such as patties, fingers, balls, etc. Finely ground marijuana leaves and twigs may be added to the resin as a binder.

A method sometimes used to produce more potent hash is by boiling ground marijuana leaves and buds in alcohol. After several hours of boiling, the alcohol and extracted resin that it contains is filtered from the vegetable matter. Finely ground marijuana leaves are added as a binder, and the alcohol is allowed to evaporate. The hash eventually solidifies and becomes hard.

The majority of hashish in the United States is imported from the countries of Pakistan, Afghanistan, Lebanon, and Morocco. There is some domestic production, but the street price for hash relative to marijuana does not make it economical. For instance, it takes no less than two pounds of marijuana to produce one pound of hash. Based on current street prices, two pounds of marijuana could be sold for around $2,400, whereas one pound of hash would bring slightly more than half that. Additionally, the THC content of hash in street samples is consistently much lower than the THC content of sinsemilla.

Hash usually has a tan, green, brown, or black color, with the darker colors generally being the more potent. It is normally very hard, and has to be cut with a knife or broken into small pieces. Hash is consumed in the same manner as marijuana. It can be smoked in a pipe or bong by itself or mixed with marijuana. Some users mix hash with food, such as fudge brownies and ingest it orally. Hash is usually packaged in plastic bags.

Average THC Content

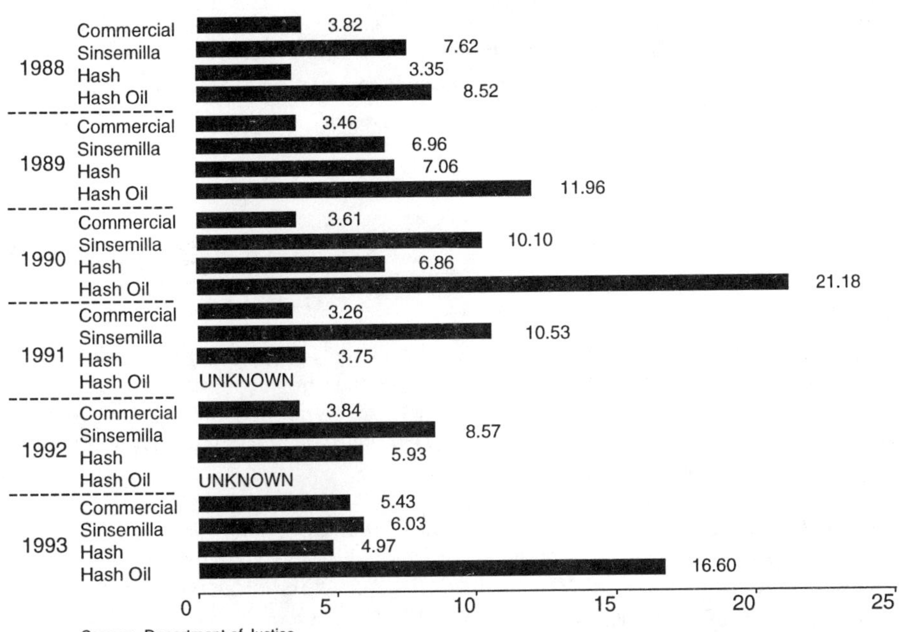

Source: Department of Justice

Hash goes by a variety of street names, such as shish, kif, charas, and nup. Names such as finger, candy bar, surf board, and patties refer to the shape in which the hash is formed. Names like Leb, blonde Lebanese, black Afghani, and Moroccan indicate the color of the hash and its country of origin. Blocks of hash are often stamped with letters and/or symbols as a trademark of the particular producer.

HASH OIL

There are many ways to produce hash oil, but the basic principle used by most operations is similar to that of percolating coffee. A basket filled with ground or chopped marijuana is suspended inside a larger container, at the bottom of which is contained a solvent, such as alcohol, hexane, chloroform, or petroleum ether. Copper tubing or similar material is arranged at the top through which cold water circulates. The solvent is heated and the vapors rise to the top where they condense, then fall into the basket of marijuana. As the solvent seeps

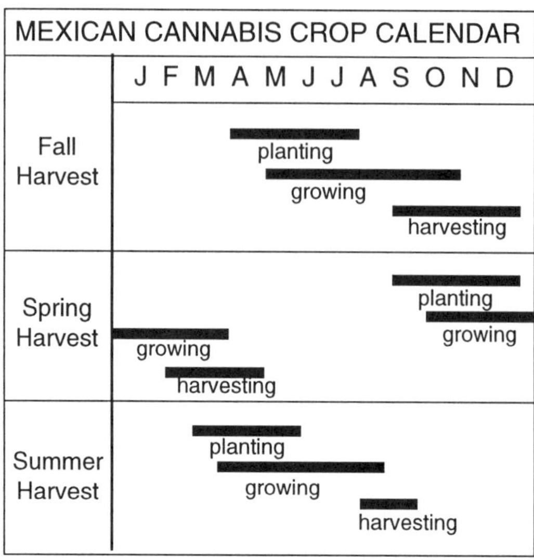

through the plant material, the THC and other soluble materials are dissolved, and the solution drops back down to the bottom of the container. Continued heating causes the process to occur over and over again. The solution becomes increasingly stronger until the plant material is exhausted of its THC. Sometimes new material is added and the same solvent reheated, yielding an even more potent solution.

Most hash oil is black in color, but honey, dark green, red, and brown colors are also seen. The color depends on the level of refinement used to produce the oil. Whereas dark colored hash is usually more potent than light colored hash, the opposite is the case with hash oil. Light colored hash oil has generally been through a more thorough refinement process than that of the black or darker colors, and is generally more potent. The potency of hash oil is adversely affected by its exposure to heat and light, so it is almost always packaged in dark colored glass vials, and is often kept in a cool environment. Hash oil normally has a very thick syrup-like consistency.

Street names for hash oil include oil and shish oil. The oil is usually either smeared on the paper used to roll a joint, or the joint is dipped into a container of the oil to enhance the joints potency. Hash oil is also smoked by itself by vaporizing it in a glass pipe, and is occasionally mixed with liquid, such as wine and taken by mouth. Like hash, a substantial amount of the hash oil in the U.S. comes from the Middle East. Jamaica is also a major supplier.

POTENCY

Marijuana buds average about 3% to 4% THC by dry weight. As a general rule, female plants contain more THC than do the male plants. THC content not only varies from plant to plant, but within individual parts of the plant as well. The following parts of the marijuana plant are

MARIJUANA

listed in order of their potency:

FLOWER CLUSTERS - The flower clusters do not look like flowers at all, but more like a clump of dense green foliage. They contain more THC than any other part of the marijuana plant. Both the male and female plants produce flower clusters, but the females is considered more potent. On the street, flower clusters are commonly called "buds". Buds range from a few inches to over 2 feet in length, and several dozen may grow on a single plant.

LEAVES - Although the leaf is the most recognizable part of the marijuana plant to most people, they take a distant second place to the buds in terms of user preference. Other than the small leaves which grow with the flower clusters, many growers discard most leaves on the plant due to a low THC content.

SEEDS, TWIGS, STALK, AND ROOT - The remainder of the plant contains only small amounts of THC. Seeds and twigs are commonly found in dried marijuana, but they are usually removed before it is smoked.

SUPPLY SOURCES

The vast majority of marijuana consumed in the United States, approximately 55%, is grown in Mexico. Thousands of tons of Mexican marijuana are smuggled into the United States every year. Of this, it is estimated that 98% enters by vehicle, and 2% by aircraft. Although it is not always considered to be the best, Mexican marijuana is readily available and affordable. It is cultivated primarily by subsistence farmers who rely on it as their only cash crop, and is often intermingled with legitimate crops such as corn and beans.

The second largest producer is America. Yearly production is estimated at approximately 35% of the total annual domestic consumption. Marijuana production in the United States has increased steadily over the years, and authorities feel this trend will continue.

Caribbean countries, primarily Belize and Jamaica, supply about 8% to 9% of the marijuana consumed in the United States. A small percentage is also smuggled from various Southeast Asian countries such as Laos, Thailand and Cambodia, as well as Africa.

MARIJUANA CULTIVATION

Tens of thousands of people grow marijuana in the United States. These growers range from those who grow only a single plant for their personal use (to avoid the risks and high price of street buys), to operations that grow hundreds or even thousands of plants. The large scale operations are profit oriented. Assuming that high quality sinsemilla sells for about $3,000.00 per pound, a professional garden of only 100 large plants could yield a profit in the area of $500,000.00 per year.

Although some cannabis plants may live for several years, it is considered an annual. After the plant matures in the fall, it develops the potent buds. The buds contain the seeds and pollen required to perpetuate the species after the plants die in early winter. When grown under ideal light and climate conditions, plants may yield not only one, but two harvests of the flower clusters in a single year.

MARIJUANA

Marijuana can be grown either indoors or out. The advantage of growing outdoors is unlimited garden sites that require minimal care and attention. The disadvantages are the possibility of discovery, theft, rodents, seasonal temperature changes, and drought. Indoor growers enjoy the advantages of security and year round growing, but often have restricted space and exorbitant lighting costs.

Marijuana can be found growing in yards, vegetable gardens, national forests, garages, basements, closets, warehouses, barns, on roof tops, and intermingled with farm crops such as corn. Marijuana is a hardy plant that grows in almost any environment, as long as it is provided with light, water, and necessary nutrients.

OUTDOOR CULTIVATION

CLIMATE: Marijuana has traditionally been thought of as a warm climate plant. However, marijuana is successfully grown in less temperate climates, such as Alaska and Canada. The warmer climates do however, offer the advantages of longer growing seasons, faster growth rates, and occasional multiple harvests of the flower clusters.

GARDEN LOCATION: Perhaps the first and most important consideration a marijuana grower has is the location of the garden. The plot must be located where it will not be easily discovered either by the police or by patch pirates (marijuana thieves). To conceal the marijuana, the grower may plant it among farm crops, in flower and vegetable gardens, or in an area with heavy natural vegetation. The grower may feel that his own property is sufficient, or that a secluded area of public or vacant land accessible only by hiking or 4-wheel drive is best. Many growers avoid putting all their eggs in 1 basket so-to-speak, and plant numerous small gardens separated from each other so that not all of the production will be lost if a plot is discovered. Regardless of where the garden is located, it must have good soil, sunlight, and adequate water for healthy plants.

SEEDS: Although light, water, and nutrients are all important in growing a potent marijuana plant, the most important single factor is the genetics of the particular seed. For this reason, good seed can bring a high price on the street.

STARTING THE SEED: Outdoor marijuana growing starts after the last frost of spring, which in most areas of the United States is about the end of April or the first part of May. Outdoor growers choose one of two ways to start growing the plant. The first is to simply plant the seed in the chosen area. The second is to plant the seed in an indoor starting box, and then transplant the seedling outdoors after the last frost. Starting the seed indoors also allows the grower to start the seed long before spring, and then transplant relatively large plants outdoors after the last frost.

WATER: Marijuana plants need plenty of water. Although the availability of water is normally not a problem for those who grow near their homes, it can be a problem for those who use public or vacant land. Experienced growers know that law enforcement officers target areas with natural streams, rivers, or springs when looking for these gardens. For this reason, many growers install elaborate watering systems, including buried water pipes and pumps to carry water to more remote and less suspect locations.

SOIL: Like any plant, marijuana needs good soil. Marijuana growers often add various fertilizers and nutrients to adjust the pH, nitrogen, potassium, and phosphorus levels of the soil.

MARIJUANA

LIGHT: Marijuana plants are almost always located where they can receive at least eight hours of direct sunlight. The more light the plants get, the faster the growth rate. To allow the plants to receive this amount of light without being seen, they are often concealed among vegetables, flowers, etc. Growers on public lands may choose a heavily wooded area, and then cut off the branches of the trees under which the marijuana has been planted.

RATE OF GROWTH: Depending on the variety of marijuana, and the nutrients, water, and light provided, a plant may grow as much as several inches every day. When grown outdoors, it usually takes about six months for most plants to mature and produce the flowering clusters. When grown under optimal indoor conditions, plants may mature and develop flower clusters in 3 months.

SECURITY: Marijuana growers go to great lengths to provide security for their gardens. In addition to planting marijuana in areas where it is not easily seen, some growers may use attack dogs, high fences, trip wires connected to explosives or alarms, steel animal traps, and fish hooks hung at eye level to keep both man and animal away. The time of outdoor harvest in late fall is when patch pirates look for opportunities. It is also the time when growers become the most protective of their cultivation sites. Growers may camp near their gardens, armed and ready to confront any would-be thieves.

HARVESTING: The flower clusters are the most potent and preferred part of the marijuana plant. These clusters are harvested after they have fully developed, which is usually around September or October. The leaves are also occasionally used and are picked from the plant throughout its growing season.

DRYING/STORAGE: After the marijuana is harvested, it is dried to eliminate the water contained in it so it can be preserved and smoked. Typical drying methods include hanging the buds on lines in open air, or placing them in an oven on low temperature. Three things will reduce the potency of dried marijuana: air, light, and heat. Once the marijuana is dried, it is typically placed in airtight bags and often stored in a cool dry place, such as a basement or refrigerator.

INDOOR CULTIVATION

Although a substantial amount of marijuana grown in the U.S. is cultivated outdoors, the trend is clearly toward the indoor operation. Growing marijuana indoors not only provides a high level of security, but also allows the grower a year-round controlled environment of temperature, light, water, and nutrients - all factors in determining a plants potency. In fact, some of the highest quality marijuana in the world comes from America's indoor operations. Basements, closets, window sills, barns, storage sheds, warehouses, and garages are all common indoor growing sites. The indoor garden may consist of only a few plants, or many as in the case of an Arizona operation which had 14,547 plants. Similarly, these gardens may be simple, utilizing sunlight from an open window or sun room, or complex operations which utilize sophisticated watering and electrical lighting systems.

Perhaps the most significant advantage of growing marijuana indoors is the ability to control the amount of light that it receives. If a marijuana plant is provided with eighteen to twenty four hours of light each day rather than the ten or twelve hours it would get outdoors, its growth rate can be greatly accelerated. Additionally, the decreasing amount of light from the sun in the fall season triggers the marijuana plant to develop its flower clusters to reproduce. This characteristic allows the indoor grower to essentially trick the plant into flowering at will, by decreasing the number of hours of light that the plant receives. Indoor growers use a wide variety of lights and lighting systems. Fluorescent, metal halide, and sodium vapor lights are all commonly used.

HYDROPONICS

Another method of growing marijuana indoors is by using hydroponics. Hydroponics is the growing of plants in a container of water with dissolved nutrients rather than in soil. The root system of the plant is supported by a medium such as rockwool, lava rock, or gravel. Although unorthodox, hydroponics is a fast and efficient way of growing many plants, including marijuana.

IDENTIFICATION AND PACKAGING

When mature, marijuana appears as a green leafy bush. Different varieties may grow from two to twenty feet in height, and have slight variations in branching configurations and leaf appearance. Probably the most distinctive aspect of the marijuana plant is the leaf. The blades of the marijuana leaf almost always consist of an odd number, such as 3, 5, 7, 9, or 11, and have a characteristically serrated edge.

At the street level, marijuana is normally a mixture of leaves, buds, small twigs, and seeds. However, because the seeds and twigs contain little or no THC, they are generally removed before the marijuana is smoked. If the sample does not have seeds, it has either been "cleaned", or is potent sinsemilla. One cannot usually tell if dried marijuana came from a male or female plant, a sativa or indica plant, was grown indoors or out, or its country of origin. Dried marijuana is typically dull green or brownish in color, and often has a very strong odor.

PACKAGING

In small amounts, marijuana can be stored in just about any type of container, but it is most often packaged in clear plastic sandwich bags or 35mm film cannisters. Large amounts, consisting of several pounds, are often packaged in plastic wrap, which serves as an air tight package to preserve the marijuana, and to contain the odor to prevent detection.

METHODS OF INGESTION

The most common way of ingesting marijuana is by smoking it. The manner in which it is smoked is one of user preference; hand rolled joints, pipes, or bongs.

Hand rolled joints using any number of brands of cigarette rolling paper is probably the most common smoking method. The marijuana is crushed with the fingers into the paper, which is rolled and twisted at each end. As the joint is smoked down, the user typically utilizes a roach clip to hold the "roach", or butt end of the joint to prevent the lips and fingers from getting burned. Electrical alligator clips and surgical hemostats are the most popular types of roach clips. The user generally holds his breath as long as possible after taking a puff to maximize the effects. Burnt marijuana has a very strong and distinctive odor.

Water pipes, or bongs, are another method used to smoke marijuana. A bong has a water chamber through which the smoke passes as it is inhaled. The water cools the smoke and removes most of the harsh water soluble chemicals. Additionally, a higher percentage of THC reaches the user with the use of a bong as compared to that of a joint.

EFFECTS

The subjective effects of marijuana can vary considerably. Some users have a slight psychedelic or hallucinatory experience, others exhilaration, others relaxation. Senses may become more acute, causing noises to become more pronounced and colors more vivid. Marijuana accentuates the feeling of hunger, causing an appetite often referred to as the "munches". A distorted sense of time and an almost uncontrollable laughter are sometimes experienced. The various effects of marijuana normally reach a peak within thirty minutes and last up to three or more hours.

The intoxicating effects of marijuana also reduce judgement and coordination. Study after study related to fatal motor vehicle accidents consistently show marijuana as a factor in a substantial number of these occurrences.

The results of a recent study to identify drivers impaired by marijuana and cocaine was reported by Daniel Brookoff, M.D., et all, in the August 25th, 1994 issue of the New England Journal of Medicine. In this study, 150 drivers who had been stopped for reckless driving agreed to submit to field urine tests for marijuana and cocaine. Reckless driving was defined as driving that would constitute probable cause to suspect intoxication. The following results were reported for the 150 drivers tested:

Category	Number	Number Arrested for Driving Under The Influence
Positive for marijuana only	50	48
Positive for cocaine only	20	20
Positive for both drugs	18	18
Negative for both drugs	62	--

The study showed that there is no typical appearance or behavior manifested by the individual under the influence of these drugs, nor are roadside alcohol tests effective in detecting drug intoxication. More importantly, there is no field test to measure the effects these drugs have on the individuals judgement and risk taking.

In another study, ten licensed pilots were given one marijuana joint containing 19 mg of THC, a relatively small amount. Twenty four hours after smoking the joint, they were tested in a flight simulator. All ten of the pilots made errors in landing, and one missed the runway completely. Similar results were reported in another test involving nine pilots. In this case they were given one marijuana joint containing 20 mg of THC, and were tested in a flight simulator twenty four hours after smoking. Seven of the nine pilots showed some degree of impairment. Only one of the pilots was aware of the fact that a joint smoked twenty four hours earlier was still effecting his performance. These, and similar tests, indicate that marijuana may impair ones ability to operate a motor vehicle long after the visible effects of the drug have worn off.

Detrimental physical and psychological effects related to marijuana use have long been argued. The immune and reproductive systems, fetal development, chromosomal damage, and brain functioning and development have all been targets of scientific study. The most conclusive of these studies relates to the lungs. Marijuana smoking poses all the threatening risks associated with cigarette smoking, including bronchitis, emphysema, and lung cancer. In fact, several studies have shown that marijuana has more than twice the amount of tar contained in an equal amount of cigarette tobacco.

An individual under the influence of marijuana may have bloodshot eyes, slowed reactions, a lack of coordination, and the strong odor of burnt vegetation. A thick white or light green coating is usually apparent on the tongue, as well as blisters on the tongue or back of throat due to the hot smoke. Marijuana also often causes the eyelids to flutter or vibrate when the eyes are closed, and reduces ones ability to cross the eyes.

MEDICAL MARIJUANA

Marijuana has been used as a medicine for thousands of years. Prior to the Marijuana Tax Act of 1937, there were roughly three dozen medicines containing marijuana marketed in the United States. Only recently has marijuana obtained its taboo and non-medicinal status. However, recent studies have concluded that marijuana can effectively treat a variety of conditions. A majority of studies completed so far indicate that marijuana may be superior to traditional drugs in the treatment of nausea and vomiting caused by chemotherapy. A survey by researchers at Harvard University, conducted in 1990, revealed that 44% of oncologists (cancer specialists) had recommended to their patients that they obtain marijuana to control the nausea caused by the chemotherapy treatment. Almost half said they would prescribe marijuana if it were legal, and over 60% were of the opinion that it was an effective drug. 70% stated that they had at least one patient who had used marijuana to control nausea. In addition to being an anti-nausea medicine, marijuana has shown a degree of effectiveness in treating glaucoma, easing muscle spasms associated with multiple sclerosis and spinal cord injuries, and appetite loss that is a side effect of AIDS and cancer therapy.

In 1990, a Federal Court of Appeals mandated that the DEA must review the current scheduling status of marijuana as a Schedule I drug, meaning it has no legitimate medical uses, and consider placing it in the Schedule II category, which would allow it to be a prescribed medicine. The ruling was not binding, and the DEA elected to keep marijuana in Schedule I. In July of 1994, the Clinton Administration announced that there would be no relaxation of the prohibition against the medicinal use of marijuana. This decision was based on a determination by the National Institute of Health that there was no clinical evidence to suggest that smoked marijuana was superior to currently available therapies.

Much of the concern over marijuana as a medicine stems from the fact that marijuana may adversely affect the body's immune system in already severely ill patients. Additionally, damage to the lungs and respiratory system caused by smoking marijuana is well established.

Much of the current research on marijuana is directed at isolating the sixty one cannabinoids it contains. These substances are found nowhere else in nature. The theory is that the therapeutic effects of these various cannabinoids could be separated from the high caused by using the natural form of the drug. However, many researchers are of the opinion that the beneficial effects of marijuana are produced by an interaction of its various chemicals, which cannot be replicated with individual application.

MARIJUANA

A synthetic form of THC, marketed under the trade name Marinol has been available since 1985. Many chemotherapy patients have remarked that this medication is simply not as effective as marijuana however. In the same Harvard study cited above, 77% of the oncologists who responded said that they believed that marijuana was more effective than the synthetic THC.

PHARMACOLOGY

The psychoactive effects of THC and the other cannabinoids in marijuana are thought to be a result of their action on dopamine, serotonin and GABA sites in the CNS and this results in euphoria, hallucinations, paranoia and abnormal thinking. THC is extremely fat-soluble and thus will concentrate in fatty areas of the body including the brain and sexual glands. PDIS (Post-Drug Impairment Syndrome) or Amotivational Syndrome are diagnosis related to marijuana's negative effects on motivation and an inability to endure life's everyday stresses. These symptoms appear to be due to physical damage to the nerve endings within parts of the brain including the "pleasure center".

▮

PCP

CSA SCHEDULE: II

ACTIVE SUBSTANCE: 1-1-phenylcyclohexyl piperidine

STREET NAMES: Ace, angel dust, animal tranquilizer, crystal, dead on arrival, DOA, dust, elephant, embalming fluid, hog, jet fuel, juice, killer joints, lovely, monkey, ozone, PCP, rocket fuel, supergrass, tac, tic, trank, and wack.

PSYCHOPHYSICAL ACTION: Dissociative anesthetic

STREET PRICES: One ounce of powder - $500.00 to $1,200.00
One ounce of liquid - $200.00 to $1,500.00
One full length cigarette saturated with liquid PCP - $30.00 to $70.00
Source: Department of Justice

HISTORY

PCP is the most common street name for the chemical known as phencyclidine. Phencyclidine was developed by the Parke-Davis Company in 1957 for use as a general anesthetic, and was tested under the trade name Sernyl. In clinical trials, it induced the desired anesthesia for surgery, but it also produced a number of postoperative problems. Upon coming out of the anesthesia, a relatively large percentage of patients experienced delirium, delusions, visual disturbances and varying degrees of psychotic behavior. While phencyclidine underwent extensive clinical tests, researchers were unable to eliminate the postoperative side effects. Because of this the drug was never marketed to the health care industry.

In 1967, Parke-Davis introduced phencyclidine to the veterinary industry for use in anesthetizing large animals. It was marketed under the trade name Sernylan. In the same year, the first illicit use of the drug occurred at a music festival in the San Francisco Bay area. It was distributed under the name PeaCe Pill. Abuse of the drug continued through the late 1970's, and in 1978 it was changed from Schedule III to Schedule II. Shortly thereafter, legitimate manufacturing of the drug was discontinued.

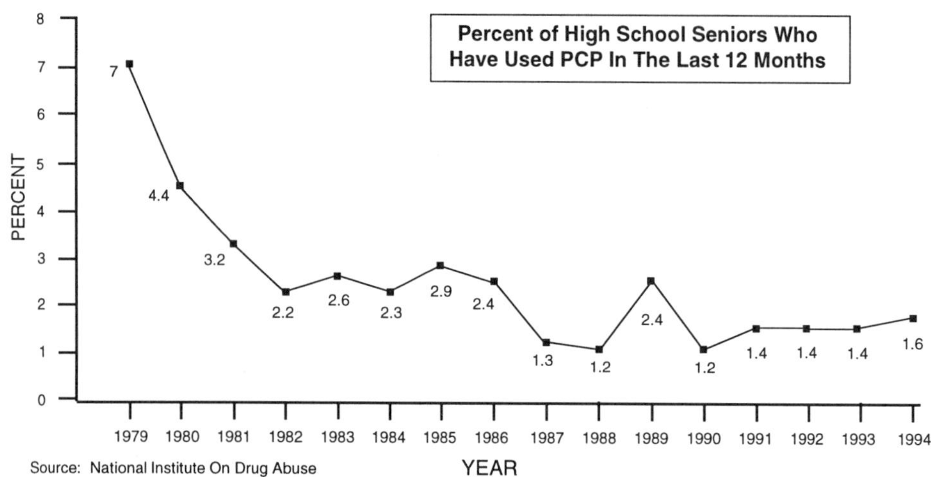

PCP

MANUFACTURING AND DISTRIBUTION

The process of manufacturing PCP is relatively simple, and generally uses the following chemicals:

Cyclohexanone
Sodium bisulfite
Phenylmagnesium bromide
Piperidine
Potassium cyanide
Bromobenzene
Ether

The synthesis consists of a two step procedure. The first step involves the manufacturing of an intermediate product known as PCC (1-piperidinylcyclohexanecarbonitrile). This product is then converted into PCP. If all impurities and chemicals used in the manufacturing process are removed, the end product is an odorless, metallic or bitter tasting, white powder. Due to makeshift manufacturing, the color of most PCP seen on the street will vary from tan to brown, and generally has a strong odor. PCP is also sold in liquid form. Due to impurities, the color of liquid PCP can range from clear to yellowish.

The manufacturing and distribution of PCP is generally controlled by inner-city gangs, and its use is most prevalent in the larger cities on the east and west coasts. The pure drug is often "cut" or diluted to a street potency by adding any of a number of substances, or by dissolving and diluting in water, acetone or ether. The drug is sold in PCP laced cigarettes ready for smoking, as well as in powder and liquid forms. The powder form of PCP is generally packaged in aluminum foil or plastic bags.

USE

One of the major problems facing the PCP user is the unknown strength, or purity, of a given dose. Quality control is unknown in the clandestine laboratories where the drug is manufactured and there are no "standards" for packaging of the product for street sale. A given dose may be nearly pure, or may have been diluted by a ratio of 20:1, 50:1 or even more.

PCP may be smoked, snorted, injected or swallowed. Smoking is the preferred method of using the drug. When smoked, the user feels the effects within two minutes. PCP is generally prepared for smoking by dissolving it in acetone, ether or other volatile liquid. It can then be sprayed or soaked onto parsley leaves, mint, or other smokeable vegetable matter. The solution is permitted to evaporate, leaving the PCP laced vegetable matter. PCP in powder form is often sprinkled on marijuana and rolled into a joint.

Regular cigarettes are also laced with PCP. Cigarettes with dark brown paper are generally used to conceal the discoloration produced by the soaking. This type of PCP laced cigarette is generally referred to as a "sherm", "shermie", or "sherm stick".

PCP

EFFECTS

PCP is a dissociative anesthetic. "Dissociative" indicates that it can induce a state of mind-body dissociation in which the user is aware of what is happening, but does not feel involved, either physically or emotionally. The user perceives themselves as an observer to their own actions. Anesthetic indicates that the drug causes insensitivity to pain. Depending on the dose, the effects of PCP can range from a pleasant feeling to mild sedation, from agitation to violent behavior, and from a total loss of sensitivity to pain to a prolonged coma.

Much has been written about the feats of incredible strength performed by individuals under the influence of PCP. Despite a number of well documented cases, there does not appear to by any medical evidence to indicate that PCP increases the users strength. At the appropriate dosage, PCP causes a total loss of sensitivity to pain, and in this condition the user is capable of feats that astound the observer. Running on two broken legs, ignoring severe burns, pulling their own teeth; the stories are endless and most are true.

Regardless of how it is taken, the physical effects of PCP are felt shortly after ingestion. When smoked the onset occurs within two to five minutes and peaks within fifteen to thirty minutes. The degree of intoxication is determined by the amount of the drug absorbed. The effects may last from one hour up to forty eight hours.

Smaller doses, generally less than 5 mg, result in a drunken state with slurred speech, numbness, and depression, often followed by stimulation. The effects of moderate doses, generally less than 10 mg, are much more pronounced and difficult to predict. Some of the more common effects at this level of ingestion are: loss of sensitivity to pain, inability to talk, increased blood pressure and heart rate, sweating, vomiting, agitation and combative behavior, muscle rigidity, lack of coordination, distorted mental images and a stupor or coma state. Higher doses can place the user in a life threatening situation, producing convulsions, respiratory depression, cardiovascular instability, and prolonged comas.

Although the PCP high usually lasts about four to six hours, PCP is stored in the fat cells of the body and released gradually over time. Because of this, varying and sporadic levels of intoxication for days, weeks, and even months after last use have been documented in PCP abusers. Unlike other hallucinogens, PCP flashbacks are true chemical flashbacks caused by residual amounts of the drug remaining in the body, and are not merely psychological.

PHARMACOLOGY

PCP is thought to stimulate alpha-adrenergic receptors, thus potentiating the effects of dopamine, epinephrine, norepinephrine and serotonin. PCP can induce a psychosis which is indistinguishable from schizophrenia and this is thought to be related to exaggerated dopamine, and possibly serotonin activity within the brain. This action also accounts for PCP's hallucinatory activity. Though not understood, PCP possesses pharmacological actions which can cause the user to commit extremely bizarre, violent acts and display almost superhuman strength. The drug's stimulant action closely resembles that of amphetamines, but paradoxically, catatonic rigidity may occur.

∎

PEYOTE

CSA SCHEDULE: I

ACTIVE SUBSTANCE: Mescaline (3,4,5-trimethoxyphenethylamine)

STREET NAMES: Buttons, cactus, cactus buttons, chief, dry whiskey, green whiskey, hikuri, mesc, mescal, mescaline, mescalito, peyote, peyotl, topi, tops.

PSYCHOPHYSICAL ACTION: Hallucinogen

STREET PRICE: $10.00 to $30.00 per button

The peyote cactus, which is botanically known as Lophophora williamsii Lemaire, is a plant which grows in northern Mexico and the southern part of Texas. Unlike most other members of the cactus family, peyote does not have spines. The top of the cactus, which is called a "button", is rounded and has a grayish-green color. It is small, averaging about one to two inches in diameter. The button contains several dozen alkaloids, the most active of which is mescaline. Perhaps due to it's scarcity, bitter taste, and difficulty in locating it, the peyote cactus has never been as common as other drugs of abuse. However, because the demand for peyote reportedly exceeds the natural supply, it is the opinion of some botanists that the peyote cactus may someday become an endangered plant. In 1991, the peyote cactus was placed on the list of endangered plants by the Mexican Government, but indigenous citizens retained the right to collect it for religious purposes.

HISTORY

The peyote cactus has been used for at least 3,000 years by Indians in Mexico. It was consumed in their religious rites, used as a medicine and used to relieve fatigue and hunger. The Spanish conquerors tried unsuccessfully to eliminate the Indians use of peyote. However, it continued and by the late 1800's the use of peyote by Indians spread into what is now the southwest United States. Non-Indians viewed the drug as devilish, and numerous attempts were made to eradicate its use. In response to the white mans attempted suppression of peyotism, the Indians organized a loose intertribal confederation in 1906. This organization, which used peyote as a religious sacrament, went through a series of evolutionary changes until in 1918 it became incorporated as the Native American Church. The Native American Church eventually won various court battles allowing its members religious use of peyote.

The use of peyote on the street did not gain much of a following until the 1950's. At that time members of the drug culture began using peyote to supplement other drugs they were taking. During the years 1967-1970, its use on the street dramatically increased when the concern over LSD-induced chromosomal damage led many users to substitute other hallucinogens for LSD. After it was learned that LSD did not cause chromosomal damage, many people returned to the cheaper and more readily available LSD. However, peyote never totally lost it's popularity with the drug culture, and it's use continues today.

SUPPLY SOURCES

Peyote grows wild in Mexico and southern Texas. Distributors licensed with the DEA and the state of Texas, of which there are currently nine, are allowed to harvest wild peyote year round for sale only to documented members of the Native American Church. In order to purchase peyote, members of the Native American Church must provide the distributor with proper documentation as prescribed by Texas drug laws. Members of the Native American Church are also allowed to harvest peyote after first providing proper documentation of their intent to the state of Texas. Virtually all of the peyote range in Texas is on privately owned land, and as a result the harvesting takes place on a land lease basis.

The cactus is harvested by cutting off only the top part, or button, leaving the root undisturbed. The root contains only trace amounts of mescaline, and it is allowed to regrow. Within three years, another button will have developed and may be large enough for harvesting. Occasionally, several buttons may grow on a single root. Documents filed by the licensed distributors show that 1,978,646 buttons were harvested in Texas in 1993. These were sold to members of the Native American Church for a total of $210,247.00, or about 10 cents each.

The most active substance in peyote, mescaline, may be chemically extracted from the button by using lye, benzene, sulfuric acid and water. When extracted and purified, mescaline crystals are small needle-shaped and translucent white in appearance. Isolating mescaline from the buttons requires substantial expertise, thus very little mescaline is seen on the street.

IDENTIFICATION

The top of a fresh peyote cactus is usually only about one to two inches in diameter, and about 1/2" to 1" tall. Most of the plant consists of a relatively large and deep root. There are no spines on the peyote cactus, but it does have short tufts of hair growing on it's top. It is often rumored that this hair contains strychnine, but it is actually cellulose.

After harvest, peyote buttons are sun dried for about seven days. When dried, the button becomes hard, and the color changes from a gray-green to a brown or tan. Dried buttons retain their potency for years. The dried buttons are sometimes ground into a powder and placed in gelatin capsules. Synthetic mescaline has also been sold on the street, but it is expensive to produce and is rarely encountered.

METHODS OF INGESTION

Peyote buttons are usually chewed and swallowed, either fresh or dried. The normal dose ranges from four to twelve buttons. Many users find the taste of peyote extremely bitter and nauseating. To overcome this objection, the buttons are sometimes ground and the powder placed into gelatin capsules. Peyote buttons are sometimes boiled to make a thick dark tea. Some users smoke peyote by grinding it and combining it with marijuana or other vegetable matter.

EFFECTS

The effects of peyote start about 1/2 to 1 hour after ingestion, and last for approximately ten to twelve hours. Physically, these effects include the following:

- increased heart rate
- increased salivation
- increased respiration
- increased perspiration
- increased body temperature
- elevated blood pressure
- muscle tension
- nausea
- vomiting
- fullness in stomach
- intoxicated like gait
- lack of coordination
- headache
- dilated pupils

PEYOTE

Because peyote is a hallucinogen, the psychological effects are considerably more significant than the physical effects. Probably the most profound psychological effect of peyote is the change it brings to visual perception. Moderate doses distort colors, making them more intense. Perception of the shape and depth of objects may be altered. The senses can become crossed in an effect known as synesthesia; sounds are heard, and colors are seen. Significant mood changes are not uncommon. As with other hallucinogenic drugs, the psychological effects of peyote are very dependent on the "set" (the user's frame of mind), and the "setting" (the location and surroundings where the drug is taken); a poor set or setting can result in a very bad experience.

As with all hallucinogens, the typical street treatment for a person having a bad experience with the drug is a "talk down". Talking down is the process of providing comforting verbal reassurance to the user, so that he may relax and not be frightened by what he is experiencing.

Addiction to peyote has not been observed in individuals who use it on a regular basis. As with other hallucinogenic drugs, the body quickly develops a tolerance to mescaline, generally within three to six days. Further use of peyote will have little effect on the user until the tolerance has been reduced by an abstinence of several days. The period of abstinence is without the usual physical addiction often seen with opiates, barbiturates, and certain other drugs.

The main dangers associated with hallucinogens such as peyote, are primarily psychological in nature. The user may experience intense anxiety or panic, disorientation, mood changes, and difficulty in distinguishing illusion from reality.

THE NATIVE AMERICAN CHURCH

Although the peyote cactus and any extract of it is a Schedule I drug, it may legally be used by members of the Native American Church. This is because of the long history of the Indians use of peyote in religious rituals, and various court rulings which have upheld members limited use of it as a constitutional right to freedom of religion. However, a 1990 court ruling on case #88-1213 by the U.S. Supreme Court in the case of Oregon Department of Human Resources v. Smith has clouded this issue. The court ruled that an individuals religious use of peyote did not place him beyond the reach of a criminal law (Oregon's law against use of peyote) as long as the law was not specifically directed at his religion. Twenty three states have laws affirming the rights of members of the Native American Church to use peyote for religious purposes. The legal status of the use of peyote by church members in the remaining twenty seven states would be questionable.

Members of the Native American Church have faith in peyote as a cure for illness, and as a means of communicating with the Great Spirit. Peyote ceremonies are held for marriages, birthdays, to cure illness, and other events that call for devout prayer. The ceremony is generally held in a teepee, with services starting at sundown. The individual who leads the ceremony is called the "roadman". He sets the pace and sequence of the worship. At the start of the ceremony, peyote buttons or peyote tea is consumed by the participants. Prayer, supplemented by drums and singing takes place throughout the night. At dawn, the worship services, which began nearly twelve hours earlier, come to an end.

PEYOTE

The use of peyote is not the only aspect of the Native American Church; it teaches brotherly love, high moral principles, and abstention from alcohol consumption. The Church claims about 250,000 members from tribes in the United States, Canada, and South America. One of the requirements for membership in the Church is that the individual be at least 25% Indian. Peyotism does not interest all Native Americans; many prefer either Christianity, or their traditional religion.

PHARMACOLOGY

Although the exact mechanism of action is unknown, the hallucinogenic and behavioral effects of mescaline appears to involve the stimulation of both serotonin and dopamine in the hippocampus, corpus striatum and cerebral cortex areas of the brain. Its actions are very similar to those distorted visual perceptions, hypersensitivity to sounds and warped thoughts and time sense associated with the use of LSD, but to a lesser degree. Its effects last up to twelve hours. Like LSD, PCP and all hallucinogens, "bad trips" as a reult of using peyote are always possible.

∎

PSILOCYBIN MUSHROOMS

CSA SCHEDULE: I

ACTIVE SUBSTANCES: Psilocybin and psilocin.

STREET NAMES: Food of the gods, funny mushrooms, happy mushrooms, magic mushrooms, mushrooms, sacred mushrooms, shrooms, teonanacatl.

PSYCHOPHYSICAL ACTION: Hallucinogen.

STREET PRICES:

Pound - $300 - $1,600	1/4 Pound - $175	Ounce - $30 - $250
1/4 Ounce - $25 - $100	Gram - $3 - $15	

Source: Department of Justice

Psilocybin mushrooms have been used for centuries by Indian cultures of Mexico and Central America. They called the mushroom "teonanacatl", meaning "food of the gods". Based on stone artifacts, psilocybin mushroom use in religious ceremonies dates back to at least 1500 B.C. The first recorded use of hallucinogenic mushrooms occurred during the coronation feast of Montezuma in 1502. However, with the introduction of Christianity to the New World, the use of these mushrooms in religious ceremonies was discouraged, and the practice was driven underground.

For centuries, the use of hallucinogenic mushrooms in Mexico went unnoticed. In 1953, a New York banker, R. Gordon Wasson, rediscovered and brought to the attention of the world the existence of a hallucinogenic mushroom cult in central Mexico. Wasson was able to obtain specimens of the mushrooms being used. A French mycologist (one who studies fungi) identified these as mushrooms of the genus psilocybe. He was also successful in cultivating this species in his laboratory, thus providing sufficient material for chemists to isolate the active substances.

Subsequently, Albert Hofmann, the discoverer of lysergic acid diethylamide (LSD), and his colleagues at the Sandoz Laboratories in Switzerland isolated two substances from the psilocybe mushrooms; psilocybin (phosphorylated 4-hydroxydimethyltryptamine), and psilocin (4-hydroxydimethyltryptamine). These substances have since been found present in numerous mushroom species of the genus Psilocybe, as well as several species of the genera Conocybe, Panaeolus, Stropharia, and Copelandia.

SUPPLY AND IDENTIFICATION

The use of psilocybin mushrooms first became popular in the United States during the 1960's, and they have remained popular ever since. Numerous species grow wild in many areas of the country, particularly on the west coast and in the southern states. In these areas, psilocybin mushrooms can be found growing virtually anywhere; in forests, grassy areas, along roads, and particularly in nutrient-rich pastures. During periods of rain between spring and fall, when the mushrooms thrive, psilocybin enthusiasts search the country side for these mushrooms. However, identifying mushrooms requires a skill and knowledge far beyond that of the average user. Psilocybin and poisonous mushrooms have very similar appearances, and people frequently pick poisonous mushrooms which were mistaken for a psilocybin variety. Poisonous mushrooms can cause liver damage or death within hours.

PSILOCYBIN MUSHROOMS

One unreliable method sometimes used to determine if a mushroom contains psilocybin is to bruise or break the mushroom, and then wait several minutes to see if the damaged area turns bluish in color. Although most species of psilocybin mushrooms exhibit a bluing effect, which is due to oxidation of the indole based substances in the mushroom, several poisonous species do so as well.

Mushrooms can also be identified by their spore print. A spore print is obtained by carefully removing the cap of the mushroom from the stem, and then placing it gill side down on paper. The spores fall from the cap and collects on the paper. Their color, along with a microscopic examination serves as an aid in identifying the species of the mushroom.

Psilocybin mushrooms are commonly grown indoors. These garage and basement operations are popular because it can be much easier to grow the mushrooms rather than search for them in the wild, and the user is not exposed to the dangers involved with picking poisonous varieties. Although the substances psilocybin and psilocin, as well as the mushrooms that contain them are illegal, the mushroom spores are not. Because of this legal loophole, psilocybin mushroom spores can be legally purchased through various sources. Kits containing everything needed to grow psilocybin mushrooms are advertised and sold in counterculture magazines. Some of these in-house growing operations are very small and designed only for personal use. Others are large profit-oriented operations growing thousands of mushrooms weekly.

Because mushrooms begin to spoil and mold soon after harvesting, they are normally preserved by drying. Once dried, psilocybin mushrooms take on a characteristically stiff and wilted appearance, and usually have a tan or brown color. Typical drying methods include putting the mushrooms in an oven on low temperature, or spreading them on a screen to dry in warm air.

At the street level, psilocybin mushrooms are normally packaged in plastic sandwich bags, and may be entirely intact, broken into small pieces, or occasionally ground into a course powder. When ground into a powder, the mushrooms may be packaged in gelatin capsules. Occasionally, regular mushrooms are laced with such drugs as PCP or LSD and sold on the street as psilocybin mushrooms to the unsuspecting user.

Another mushroom, which is of the genus Amanita, should not be confused with the psilocybin varieties. Amanita mushrooms are also abused as hallucinogens, but contain the toxic substances muscimol and ibotenic acid rather than psilocybin. The margin between a hallucinogenic dose and death with these mushrooms is very narrow. They grow in various parts of the country, and appear with a brown, red, yellow or orange cap with white warts.

METHODS OF INGESTION

Psilocybin mushrooms are usually eaten, either fresh or dried. They are also occasionally used to brew a tea. Due to an acrid taste, the mushrooms are sometimes ground to a powder and placed in gelatin capsules. Psilocybin mushrooms are sometimes used in recipes in lieu of regular mushrooms. A dose consists of one or more mushrooms (which includes both the stem and cap), depending on the mushrooms size and potency, and the users tolerance.

PSILOCYBIN MUSHROOMS

EFFECTS

Psilocybin mushrooms contain the chemicals psilocybin, and to a lesser extent psilocin. Upon ingestion, the body apparently converts the psilocybin to psilocin, making the latter primarily responsible for the hallucinogenic effects. Psilocybin mushrooms produce a range of effects similar to those produced by LSD, however the potency of LSD is considerably greater. In small amounts there may be only a slight stimulant effect, slightly increased pulse and blood pressure, and dilated pupils. As the dosage increases, sight and sound become distorted, and feelings of excitement or anxiety may take place. Large amounts produce hallucinations. In a clinical setting, Dr. Leo E. Hollister of the Palo Alto Veteran's Hospital described the pattern of effects on volunteer subjects given doses of psilocybin as follows:

> First 30 minutes—Dizziness, light-headedness or giddiness, weakness, muscle aching and twitching, shivering, nausea, abdominal discomfort, anxiety, tension, restlessness, numbness of the tongue, lips or mouth, heaviness or lightness of the extremities.
>
> 30 to 60 minutes—Blurred vision, brighter colors, longer afterimages, sharp definition of objects, visual patterns (eyes closed), increased acuity of hearing, yawning, tearing, facial flushing, sweating, dreamy state, loss of attention and concentration, slow thinking, feelings of unreality, depersonalization, incoordination, difficult and tremulous speech.
>
> 60 to 90 minutes—Increased visual effects (colored patterns and shapes, generally pleasing, sometimes frightening, most often with eyes closed, occasionally superimposed upon objects in field of vision), undulation of viewed surfaces, distance perception impaired, euphoria, general stimulation, ruminative state, slowed passage of time.
>
> 90 to 120 minutes—Continuation of many of the above effects in varying degrees, especially introspective state, increased bodily sensations and mental perceptions.
>
> 120 to 180 minutes—Waning of previously described effects.
>
> 180 to 300 minutes—Nearly complete resolution of drug-induced effects.

Other effects reported, although not as frequently as those outlined above included: decreased salivation and appetite, transient sexual feelings and synesthesias (e.g.,"seeing" sounds and "hearing" colors).

The main dangers associated with psilocybin mushrooms, as well as the other hallucinogens, are primarily psychological in nature. The user may experience a bad trip; intense anxiety, panic or fear, disorientation, mood changes, and difficulty in distinguishing fantasy from reality. The typical street treatment for a person having such an experience is to provide a nonthreatening environment and reassure the individual that the effects of the drug will wear off shortly, and he will return to normal.

Addiction to psilocybin has not been observed in individuals who ingest the mushrooms on a regular basis. The body develops rapid tolerance to psilocybin, and further use will have little effect until the tolerance has been reduced by a period of abstinence of several days.

PSILOCYBIN MUSROOMS

PHARMACOLOGY

Psilocybin is similar in action to mescaline and LSD. Its action appears to be related to the inhibition of serotonin within the areas of the brain known as the hippocampus, corpus striatum and cerebral cortex resulting in certain sensory neurons to go "unchecked" and increase their electrical firing. This action results in the perceptual and thought distortions which are the basis for hallucinations. It is less potent than LSD and its hallucinogenic effects last up to six hours.

SLANG

ABE - Five dollars worth of a drug. Derived from the picture of Abraham Lincoln on the five dollar bill.
ACAPULCO GOLD - High grade Mexican grown marijuana.
ACCESSORIES - Items with which drugs are used, such as a pipe, syringe, etc.
ACE - 1. A marijuana joint. 2. Street name for PCP.
ACETIC ANHYDRIDE - A chemical regulated by the Chemical Diversion and Trafficking Act of 1988 as an essential chemical, and which is sometimes used in the synthesis of heroin and other illicit drugs.
ACETONE - A chemical regulated by the Chemical Diversion and Trafficking Act of 1988 as an essential chemical, and which is sometimes used in the synthesis of methamphetamine and other illicit drugs. Acetone vapors are also inhaled for the euphoric producing effects.
ACID - Street name for LSD.
ACID CUBE - A sugar cube laced with LSD.
ACID HEAD - An LSD user.
ACTION - The use or sale of drugs.
AD - A drug addict.
ADAM - Street name for the drug MDMA.
ADDICT - A person who is physically and/or mentally habituated to a drug.
ADDICTION - A psychological and/or physical compulsion to take a drug on a continuous or periodic basis in order to experience the drugs effects, and sometimes to avoid the discomfort of its absence. A person may be addicted to more than one drug.
ADULTERANT - A substance added to a drug to increase the drugs volume. An adulterant usually has an appearance similar to, but costing much less than the drug to which it is added. This allows the seller to increase profits by replacing a portion of the original drug with the less expensive adulterant.
ADULTERATE - To make a drug impure by adding a less desirable and generally less expensive substance. The purpose of adulterating a drug is to increase the sellers profits. Occasionally drugs are adulterated with a more active substance in order to increase the drugs potency.
AFGHANI - Drugs that originate from the country of Afghanistan. Afghani usually refers to marijuana or hash, but may also refer to opium or heroin.
AFRICAN LSD - See **IBOGAINE**.
APHRODISIAC - A food, drug, or other substance that arouses, or is reputed to arouse sexual desire. Drugs such as cocaine and MDA are often considered aphrodisiacs.
ALICE B. TOKLAS BROWNIES - An antiquated term for fudge brownies containing marijuana. Named after the individual who supposedly developed the recipe.
ALKALOID - The active ingredients in plants which usually produce psychoactive, or mind altering effects. Most medicinal and toxic plants, as well as hallucinogenic plants owe their biological activity to alkaloids. Examples of alkaloids include cocaine, morphine, and codeine. THC, the primary psychoactive substance in marijuana is an exception. The term is also applied to synthetic alkaloids which have structures similar to natural plant alkaloids.
ALPHA-METHYLFENTANYL - The first of many analogs of the prescription drug fentanyl discovered being used on the street. It is produced by illicit chemists, and sold in powder form under such names as China white and synthetic heroin. It is several times more potent than heroin itself, and has caused numerous overdose deaths.
AMANITA MUSCARIA - A large toxic mushroom with a red, orange, or yellow cap with white spots. It is native to North America, and is sometimes abused as a hallucinogen. Commonly referred to as “fly agaric”. The active substances are muscimol and ibotenic acid.
AMF - Street name for the illicit synthetic drug alpha-methylfentanyl.
AMINE - An organic derivative of ammonia and a basic functional molecular group that is one of the fundamental building blocks of biochemistry. It is the basic part of amino acid compounds and is a component of many natural and synthetic drugs such as amphetamine.
AMPED - High on amphetamines.
AMPHETAMINE - A name given to a category of stimulant drugs having similar chemical formulas; amphetamine sulfate, dextroamphetamine sulfate, and methamphetamine hydrochloride. They basically variate from each other only in their potency (amphetamine sulfate being the least potent, and methamphetamine being the most) and manufacturing process. Amphetamines were at one time the most commonly prescribed drugs, but are now strictly controlled and prescribed

SLANG

for very selected medical conditions, such as severe obesity and narcolepsy. Amphetamines, particularly methamphetamine, are commonly manufactured in clandestine laboratories and sold through illicit channels in powder, tablet and liquid form.

AMPHETAMINE SULFATE - Amphetamine was first used in the early 1930's as an inhaler decongestant and in the treatment of narcolepsy. During World War II, it was used by troops to counteract fatigue. Today it is occasionally prescribed for conditions such as attention deficit disorder, narcolepsy, and severe obesity. Amphetamine sulfate is also illicitly manufactured, but to a much lesser degree than is the more potent methamphetamine.

AMYL NITRITE - A clear yellow liquid sold in small cloth covered glass vials, which when broken, release fumes that are inhaled. Inhaling these fumes causes a brief but powerful "rush". It is a prescription drug used legitimately to treat coronary artery disease, but it is also widely abused due to its euphoric effects. Often referred to on the street as amys, amyls, bolt, pearls, poppers, rush, and snappers.

AMYLS, AMYS - Street name for the prescription drug amyl nitrite.

ANABOLIC STEROIDS - By definition, and anabolic steroid is any drug or hormonal substance, chemically and pharmacologically related to testosterone (other than estrogens, progestins, and corticosteroids) that promotes muscle growth. Anabolic steroids are more correctly referred to as anabolic-androgenic steroids; "anabolic" referring to a tissue building effect, and "androgenic" referring to masculinizing effects. Steroids are widely abused by athletes attempting to increase their performance, strength, or muscle size. Medically, they are used as a treatment for some types of anemia, osteoporosis, and other conditions.

ANALGESICS - A classification of drugs that produce relief from sensitivity to pain. The most common controlled analgesic is codeine.

ANALOG - A synthetic drug produced by making a small change in the chemical structure of the parent drug. Also referred to as "designer drugs", analogs have included such drugs as alpha-methylfentanyl, MDA, and MDMA. An analog can be many times more potent than the drug it was patterned after.

ANDROGEN DRUGS - Drugs which cause the development of masculine features, such as an increase in body hair, deepening of the voice, etc. Anabolic steroids are androgen drugs.

ANESTHETIC - A drug which abolishes the sensation of pain. An anesthetic can be local, affecting only the area to which it is administered, or general, affecting the entire body, often producing loss of consciousness. Local anesthetics include such drugs as cocaine, tetracaine, benzocaine, and lidocaine. General anesthetics include such drugs as morphine sulfate, fentanyl citrate, and ketamine.

ANGEL DUST - Street name for many drugs, particularly PCP.

ANIMAL TRANK - Street name for PCP.

ANORECTIC DRUG - A drug which is used to treat obesity by decreasing appetite.

ANTHRANILIC ACID - A chemical regulated by the Chemical Diversion and Trafficking Act of 1988 as a precursor chemical, and which is sometimes used as in the synthesis of illicit drugs.

ANTIDEPRESSANT - A classification of drugs which are medically used to improve mood in severely depressed patients.

ANTIFREEZE - Street name for heroin.

ARMY DISEASE - An expression often used as a synonym for morphine addiction after the Civil War. Also called "soldier's illness". During the Civil War the hypodermic needle was first used to inject morphine, which was used indiscriminately as an analgesic. Because only soldiers were so widely affected, the addiction became known as the army disease.

ARTILLERY - Street name for apparatus used to inject drugs, such as a needle/syringe, tourniquet, cooker, etc.

ASTRO TURF - Street name for marijuana.

AUTHOR - An individual who has the wherewithal to write illegal prescriptions for drug abusers.

BAD TRIP - An unpleasant drug experience, usually involving a hallucinogenic drug.

BADOH NEGRO - A variety of the morning glory plant, the seeds of which contain d-lysergic acid amide, a substance chemically similar to LSD which may cause mild hallucinations when ingested.

BAG - A generic term for a package containing any amount of a drug.

BALL - Street name for Mexican tar heroin.

SLANG

BALLOON - A balloon which is used as a package for heroin. The balloons are sometimes swallowed to smuggle the drug or if an arrest seems likely, and are later retrieved by defecation.
BANG - Injecting a drug.
BARBS, BARBIES - Street name for barbiturates.
BARBITURATE - Barbiturates are a group of sedative/hypnotic drugs which relieve tension and anxiety. They are commonly prescribed as sleeping pills, and are widely abused. Examples of barbiturates include phenobarbital, amobarbital, mephobarbital, metharbital, pentobarbital, and secobarbital. The effects of barbiturates may last anywhere from 3 to 12 hours.
BARREL - Antiquated street name for LSD.
BASA - Spanish word for base.
BASE - 1. Street name for cocaine freebase. 2. An intermediate product in the refinement of cocaine. Base, in terms of the refinement process of cocaine, contains a number of chemicals and is characteristically different than the base product that is typically used in the United States.
BASEBALL - Street name for cocaine freebase.
BASEBALLING, BASING - The process of converting cocaine hydrochloride, the type used for snorting, to a smokeable freebase form.
BASUCO - Spanish street name for an off-white to light brown putty-like substance which is an intermediate product in the refinement of cocaine. It contains impurities such as kerosene, sulfuric acid, and sodium carbonate. Because of it's relatively low price, it is very accessible to low income groups. It is usually smoked with tobacco, and it's use is limited primarily to South America where it is also known as "basa".
BATU - Street name for a smokeable, highly pure form of methamphetamine, more commonly referred to as "ice".
BEAMIN - High on cocaine
BEANS - Street name for the prescription drug Dexedrine.
BELLADONA - An extract from the leaves and roots of the deadly nightshade (Atropa belladonna) plant, which contains the alkaloids hyoscyamine and scopolamine. It is native to parts of Europe and Asia, and has been naturalized in the United States. It has been used in medicine since ancient times, and today is used medically to treat such conditions as digestive disorders and motion sickness. Belladonna is sometimes abused as a hallucinogen by smoking or swallowing the crushed leaves or roots, but doses sufficient for this purpose could be fatal.
BELLY HABIT - Level of drug addiction at which withdrawal would result in stomach cramps or other severe physical effects.
BELT - The onset of the effect, or "rush", of a drug.
BENNIES - Street name for the prescription drug Benzedrine, a stimulant no longer manufactured.
BENT - A drug high.
BENZ - Street name for the prescription drug Benzedrine, a stimulant no longer manufactured.
BENZEDRINE - Benzedrine was a prescription brand of amphetamine sulfate widely abused until it's manufacture was discontinued.
BENZOCAINE - A local anesthetic sometimes used as a cut in drugs which have a similar appearance, such as cocaine.
BENZODIAZEPINE - A family of drugs used for the control of symptoms due to stress and anxiety. They slow mental activity, reduce feelings of anxiety, relax muscles, and induce sleep. Common examples of prescription drugs in the benzodiazepine class are Librium, Valium, Restoril, Ativan, and Xanax.
BENZYL CHLORIDE - A chemical regulated by the Chemical Diversion and Trafficking Act of 1988 as an essential chemical, and which is sometimes used in the manufacturing of methamphetamine and other illicit drugs.
BENZYL CYANIDE - A chemical regulated by the Chemical Diversion and Trafficking Act of 1988, as a precursor chemical, and which is sometimes used in the manufacturing of methamphetamine and other illicit drugs.
BERNICE - Street name for cocaine.
BETAL NUT - A nut from the areca palm tree that, when combined with catechu gum from the acacia tree and burnt lime has a mild stimulant effect. Prolonged use causes the teeth and gums to develop dark red stains. Use of betal nut is common in certain Asiatic countries.
BHANG - 1. Street name for marijuana. 2. Hindu word for food or drink which contains marijuana.

SLANG

BIG C - Street name for cocaine.
BIG CHIEF - Street name for peyote.
BIG D - Street name for LSD.
BIG DADDY - Street name for heroin.
BIG H - Street name for heroin.
BIG HARRY - Street name for heroin.
BIG MAN - A high level drug dealer.
BINDLE - Paper folded in an envelope fashion to hold a powdered drug.
BING - Street name for heroin.
BINGE - A period of several hours, or even several days of constant drug use.
BLACK AND WHITES - Street name for the prescription drug Biphetamine in a 12.5 mg black and white capsule.
BLACK BEAUTIES, BLACK BIRDS, BLACK MOLLIES - Street name for the prescription drug Biphetamine in a 20 mg solid black capsule.
BLACK HEROIN - Street name for Mexican tar heroin.
BLACK TAR - Street name for Mexican tar heroin.
BLANK - A substance added to a drug as an adulterant.
BLASTED - A drug high.
BLOND - Light colored, and generally low quality hash from the Middle East.
BLOTTER - Street name for LSD.
BLOTTER ACID - Street name for blotter (absorbent) paper impregnated with LSD. Blotter paper usually appears in sheets consisting of several small perforated squares, often called "tickets", each containing a dose of LSD. The sheets typically have variously colored designs printed on them as a trademark of the particular distributor. The paper is placed on the tongue to absorb the LSD.
BLOW - 1. Street name for cocaine. 2. The act of snorting a drug.
BLOW THE VEIN - Causing a vein to collapse by repeated drug injections.
BLOWN AWAY - A drug high.
BLUE ANGELS, BLUE BULLETS, BLUE DEVILS, BLUE DOLLS, BLUES - Street name for the prescription drug Amytal Sodium in a blue capsule form.
BLUE HEAVEN - Street name for LSD.
BLUE STAR - One of several varieties of the morning glory plant, the seeds of which contain d-lysergic acid amide, a substance chemically similar to LSD. The seeds can produce mild hallucinations when ingested.
BLUNT - A large marijuana joint wrapped with a tobacco leaf.
BODY BAG - Street name for heroin.
BODY CARRIER - A person who smuggles drugs by concealing it in their clothing or by taping it to their body.
BODY PACKER - One who swallows balloons or condoms containing drugs for the purpose of smuggling. Later retrieved by defecation. Occasionally, the drug packages are placed into body cavities, and have also been implanted into surgical incisions of the legs.
BOGART - Unwilling to share a marijuana joint with others.
BOLIVIAN - A very pure form of cocaine with dense crystals. Commonly called "Bolivian rock" or "Bolivian flake", it refers to the style and not necessarily the country of origin.
BOLSA - Spanish word for bag. Usually refers to a small bag of heroin.
BOLT - Street name for the prescription drug amyl nitrite.
BOMBED - A drug high.
BONG - A marijuana smoking pipe that contains a water chamber through which the smoke passes, cooling it and making it less irritating. Marijuana bongs appear in a wide variety of shapes and sizes. Other terms for a bong: hooka, one hitter, party bowl, and water pipe.
BOWL - A marijuana pipe.
BOY, BOY JIVE - Street name for heroin.
BRICK - A compressed brick shaped quantity of marijuana or hash.
BRODY - Acting ill to obtain a prescription for a drug.
BROMO - Street name for the hallucinogenic drug 2C-B (4-bromo-2,5-dimethoxyphenethylamine).
BROOM - A member of the bean family with blossoms that are dried and smoked for the reported intoxicating effects.

SLANG

BROTHER - Street name for heroin.
BROWN, BROWN HEROIN, BROWN STUFF, BROWN SUGAR - Heroin which is brown in color. The brown color is generally due to impurities left by make-shift manufacturing processes. Brown heroin is normally associated with a Mexican origin, as opposed to white heroin, which is normally associated with Asia. However, powdered heroin can range in color from very white to dark brown regardless of the country of origin.
BROWNIES - 1. Fudge brownies which contain marijuana. 2. Street name for the prescription drug Dexedrine.
BUD - A cluster of flowers on a marijuana plant. The bud is high in THC content and is the part of the marijuana plant that is normally used for smoking. Several dozen buds may grow on an individual marijuana plant.
BUDA - A marijuana joint containing crack.
BUDDHA STICK - Potent marijuana grown in Southeast Asia which is traditionally wrapped around a bamboo stick 4" to 10" in length. More commonly referred to as a "Thai stick". The Thai stick itself is not smoked, the marijuana is removed and used in joints or smoked in a pipe.
BUFF - 1. The act of adulterating a drug. 2. A substance added to a drug as an adulterant.
BUFOTENINE - A hallucinogenic drug chemically related to DMT. It can be derived from various West Indian and South American plants. Bufotenine is a substance which is also part of a defensive secretion given off by certain toads.
BULLET - A bullet shaped vial used to snort a powdered drug.
BUM, BUMMER - A bad drug experience.
BUNK - Low quality drugs.
BURNED - Cheated on a drug deal.
BURNOUT - A lethargic attitude developed by frequent drug users.
BUSH - Street name for marijuana.
BUSINESS MANS HIGH, BUSINESS MANS LUNCH, BUSINESS MANS SPECIAL - Street name for the drug DMT (dimethyltryptamine). So called because the effects of DMT generally last one hour or less.
BUTTON - The top of the peyote cactus. The buttons contain the hallucinogenic drug mescaline, and are often consumed by chewing, but may also be used to brew a tea, or ground and placed into gelatin capsules. Buttons usually have a diameter about the size of a quarter.
BUZZ - A drug high.
C - Street name for cocaine.
CABALLO - Spanish street name for heroin.
CACHE - A hidden supply of drugs.
CACTUS - Street name for the peyote cactus.
CACTUS BUTTON - Street name for the top of the peyote cactus.
CADET - A new or inexperienced drug user.
CAFFEINE - Caffeine is a white, bitter, crystalline substance sometimes used as a cut in drugs which have a similar appearance, such as heroin.
CAINE - Street name for cocaine.
CALAMUS - A palm plant, the leaves of which are ingested as a mild stimulant. Calamus grows wild in various parts of the United States.
CALIFORNIA POPPY - The state flower of California. It is often rumored that this poppy contains opium, but in fact does not contain any psychoactive drug.
CALIFORNIA SUNSHINE - Street name for LSD.
CAMEL - A drug transporter.
CAN - One ounce of marijuana.
CANDY - Term for drugs in general.
CANDY BAR - Hashish pressed in a candy bar-like shape.
CANDY MAN - A drug dealer.
CANNABIDIOL (CBD) - One of the cannabinoids found in the marijuana plant. It is not psychoactive, but reportedly enhances the effect of THC.
CANNABINOIDS - A series of chemical substances found only in the marijuana plant, the most psychoactive of which is THC.
CANNABINOL (CBN) - A cannabinoid produced from the oxidation of THC in the drying, processing, and storage of marijuana. It has little or no psychoactive effect.

SLANG

CANNABIS - Marijuana.
CAP - 1. To buy drugs. 2. A capsule containing a drug.
CARGA - Spanish street name for heroin.
CARRIER - A drug transporter.
CARRY - To possess drugs.
CARTWHEELS - Street name for amphetamine tablets.
CAT - 1. Street name for heroin. 2. Street name for methcathinone.
CATNIP - A plant that when dried, is sometimes used to adulterate marijuana. Inferior marijuana is sometimes referred to as catnip.
CECIL - Street name for cocaine.
CENT - Drug culture term for one dollar.
CENTRAL NERVOUS SYSTEM (CNS) - The brain, brain stem, and spinal cord. The primary bodily system affected by psychoactive drugs.
CHALICE - A marijuana pipe.
CHALK - Street name for amphetamines.
CHAMBER PIPE - A marijuana smoking pipe which has a chamber between the bowl and the mouth piece. Marijuana is placed into the chamber and acts as a filter. In this fashion, the marijuana in the chamber collects some of the potent resin of the marijuana being smoked.
CHANDU - Asian term for smoking opium.
CHAPAPOTE - Spanish street name for Mexican tar heroin.
CHARAS - Hindu word for hashish or marijuana.
CHARGE - The onset of the effect, or "rush" of a drug.
CHARLIE - Street name for cocaine.
CHASING AND BASING - Smoking a combination of heroin and freebase cocaine.
CHASING THE DRAGON - The heating of heroin on a piece of aluminum foil over an open flame, and inhaling the rising wisps of smoke through a straw or similar device.
CHEAP BASING - The process of converting cocaine hydrochloride, the form used for snorting, to crack, a freebase form used for smoking.
CHICK - Street name for cocaine.
CHICKLOSA - Spanish street name for tar heroin.
CHIEF - Street name for peyote.
CHIEN - Asian measurment of 700 grams.
CHILLUM - A cone shaped marijuana/hash pipe.
CHINA MAN - Street name for heroin.
CHINA WHITE - 1. Street name for synthetic heroin (alpa-methylfentanyl). 2. Very pure Southeast Asian heroin.
CHIPPER - An occasional user of heroin.
CHIVA, CHIVO - Spanish street name for Mexican tar heroin.
CHLORAL HYDRATE - A sedative/hypnotic drug used mainly as a short term treatment for insomnia. The combination of chloral hydrate and an alcoholic beverage is known as a Mickey Finn or a knockout drop.
CHOCOLATE - Street name for Mexican tar heroin.
CHOI - Asian measurment of 1.6 kilograms of opium or opium products.
CHOP - The act of adulterating a drug.
CHRISTMAS TREES - 1. Street name for the prescription drug Dexedrine. 2. Street name for the prescription drug Tuinal.
CHRONIC - Potent marijuana.
CLANDESTINE - Something done in secrecy or concealment.
CLARITY - Street name for the drug MDMA.
CLEAN - 1. The removal of the non-potent stems and seeds from dried marijuana. 2. Not using or not possessing drugs.
CLEAR LIGHT - Street name for small, usually square pieces of gelatin which contain LSD.
CLIP - A gripping device, usually an electrical alligator clip or surgical hemostat, which holds the end of a marijuana joint while being smoked. This allows the joint to be smoked almost completely without burning the lips or fingers.
CLOROX TEST - A street test which involves placing a small amount of cocaine in a glass containing

Clorox bleach. The purity of the cocaine is indicated by the manner in which it and any cuts dissolve.

CNS - Abbreviation for central nervous system.

COASTING - The lethargic feeling experienced after using heroin.

COCA - A bush that is native to the mountainous regions of South America, as well as parts of Africa and Indonesia. The leaves of the coca bush contain small amounts of the alkaloid cocaine, and have been chewed for centuries by the Indians of Peru and Bolivia for various social, religious, and medicinal reasons. 300 pounds of coca leaves can usually produce about 1 to 2 pounds of the finished cocaine hydrochloride product.

COCAINE - A powerful stimulant contained in the leaf of the coca bush, which is cultivated chiefly in the South American countries of Peru, Bolivia and Colombia. Widespread use of cocaine first occurred in America in the late 1800's. By the end of the century, cocaine was firmly in the mainstream of popular acceptance as a harmless and pleasant stimulant. Within a few years of increasingly widespread use, the destructive nature of the drug became evident. Beginning with the passage of the Harrison Narcotic Act of 1914, Congress took a series of steps restricting the drugs distribution. Today, cocaine is still used as a local anesthetic for certain medical procedures, but it has been replaced to a large degree by various synthetic drugs. It is widely abused, and generally appears in the illicit market as a white crystalline powder, which is commonly snorted, but which may also be dissolved in water and injected. Cocaine also appears in freebase form as either freebase crystals or crack, both of which are smoked.

COCAINE BLUES, COCAINE CRASH - The depression experienced after the cocaine "high" has diminished.

COCAINE FREEBASE - The result of a chemical process whereby cocaine hydrochloride, the type used for snorting, is converted to a base by "freeing" the cocaine from the hydrochloride part of the molecule. This allows the cocaine to be smoked (the hydrochloride form cannot be smoked without destroying most of it at smoking temperatures). Freebase cocaine can be prepared in 2 ways, as either freebase crystals or crack. The preparation of freebase crystals involves dissolving the cocaine hydrochloride in water, converting the hydrochloride to the alkaloid form by addition of a strong base, such as sodium or ammonium hydroxide, extraction of the alkaloid with an organic solvent, such as petroleum ether, and crystallization of the freebase. This method effectively removes most of the adulterants commonly added to cocaine but is a hazardous method due to the volatile chemicals involved. Crack is produced by dissolving the cocaine hydrochloride in water with baking soda and then heating the mixture. The mixture coalesces into a soft mass which hardens when dried. Unlike the previous method, crack contains most of the adulterants that were in the cocaine hydrochloride. Crack and freebase crystals are usually smoked in glass pipes. The glass pipe has a bowl fitted on it with one or more fine mesh metal screens, which support the cocaine. The user heats the side of the bowl with a small butane torch or lighter, vaporizing the drug, which is then inhaled through the pipe.

COCAINE HYDROCHLORIDE - The form of cocaine typically seen on the street. It almost always appears as a white or off white crystalline powder which is snorted for ingestion.

CODEINE - A derivative of opium which is used to relieve mild to moderate pain, and to control coughing and diarrhea.

COKE - Street name for cocaine.

COKE BUGS - The sensation a cocaine user has that bugs are crawling on or under the skin.

COKE HEAD - A user of cocaine.

COKE SPOON - A very small spoon used for snorting cocaine. Coke spoons are about 2 inches in length, and are often made into jewelry such as earrings and necklaces.

COLA - A cluster of buds on a branch of a marijuana plant.

COLD SHOT - An injection of a fake or heavily adulterated drug which has little or no effect.

COLLAPSED VEIN - A condition not uncommon to people who inject drugs, caused by repeated injections in a vein and often precipitated by contaminants in the drug and unsanitary procedures. After a regularly used vein collapses, other veins are sought in new areas of the body, including the arms, hands, legs, feet and neck.

COLOMBIAN - Drugs which originate from Colombia, particularly marijuana.

COME DOWN - The return to normal mind and body after the effects of a drug begin to diminish.

COME-ON - The onset of the effect, or "rush" of a drug.

SLANG

COMPREHENSIVE DRUG ABUSE PREVENTION AND CONTROL ACT OF 1970 -Better known as the Controlled Substances Act of 1970. It is the Federal law which provides the basis for reducing the consumption of illegal drugs. It provides the mechanisms for reducing the availability of controlled substances, the procedures for bringing a substance under control, the criteria for determining control requirements, and also the obligations incurred by international treaty arrangements. It also provides for the registration of drug handlers, record keeping requirements, quotas on manufacturing, restrictions on distribution and dispensing, limitations on imports and exports, conditions for storage of drugs, reports of transactions to the government, and penalties for illegal acts.

CONDUCTOR - An experienced individual who talks down a person having a bad experience involving a hallucinogenic drug. The conductor provides comforting verbal support.

CONNECT - To buy drugs.

CONNECTION - A drug dealer.

CONTACT - A drug dealer.

CONTACT HIGH - 1. Phenomenon whereby an individual is affected by the second hand smoke of a drug being smoked in close proximity. Contact high has also been used to describe the phenomenon whereby a drug-free individual believes he is experiencing the effect of a drug used by another, reportedly by simply observing the intoxicated state of the other individual.

CONTROLLED SUBSTANCES ACT OF 1970 - See **COMPREHENSIVE DRUG ABUSE PREVENTION AND CONTROL ACT OF 1970.**

COOK - 1. To prepare a drug for injection. This is usually performed by mixing a small amount of the drug with water in a "cooker", such as a spoon, and then heating the spoon from below with a cigarette lighter to help further dissolve the drug. The drug is then drawn into a syringe. 2. The manufacturing of illicit drugs.

COOKED - A drug high.

COOKER - 1. Any small heat resistant container in which a drug is dissolved in water and heated, most often a common metal spoon. 2. A person who manufactures illicit drugs.

COP, COPPING - To buy drugs.

COPPING AREA - A location where drugs are sold.

COPILOT - 1. An experienced individual who talks down a person having a bad experience involving a hallucinogenic drug. The copilot provides comforting verbal support. 2. Street name for amphetamine tablets.

CORINE - Street name for cocaine.

COTTON - A piece of cotton used to filter the impurities from a liquid drug while it is being drawn into a syringe. The cotton is kept after use because it retains a small amount of the drug, which can be extracted by soaking the cotton in water if the user is unable to obtain additional drugs.

COTTON FEVER, COTTON POISONING - Chills and fever resulting from inadvertently injecting fiber of filter cotton into the blood stream. It usually appears about 2 hours after injecting the drug and continues for about 3 hours.

COTTON HEAD, COTTON PICKER - A person who uses the residual amounts of a drug remaining in a piece of cotton previously used to filter a liquid drug while being drawn into a syringe.

COUNTERCULTURE - A term coined in the 1960's that describes a culture whose members reject key norms and values of the larger society.

COURIER - A drug transporter.

CRACK - Street name given to cocaine that has been processed from cocaine hydrochloride, the type used for snorting, to a base by mixing the cocaine with baking soda in water, and heating the mixture to remove the hydrochloride. The freebase cocaine precipitates and coalesces into a soft mass that becomes hard after it dries. The process does not necessarily result in purer cocaine. This is performed to transform the powdered cocaine, which cannot be smoked without destroying most of it, into a form that has a lower melting point and can be effectively smoked. Crack is sold in the form of off-white solid chunks called "rocks". The term crack supposedly came about by the crackling sound that is heard when it is smoked.

CRACK FACTORY - House, apartment, or structure where crack is manufactured.

CRACK HOUSE - A dwelling where crack is sold and used.

CRACK METH - Street name for a smokeable, highly pure form of methamphetamine, more commonly referred to as "ice".

SLANG

CRACK SPOT - A location where crack can be purchased but not used. As opposed to "crack house".
CRANK - Street name for methamphetamine.
CRANK BUGS - The sensation a methamphetamine user has of bugs crawling on or under the skin.
CRAP - 1. Street name for heroin. 2. Low quality drugs.
CRASH - The coming down from a drug high, characterized by depression and/or physical exhaustion.
CRISTY - Street name for methamphetamine.
CROAKER - Drug users term for a medical doctor.
CROKE - Street name for a combination of cocaine and methamphetamine.
CROSS TOLERANCE - A condition in which tolerance to one drug often results in a tolerance to a chemically similar drug.
CRYSTAL - 1. Street name for methamphetamine. 2. Street name for PCP.
CRYSTAL METH - Street name for a smokeable, highly pure form of methamphetamine, more commonly referred to as "ice".
CUBE - Street name for LSD.
CUT - 1. The act of adulterating a drug. 2. A substance added to a drug as an adulterant.
CYCLING - Cycling is a process of alternating steroid use over a period generally lasting 3 to 12 weeks. For example, steroid A may be taken for 3 weeks and then steroid B is taken for 3 weeks. This is an attempt to maximize the steroids effects and also to minimize side effects caused by any one steroid.
D - Street name for LSD.
DABBLER - An occasional user of drugs.
DAGA - Street name for marijuana.
DAMA BLANCA - Spanish street name for cocaine.
DART - Street name for a needle/syringe.
DATURA - Any plant of the genus Datura. Some varieties are commonly called jimson weed, thornapple, belladonna, and wolfbane. The leaves and roots of these plants are sometimes smoked or seeped into a tea, with possible hallucinogenic but toxic effects.
DAVA - Street name for heroin.
DAWN - Acronym for The Drug Abuse Warning Network. A federally funded large scale drug abuse data collection system, utilizing approximately 700 medical examiners and hospital emergency rooms to collect data on drug abuse patterns.
DEA - Drug Enforcement Administration.
DEAD ON ARRIVAL - 1. Street name for PCP. 2. Street name fer heroin.
DEADLY NIGHTSHADE - A plant (Atropa belladonna), the leaves and roots of which contain atropine, scopolamine, and other substances, cumulatively referred to as "belladonna". It is native to parts of Europe and Asia, and has been naturalized in the United States. Belladonna has been used in medicine since ancient times, and today is sold as a prescription drug used primarily to treat digestive disorders. Belladonna is sometimes abused as a hallucinogen by smoking or swallowing the crushed leaves and roots, but doses sufficient for this purpose could be fatal.
DEAL - To peddle or sell drugs.
DEALER - An individual who sells drugs.
DEALERS HABIT - A heavy addiction to a drug.
DECK - A retail package of heroin.
DECRIMINALIZATION - The legal process of revising drug laws by replacing the criminal penalties (possible imprisonment) with civil penalties (fines without possible imprisonment). Many are of the opinion that marijuana should be decriminalized as imprisonment is too harsh for marijuana violations. Decriminalization is not legalization (legally sanctioned).
DELTA-9-TETRAHYDROCANNABINOL - (THC). One of the cannabinoids found in the marijuana plant. It is responsible for most of the psychoactive effect of marijuana.
DEPENDENCE - A state of psychic or physical dependance or both on a drug, arising in a person following administration of that drug on a periodic or continuous basis.
DEPRESSANT - A drug which depresses the central nervous system, resulting in sedation and a decrease in bodily activity. Not to be confused with the psychological state of depression, these

drugs can in fact be mood elevators by lowering inhibitions. Depressants include barbiturates, sedative-hypnotics, narcotic analgesics, and tranquilizers.

DESIGNER DRUG - See **ANALOG**.

DET - Diethyltryptamine. A fast acting synthetic hallucinogenic drug similar to DMT. It is produced in both liquid and powder forms, and is generally added to vegetable matter and smoked.

DEVELOPING PAPER - Cigarette paper used to make a marijuana joint.

DEX, DEXIES - Street name for the prescription drug Dexedrine.

DEXTROAMPHETAMINE SULFATE - A central nervous system stimulant. Dextroamphetamine is manufactured as the prescription drug Dexedrine, and is prescribed for narcolepsy, hyperactivity in children, and occasionally for obesity. Like the other amphetamines, dextroamphetamine is commonly abused.

DIACETYLMORPHINE - Heroin.

DIESEL - Street name for heroin.

DILUENT - A substance which has little or no psychoactive effect that is added to a drug as a cut.

DILLIES - Street name for the prescription drug Dilaudid.

DIME - Ten dollars worth of a drug.

DIMETHYLTRYPTAMINE - See **DMT**.

DIPPING - The dipping of blotter paper into a liquid LSD solution.

DIRTY - Carrying or using drugs.

DIRTY BASING - See **CHEAP BASING**.

DIRTY URINE - Positive test results for the presence of drugs in a urine specimen indicating drug use by the subject.

DITCH WEED - Low quality marijuana.

DIVERSION - The transfer of any controlled substance from a legal to an illegal channel of distribution or use.

DMT - Dimethyltryptamine. A hallucinogenic drug with effects similar to LSD. Often referred to on the street as "business mans high", "business mas lunch", or "business mans special", because the effects generally last one hour or less. It can be derived from various South American and west Indian plants, but its use in the United States is generally in a synthetic form. DMT is sold either as a liquid or powder, and may be snorted or injected, but is usually added to dry vegetable matter and smoked.

DO A LINE - To snort a line of a powdered drug.

DOA - (Dead On Arrival). Street name for PCP.

DOB - 2,5-dimethoxy-4-bromoamphetamine. One of the many MDA-like compounds found on the illicit market.

DOCTOR - 1. Street name for the drug MDMA. 2. Street name for the prescription drug meperidine.

DOCTOR FEELGOOD - A doctor who prescribes drugs to drug abusers.

DOJE - Street name for heroin.

DOLLAR - One hundred dollars worth of a drug.

DOLLIES, DOLLS - Street name for the prescription drug Dolophine (methadone).

DOM - (2,5-dimethoxy-4-methylamphetamine). A synthetic hallucinogen which was developed in 1964, and introduced to the counter culture at the first hippie "love-in" in 1967 under the name STP, which has been said to stand for serenity, tranquility and peace. In larger doses, it produces an intense hallucinogenic trip similar to LSD, but with much longer effects.

DOOBIE - A marijuana joint.

DOOJEE - Street name for heroin.

DOORS AND FOURS - A combination of the prescription drugs Doriden (glutethimide) and 60 mg codeine tablets.

DOPE - Term for drugs in general.

DOPE HEAD - A heavy user of drugs.

DOPED-UP - A drug high.

DOPER - A heavy user of drugs.

DOSE - 1. Street name for LSD. 2. The quantity or amount of a drug that is taken.

DOSING - Placing LSD on a medium, such as blotter paper or sugar cubes.

DOT - Street name for LSD.

DOUBLE TROUBLE - Street name for the prescription drug Tuinal.

SLANG

DO UP - To inject a drug.
DOWNER, DOWNIE - 1. Street name for a drug which has a depressant effect. 2. A bad drug experience.
DOWNTOWN - Street name for heroin.
DRAG - 1. A marijuana joint. 2. A bad drug experience.
DRAGON CHASING - The heating of heroin on a piece of aluminum foil over an open flame, and inhaling the rising wisps of smoke through a straw or similar device.
DRIVERS - Street name for amphetamines.
DROP - to take a drug orally, as opposed to snorting, injecting, or smoking.
DROP A DIME - To be an informer. To drop a dime in a pay phone and call narcotic officers.
DRUG - In general use, there is little consistency in popular conceptions of what a drug is. Many equate drugs only with the illicit substances used recreationally, such as heroin or cocaine, viewing them as fundamentally different and more harmful than the licit substances used recreationally, such as alcohol and tobacco, or the so called medical drugs, such as the tranquilizers and barbiturates.
DRUG ENFORCEMENT ADMINISTRATION - The lead agency in drug suppression programs at both the national and international levels. The DEA was established in the Department of Justice in 1973, replacing the Bureau of Narcotics and Dangerous Drugs. The DEA was created to enforce the controlled substances laws and regulations of the United States.
DRUGGIE - A heavy user of drugs.
DRY - 1. Not using drugs. 2. A situation in which drugs are not available.
DRY WHISKEY - Street name for peyote.
DUBIE - A marijuana joint.
DUFF - The powdered portion of cocaine, as opposed to the chunks or flakes.
DUJEE - Street name for heroin.
DUMMY - 1. The act of adulterating a drug. 2. A substance added to a drug as a cut.
DUST - Street name for many drugs in powder form, such as heroin or cocaine, but most often refers to PCP.
DUSTER - 1. A marijuana joint which contains PCP or heroin. 2. A user of PCP.
DYNAMITE - Street name for heroin.
DYNO - 1. High quality drugs. 2. Street name for heroin.
E, ECSTASY - Street name for the drug MDMA.
EIGHT BALL - 1/8 ounce of cocaine.
EIGHTH - 1/8 ounce or 1/8 gram of a drug.
ELEPHANT - Street name for the drug PCP.
EMBALMING FLUID - (Formaldehyde). 1. A chemical that is sometimes abused by inhaling the fumes, or added to marijuana to produce joints known as "clickems", or "clickers". 2. Street name for the drug PCP.
EMBROIDERY - See **TRACKS**.
EMERALD TRIANGLE - An area of California which includes Humbolt, Trinity, and Mendocino counties, where substantial marijuana growing occurs.
EMMA - Street name for morphine.
EPHEDRINE - A chemical regulated by the Chemical Diversion and Trafficking Act of 1988 as a precursor chemical, and which is sometimes used in the manufacturing of methamphetamine.
EQUIPMENT - Apparatus to use drugs, such as a syringe, pipe, etc.
ERGONOVINE - A chemical regulated by the Chemical Diversion and Trafficking Act of 1988 as a precursor chemical, and which is sometimes used in the synthesis of LSD.
ERGOT - A fungus which grows on rye, wheat and other grasses. It is a source for lysergic acid, which in turn is used in the manufacturing of LSD.
ERGOTAMINE - A chemical regulated by the Chemical Diversion and Trafficking Act of 1988 as a precursor chemical, and which is sometimes used in the synthesis of LSD.
ERYTHROXYLON COCA - Botanical name for the coca plant, the source of cocaine.
ESSENCE - Street name for the drug MDMA.
ESSENTIAL CHEMICAL - A chemical that is used as a solvent, reagent, or catalyst in the manufacturing of a controlled substance.
ESTUFFA, ESTUFFAN - Spanish street name for heroin.

SLANG

ETHYL ETHER - A chemical regulated by the Chemical Diversion and Trafficking Act of 1988 as an essential chemical, and which is sometimes used in the manufacture of illicit drugs.

ETORPHINE - A derivative of opium, several times more potent than morphine. It is currently used as an animal tranquilizer, and is marketed as M99.

EUPHORIA - 1. A sense of extreme well being and optimism, often accompanied by heightened physical activity, which may be experienced in some drug induced states. 2. Street name for the hallucinogenic drug 4-methylaminorex.

EVE - Street name for the drug MDE (3,4-methylenedioxy-n-ethylamphetamine).

EYE ACID - Liquid LSD dripped onto the eye.

FALSE NEGATIVE - A test result that indicates the absence of a drug when in fact it is present.

FALSE POSITIVE - A test result that indicates the presence of a drug when in fact it is absent.

FENDER BENDER - Street name for the prescription drug secobarbital sodium.

FENTANYL - A short acting synthetic narcotic analgesic commonly used in surgeries in the United States. Numerous analogs of this drug have been illegally produced and sold/used under many names, including alpha-methylfentanyl, 3-methylfentanyl, China white, Persian white, and synthetic heroin.

F-40 - Street name for the prescription drug Seconal.

FIENDING - Acute crack binging.

FINGER - 1. An amount of hash roughly the shape of a finger. 2. Condoms filled with drugs and swallowed or hidden in body cavities for smuggling.

FIRE-A-LINE - To snort a line of a powdered drug.

FIREBALL - 1. A combination of cocaine and PCP. 2. A combination of cocaine and heroin.

FIRED UP - A drug high.

FIT - Street name for apparatus used to inject drugs, such as a syringe, tourniquet, cooker, etc.

FIVE CENT BAG - Five dollars worth of a drug.

FIX - A dose of a drug, most often in reference to an injection of heroin.

FIXER - A drug dealer.

FLAG - Show of blood drawn back into a syringe by an intravenous drug user before injecting a drug. Shows that the needle has penetrated a vein.

FLAKE - Small flaky crystals of cocaine, as opposed to the powder or rocks. Flake is considered to be of high quality, but is rarely seen on the illicit market.

FLASH - The onset of the effect, or “rush” of a drug.

FLASHBACK - An involuntary recurrence of a hallucinogenic drug experience days, months, or even years after the drug was last taken. The mechanism responsible for flashbacks is not understood, but it is believed they are similar to deja vu. There appears to be a relationship between the amount and the number of times hallucinogenic drugs are taken and the occurrence of flashbacks. Flashbacks may involve any of the senses, including taste, smell, hearing, and sight. Flashbacks may be pleasant or terrifying. PCP, which is stored in the fat cells of the body, produces true chemical flashbacks as it is slowly metabolized by the body.

FLUFFING - The process of chopping a powdered drug, such as cocaine, with a razor blade to break any large pieces, and then pushing the powder through a fine mesh stocking. This can result in increasing the volume of the drug by as much as 50% to 100%.

FLUSH - The onset of the effect, or “rush” of a drug.

FLY AGARIC - A large, very toxic mushroom with a red, orange, or yellow cap with white spots. It is native to North America, and is sometimes abused as a hallucinogen. The active hallucinogenic substances are muscimol and ibotenic acid.

FLYING SAUCERS - A variety of the morning glory plant with white striped blue flowers, the seeds of which contain d-lyseric acid amide, a substance chemically similar to LSD. The seeds can produce mild hallucinations when ingested.

FOIL - Aluminum foil used as a package for a small amount of a drug.

FOIL BURN TEST - A street test to determine the purity of cocaine. A small amount of cocaine is placed on aluminum foil and melted over an open flame. Pure cocaine will usually leave an amber colored residue, whereas adulterated cocaine will leave various colored residues depending on the cuts present.

FOILING - Smoking a drug by placing it on a piece of aluminum foil which is heated by an open flame held beneath it, and inhaling the rising vapors.

SLANG

FORMALDEHYDE - 1. A chemical that is sometimes abused by inhaling the fumes, or added to marijuana to produce joints known as "clickems", or "clickers". 2. Street name for the drug PCP.
FORMICATION - The sensation of insects crawling under the skin. Formication is sometimes experienced by individuals under the influence of such drugs as cocaine and methamphetamine.
4'S - Street name for prescription codeine tablets stamped with the number 4, designating a strength of 60 mg.
FOURS AND DOORS - A combination of the prescription drugs Doriden (glutethimide) and 60 mg codeine tablets.
FREAK - A frequent user of drugs.
FREEBASE - Street term for the alkaloid form of a drug. Usually used in reference to cocaine or heroin.
FRIED - 1. A drug high. 2. The state of burnout by a frequent user of drugs.
FUETE - Syringe.
FUNK - Street name for heroin.
FUNNY BROWNIES - Fudge brownies containing marijuana.
FUNNY MUSHROOMS - Street name for hallucinogenic mushrooms.
GANJA - Hindu word for marijuana.
GARBAGE - 1. Street name for heroin. 2. Low quality drugs.
GAS - Street name for nitrous oxide.
GATEWAY DRUGS - Drugs that are perceived by a portion of the population as being safe to use, such as alcohol or marijuana, but which may lay the foundation for trying more dangerous drugs, such as cocaine, heroin, etc.
GET DOWN - To inject heroin.
GET OFF - The onset of the effect, or "rush" of a drug.
GHOSTBUSTER - A mixture of cocaine and PCP.
GIRL - Street name for cocaine.
GLASS - Street name for a smokeable, highly pure form of methamphetamine, more commonly referred to as "ice".
GLASSWARE - Items made of glass to manufacture or use drugs, such as a glass bong or glass beaker.
GLOBO - Street name for heroin.
GLUCOSE - A sugar sometimes used as an cut in drugs which have a similar appearance, such as cocaine.
GO, GO FAST - Street name for amphetamines.
GOLDEN CRESCENT - A major opium producing area of Southwest Asia which encompasses portions of Pakistan, Iran, and Afghanistan.
GOLDEN TRIANGLE - A major opium producing area of Southeast Asia which encompasses portions of Burma, Laos, and Thailand.
GOMA, GOMERO - Spanish street name for Mexican tar heroin.
GOOB - Street name for methcathinone
GOOBER - A marijuana joint.
GOOF BALLS - Street name for the prescription drug glutethimide.
GRAM - Typical street level sale for cocaine and other drugs. The basic metric weight level, which is approximately 1/28 of an ounce.
GRASS - Street name for marijuana.
GRASS BROWNIES - Fudge brownies which contain marijuana.
GRAVEL - Street name for crack
GREEN FROGS - Street name for chloral hydrate..
GREEN MEANIES - Street name for chloral hydrate.
GREEN WHISKEY - Street name for peyote.
GRIFA - Spanish street name for marijuana.
GROUND CONTROL - An experienced individual who talks down a person having a bad experience involving a hallucinogenic drug, by providing comforting and personal verbal support.
GUM, GUMBALL - Street name for Mexican tar heroin.
GUN - Street name for a needle/syringe.
GUTTER - The vein of the inside elbow typically used to inject drugs.

SLANG

H - Street name for heroin.
HABIT - 1. A drug addiction. 2. A drug users term for his drug of choice.
HALF - One half ounce or one half gram of a drug.
HALF LIFE - Amount of time required for the body to eliminate 50% of a drug from the blood stream.
HALLUCINATION - A sensory experience of something that does not exist outside of the mind. A hallucination may involve any of the senses, including sight, smell, hearing, taste and touch. Hallucinogenic drugs usually produce what are referred to as pseudo-hallucinations; hallucinations in which the user knows that what he is seeing, hearing, tasting, etc., is not real but a product of the drug.
HALLUCINOGEN - A natural or synthetic drug which can be expected to cause hallucinations when ingested. Hallucinogens can cause profound perceptual changes in any of the senses, including sight, hearing, taste, and smell. They are also variously known as psychedelic drugs. Although other drugs, such as marijuana and alcohol may produce hallucinations if a very high dose is used, they are not classified as hallucinogens because this is not the usual effect expected or experienced. The results of the use of a hallucinogen are variable, a "good trip", or a "bad trip" may be experienced by the same person on different occasions. Flashbacks, or recurring drug-free hallucinations may also be experienced by users of hallucinogens. Common examples of hallucinogens are LSD, peyote, psilocybin mushrooms, PCP, and MDMA.
HANYAK - Street name for a smokeable, highly pure form of methamphetamine, more commonly referred to as "ice".
HARD DRUGS - An ambiguous term generally used to describe cocaine and the narcotic drugs, such as heroin and morphine.
HARD STUFF - Street name for heroin.
HARRY - Street name for heroin.
HARVEY WALLBANGER - A combination of the drugs STP and LSD.
HASH, HASHISH - The drug-rich resinous secretions of the marijuana plant, which are collected, dried, and then compressed into a variety of forms, such as balls, cakes, patties, or oblong fingers. Hash varies widely in color, from tan to black, and usually has a hard consistency. Hash is either smoked by itself or mixed with marijuana.
HASH OIL - A refined oily extract of the marijuana plant that contains a higher concentration of THC than the other forms of marijuana. It is a thick liquid, and is almost always brown or black in color depending on the refinement process. Hash oil is typically added to marijuana, or smeared on the paper used to roll a joint to enhance the potency of the marijuana.
HAWAIIAN SALT - Street name for a smokeable, highly pure form of methamphetamine, more commonly referred to as "ice".
HAWAIIAN SUNSHINE - Street name for LSD.
HAWAIIAN WOODROSE SEEDS - Seeds of the Hawaiian woodrose plant contain d-lysergic acid amide, a substance chemically similar to LSD which can produce mild hallucinations when ingested. There are 2 related varieties, the Hawaiian baby, and large woodrose, both of which are commonly sold in counter-culture magazines.
HAY - Street name for marijuana.
HEAD - A heavy user of drugs.
HEAD SHOP - A retail drug paraphernalia store.
HEARTS - Street name for the prescription drug Dexedrine.
HEAVENLY BLUE - 1. A variety of the morning glory plant with large blue flowers, the seeds of which contain d-lysergic acid amide, a substance chemically similar to LSD. 2. Street name for LSD.
HEMP - A term often used for cannabis in general, but more specifically for cannabis plants low in THC harvested for their fiber or seed.
HER - Street name for cocaine.
HERB - Street name for marijuana.
HEROIN - Heroin comes from the German word "heroisch" meaning large or powerful. It is a drug derived from morphine, which is extracted from opium. Ironically, heroin is reported to have been once used as a non-addictive substitute for morphine addiction. It is seen on the street as a powder which may vary in color from white to brown, depending on its refinement process and any adulterants. It is also seen in a tar form, which can vary in consistency from hard to gummy, and in color from brown to black. Heroin is usually dissolved in water and injected, but is also

smoked and snorted. The DEA has designated 4 stages of heroin refinement: heroin #1, heroin #2, heroin #3 and heroin #4. Heroin #1 is basically crude morphine base. Heroin #2 is a further refined product of heroin #1. Heroin #3, or "smoking heroin", is in turn a more refined product than heroin #2, and is probably the most common type seen on the street. Heroin #4, or "injectable heroin" is the most refined.

HGH - See **HUMAN GROWTH HORMONE.**

HIERBA - Spanish street name for marijuana.

HIGH - The effects of drug use which the user feels as pleasurable. Other terms describing a high: bent, blasted, blown away, bombed, cooked, doped up, fired up, fried, jacked up, loaded, smashed, spaced out, stoned, wasted, and wired.

HIKURI - Street name for peyote.

HIM - Street name for heroin.

HIROPON - Street name for a smokeable, highly pure form of methamphetamine, more commonly referred to as "ice".

HIT - 1. A dose of a drug. 2. The act of adulterating a drug. 3. The onset of the effect, or "rush" of a drug.

HIT UP - To inject a drug.

HOG - Street name for PCP.

HOLD - To possess drugs.

HOMBRE - Spanish street name for heroin.

HONEY OIL - Purified hash oil which has a light brown translucent color.

HOOKA - A marijuana bong.

HOOKED - Addicted to a drug.

HORN - To snort a powdered drug.

HORSE - Street name for heroin.

HOT BOX - A device which melts a drug and determines the melting point of the drug and any adulterants. Used on the street by dealers to determine a drugs purity.

HOT ICE - Street name for a smokeable, highly pure form of methamphetamine, more commonly referred to as "ice".

HOT SHOT - 1. An injection of a drug with a purity much higher than expected, which may cause an overdose and possibly death. 2. A bag of poisoned heroin sold to kill an informer.

HOUSE - A dwelling where drugs are sold and/or used.

HUATARI - Indian name for peyote.

HUBBA - Street name for cocaine freebase.

HUFFER - A person who inhales substances such as glue or paint to get high.

HUFFING - Inhaling substance fumes through an open mouth rather than through the nose.

HUG DRUG - Street name for the drug MDMA or MDA

HUMAN GROWTH HORMONE - A substance produced by the body's pituitary gland which stimulates normal body growth. In the past, the only source for HGH was pituitary glands of human cadavers. It is now produced synthetically as the drugs Protropin and Humatrope. HGH is prescribed to children who have a growth failure (dwarfism) due to a pituitary gland disorder. It increases both the size and number of skeletal muscle cells, and hence allows some children to grow to a normal size. HGH is widely abused by athletes attempting to increase their muscle strength and size. HGH can have serious side effects, including acromegaly, a condition characterized by an enlarged skull, jaw, hands, feet, nose, ears, and widely separated teeth. HGH is not an anabolic steroid.

HUNGRY CROAKER - A doctor who prescribes drugs to drug abusers.

HUSTLE - An individuals methods of obtaining money illegally, such as through prostitution or theft.

HYDRIODIC ACID - A chemical regulated by the Chemical Diversion and Trafficking Act of 1988 as an essential chemical, and which is sometimes used in the synthesis of illicit drugs.

HYDROPONICS - The cultivation of plants in water containing dissolved nutrients, rather than in soil. The plants root system is supported by a porous material such as lava rock or rockwool. Hydroponics is a common growing method used by indoor marijuana growers due to its ability to greatly increase the growth rate of plants.

HYPE - 1. An injection of a drug. 2. A person who injects drugs. 3. Street name for a needle/syringe.

HYPE STICK - Street name for a syringe.

SLANG

HYPNOTIC DRUG - A drug which induces sleep.

IBOGAINE - Ibogaine is a substance contained in the roots of the Tabernanthe iboga plant, which is native to Africa. It is a hallucinogen, and is used primarily in Africa for ceremonial purposes. It is listed in the CSA as a Schedule I drug.

ICAR - Acronym for the International Cannabis Alliance for Reform. An international organization of cannabis law reform groups which promote the idea of legalizing marijuana.

ICE - Street name for a smokeable, highly pure form of methamphetamine. Also referred to as batu, crack meth, glass, hanyak, Hawaiian salt, hiropon, kak sonjae, quarty, shabu, and snot.

ILLICIT - Not legally permitted.

IMPORT STEP - The point at which an imported drug is first adulterated after it is brought into the United States.

INDICA - A variety of marijuana which is often considered to be more potent than the other two varieties, sativa and ruderalis.

INHALANTS - Substances which give off vapors or fumes that are inhaled for a high. There are 4 basic classes of inhalants: 1) volatile solvents, including glue, lighter fluid, paint thinners, degreasing compounds, and gasoline; 2) aerosols, including hair sprays, vegetable frying pan lubricants, and spray paints; 3) anesthetics, including ether, chloroform, and nitrous oxide; 4) volatile nitrites, including amyl nitrite and butyl nitrite. Inhalant vapors can be sniffed through the nose, or "huffed" through the mouth, the effects lasting anywhere from a few minutes to several hours. Inhalants are often abused by adolescents because of their low cost and easy availability.

INHALATION - To inhale, or snort a drug.

INHALER - A small bullet shaped vial attachment used to snort a powdered drug, usually cocaine.

INOSITOL - Vitamin B powder. It is sometimes used as an cut in drugs which have a similar appearance, such as cocaine.

INJECTION - To force a liquid substance into the body with the use of a syringe. An injection may be made in a vein (mainlining), in a muscle (muscling), or directly under the surface of the skin (skin popping).

INSUFFLATE - To inhale a powdered or gaseous drug through the nose.

INTRAMUSCULAR INJECTION - An injection into a muscle. Often referred to as "muscling".

INTRAVENOUS INJECTION - An injection into a vein. Often referred to as "mainlining".

J - 1. A marijuana joint. 2. Street name for marijuana.

JAB - To inject a drug.

JACKED-UP - A drug high.

JAMAICAN - Marijuana originating from Jamaica.

JANE - Street name for marijuana.

JARWEED - Street name for marijuana.

JAY - Street name for marijuana.

JELLY BEANS - Street name for the prescription drug chloral hydrate.

JET FUEL - Street name for PCP.

JIMSON WEED - See **DATURA.**

JIN - Asian measurment of 500 grams.

JIVE - 1. Street name for marijuana 2. Street name for heroin.

JOI - Asian measurment of 1.6 kilograms

JOINT - A marijuana cigarette. Other terms for a marijuana joint: ace, doobie, drag, goober, j, reefer, smoke, and roach.

JOLT - The onset of the effect, or "rush" of a drug.

JONES - A drug addiction.

JOY POPPING - 1. Injecting a drug directly beneath the surface of the skin, rather than in a vein (mainlining), or muscle (muscling). 2. Occasional use of heroin.

JUANITA - Street name for marijuana.

JUGGLER - A drug dealer.

JUICE - 1. Street name for steroids. 2. Street name for PCP. 3. Street name for methadone.

JUICING - Using steroids.

JUMBO - A large vial of crack.

JUNK - 1. Street name for heroin. 2. General term for drugs.

SLANG

JUNKIE - A drug addict, particularly one addicted to heroin.
JUNK WEED - Low quality marijuana.
K - Street slang for kilogram; metric equivalent of 2.2 pounds.
KAKSONJAE - Street name for a smokeable, highly pure form of methamphetamine, more commonly referred to as "ice".
KALI - Jamaican term for high quality marijuana.
KAVA KAVA - A shrub native to the South Pacific and Hawaiian islands, the roots of which contain several substances which act as mild stimulants. The root is sold in counter-culture magazines in either a dried root form or capsules.
KETAMINE - A close relative of PCP. It is available by prescription and is used to control severe pain. It is sold as a liquid for injection, but is also sometimes evaporated to a crystal and smoked, snorted, or swallowed by abusers.
KICK - The onset of the effect, or "rush" of a drug.
KIF, KIEF - Street name for marijuana.
KILLER JOINT - 1. A marijuana joint containing PCP. 2. A marijuana joint with very potent marijuana.
KILLER WEED - 1. Marijuana which has had PCP added to it. 2. Very potent marijuana.
KILOGRAM - Metric equivalent of 2.2 pounds. Standard quantity package amount for many drugs. Also referred to as k, kee, ki, and kilo.
KIND - KIND BUD - Street names for marijuana.
KINDLING - Increased sensitivity, or a form of reverse-tolerance of long term users of cocaine to certain effects of the drug. Small doses can produce results, such as an overdose, normally expected from larger doses.
KIT - 1. Items with which drugs are used, such as a syringe, pipe, etc. 2. A set of glassware items used to manufacture drugs in an illicit laboratory.
KJ - Street name for PCP.
KNOCKOUT DROPS - Street name for the prescription drug chloral hydrate.
KONA GOLD - A variety of marijuana grown in Hawaii.
KOOLS - Marijuana or tobacco cigarettes laced with PCP.
KRYSTAL - 1. Street name for PCP. 2. Street name for methamphetamine.
KUSH - Street name for marijuana.
L - Street name for LSD.
LACE - To add one substance to another. An example would be to add, or lace a sugar cube with LSD.
LACTOSE - A milk sugar sometimes used as a cut in drugs with a similar appearance, such as cocaine.
LADY, LADY SNOW - Street name for cocaine.
L.A. GLASS, L.A. ICE - Street name for a smokeable, highly pure form of methamphetamine, more commonly referred to as "ice".
L.A. TURNAROUNDS - Street name for amphetamines.
LAUGHING GAS - Slang for nitrous oxide.
LEAF - Street name for marijuana, and occasionally cocaine.
LEAPERS - Street name for amphetamines.
LEB, LEBANESE - Hash produced in Lebanon.
LEMMON DOPE - Street name for heroin.
LET DOWN - The coming down from a drug high, characterized by feelings of dullness, tenseness, and edginess.
LETTUCE OPIUM - Street name for lactucarium, a chemical substance contained in certain varieties of lettuce. It has been reported that ingestion of lactucarium produces a mild sedative effect.
LIBERTY CAPS - Street name for the hallucinogenic Psilocybe semilanceata mushroom.
LIBS - Street name for the prescription drug Librium.
LID - One ounce of marijuana.
LIDOCAINE - A local anesthetic sometimes used as a cut in drugs which have a similar appearance, such as cocaine.
LIGHTWEIGHTING - The act of adulterating a drug.
LINE - 1. A thin line of a powdered drug, such as cocaine, that the user snorts. The line is usually

about 1/8 inch wide and 1 to 2 inches long, and is placed on a flat non-porous surface such as a mirror. 2. A vein into which a drug is injected. Abbreviation of mainline.

LOADED - A drug high.

LOADS - A combination of the prescription drugs glutethimide and codeine.

LOCO WEED - Street name for marijuana.

LORDS - Street name for the prescription drug Dilaudid.

LOVE DRUG - Most often a street name for the drug MDMA, but it has also been used as a street name for cocaine, MDA, MMDA, and methaqualone.

LOVELIES - Marijuana or tobacco cigarettes laced with PCP.

LSD - D-lysergic acid diethylamide. A synthetic hallucinogenic drug derived from lysergic acid. LSD was first synthesized in 1938, but its effects were not discovered until 1943 when a chemist accidentally ingested a minute quantity. In its original state LSD is a colorless and odorless crystal. It is an extremely potent drug, requiring only a very small amount to induce a "trip". One ounce is enough to provide up to about 500,000 doses. It is almost always taken orally. A dose can be soaked into almost any medium, such as a sugar cube, toothpick, gelatin, blotter paper, etc. A LSD dose can last anywhere from 2 to 12 hours.

LUDES - Street name for methaqualone.

LYSERGIC ACID - A substance obtained from ergot alkaloids or made synthetically. Used in the manufacture of LSD.

LYSERGIC ACID AMIDE - A chemical found in the seeds of certain morning glory and woodrose plants which can produce mild hallucinations when ingested.

LYSERGIC ACID DIETHYLAMIDE - See **LSD**.

M - 1. Street name for marijuana. 2. Street name for morphine. 3. Street name for the drug MDMA.

M & M - Street name for the drug MDMA.

MADJUN - A Turkish food which contains marijuana.

MAGIC MUSHROOMS - Street name for hallucinogenic mushrooms.

MAINLINING - To inject a drug into a vein.

MAKE A BUY - To buy drugs.

MAKE A CONTACT - To buy drugs.

MAN - A drug dealer.

MANICURE - 1. Removal of loose and extraneous leaves from the bud of the marijuana plant. 2. The removal of the non-potent seeds and stems from dried marijuana.

MANNITE - See **MANITOL**.

MANNITOL - A mild baby laxative which is probably the most common cut used in cocaine.

MARIJUANA - The term marijuana is used to refer to the cannabis plant and to any part or extract of it that produces psychophysical changes. It is cultivated in many parts of the world. Once dried it appears brown, green, or gold in color, and it often has a very strong odor. The main active substance in marijuana is tetrahydrocannabinol (THC). THC is not evenly distributed throughout the plant, but varies in decreasing order of concentration as follows: resin, female flower, male flower, and leaves. The seeds and stems contain little or no THC.

MARKS - See **TRACKS**.

MARY JANE - Street name for marijuana.

MARY WARNER - Street name for marijuana.

MAUI WOWIE - Hawaiian grown marijuana.

MDA - 3,4-methylenedioxyamphetamine. Often referred to on the street as the "Mellow Drug of America". It is a synthetic hallucinogen which can produce effects similar to LSD.

MDM - Street name for the drug MDMA.

MDMA - 3,4-methylenedioxy-n-methylamphetamine. A synthetic hallucinogen with amphetamine like properties. It is usually sold on the street in a white tablet or white crystalline powder form, but a reddish or brownish color is also seen and is due to makeshift manufacturing.

MELLOW DRUG OF AMERICA - Street name for the drug MDA.

MELTING POINT TEST - A street test for cocaine which utilizes the fact that cocaine and its common adulterants have different melting points. The cocaine is heated and the temperature at which it, or its adulterants melt is evaluated.

MENIT, MENITA - Alternate spelling for mannitol.

MESC - Street name for the peyote cactus or mescaline.

SLANG

MESCAL - 1. Often used synonymously with the peyote cactus and mescaline. 2. The very toxic mescal bean, found on a shrub which grows in the southwest United States and Mexico, which reportedly can produce hallucinations when ingested. 3. A popular alcoholic drink in Mexico.

MESCAL BUTTON - Street name for the top of the peyote cactus.

MESCALINE - The hallucinogenic alkaloid contained in the peyote cactus. It has also been produced synthetically. The effects of mescaline may last up to 12 hours.

MESCALITO - Street name for peyote.

METABOLITE - The substance(s) produced by the body breaking down, or metabolizing a drug. In some cases the metabolite, rather than the drug itself is responsible for the drugs effect. Metabolites can be detected in blood and urine, and are the basis for many drug tests.

METH - Street name for methamphetamine.

METHADONE - A synthetic narcotic used in the treatment of heroin addiction because 1) it prevents heroin withdrawal symptoms; 2) it fulfils the addicts need for the drug; 3) at sufficiently high doses it blocks the effects of heroin through cross tolerance, thus a shot of street heroin while undergoing methadone treatment will probably give no pleasurable effect; 4) it is a longer acting drug than heroin, the average dose lasting about 24 hours; 5) it is effective orally, thus breaking the ritual of injection; and 6) it can be dispensed at a treatment center. The ultimate aim is to wean addicts from heroin and the heroin lifestyle, and allow them to adjust to a new lifestyle through which they can then withdraw from methadone and live drug free. Methadone is also used to relieve severe pain, and is manufactured in injection, tablet and oral liquid forms.

METHAMPHETAMINE HYDROCHLORIDE - A central nervous system stimulant similar to amphetamine sulfate, but much more potent. The favored drug among habitual amphetamine users, who frequently take it by intravenous injection. Methamphetamine hydrochloride is legally manufactured as the prescription drug Desoxyn, which is used to treat obesity and attention deficit disorder in children. Illicit methamphetamine is sold on the street in powder, liquid and tablet form.

METHANOL TEST - A street purity test which involves placing a small amount of cocaine in a glass containing methanol (methyl alcohol). The purity of the cocaine is determined by the manner in which the cocaine and any adulterants dissolve.

METHAQUALONE - A powerful sedative/hypnotic prescription drug widely abused in the United States until legal production was ceased in 1984. Most methaqualone currently sold on the street is counterfeit, containing such drugs as diazepam or phenobarbital. There is a small amount of domestic illicit manufacture of methaqualone, and some smuggling from countries where it is still legally manufactured. Methaqualone is sometimes referred to on the street as ludes and a former brand name, Qualude.

METHYL ETHYL KETONE - (2-butanone, MEK). A chemical regulated by the Chemical Diversion and Trafficking Act of 1988 as an essential chemical, and which is sometimes used in the manufacturing of illicit drugs.

MEXICAN BROWN HEROIN - A brown colored powder heroin produced in Mexico. The brown color is due to impurities resulting from poor refinement techniques. Although Asian heroin is occasionally seen with a brown color, brown heroin is normally associated with a Mexican origin.

MEXICAN MUD - Street name for Mexican tar heroin.

MEXICAN REDS - Seconal tablets manufactured in Mexico.

MEXICAN TAR HEROIN - A crude form of heroin produced in Mexico. Consistency varies from sticky to hard, and the color from black to brown. Purity generally ranges from 20% to 80% - substantially higher than the purity normally encountered with powdered heroin. It is usually dissolved in water and injected.

MICKEY FINN - A combination of the prescription drug chloral hydrate and an alcoholic drink.

MICRODOTS, MICROTABS - Street name for very small (less than 1/8 inch across) LSD tablets.

MIERDA - Spanish street name for heroin.

MIKE - Street name for microgram, a measurement equal to one millionth of a gram. Used in reference to the potency of an LSD dose.

MICAGE - The microgram potency of LSD.

MIOSIS - Constriction of the pupils, such as that caused by bright light. Miosis can be caused by narcotic drugs such as heroin and codeine.

MISS EMMA - Street name for morphine.

MJ - Street name for marijuana.

MMDA - 3-methoxy-4,5-methylenedioxyamphetamine. One of the many phenethylamines available on the illicit market.

M99 - See **ETORPHINE**.

MONKEY - Street name for the drug PCP.

MONKEY ON MY BACK - A drug addiction.

MORNING GLORY - A common decorative garden plant with twining vines, having funnel shaped variously colored flowers that close late in the day. The seeds of a number of varieties contain d-lysergic acid amide, a chemical similar to LSD. The seeds can produce mild hallucinations when ingested. Varieties with the highest d-lysergic acid amide content are heavenly blue, pearly gates, flying saucers, wedding bells, summer skies, and blue star.

MORPHINE - Morphine is the principle active ingredient in opium. Raw opium is composed of approximately 10% morphine by weight. Isolated in 1803 and named after Morpheus, the Greek god of dreams, morphine first received widespread use in the United States during the Civil War. It is often considered to be superior to all other drugs for relief of pain, but is very addictive, and its medical use is strictly controlled.

MOTA - Spanish street name for marijuana.

MOTHER OF PEARL - Street name for highly pure Peruvian flake cocaine.

MPPP - A designer drug derived from the prescription drug meperidine, a synthetic narcotic analgesic. MPPP is seen as a powder on the street, and produces heroin-like effects.

MPTP - A neurotoxic substance created by the improper synthesis of the designer drug MPPP. MPTP has been linked to a Parkinson's-like disease, which is caused by degeneration or damage to certain nerve cells in the brain. The disease is characterized by muscle rigidity, slow body movement, an unbalanced walk, and even paralysis. There is no cure.

MUD - Street name for Mexican tar heroin.

MULA - A cocaine adulterant or cut.

MULE - A person who transports drugs.

MUNCHIES - The hunger experienced after using marijuana.

MUSCLING - Injecting a drug into a muscle, as opposed to a vein.

MUSHROOMS - Street name for hallucinogenic mushrooms.

MYDRIASIS - Dilation (enlarging) of the pupils of the eyes, such as that which occurs naturally in the dark. Certain drugs also cause dilation of the pupils, such as cocaine and many of the hallucinogens.

MYRISTICA OIL - A constituent of nutmeg and related plants which reportedly contain small amounts of substances similar to the drug MDA.

N-ACETYLANTHRANILIC ACID - A chemical regulated by the Chemical Diversion and Trafficking Act of 1988 as a precursor chemical, and which is sometimes used in the manufacturing of illicit drugs.

NARC - A narcotics officer.

NARCOTIC - The term narcotic usually refers only to the opiates and opioids, such as heroin, codeine, and morphine. Narcotic has also often been used synonymously for illegal drugs, or any street drug used recreationally that produces sleep or hallucinations and/or appears addicting or harmful. The United States Code also includes cocaine under the category of narcotic.

NARCOTIC ANALGESIC - A narcotic analgesic is a morphine related drug that relieves or allays pain. Some drugs which fall into this category are codeine, opium, and meperidine (Demerol).

NARCOTIC ANTAGONIST - A drug that blocks or counteracts the effects of the opiate drugs. They are used both to treat narcotic addiction and the effects of narcotic overdose. The narcotic antagonist drugs include naloxone and naltrexone.

NATIVE AMERICAN CHURCH - A religion existing among Native Americans that combines elements of Christianity, native religious rites, and the ritual use of peyote. Peyote use first became apparent among the tribes of the United States in the latter part of the 19th century, when it was used in religious rites and to heal the sick. Gradually a religion developed around the use of the cactus that combined elements of Christianity with the vision-quest ritual typical of the plains Indians. The religion teaches brotherly love, high moral principles, abstention from alcohol consumption, and considers peyote a sacrament through which God is manifested. The religion was first organized in 1918, and has a membership that exceeds 250,000. Membership is limited to those individuals who are at least 25% Native American.

NEBBIES - Street name for the prescription drug Nembutal.

NEEDLE FREAK - 1. One who's preferred method of taking drugs is by injection; occasionally to the point where the enjoyment of injection exceeds the enjoyment of the effect of the drug. 2. One who's drugs of choice are those that are injected.

NEXUS - Street name for methcathinone.

NICKEL - Five dollars worth of a drug.

NIEVE - Spanish street name for cocaine.

NITROGEN MONOXIDE - See **NITROUS OXIDE**.

NITROUS OXIDE - Nitrous oxide is the most common anesthetic gas, used mainly by dental offices. It is also sold in small metal cylinders for use as a propellant with whipping cream cannisters. When used therapeutically, the effects are those of anesthesia and analgesia. In recreational use, its effects are closer to those of the vaporous anesthetics ether and chloroform, making the user giddy or exhilarated for about 5 minutes. Occasionally hallucinations may occur. Excessive doses may cause nausea, vomiting, or unconsciousness because of lack of oxygen. Discovered in the 1770's by Joseph Priestley, but not used as an anesthetic until the middle of the 19th century, it was the first effective modern anesthetic, followed by ether and chloroform. Called "laughing gas", or "gas" on the street, it is abused for its mood altering capability.

NOD - The stuporous state characterized by a bowed head and drooping eyelids. Experienced by heroin and high dose methadone users after the drugs initial euphoric effects have diminished.

NORML - Acronym for National Organization for the Reform of Marijuana Laws. NORML actively lobbies for the legalization of marijuana, recognition of the medical uses of marijuana, and destruction of criminal records for marijuana law offenders. NORML policies however, are against the abusive use of all drugs, the use of marijuana by children, and driving while under the intoxicating effects of marijuana or any other drug.

NORPSEUDOEPHEDRINE - A chemical regulated by the Chemical Diversion and Trafficking Act of 1988 as a precursor chemical, and which is sometimes used in the manufacturing of amphetamines and other illicit drugs.

NORTHERN LIGHTS - A potent variety of marijuana.

NOSE CANDY, NOSE POWDER, NOSE STUFF - Street name for cocaine.

NOVICE - An occasional user of drugs.

NUAI - Asian measurment of 700 grams.

NUKING THE COCAINE - Using a microwave oven as a heat source to catalyze the conversion of baking soda and cocaine hydrochloride, the type used for snorting, into crack.

NUP - High quality hash produced in India.

NUTMEG - Common nutmeg, like that found in most kitchens, is sometimes abused as a minor hallucinogen. Although consuming amounts sufficient to cause any effects will also cause nausea and vomiting. Nutmeg also contains many of the precursors to the MDA related compounds.

NYSTAGMUS - The involuntary jerking of the eyes as they move vertically or horizontally, or when held to the extreme edge of the eye socket. Nystagmus is an indication of recent use of certain depressant and inhalant drugs, and PCP. The test is commonly used by police officers in determining an individuals drug or alcohol intoxication.

O - Street name for opium.

O.D. - Abbreviation for overdose.

OIL - Street name for hashish oil.

OLOLIUQUI - A variety of the morning glory plant with seeds that contain d-lysergic acid amide, a substance chemically similar to LSD that may produce mild hallucinations when ingested.

ONE HITTER - 1. A marijuana bong. 2. A small baseball bat shaped marijuana pipe.

OPIATES - Specifically refers to natural drugs which are refined from opium; morphine and codeine. Sometimes generally used to refer to opium, opium alkaloids and their derivatives, and the synthetic opioids as a whole.

OPIOIDS - Synthetic drugs which are manufactured to resemble the natural opiates in action and effect. These include such drugs as methadone and fentanyl.

OPIUM - A bitter, strongly addictive drug prepared from the dried sap of the opium poppy (Papaver somniferum), from which all opiate drugs are derived. Opium has been used for centuries as a medicinal and recreational drug. The development of more effective opiates and opioids has now virtually eliminated its use medically, and recreational opiate users more often abuse heroin.

OPIUM POPPY - The scientific name of the opium poppy is Papaver Somniferum, which means "the poppy that brings sleep". The seed pod is cut, permitting a resinous substance to ooze out of the incision. This substance is opium, from which several drugs are obtained, such as morphine, heroin and codeine.

ORANGE HEARTS - Street name for the prescription drug Dexedrine.

OTC - Abbreviation for over-the-counter. Drugs which may be purchased without a prescription, such as common aspirin.

OUNCE MAN - A drug dealer.

OUTFIT - Street name for apparatus used to inject drugs, such as a syringe, tourniquet, cooker, etc.

OVERAMPED - A drug overdose normally associated with the use of an amphetamine or cocaine.

OVERDOSE - An excessive ingestion of drugs which causes illness or death.

OVER-THE-COUNTER - Drugs that can be legally purchased without a prescription, such as common aspirin.

OWSLEY - Antiquated street name for LSD.

O-Z - One ounce of a drug.

OZONE - Street name for the drug PCP.

PAKALOLO - Street name for marijuana.

PANAMA GOLD - Potent marijuana from Panama.

PANAMA RED - Marijuana from Panama which has a reddish hue.

PANTHER - Street name for a very toxic mushroom, amanita pantherina, which is native to North America. It is sometimes abused as a hallucinogen. It generally has a brownish cap with white warts, and contains the hallucinogenic substances muscimol and ibotenic acid.

PAPAVER SOMNIFERUM - Botanical name for the opium poppy plant, source for opium and other narcotic drugs.

PAPER - 1. A folded piece of paper containing a small amount of a drug. 2. LSD blotter paper. 3. Rolling papers used to make a marijuana joint.

PAPER ACID - Street name for blotter paper impregnated with LSD.

PARENTERAL - Taking a drug by injection.

PARAPHERNALIA - As defined by Title 21 of the United States Code, drug paraphernalia means "any equipment, product, or material of any kind which is primarily intended or designed for use in manufacturing, compounding, converting, concealing, producing, processing, preparing, injecting, ingesting, inhaling, or otherwise introducing into the human body a controlled substance, possession of which is unlawful under the Controlled Substances Act...".

PARAQUAT - A herbicide that was sprayed over illicit marijuana fields in Mexico in the mid-1970's at the urging of the U.S. government.

PARTY BOWL - A marijuana bong.

PASTA - Spanish word for paste.

PASTE - An off-white to light brown putty-like substance, which is an intermediate product in the refinement of cocaine. It contains impurities such as kerosene, sulfuric acid, and sodium carbonate. Because of its relatively low price, paste is very accessible to low income groups. It is usually smoked with tobacco, and is used primarily in South America.

PATCH PIRATES - Individuals who steal from unattended marijuana gardens.

PATTIES - Hashish formed into the shape of a patty.

PAWN - Low level drug dealer.

PCE - (N-ethyl-1-phenylcyclohexylamine). An analog of the drug PCP.

PCP - Street name for the drug phencyclidine. Originally developed as a human anesthetic, but the use was discontinued due to undesirable side effects. It was used in veterinary medicine until 1978. It is a very strong disassociative hallucinogen, rendering the user insensitive to pain during the period of intoxication. Synthesis is relatively simple for todays illicit manufacturers. In its pure form, it is a white crystalline powder that readily dissolves in water. Most PCP contains contaminants resulting from its makeshift manufacture, causing the color to range from tan to brown. The liquid form of PCP remains the most commonly encountered, although it is also sold in tablets, capsules, and as a powder. PCP is typically applied to a leafy material such as mint, parsley, or marijuana and smoked. Commercially manufactured cigarettes are also adulterated by dipping them in liquid PCP.

PDR - Abbreviation for Physicians Desk Reference. A publication sometimes used by drug abusers to gather information on prescription drugs.

PEACE WEED - Street name for marijuana which has been laced with PCP.

PEACH HEARTS - Street name for the prescription drug Dexedrine.

PEANUT BUTTER SPEED - Street name for methamphetamine.

PEARLY GATES - 1. A variety of the morning glory plant with large white flowers, the seeds of which contain d-lysergic acid amide, a substance chemically similar to LSD. The seeds can produce mild hallucinations when ingested. 2. Street name for LSD.

PEBBLES - Small rocks of crack.

PEDAZO - Spanish street name for heroin.

PELLETS - 1. Street name for LSD. 2. Street name for the prescription drug Ritalin.

PEP PILLS - Street name for amphetamine tablets.

PER - Street abbreviation for prescription.

PERCS - Street name for the prescription drug Percodan.

PERICO - Spanish street name for cocaine.

PERSIAN BROWN - Heroin from Southwest Asia that has a tan or light brown color.

PERSIAN WHITE - 1. Street name for synthetic heroin (alph-methylfentanyl). 2. Street name for white Asian heroin.

PERUVIAN FLAKE - A very pure form of cocaine hydrochloride consisting of thin pearly iridescent crystals. Peruvian flake refers to the style of cocaine, not necessarily the country of origin.

PERUVIAN PINK - Cocaine hydrochloride with thin, slightly pink crystals.

PERZE - Street name for Southwest Asian heroin.

PETROLEUM ETHER - A highly flammable chemical used in the manufacture and purification of a number of drugs.

PEYOTE BUTTONS - The top of the peyote cactus. The buttons contain the hallucinogenic drug mescaline, and are usually consumed by chewing, but may also be used to brew a tea, or are ground up and placed into gelatin capsules.

PEYOTE CACTUS - A small, spineless cactus indigenous to Mexico, northern South America, and the extreme southwest United States. The peyote cactus contains the hallucinogenic substance mescaline. Its hallucinogenic properties were known to the Aztecs, who considered it divine and called it "peyotl". During the 19th century, use spread among Native Americans who used it in their religious rites as an aid to their traditional search for divine visions, and to heal the sick. Eventually this use developed into a religion incorporating elements of Christianity, which is now known as the Native American Church. As a crucial sacrament of this church, legal use of peyote is limited only to bonafide members.

PEYOTL - Indian name for the peyote cactus.

PHARMACOLOGY - The study of the effect of drugs on the living organism.

PHENCYCLIDINE - See **PCP.**

PHENETHYLAMINES - Amphetamine related compounds.

PHENNIES, PHENOS - Street name for the prescription drug phenobarbital.

PHENYLACETIC ACID - A chemical regulated by the Chemical Diversion and Trafficking Act of 1988 as a precursor chemical, and which is sometimes used in the manufacturing of methamphetamine and other illicit drugs.

PHENYLPROPANOLAMINE - A chemical regulated by the Chemical Diversion and Trafficking Act of 1988 as a precursor chemical, and which is sometimes used in the manufacturing of amphetamines and other illicit drugs.

PHP - (1-(1-phenylcyclohexyl)-pyrrolidine). An analog of the drug PCP.

PIECE - 1 gram or 1 ounce of a drug.

PIEDRA - Spanish street name for crack.

PIN - 1. Street name for a needle/syringe. 2. A very thin marijuana joint.

PINCH HITTER - A small baseball bat shaped marijuana pipe.

PINK HEARTS - 1. Street name for legal caffeine tablets which are heart shaped. 2. Street name for the prescription drug Preludin. 3. Street name for the prescription drug Benzedrine, a stimulant no longer manufactured.

SLANG

PINK LADIES, PINKS AND GRAYS - Street name for the prescription drug Darvon.

PINNED - Refers to constricted pupils resulting from the recent use of a narcotic, such as heroin, morphine, etc.

PIPE - Street name for a vein used to inject a drug.

PIPERIDINE - A chemical regulated by the Chemical Diversion and Trafficking Act of 1988 as a precursor chemical, and which is sometimes used in the manufacturing of PCP.

PITZU - Crude morphine base.

PLATA O PLOMO - Spanish for "silver or lead". South American drug culture phrase which means that one will either accept a bribe or be killed.

PLATEAUING - The point at which steroid use no longer produces desired gains. The user then resorts to increasing the dose, the number of drugs, or both.

PMA - Street name for the hallucinogenic drug 4-methoxy-amphetamine.

POINT - Street name for a needle/syringe.

POLVO - Spanish street name for cocaine.

POLYDRUG USE - The use of more than one drug.

PONG - Asian measeurment of 375 grams.

POOR MANS ACID - Street name for morning glory seeds.

POOR MANS SPEEDBALL - A combination of cocaine and amphetamine.

POP - 1. The swallowing of a tablet or capsule. 2. The injecting of a drug directly beneath the surface of the skin, as opposed to a vein (mainlining), or muscle (muscling).

POPPERS - Street name for the prescription drug amyl nitrite.

POPPING - 1. Swallowing a drug. 2. The injecting of a drug directly beneath the surface of the skin, as opposed to a vein (mainlining), or a muscle (muscling).

POPPY - See **OPIUM POPPY**.

POPPY STRAW - The entire cut and dried plant material of the opium poppy, other than the seeds.

POT - Street name for marijuana.

POTASSIUM PERMANGANATE - A chemical regulated by the Chemical Diversion and Trafficking Act of 1988 as an essential chemical, and which is sometimes used in the processing of cocaine.

POTENCY - The relative strength of a drug.

POTENTIATION - The ability of one drug to increase the activity of another drug taken simultaneously. The overall effect of the drugs taken together is greater than the total effects of each drug taken alone. Also known as an "additive effect".

POTHEAD - A user of marijuana.

POT PILLS - Gelatin capsules for oral ingestion which contain any number of preparations mixed with hash oil.

PRECURSOR CHEMICAL - A chemical that is used in manufacturing a controlled substance, and is critical to the creation of the controlled substance.

PRESCRIPTION - The written direction for the preparation, obtaining, and use of a medicine. Can also refer to the prescribed medicine itself.

PRESENCE - Street name for the drug MDMA.

PROCAINE - A local anesthetic sometimes used to adulterate drugs which have a similar appearance, such as cocaine.

PRODUCTO - Spanish street name for cocaine.

PSEUDOEPHEDRINE - A chemical regulated by the Chemical Diversion and Trafficking Act of 1988 as a precursor chemical, and which is sometimes used in the manufacturing of illicit drugs.

PSEUDO-HALLUCINATION - A hallucination the individual knows it is not real, but is a result of drug use. Most drug induced hallucinations are of this type.

PSILOCYBE - A genus of mushroom which consists of many species, most notably Psilocybe cubensis and Psilocybe cyanescens. These mushrooms contain the hallucinogenic substances psilocybin and psilocin.

PSILOCYBIN - The hallucinogenic substance found in a number of species of mushrooms. Ingestion of mushrooms containing psilocybin, which is converted to psilocin in the body, produces a hallucinogenic experience similar to, but much milder than LSD.

PSILOCIN - A hallucinogenic substance which, in addition to psilocybin, is found in a number of species of mushrooms, but in a smaller concentration. However, because psilocybin is converted to psilocin in the body, psilocin is responsible for most of the hallucinogenic effect.

SLANG

PSYCHEDELIC - Refers to hallucinogenic drugs themselves, or the mind-altering and increased sensory perception effects of hallucinogenic drugs.

PSYCHOACTIVE - Having a significant effect on mood or mental state.

PSYCHOPHYSICAL - Mind and body.

PSYCHOSIS - A mental disorder in which the individual loses contact with reality. The term is often used with particular drugs that are abused, such as cocaine psychosis, steroid psychosis, amphetamine psychosis, etc.

P2P - (phenylacetone). A chemical used in the manufacture of amphetamines.

PUNTA ROJA - A potent variety of marijuana from Colombia.

PUSHER - A drug dealer.

QUALUDE - Trade name for methaqualone when it was a legal prescription drug. Now used as a street name for illicit methaqualone.

QUARTER - 1. Twenty five dollars worth of a drug. 2. A quarter ounce or quarter gram of a drug.

QUARTY - Street name for a smokeable, highly pure form of methamphetamine, more commonly referred to as "ice".

QUININE - A white crystalline alkaloid derived from cinchona bark. It is sometimes used as cut in drugs that have a similar appearance, particularly heroin.

RAGWEED - Low quality marijuana.

RAILS - Parallel lines of a powdered drug prepared for snorting.

RAINBOWS - Street name for the prescription drug Tuinal.

RAVE - A large party that often includes the use of hallucinogens, particularly LSD or MDMA.

READER - A fraudulent prescription for drugs.

RED AND BLUES - Street name for the prescription drug Tuinal.

RED OIL - Red colored hash oil.

REDS, RED BULLETS, RED DEVILS, RED BIRDS - Street name for the prescription drug secobarbital sodium.

REEFER - 1. Street name for marijuana. 2. A marijuana joint. 3. A marijuana joint which has had hash oil added to it.

REGISTER - Show of blood drawn back into a syringe by an intravenous drug user before injecting a drug. Shows that the needle has penetrated a vein.

RESIN - The viscous secretions of the marijuana plant. Marijuana resin consists of millions of sticky microscopic glands which form on the outer surface of the plant, and contain THC, the main psychoactive substance of marijuana.

RIG - Street name for a needle/syringe.

RIPDOWN - Approximately 3 $^{1}/_{2}$ grams of a drug.

RIPPED - A drug high.

ROACH - 1. A marijuana joint. 2. The butt end of a marijuana joint which is saved and combined with others to make new joints.

ROACH CLIP - A gripping device, usually an electrical alligator clip or surgical hemostat, which holds the end of a marijuana joint while being smoked. This allows the joint to be smoked almost completely without burning the lips or fingers.

ROADMAN - The Indian leader at a peyote ceremony.

ROCA - Spanish street name for crack.

ROCK - 1. Street name for crack. In some areas, rock is used to describe chunks of powdered cocaine HCl.

ROCK COCAINE - Physical form of cocaine which consists of chunks or rocks, as opposed to flake or powder. The cocaine rocks are typically about the size of a pencil eraser, and are chopped up and snorted. In most areas, the term "rock cocaine" is not the same as "rock" (crack).

ROCK UP - Street name for the process of converting cocaine hydrochloride, the type used for snorting, to crack, a type used for smoking.

ROCKET FUEL - Street name for the drug PCP.

ROID RAGE - A violent temperament displayed by some individuals who use steroids.

ROIDS - Slang for steroids.

ROLLING PAPER - Cigarette paper used to make a marijuana joint.

ROPE - Street name for marijuana.

ROXANNE - Street name for crack.

SLANG

ROYAL BLUE - Street name for LSD.
RUDERALIS - A variety of marijuana native to Russia which has a very low THC content. Sparsely branched, 1 foot to 4 feet in height. Very rare in the United States.
RUFUS - Street name for heroin.
RUN - 1. A period of several hours, or even several days of constant drug use. 2. The transportation of drugs.
RUNNER - One who transports drugs.
RUSH - 1. The initial onset of effect of a drug prior to the high. The "high" is more prolonged than the "rush". 2. Street name for the prescription drug amyl nitrite.
SAN PEDRO CACTUS - A cactus native to South America which grows to heights of 15 feet. Like the peyote cactus, san pedro contains the hallucinogenic substance mescaline, but in a smaller concentration.
SANDOZ - Street name for LSD. Sandoz Laboratories of Switzerland was the original producer of LSD.
SAN ISIDRO - Street name for the Psilocybe cubensis mushroom.
SANTA MARTA GOLD - A potent, light brown colored variety of marijuana from Colombia.
SATCH COTTON - A piece of cotton used to filter the impurities out of a liquid drug while it is being drawn into a syringe. The cotton is kept after use because it retains a small amount of the drug, which can be extracted if the abuser is unable to obtain additional drugs.
SATIVA - 1. Street name for marijuana. 2. A variety of marijuana with heavy branching, growing to a height of 6 feet or more.
SATURDAY NIGHTER - An occasional user of drugs.
SCARS - See **TRACKS**.
SCAT - Street name for heroin.
SCHEDULED DRUGS - Scheduled drugs are those drugs which are considered to have an abuse potential, and are controlled under the Controlled Substances Act of 1970.
SCHMECK - Street name for heroin.
SCHOOL BOY - Street name codeine.
SCORE - To buy drugs.
SCREENS - Small round brass or stainless steel screens used to hold a drug in a pipe while being smoked.
SCRIBE - A person who has the wherewithal to write illegal prescriptions for drug abusers.
SCRIPT - Slang for a drug prescription.
SCRIPT DOCTOR - A doctor who prescribes drugs to drug abusers.
SECCIES - Street name for the prescription drug Seconal Sodium.
SEDATIVE - A drug which relaxes, calms, or sooths the body or mind.
SEDATIVE/HYPNOTIC - A classification of depressant drugs with such primary effects as calming, sedation, or induction of sleep. The sedative/hypnotics are usually divided into 4 categories: 1) barbiturates, 2) alcohol, 3) antianxiety tranquilizers, 4) nonbarbiturate drugs.
SENS - Slang for sinsemilla.
SENSITIZATION - The reverse of drug tolerance. The effect of increased responsiveness with prolonged use of a drug, rather than decreased effect with prolonged use.
SET - The mental state or attitude a person has when using a hallucinogenic drug. The set may influence the reaction to the drug.
SETS - 1. A combination of the prescription drugs glutethimide and codeine. 2. A combination of the prescription drugs Talwin (pentazocine), and PBZ (tripelennamine).
SETTING - The physical environment in which drug use takes place. Some researchers hold that the set and setting determine whether a drug experience will be good or bad.
SHABU - Street name for a smokeable, highly pure form of methamphetamine, more commonly referred to as "ice".
SHAKE - The leaves of the marijuana plant, as opposed to the buds.
SHAVE - The act of adulterating a drug.
SHE - Street name for cocaine.
SHEET ACID - Blotter paper form of LSD.
SHERMANS, SHERMIES, SHERMS - A cigarette brand with dark paper wrapping which is laced with liquid PCP by abusers. The dark paper helps conceal the fact that the cigarette has been dipped in a liquid.

SLANG

SHIT - 1. Street name for heroin. 2. Low quality drugs.
SHOOT, SHOOT UP - To inject a drug.
SHOOTING GALLERY - Place where drugs are regularly injected, such as a certain residence or building.
SHORT COUNT - An amount of a drug received, less than that which was paid for.
SHOTGUN - A person who follows a drug transporter (mule) to ensure the drugs are delivered.
SHOTGUNNING - An athletes term for using any steroid available.
SHOVE - To sell drugs.
SHROOMS - Street name for hallucinogenic mushrooms.
SHROOMING - Using hallucinogenic mushrooms.
SID - Street name for LSD.
SIDE EFFECTS - All actions produced by a drug with the exception of the specific action for which the drug was administered.
SINS - Slang for sinsemilla.
SINSEMILLA - Spanish for "without seed". Sinsemilla is the technique of separating male marijuana plants from the female plants to prevent their pollination. Keeping the female plants unpollinated allows increased production of resin, which contains a high concentration of THC. If the female plant becomes fertilized, it devotes a large part of its chemical energies to making seeds, and in the process lowers its resin production. The growth of sinsemilla requires the identification and weeding out of the male plants before they begin pollination.
SKAG - Street name for heroin.
SKIN POPPING - Injecting a drug directly under the surface of the skin, rather than in a vein or in a muscle. This may be performed by addicts who's veins in common injection sights have collapsed.
SKUNK - Marijuana which has a heavy pungent odor.
SLAB - A large piece of crack.
SLAMMING - To inject a drug.
SLEEPERS - Street name for tranquilizers.
SMACK - Street name for heroin.
SMECK - Street name for heroin.
SMASHED - A drug high.
SMOKE - Street name for marijuana.
SNAPPERS - Street name for the prescription drug amyl nitrite.
SNIFFING - Inhaling drugs through the nose.
SNORT - 1. To inhale a powdered drug through the nostrils. Other terms to describe snorting: blow, blowing, do a line, fire a line, horning, sweep, toot, and tooting. 2. Street name for cocaine.
SNOT - 1. Street name for smokeable methamphetamine (ice). 2. Street name for cocaine.
SNOW - Street name for cocaine.
SNOW BUGS - The sensation a cocaine user has that bugs are crawling on or under the skin.
SNOW PAPER, SNOW SEAL - A folded piece of paper containing a small amount of cocaine. Also referred to as a "bindle".
SNUFF SPOON - See **COKE SPOON**.
SOFT DRUGS - A vague, imprecise term that is sometimes used to refer to all drugs other than those which can easily cause addiction, such as the opiates.
SOLES - Hash formed into a semi-circular shape.
SOURCE - A drug dealer.
SPACED OUT - A drug high.
SPEED - Street name for amphetamines.
SPEEDBALL - A combination of an upper and a downer. Most often an injected mixture of heroin and cocaine, but may include the combination of heroin with amphetamine. Speedball is also used as a street name for the smoked combination of heroin and crack.
SPECTRUM - Street name for the drug 2C-B.
SPEED LAB - Facility where amphetamines are illegally manufactured.
SPIKE - Street name for a needle/syringe.
SPLASH - Placing LSD on a medium, such as toothpicks or blotter paper.
SPLIFF - A marijuana joint.

SLANG

SPOON - 1. A small spoon used to snort a powdered drug. 2. A spoon used to heat and dissolve a powdered drug in water for injection. 3. An imprecise quantity of a drug, ranging from 1/2 gram to 2 grams.
SPORE - The reproductive body of a mushroom.
SPOTS - Street name for LSD.
STACKING - The concurrent use of two or more different steroids.
STAR - Street name for methcathinone.
STAR DUST - Street name for cocaine.
STASH - A secure location where drugs are kept.
STASH MAN - A drug dealer.
STEP ON - The act of adulterating a drug.
STEROID BLOAT - A water retention effect caused by steroid use. Steroid users often take diuretic drugs to help remove excess water from the body.
STEROIDS - See **ANABOLIC STEROIDS**.
STICK - A marijuana joint.
STIMULANTS - A major classification of drugs that stimulate or accelerate the central nervous system.
STINK WEED - Street name for marijuana.
STOFFA - Spanish slang for heroin.
STONED - A drug high.
STP - See **DOM**.
STRETCH - The act of adulterating a drug.
STRUNG OUT - 1. The sickly appearance of long term drug users. 2. A drug addict going through withdrawal symptoms.
STUFF - General term for drugs, particularly heroin.
STUPOR - A state of semi-consciousness in which the individual is unaware of what is going on in his or her surroundings.
SUBCUTANEOUS - Injecting a drug directly under the surface of the skin, rather than in a vein or a muscle. Referred to on the street as “popping”, “joy popping”, or “skin popping”. This may be performed by an addict who’s veins of common injection have collapsed.
SUCROSE - A sugar which is sometimes used to adulterate drugs which have a similar appearance, such as cocaine.
SUGAR - Street name for heroin.
SUGAR DOWN - The act of adulterating a drug.
SUMMER SKIES - One of several varieties of the morning glory plant, the seeds of which contain d-lysergic acid amide, a substance chemically similar to LSD. The seeds can produce mild hallucinations when ingested.
SUNSHINE - Street name for LSD.
SUPER COKE - Street name for crack.
SUPER GRASS - 1. Very potent marijuana. 2. Marijuana which contains PCP.
SUPER ICE - Street name for a smokeable highly pure form of methamphetamine, more commonly referred to as “ice”.
SUPER JOINT - 1. A marijuana joint laced with PCP. 2. A joint containing very potent marijuana.
SUPER K - Street name for the prescription drug ketamine.
SUPER WEED - 1. Marijuana which contains PCP. 2. Very potent marijuana.
SUPPLIER - A drug dealer.
SUPPLIES - Items with which drugs are used, such as a syringe, pipe, etc.
SURF BOARDS - Hash formed into a thin oblong shape.
SWALLOWER - A person who swallows drugs in rubber packages for the purpose of smuggling, which are later retrieved by defecating.
SWEEP - To snort a drug.
SYNESTHESIA - Term used to describe perceptual distortions brought on by hallucinogenic drugs. Sound can be “seen”, colors can be “heard”, etc.
SYNTHETIC HEROIN - Street name for the fentanyl analogs, which can be several times more potent than heroin itself.

SLANG

SYRINGE - A device for pumping liquids through a small aperture into the body. A syringe may be in the form of a common medical syringe, a make-shift type which utilizes a hypodermic needle attached to the rubber bulb of a baby's pacifier, or other similar device.
T - Street name for the prescription drug Talwin.
TABS - 1. Street name for LSD. 2. Street name for a drug tablet.
TAC - Street name for PCP.
T's and B's, T's and BLUE's - A combination of the prescription drugs Talwin (pentazocine), and PBZ (tripelennamine). The tablets are dissolved in water and injected as a heroin substitute.
TAKE OFF - The onset of effect or "rush" of a drug.
TALK DOWN - The process of providing comforting and personal verbal support to a person having a bad experience with a hallucinogenic drug. The talking down continues until the person overcomes the difficulty, or returns to a normal state of mind.
TAR - Street name for Mexican tar heroin.
TASTE - To sample a drug before buying it.
TATTOOING - See **TRACKS**.
TCP - 1[1-(2-thienyl-cyclohexyl)]piperidine. An analog of the drug PCP.
TEA - Street name for marijuana.
TEDDIES AND BETTIES - See **T's and B's**.
TEMPLE BALLS - Round balls of hash from Nepal, which often contain small amounts of opium.
TEN CENT BAG - Ten dollars worth of a drug.
TEN CENT PISTOL - A bag of poisoned heroin sold to a suspected informer.
TEONANACATL - Indian word for psilocybin mushrooms, meaning "food of the gods".
TETRACAINE - A local anesthetic sometimes used as an cut in drugs which have a similar appearance, such as cocaine.
TETRAHYDROCANNABINOL - See **THC**.
TEXAS TEA - Street name for marijuana.
THAI STICK - Potent marijuana grown in Thailand and its neighboring countries, which is wrapped around a bamboo stick 4 to 10 inches in length. The Thai stick itself is not smoked, the marijuana is separated and made into joints or smoked in a pipe.
THC - Delta-9-tetrahydrocannabinol. One of the cannabinoids found in the marijuana plant. It is responsible for most of the psychoactive effect of marijuana. Marijuana generally contains anywhere from less than 1% to 10% THC, but averages around 2% or 3%.
THORNAPPLE - See **DATURA**.
3's - Street name for prescription codeine tablets stamped with the number 3, designating the strength.
3,4-METHYLENEDIOXYPHENYL-2-PROPANONE - A chemical regulated by the Chemical diversion and Trafficking Act of 1988 as a precursor chemical, and which is sometimes used in the manufacturing of illicit drugs.
THRESHOLD DRUGS - Drugs that are perceived by a portion of the population as being safe to use, such as alcohol or marijuana, but which may lay the foundation for trying more dangerous drugs, such as cocaine, heroin, etc.
THRUSTERS - Street name for amphetamines.
TICKETS - Small perforated squares of blotter paper which contain doses of LSD.
TIE - A tourniquet device, such as a belt or string used to help locate a vein and inject a drug.
TIE OFF - Applying pressure to a vein to make it rise for an injection.
TITRATION - Controlling the dose of a drug by the amount of the drug ingested.
TMA - Trimethoxyamphetamine. One of the many MDA-like compounds.
TOKE - To take a puff from a joint or pipe.
TOKER - One who smokes marijuana.
TOLERANCE - The body's resistance to the effects of a drug. As a person's tolerance to a drug increases with continued use, he or she needs progressively higher doses to obtain the desired effects.
TOLUENE - A chemical regulated by the Chemical Diversion and Trafficking Act of 1988 as an essential chemical, and which is sometimes used in the manufacturing of illicit drugs.
TOOLS - Items with which drugs are used, such as a syringe, pipe, etc.
TOOT - 1. Street name for cocaine. 2. The act of snorting a drug.

SLANG

TOOTER - A straw, rolled up paper currency, or similar device used to snort a powdered drug.
TOOTSIE ROLL - Street name for Mexican tar heroin.
TOPI - Street name for peyote.
TOPS - Street name for the buttons of the peyote cactus.
TOPS AND BOTTOMS - See **T's and BLUE's**.
TOYS - Items with which drugs are used, such as a syringe, pipe, etc.
TPCP - 1[1-(2-thienyl-cyclohexyl)]piperidine. An analog of the drug PCP.
TRACKS - Hypodermic needle marks. In more severe cases of drug addiction, individuals may have scars, scar tissue, and abscesses over major veins as a result of repeated injections. An injection can be made virtually anywhere on the body, but the inside elbow area is the most common. Needle marks are a readily visible indicator of sustained illicit drug use, and are often tattooed over or covered with long sleeves in an attempt to conceal them.
TRAFFICKING - The obtaining, transporting, and selling of illicit drugs for commercial purposes.
TRANK - Street name for the drug PCP.
TRANQUILIZER - A drug which has a sedative, calming, or muscle relaxing effect. Tranquilizers are classified into 2 categories; antianxiety tranquilizers, which are used for sedation, and antipsychotic tranquilizers, which are used for treatment of psychiatric problems.
TRAVEL AGENT - 1. An LSD dealer. 2. An experienced individual who talks down a person having a bad experience involving a hallucinogenic drug by providing comforting and personal verbal support.
TREAT - A dose of heroin.
TRIP - A drug use experience.
TRUCK DRIVERS - Street name for amphetamines.
TUIES - Street name for the prescription drug Tuinal.
TURKEY TROTS - See **TRACKS**.
TWEAKED - A methamphetamine high.
2-BUTANONE - A chemical regulated by the Chemical Diversion and Trafficking Act of 1988 as an essential chemical, and which is sometimes used in the manufacturing of illicit drugs.
2-CB - 2,5-dimethoxy-4-bromo-phenethylamine. A hallucinogenic drug with an effect similar to mescaline.
U4EUH - Street name for the hallucinogenic drug 4-methyl aminorex.
UNCUT - A drug to which an adulterant has not been added.
UNDERGRAD - An occasional user of drugs.
UPPERS, UPS - Street name for a stimulant drug, most often referring to amphetamines.
UPTOWN - Street name for cocaine.
URINALYSIS - In the drug abuse field, urinalysis is the testing for the presence of illicitly used drugs.
V, VALS - Street name for the prescription drug Valium.
VENOUS THROMBOSIS - Swollen and blocked condition of the veins resulting from repeated drug injections.
VENUS - Street name for the drug 2C-B.
VISS - Burmese measurment of 1.6 kilograms oh opium or opium products.
WACK - 1. Street name for the drug PCP. 2. The act of adulterating a drug. 3. A substance added to a drug as an adulterant.
WACKY WEED - Street name for marijuana.
WAKE-UPS - Street name for amphetamines.
WASTED - A drug high.
WATER - Street name for methamphetamine.
WATER PIPE - A smoking pipe which utilizes a water chamber to cool the smoke. Many drugs which are smoked, such as marijuana and crack are often smoked in a water pipe. More often referred to as a bong.
WAVY CAPS - Street name for the hallucinogenic Psilocybe cyanescens mushroom.
WEDDING BELLS - A variety of the morning glory plant with large pink flowers, the seeds of which contain d-lysergic acid amide, a substance chemically similar to LSD. The seeds can produce mild hallucinations when ingested.
WEDGE - 1. Street name for LSD. 2. A combination of STP and LSD.
WEED - Street name for marijuana.

SLANG

WEEKENDER - An occasional user of drugs.
WEST COAST PELLETS - Street name for the prescription drug Ritalin.
WET DADDY - Street name for a marijuana joint laced with PCP.
WHITE - Street name for cocaine.
WHITE CROSSES - 1. Antiquated street name for illicit amphetamine tablets. 2. Street name for legal caffeine or ephedrine tablets which are white and double scored on one side.
WHITE GIRL - Street name for cocaine.
WHITE LADY - Street name for cocaine.
WHITE PIPE - Street name for cocaine freebase.
WHITE STUFF - Street name for heroin or cocaine.
WHITE TORNADO - Street name for cocaine freebase.
WHITES - Street name for illicit amphetamine tablets..
WINDOW PANE - Street name for small, usually square pieces of gelatin which contain LSD.
WIPED OUT - A drug high.
WIRE - Street name for methamphetamine.
WIRED - A drug high.
WITHDRAWAL - The psychological and physical trauma that develop upon discontinuation of a drug to which one has become addicted.
WOODROSE SEEDS - Seeds of the woodrose plant contain d-lysergic acid amide, a substance chemically similar to LSD which can produce mild hallucinations when ingested.
WONDER - Street name for methcathinone.
WORKS - Street name for apparatus used to inject drugs, such as a syringe, tourniquet, cooker, etc.
X, XTC - Street name for the drug MDMA.
YELLOWS, YELLOW BULLETS, YELLOW JACKETS - Street name for the prescription drug Nembutal.
YAGE - A hallucinogen derived from the ayahuasca vine of the Amazon forests.
YERBA - Spanish street name for marijuana.
YOHIMBINE - An alkaloid of the bark of the West African Corynanthe yohimbe tree. It is sometimes abused due to its stimulant and aphrodisiac properties.
YUPPIE DRUG - Street name for the drug MDMA.
Z - One ounce of a drug.
ZACATE - Spanish street name for marijuana.
ZEN - Street name for the drug MDMA.
ZIP - Street name for amphetamines.

SUGGESTED READING

Cherniak, L., The Great Books of Cannabis, Tasa International, P.O. Box 154, Station "B", Toronto, Ontario, Canada M5T 2T3, 1983

DeKorne, J., Psychedelic Shamanism, Loompanics, Port Townsend, 1994

Dolan, E., Drugs in Sports, Franklin Watts, New York, 1986

Eisner, B., Ecstasy The MDMA Story, Ronin Publishing, Inc., Berkeley, 1989

Fester, U., Secrets of Methamphetamine Manufacture - Third Edition, Loompanics, Port Townsend, 1991

Frank, M., Marijuana Grower's Insider's Guide, Red Eye Press, Los Angeles, 1988

Frank, M., and Rosenthal, E., Marijuana Growers Guide, Red Eye Press, Los Angeles, 1990

French, S., The Complete Guide To The Street Drug Game, Lyle Stuart, Inc., Secaucus, 1980

Goldstein, A., M.D., Addiction, W.H. Freeman and Co., New York, 1994

Griffith, W., Opium Poppy Garden, Ronin Publishing, Inc., Berkeley, 1993

Herer, J., The Emporer Wears No Clothes, HEMP/Queen of Clubs Pblng, Van Nuys, 1993

Hofmann, A., LSD My Problem Child, Jeremy P. Tarcher, Inc., 1983

Hogshire, J., Opium for the Masses, Loompanics Unlimited, Port Townsend, 1994

Inaba, D., Pharm. D., and Cohen, W., Uppers, Downers, All Arounders, Cinemed Inc., Ashland, 1990

Kirsch, M., Designer Drugs, Comp Care Publications, Minneapolis, 1986

Lassen, G., The Secret Garden Marijuana, Redwood Press, San Carlos, 1986

Lee, D., Cocaine Consumers Handbook, What If?, San Rafael, 1985

Long, H., Getting Started in the Illicit Drug Business, Loompanics Unlimited, Port Townsend, 1988

Maisto, S., et al., Drug Use and Misuse, Holt, Rinehart and Winston, Inc., Chicago, 1991

Miller, G., Drugs and The Law, Gould Publications, Altamonte Springs, 1992

Nimble, J., Construction and Operation of Clandestine Drug Laboratories, Loompanics, Port Townsend, 1986

Nuckols, C., Cocaine From Dependency to Recovery, TAB Books, Blue Ridge Sum, 1989

SUGGESTED READING

O'Brien, R., et al., The Encyclopedia of Drug Abuse, Facts on File, New York, 1992

Oss, O., and Oeric, O., Psilocybin, Lux Natura, Berkeley, 1986

Ott, J., Hallucinogenic Plants of North America, Wingbow Press, Berkeley, 1979

Psychedelics Encyclopedia, Ronin Publishing, Inc., Berkeley, 1992

Radcliffe, A., M.D., et al., Pharmer's Almanac, MAC Publishing, Denver, 1990

Raye, D., Pipe Dreams An Inside Look at Free-Base Cocaine, Family Publishing Company, 1980

Restak, R., M.D., Receptors, Bantam Books, New York, 1994

Rosenthal, E., Marijuana Question? Ask Ed, Quick American Publishing Company, San Francisco, 1987

Rosenthal, E., Closet Cultivator, Last Gasp of S.F., San Francisco, 1991

Saunders, N., Nicholas Saunders, London, 1993

Seymour, R., and Smith, D., M.D., Guide to Psychoactive Drugs, Harrington Park Press, New York, 1987

Shulgin, A., and Shulgin, A., PIHKAL A Chemical Love Story, Transform Press, Berkeley, 1992

Smith, M., Psychedelic Chemistry, Loompanics Unlimited, Port Townsend, 1981

Stafford, P., Psychedelics Encyclopedia, Ronin Publishing, Inc., Berkeley, 1992

Stamets, P., Growing Gourmet and Medicinal Mushrooms, Ten Speed Press, Berkeley, 1994

Starks, M., Marijuana Chemistry, Ronin Publishing, Inc., Berkeley, 1990

Stevens, J., and Gee, R., How to Identify and Grow Psilocybin Mushrooms, Sun Magic Publishing, Seattle, 1987

Strausbaugh, J., and Blaise, D., Drug User, Blast Books, Inc., New York, 1991

Storm, D., Marijuana Hydroponics, And/Or Books, Berkeley, 1991

Weil, A., M.D., and Rosen, W., Chocolate to Morphine - Revised and Updated, Houghton Mifflin Co., Boston, 1993

Westermeyer, J., Poppies, Pipes, and People, University of California Press, Ltd., 1982

DURATION OF DETECTABILITY OF DRUGS IN URINE

DRUG	RETENTION TIME DURING WHICH DETECTABLE
Amphetamine/methamphetamine	12-72 hours
Barbiturates	
Amobarbital	2-4 days
Butalbital	2-4 days
Pentobarbital	2-4 days
Phenobarbital	Up to 30 days
Secobarbital	2-4 days
Benzodiazepines	
Diazepam (Valium)	Up to 30 days
Chlordiazepoxide (Librium)	Up to 30 days
Cocaine Metabolites	12-72 hours
Cannabinoids (Marijuana)	
Single use	3 days
Moderate smoker (4 times/week)	5 days
Heavy smoker (daily)	10 days
Chronic smoker	21-27 days
Methadone	1-4 days
Opiates	
Codeine	2-4 days
Hydromorphone (Dilaudid)	2-4 days
Morphine/Heroin	2-4 days
PCP	
Casual use	Up to 5 days
Chronic use	Up to 14 days

Note: Retention times may vary depending on variables including drug metabolism and half-life, patients physical condition, fluid intake, and method and frequency of ingestion.

Sources: National Institute on Drug Abuse and PharmChem Laboratories.

WEIGHT CONVERSION CHART

1 microgram	= 0.000001 gram		
1 milligram	= 0.001 gram	= 0.01543 grain	
1 centigram	= 0.01 gram	= 0.1543 grain	
1 grain	= 0.06479 gram	= 0.03657 dram	
1 decigram	= 0.10 gram	= 1.543 grains	= 0.05644 dram
1 gram	= 15.4324 grains	= 0.56438 dram	= 0.03527 ounce
1 dram	= 1.771 grams	= 27.343 grains	= 0.0625 ounce
1 dekagram	= 10 grams	= 5.6438 drams	= 0.3527 ounce
1 ounce	= 28.349 grams	= 437.5 grains	= 16.0 drams
1 hectogram	= 100 grams	= 1543 grains	= 3.527 ounces
1 pound	= 453.592 grams	= 16 ounces	= 0.4536 kilograms
1 kilogram	= 1000 grams	= 35.273 ounces	= 2.2046 pounds

TO CONVERT

Drams to grains	multiply	Drams X 27.343 = grains
Drams to grams	multiply	Drams X 0.56438 = grams
Drams to ounces	multiply	Drams X 0.0625 = ounces
Drams to pounds	multiply	Drams X 0.0039 = pounds
Drams to kilograms	multiply	Drams X 0.00177 = kilograms
Grains to grams	multiply	Grains X 0.06479 = grams
Grains to drams	multiply	Grains X 0.03657 = drams
Grams to grains	multiply	Grams X 15.4324 = grains
Grams to drams	multiply	Grams X 0.56438 = drams
Grams to ounces	multiply	Grams X 0.03527 = ounces
Grams to pounds	multiply	Grams X 0.002205 = pounds
Grams to kilograms	multiply	Grams X 0.001 = kilograms
Kilograms to grains	multiply	Kilograms X 15432 = grains
Kilograms to drams	multiply	Kilograms X 564.383 = drams
Kilograms to grams	multiply	Kilograms X 1000 = grams
Kilograms to ounces	multiply	Kilograms X 35.273 = ounces
Kilograms to pounds	multiply	Kilograms X 2.2046 = pounds
Ounces to grains	multiply	Ounces X 437.5 = grains
Ounces to drams	multiply	Ounces X 16 = drams
Ounces to grams	multiply	Ounces X 28.3495 = grams
Ounces to pounds	multiply	Ounces X 0.0625 = pounds
Ounces to kilograms	multiply	Ounces X 0.028350 = kilograms
Pounds to grains	multiply	Pounds X 7,000 = grains
Pounds to drams	multiply	Pounds X 256 = drams
Pounds to grams	multiply	Pounds X 453.592 = grams
Pounds to ounces	multiply	Pounds X 16 = ounces
Pounds to kilograms	multiply	Pounds X 0.4536 = kilograms

Drug Identification Bible

Dear Customer,

Thank you for purchasing the 2nd Edition of the Drug Identification Bible. I'm confident you will find that the DIB is the most complete and comprehensive reference available for drug identification. There is simply no other source found anywhere that illustrates more DEA controlled prescription drugs (pages 182 thru 228), or illicit drugs (pages 295 thru 362).

Additionally, no other source provides such a complete and up-to-date tablet and capsule imprint listing (pages 6 thru 191), which allows you to identify more than 9,000 prescription and over-the-counter medications. Street slang (pages 423 thru 454) and street prices and purities (pages 363 thru 422) are some of the other useful information you will find in the DIB.

If you have any comments or suggestions about the DIB we would be happy to hear from you.

Best regards,

Tim Marnell

Tim Marnell
Editor

Box 480244 Denver, Colorado 80248
TEL 1-800-772-2539 FAX 1-800-852-7870